Understanding Neural Plasticity

Understanding Neural Plasticity

Editor: Ryder Dixon

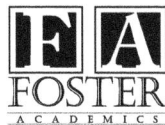

FA FOSTER
ACADEMICS

www.fosteracademics.com

www.fosteracademics.com

FA
FOSTER
ACADEMICS

Cataloging-in-Publication Data

Understanding neural plasticity / edited by Ryder Dixon.
    p. cm.
Includes bibliographical references and index.
ISBN 978-1-63242-731-1
1. Neuroplasticity. 2. Developmental neurobiology. 3. Neurophysiology. I. Dixon, Ryder.
QP363.5 .U54 2019
612.8--dc23

Foster Academics,
118-35 Queens Blvd., Suite 400,
Forest Hills, NY 11375, USA

ISBN 978-1-63242-731-1 (Hardback)

Contents

Preface

Neural plasticity refers to the ability of the brain to change throughout its lifetime. This change is expressed in terms of change in the proportion of grey matter, strengthening or weakening of synapses and the transfer of functions to different locations. Such changes can be witnessed at the microscopic level of neurons to large-scale changes such as cortical remapping during an injury. Evidence shows that the plasticity of the developing brain is more than an adult brain. An important aspect of neuroplasticity is the transfer of brain activity from one location to the other. This occurs during repair from brain injury and serves as the basis of the treatment of acquired brain injuries. Rehabilitation techniques supporting neural plasticity are being explored. The topics included in this book on neural plasticity are of utmost significance and bound to provide incredible insights to readers. It includes some of the vital pieces of work being conducted across the world, on various topics related to neural plasticity. It is a vital tool for all researching and studying this field.

This book is a result of research of several months to collate the most relevant data in the field.

When I was approached with the idea of this book and the proposal to edit it, I was overwhelmed. It gave me an opportunity to reach out to all those who share a common interest with me in this field. I had 3 main parameters for editing this text:

1. Accuracy – The data and information provided in this book should be up-to-date and valuable to the readers.

2. Structure – The data must be presented in a structured format for easy understanding and better grasping of the readers

3. Universal Approach – This book not only targets students but also experts and innovators in the field, thus my aim was to present topics which are of use to all

Thus, it took me a couple of months to finish the editing of this book.

I would like to make a special mention of my publisher who considered me worthy of this opportunity and also supported me throughout the editing process. I would also like to thank the editing team at the back-end who extended their help whenever required.

Editor

Drosophila: An Emergent Model for Delineating Interactions between the Circadian Clock and Drugs of Abuse

Aliza K. De Nobrega and Lisa C. Lyons

Department of Biological Science, Program in Neuroscience, Florida State University, Tallahassee, FL 32306, USA

Correspondence should be addressed to Lisa C. Lyons; lyons@bio.fsu.edu

Academic Editor: Harry Pantazopoulos

Endogenous circadian oscillators orchestrate rhythms at the cellular, physiological, and behavioral levels across species to coordinate activity, for example, sleep/wake cycles, metabolism, and learning and memory, with predictable environmental cycles. The 21st century has seen a dramatic rise in the incidence of circadian and sleep disorders with globalization, technological advances, and the use of personal electronics. The circadian clock modulates alcohol- and drug-induced behaviors with circadian misalignment contributing to increased substance use and abuse. Invertebrate models, such as *Drosophila melanogaster*, have proven invaluable for the identification of genetic and molecular mechanisms underlying highly conserved processes including the circadian clock, drug tolerance, and reward systems. In this review, we highlight the contributions of *Drosophila* as a model system for understanding the bidirectional interactions between the circadian system and the drugs of abuse, alcohol and cocaine, and illustrate the highly conserved nature of these interactions between *Drosophila* and mammalian systems. Research in *Drosophila* provides mechanistic insights into the corresponding behaviors in higher organisms and can be used as a guide for targeted inquiries in mammals.

1. Introduction

1.1. Alcohol and Drug Abuse. The long-term chronic abuse of alcohol and other drugs has adverse consequences for individual health, society, and the economy [1–3]. Alcohol is one of the most commonly used and abused drugs in the United States [4] and the world [5]. As of 2014, 17 million Americans have an alcohol use disorder (AUD) representing 79% of the people diagnosed with substance use disorders, and additional 2.6 million (12.1%) have comorbid AUD and illicit drug use disorder [4]. Alcohol and other drugs of abuse collectively account for ~75,000 deaths annually in the US [6, 7]. In the United States, the health and economic costs associated with alcohol abuse are estimated at approximately $223 billion annually [1] with costs associated with other drugs of abuse including tobacco, illicit drugs, and prescription opioids collectively estimated at approximately $571.6 billion annually [8–10]. In the past few years, cocaine use has reemerged as a public health problem with a 26% increase in the number of new users in 2015 compared to 2014, with the greatest increase in users occurring among young adults [11]. Understanding the factors that contribute to alcohol and substance abuse and addiction and drug pathologies is critical for the development of therapies for the prevention and treatment of substance abuse disorders.

1.2. The Link between the Circadian Clock and Drug Use. From bacteria to humans, circadian clocks regulate cellular, physiological, and behavioral rhythms in coordination with the natural light-dark cycle (Figure 1). In addition to light, entrainment of the peripheral circadian system can be mediated by food intake schedules, exercise, or social activity [12–14]. The circadian clock modulates rhythms in metabolism, gene expression, hormone production, cell regeneration, and brain wave activity [15–17]. In the past two decades, the importance of the circadian clock in modulating alcohol and drug use and the associated pathologies has become more apparent (Figure 2). Individuals with an evening chronotype, the behavioral pattern reflecting an individual's circadian phase, exhibit higher levels of alcohol

(a)

(b)

(c)

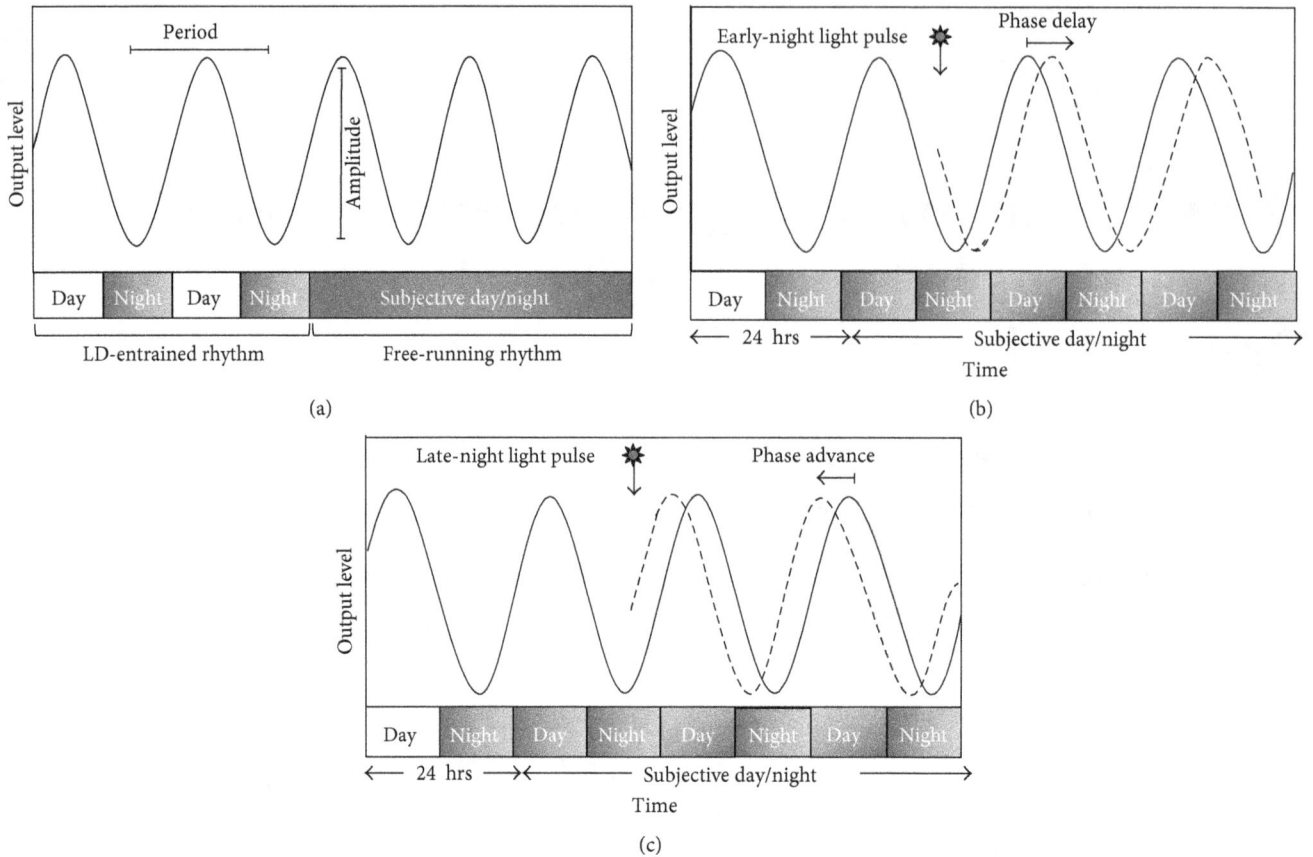

FIGURE 1: Measures of the circadian rhythm. (a) Cycles of peaks and troughs of activity occur at approximately 24-hour intervals. The period of the cycle is the time between successive peaks (or troughs) of activity whereas the extent of the increase or decrease in activity represents the amplitude of the cycle. (b) An early-night light pulse results in a phase delay. (c) A late-night light pulse results in a phase advance.

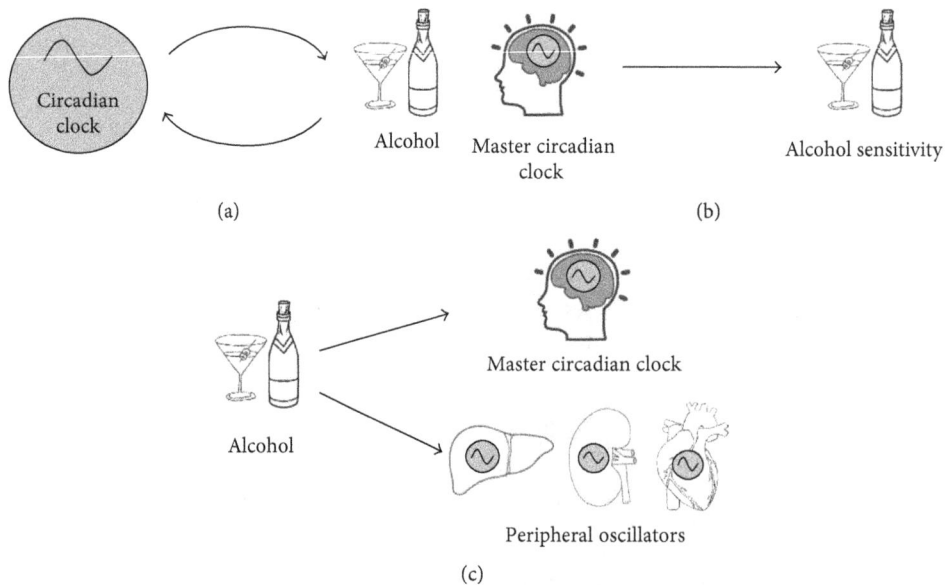

(a)

(b)

(c)

FIGURE 2: The bidirectional relationship between the circadian clock and alcohol. (a) The circadian clock modulates alcohol sensitivity and alcohol consumption. Alcohol acts upon circadian oscillators to affect phase shifting of oscillators as well as expression patterns of circadian genes leading to circadian dysfunction. (b) The master circadian clock in the brain modulates the behavioral sensitivity to alcohol including hyperactivity, sedation, recovery, and tolerance. (c) Alcohol affects the master circadian clock in the SCN as well as in peripheral oscillators in the liver, kidney, and heart.

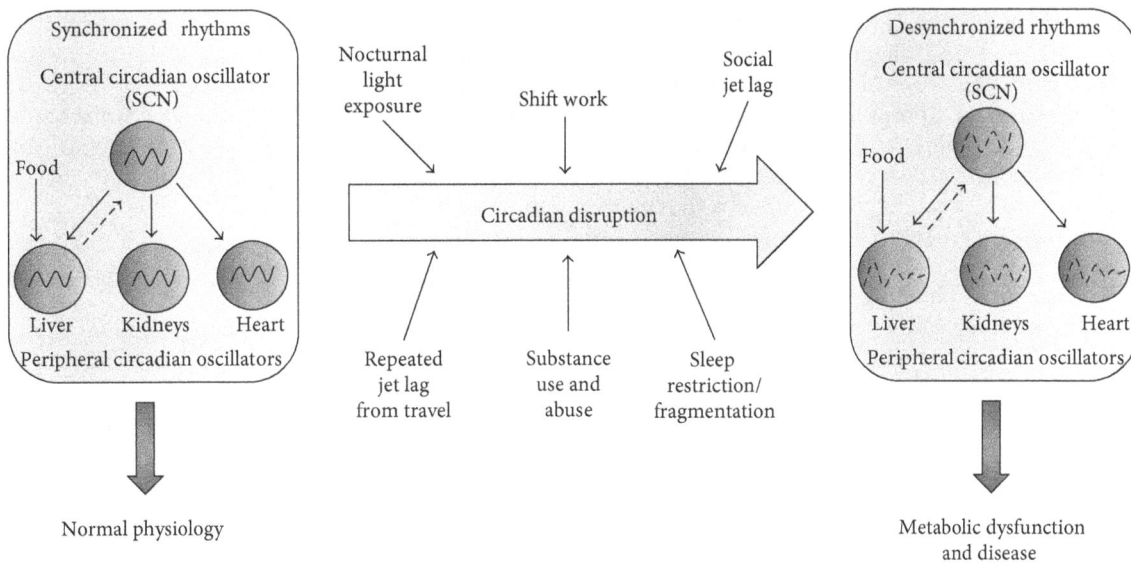

FIGURE 3: Central and peripheral circadian regulation of metabolic function. Under normal conditions, the central circadian oscillator in the SCN is entrained by light and synchronizes peripheral oscillators. Meal timing can also entrain the liver oscillators. Environmental perturbations such as shift work, jet lag, sleep restriction, and substance abuse create misalignment between the SCN and the peripheral oscillators resulting in metabolic syndromes and disease.

use [18, 19] and increased drug use [20, 21]. Recent research using functional imaging has shown that evening chronotypes have altered neural responses to reward compared to morning chronotypes with increased activity in the ventral striatum and decreased reactivity in the medial prefrontal cortex [22] which has previously been associated with increased alcohol consumption [23].

1.3. Circadian Misalignment. Impairments of the circadian system or desynchronization adversely affects individual health with increased risk of obesity, diabetes, cardiovascular diseases, cancer, and mood disorders [24–28] (Figure 3). Recently, research in animal models and humans has linked circadian dysfunction with increased risk of drug and alcohol abuse. Drug abuse and drug-related pathologies appear higher in populations in which circadian misalignment and sleep deprivation are common [3, 29] including shift workers [30–32] and aging individuals [33]. These substance abuse issues are expected to escalate with increases in the aging population and the proportion of people working extended and rotating shifts [34–36]. Drug abuse and alcohol abuse affect the functioning of the circadian system with the subsequent circadian dysfunction increasing the risks and harms of drug abuse. In this review, we will discuss factors contributing to the increase in sleep and circadian disorders and focus on *Drosophila* as a model for investigating the bidirectional interactions between the circadian clock and drug use.

2. Factors Contributing to the Increase in Circadian and Sleep Disorders

2.1. Work Schedules. In the past few decades, the number of individuals affected by circadian or sleep disorders has rapidly risen [37]. Insufficient sleep is a pervasive problem affecting approximately 30% of adults and 60% of adolescents [38]. Technological advances and globalization have driven changes in occupational and professional practices with a greater number of individuals working extended hours and shift work. In the United States and other developed countries, approximately 15–30% of the population work irregular or shift work schedules [36, 38] contributing to increased circadian and sleep disorders. Individuals working longer days and extended work weeks have become increasingly more common with more than 18% of the people in the United States working more than 48 hours per week [36]. These problems are compounded by poor entrainment of the circadian clock in modern societies.

2.2. Circadian Entrainment and Artificial Light at Night. The circadian system and sleep profiles evolved in coordination with the natural light-dark cycles with light providing the strongest zeitgeber or entrainment signal to the circadian oscillator. With the majority of the world's population now living in urban environments [39], artificial indoor lighting substitutes for the natural light-dark cycle entrainment of the circadian clock. Studies in the United States, Canada, and England found that individuals spend less than 12% of their time outside or less than 1-2 hours per day overall [40–43]. As indoor light levels (100–300 lux) are orders of magnitude lower than those of direct sunlight (10,000 lux range), decreased time outdoors results in weaker signals to the circadian clock and poorer entrainment [44]. In contrast to light signals during the day, light at night shifts the phase of the circadian clock (Figures 1(b) and 1(c)). It has been estimated that 99% of individuals living in the United States and Europe and 80% of the people worldwide experience significant light pollution at night [45, 46]. During the night, light from a full moon is less than 1.0 lux of light, usually 0.1–0.3 lux [45]. However, artificial light at night is considerably higher from a variety of sources including outdoor lighting estimated at 5–15-lux light exposure, indoor evening lighting at 100–200-lux light exposure, and personal electronic use ranging up to 100-lux light exposure [45]. In the past decade, the shift from the use of incandescent light bulbs to the use of fluorescent and LED lights with shorter wavelengths increases the potential for circadian disruption at night as melanopsin, the circadian photopigment, is particularly sensitive to shorter-wavelength blue light [47, 48]. Increased exposure to artificial light at night has been associated with increased risk of cancer, diabetes, obesity, and mood and behavioral disorders [45, 49–51]. Increased artificial light at night [46, 52] combined with reduced individual exposure to daytime sunlight [43] contributes to weakened circadian entrainment and circadian dysfunction. Poor entrainment and low-level circadian function make it more difficult to maintain synchronization of central and peripheral circadian clocks in the face of circadian perturbation.

2.3. Evening Chronotype. An individual's chronotype may also increase the risk of circadian desynchronization. Individuals with evening chronotypes are prone to even greater late-night phenotypes with less exposure to sunlight and more reliance on artificial lighting compounding the problem [53]. The phase of the circadian clock changes with development and aging. Whereas young children have a morning chronotype, in teenagers and young adults, the biological clock is naturally shifted by several hours resulting in the prevalence of evening chronotypes in this age group [54–56]. Fixed work and school schedules compound the problem of circadian dysfunction in individuals with an evening chronotype.

2.4. Personal Electronics. The use of personal electronics and shifts in activity patterns between weekdays and weekends strongly contribute to the rise in circadian and sleep disorders. The use of smartphones and personal electronics at night has further potentiated circadian disorders and associated problems by increasing exposure to light during the night [45, 57, 58]. Computer and cell phone use at night by adolescents has been correlated with decreased weekday sleep [59]. Teenagers and young adults are particularly susceptible to smartphone dependence [60], with more than 50% of adults and approximately 75% of children and adolescents exhibiting signs of dependence upon their smartphones including anxiety [61]. Smartphone dependence appears almost universal around the world contributing to sleep disorders and poor sleep quality in teenagers, college students, and adults [62, 63].

2.5. Social Jet Lag. Social jet lag, defined as a change in activity/rest patterns between workdays and free days, results in individuals continuously undergoing shifts to their circadian clock and a perpetual state of circadian misalignment as peripheral circadian oscillators have insufficient time to resynchronize prior to the next phase shift (Figure 3). Social jet lag is prevalent in adults and adolescents, particularly in individuals with an evening chronotype, with estimates of social jet lag affecting almost 70% of individuals [64]. Social jet lag has been correlated with increased obesity [65], diabetes, cardiac function and heart disease [66, 67], and depression [68]. Higher levels of alcohol use observed in individuals with evening chronotypes may be compounded by social jet lag [18].

3. *Drosophila* as a Versatile Model System

3.1. Advantages of Drosophila. Drosophila is an excellent model system for dissecting the bidirectional connections between the circadian clock and drugs of abuse as the signaling pathways that regulate reward processes, addiction, and circadian function are highly conserved between *Drosophila* and mammals [69–71]. The free-running period in *Drosophila* is approximately 24 hours with flies exhibiting crepuscular activity under laboratory conditions including dawn anticipatory activity [72, 73]. The relatively short life cycle, the ability to generate large populations in a short time period, and the low cost of culture and maintenance in *Drosophila* permit complex genetic experiments to be completed in a fraction of the time it would take in vertebrate models [74, 75]. Powerful neurogenetic techniques including forward genetic screens, reverse genetic techniques with genome-wide RNAi lines available, and optogenetic monitoring to assess individual neuronal changes using voltage or calcium sensors have enhanced the utility of the *Drosophila* model [76–81]. *Drosophila* also provides an excellent model to study the complexity of the aging process, offering the ability to characterize single-gene mutations that extend or shorten lifespan [82–85]. Similar to mammals, *Drosophila* shows declines with aging in functional and behavioral performance including sensory functions [86, 87], circadian and sleep-like behavior [88–92], learning and memory [93–95], locomotion [96–98], and organ function [99–101].

3.2. Conservation between Drosophila and Mammals. The physiological mechanisms underlying most biological processes between *Drosophila* and mammals are remarkably well conserved despite the obvious differences in anatomical structure and complexity [102, 103]. The fly genome contains approximately 14,000 genes, and it is estimated that nearly 75% of the genes implicated in human diseases have functional orthologs in the fly, with 80 to 90% similarity in conserved functional domains at the nucleotide level or protein sequence [104–106]. Anatomically, *Drosophila* has functional equivalents of the mammalian heart [107–109], lung [110, 111], kidney [112, 113], gut [114–116], and reproductive tract [117, 118].

Despite the considerable neuroanatomical differences between flies and mammals, the molecular, cellular, genetic, and electrophysiological properties underlying neuronal behavior and synaptic plasticity also are well conserved [119, 120]. The approximately 100,000 neurons constituting the fly brain form discreet networks that regulate complex behaviors such as sleep [121–123], learning and memory [124, 125], grooming and feeding [69, 126–129], circadian rhythms [130–134], aggression [135, 136], and courtship [137, 138]. The fundamental mechanisms comprising the homeostatic systems and neurochemical circuits are also conserved between *Drosophila* and mammals [69, 139, 140]. At the molecular level, neurotransmission also appears highly conserved from *Drosophila* to mammalian species with classical neurotransmitters including acetylcholine, GABA, glutamate, dopamine, octopamine, serotonin, histamine, and peptide neurotransmitters such as neuropeptide Y/neuropeptide F and insulin-like peptides common to both [69, 141, 142].

The striking mechanistic similarities to mammals have propelled *Drosophila* to the forefront as a competitive model to investigate the link between the circadian system and drug sensitivity, abuse, and addiction. In this review, we highlight *Drosophila* research revealing the interactions between the circadian clock and two drugs of abuse, alcohol and cocaine, and the parallels to mammalian systems.

4. *Drosophila* as a Model for the Circadian Clock

Since the 1950s and the pioneering work of Colin Pittendrigh, *Drosophila* has been a prominent model for research defining the conceptual, functional, and molecular basis of the circadian clock [143–147]. The circadian clock in *Drosophila* modulates a broad spectrum of physiological and behavioral processes including locomotor activity, sleep patterns, courtship, learning and memory, feeding behavior, chemosensation, and immune responses [148–157]. As in mammals, the *Drosophila* circadian oscillators also coordinate rhythms in peripheral organs, such as olfactory and gustatory sensitivity rhythms [158–160] and the mitotic response of gut stem cells to damage [161].

Konopka and Benzer isolated the first clock gene mutants in 1971 using forward genetics in *Drosophila* and analysis of the period length of the circadian rhythm in eclosion [162]. Flies with mutations in the gene *period* (per^L, per^S, and per^{01}) exhibit rhythms in eclosion that are longer, shorter, or arrhythmic, respectively [162]. Identification of *per* spawned additional genetic screens for components of the circadian clock leading to the discovery of *timeless*, *clock*, *cycle*, *doubletime*, *shaggy*, *casein kinase 2* subunits, and *cryptochrome* [163–172]. These studies and subsequent identification of the corresponding genes facilitated research in mammalian systems leading to the discovery of mammalian *per* and *clock* genes, the first circadian genes identified and sequenced in mice [173–175].

The *Drosophila* central brain circadian system comprises approximately 150 clock neurons organized into a network of oscillators: the small and large ventral lateral neurons which control the morning peak of activity and the lateral dorsal and dorsal neurons that control the evening peak of activity [176, 177]. Circadian rhythms generated by both the *Drosophila* and mammalian clock are driven by interlocking autoregulatory transcriptional/translational feedback loops along with posttranscriptional regulatory elements that facilitate the rhythmicity of the clock and generate the 24-hour period [176, 178–183]. Figure 4 provides an

overview of the molecular clock in *Drosophila* and mammals. As additional information on the molecular mechanisms of the core circadian oscillators in *Drosophila* and mammals is provided in many excellent reviews [176, 184–186], we only briefly describe the core clock mechanism below.

In *Drosophila*, the positive regulatory elements in the core oscillator are the basic-helix-loop-helix transcriptional elements *clock* (*clk*) and *cycle* (*cyc*) which form a heterodimer and bind to the *per* and *timeless* (*tim*) DNA promoters to activate transcription of the core circadian genes, *per* and *tim* [166, 167, 171], and hundreds of clock-controlled output genes [187, 188]. Monomers of the PER protein are unstable, phosphorylated by *doubletime* (DBT), and targeted for degradation. As dTIM and dPER levels rise, they form a dTIM/dPER/DBT complex which translocates to the nucleus and binds to the dCLK/dCYC complex [165, 172, 189], thereby inhibiting transcription of the *per* and *tim* genes [182, 189]. In mammals, the positive regulatory elements are the transcriptional elements CLOCK (CLK) and BMAL1 (instead of CYC) which form a heterodimer to activate transcription of the clock genes: three orthologs of *period* (m*Per1*, m*Per2*, and m*Per3*) and two *cryptochrome* genes (m*Cry1* and m*Cry2*) as well as other clock-controlled genes [190, 191]. Following translation of the proteins mPER and mCRY, the proteins dimerize to mediate stability and nuclear translocation and then interact with the mCLK/mBMAL1 complex in the nucleus, inhibiting further transcriptional activation [191]. In flies as in mammals, posttranscriptional elements are necessary for the regulation of protein stability, nuclear entry, and fine-tuning of period length [170, 189, 192]. These include the kinases *doubletime* (DBT), the homolog to mammalian *casein kinase 1 epsilon* (CK1E) [172] which targets dPER for phosphorylation and subsequent degradation [165], and dSHAGGY, a homolog to the mammalian glycogen synthase kinase-3 (mGSK3) [193] which aids in nuclear translocation of the dTIM/dPER/dDBT complex [170, 189, 192]. The above provides a brief outline of the core circadian oscillator with more detailed descriptions of the circadian oscillator and its components in *Drosophila* and mammalian models available in several recent review articles [176, 180, 189, 194].

5. *Drosophila* as a Model for Studies of Alcohol Neurobiology

5.1. Alcohol-Induced Behaviors. As a model system, *Drosophila* has exemplified the value of invertebrate research and its parallels and conversion into meaningful knowledge in mammalian systems particularly for studies of drugs of abuse [139, 195, 196]. See Table 1 for comparisons of drug-induced behaviors and assays used in *Drosophila* and rodent models. Stereotypical behaviors associated with alcohol exposure are conserved between flies, rodents, and humans [74, 139, 197] including hyperactivity in response to low concentrations of alcohol followed by loss of motor control as alcohol exposure progresses [139, 198–200]. Prolonged exposure to alcohol results in the development of functional tolerance, sedation, and eventually death [139, 198–200]. Similar to mammalian species, *Drosophila* also exhibits sex

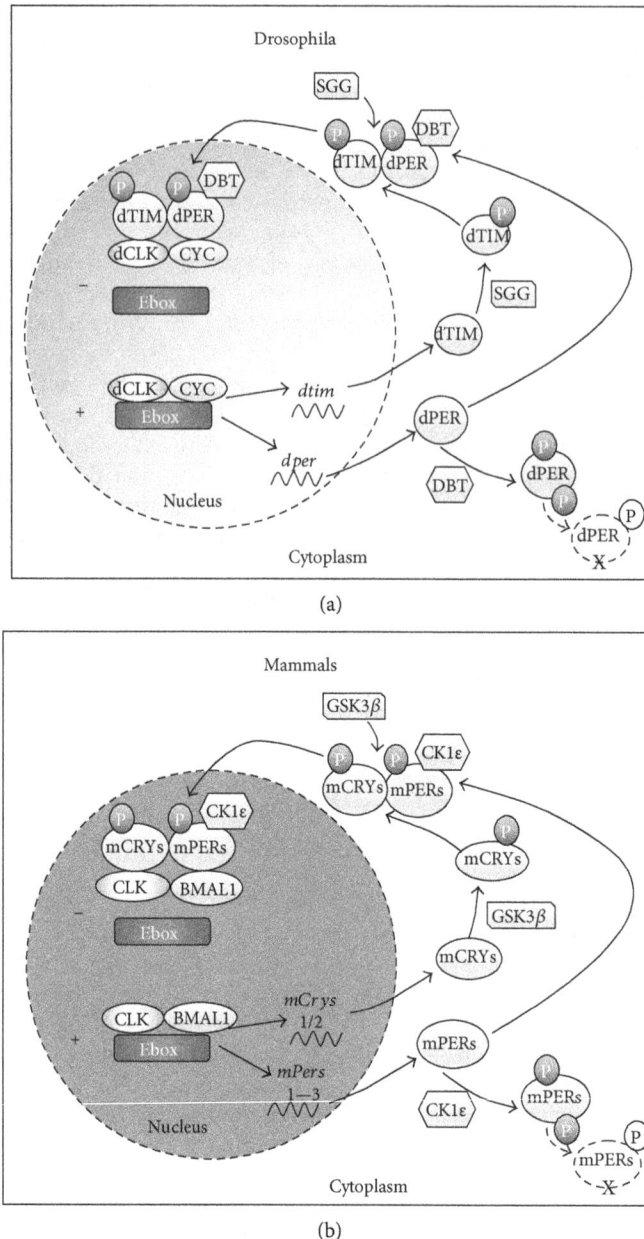

FIGURE 4: The molecular clocks of *Drosophila* (a) and mammals (b). (a) In *Drosophila*, dCLK and CYC form a dimer, which binds to the E boxes in the promoter of *per* and *tim* as well as to other clock-controlled genes to facilitate transcription. PER and TIM proteins form a complex and translocate into the nucleus providing negative feedback to inhibit dCLK-CYC DNA binding. Phosphorylation mediated by DBT and SGG regulates protein–protein interactions, nuclear translocation, and degradation. (b) In mammals, the transcription factors BMAL1 and CLK form a dimer that binds to E boxes in the promoter of *mPer* and *mCry*. mPER and mCRY proteins form dimers, enter the nucleus, and inhibit the BMAL1-CLK activity. Phosphorylation mediated by CK1 and GSK3 regulates protein–protein interactions, nuclear translocation, and degradation.

differences in alcohol sensitivity with males less sensitive to the acute behavioral effects of alcohol but more susceptible to alcohol-induced mortality than females [201, 202].

The molecular and neural mechanisms underlying alcohol-induced behavioral changes appear conserved between flies and mammals [69, 198, 199, 203] making *Drosophila* a practical model for studying the development of functional tolerance, addiction, and reward pathways. Functional tolerance includes the development of rapid and chronic tolerance due to changes in neuronal plasticity

rather than changes in the absorbance and metabolism of alcohol [204–206]. Like higher vertebrates, flies develop rapid tolerance following a single alcohol exposure and chronic tolerance with multiple or prolonged alcohol exposure [71, 139, 200]. *Drosophila* demonstrates a preference for alcohol-containing food over non-alcohol-containing food [198, 207–209], although the question has arisen as to whether the underlying preference is due to its caloric value [210]. Recent research has shown that the preference for and voluntary consumption of alcohol in *Drosophila* are

TABLE 1: Behavioral measures and assays of drug addiction in *Drosophila* and rodents.

Behavior	Assay	Examples of research studies	
		Drosophila	*Rodents*
Reward/preference Induced state that leads to conditioned reinforced behavior	(1) Self-administration (2) Electrical stimulation (3) Conditioned place preference (4) Conditioned taste preference (5) Conditioned taste avoidance	(1) [198, 207, 211] (2) [200] (3) [198, 200] (4) [198, 398] (5) [198]	(1) [399] (2) [400, 401] (3) [402, 403] (4) [399, 404] (5) [405, 406]
Drug seeking Affective state inferred from increased behavioral responses to drugs, drug-associated cues, or stress	(1) Self-administration (2) Electrical stimulation	(1) [198] (2) [200]	(1) [407, 408] (2) [409, 410]
Functional tolerance Adaptations in neural function *Rapid tolerance* Following a single acute exposure when drug has metabolized *Chronic tolerance* Following prolonged or repeated drug exposures	(1) Injection behavioral assays (2) Self-administration (3) Sedation and negative geotaxis assay	(1) [228] (2) — (3) [204, 205, 280]	(1) [405, 411] (2) [412] (3) [413, 414]
Sensitization Increased motor-stimulant response following repeated drug exposures	(1) Locomotor activity test	(1) [332, 334, 415, 416]	(1) [324, 417–420]
Withdrawal Aversive state that motivates drug seeking	(1) Conditioned place aversion (2) Sedation and negative geotaxis (3) Self-administration	(1) — (2) [421, 422] (3) —	(1) [423] (2) [424, 425] (3) [426, 427]
Relapse/reinstatement Spontaneous recovery of drug seeking after abstinence or extinction of behavior may be triggered by cues previously paired with drug use or stress	(1) Self-administration (2) Electrical stimulation (3) Injections	(1) [198, 428] (2) — (3) —	(1) [429, 430] (2) [431, 432] (3) [433]

experience-dependent based upon previous alcohol exposure [211] and independent of caloric, gustatory, or olfactory biases for alcohol [209]. *Drosophila* also exhibits alcohol addiction-like behavior preferring alcohol-containing food even when accompanied by a noxious stimulus as well as relapse-like behavior with high levels of alcohol consumption after alcohol deprivation [198, 208].

5.2. Molecular Pathways in Alcohol Responses. The power of genetic approaches in *Drosophila* has facilitated the identification of molecular and cellular mechanisms that mediate alcohol-induced behavior and neural plasticity [212, 213] with many of the identified genes and molecular pathways playing a similar role in mammalian responses to alcohol [214, 215].

5.2.1. cAMP-PKA Pathway. Mutagenesis studies in flies have provided substantial evidence for the role of the cAMP-protein kinase A pathway in alcohol-induced behavioral responses including the adenylyl cyclase-encoding gene, *rutabaga*; the cAMP phosphodiesterase-encoding gene, *dunce*; and the PKA-C1-encoding gene, *dco* [216]. Increased sensitivity to alcohol-induced sedation is observed in *rutabaga* flies although *dunce* mutant flies exhibit sensitivity to alcohol-induced sedation similar to wild-type flies [216]. Flies with mutations in PKA show altered alcohol sensitivity with mutations in the catalytic subunit (*dco* mutation) making them more sensitive to the sedating effects of alcohol

[216] while flies with a mutation in the RII subunit of PKA exhibit reduced sensitivity to alcohol-induced sedation [217]. The preference for alcohol self-administration and potentially the processing of its reward salience are also dependent upon adenylyl cyclase activity [209]. The role of cAMP-PKA signaling in alcohol neurobiology appears conserved across species. Genetic downregulation of the cAMP-PKA pathway in mice through manipulation of G protein transduction increases sensitivity to ethanol while upregulation of adenylyl cyclase activity reduces the sensitivity of mice to alcohol-induced sedation [218]. Mice with a knockout mutation in the RIIβ subunit of PKA exhibit lowered alcohol sensitivity [219] similar to what is observed in flies. The PACAP-like analog *amnesiac* encodes a putative neuropeptide which may trigger the cAMP-PKA pathway via adenylate cyclase activity [220]. Flies with mutations in the *amnesiac* gene also exhibit increased sensitivity to the sedative effects of alcohol [216]. Thus, the cAMP-PKA pathway appears to be a key regulator in behavioral alcohol sensitivity and the preference for alcohol across species.

5.2.2. The LMO-ALK Axis. *Drosophila* LIM-domain only (*dLmo*), also known as Beadex, encodes a transcriptional regulator that affects behavioral responses in the adult fly to alcohol and cocaine. In flies, decreased *dLmo* levels increase alcohol sensitivity with flies sedating more quickly while increased *dLmo* decreases sensitivity to alcohol sedation [221]. Similarly, mice with reduced expression of *Lmo3* exhibit increased sensitivity to the sedating effect of alcohol [221, 222]. *Lmo3*-null mice also drink more alcohol in the "drinking in the dark" test compared to wild-type mice [222]. In a microarray analysis for gene targets with inverse expression of the *Bx* repressor, the *Drosophila* homolog of *anaplastic lymphoma kinase* (*dAlk*) was found to be negatively regulated by *dLmo* [221]. Flies with mutations in dAlk show increased resistance to alcohol-induced sedation [223]. *dAlk* has been shown to modulate *Erk* activity in the fly brain and likely influences sensitivity to alcohol via *Erk* signaling [224]. Similarly, rodent and human orthologs of *dAlk* include *Bx* (*Lmo4*) and *Alk* that have been shown to modulate alcohol sensitivity and consumption and may be involved in alcohol dependence [223, 225–227]. *Alk*-knockout mice also show higher alcohol consumption compared to wild-type mice [223].

5.2.3. GABA Neurotransmission. The effects of alcohol on neurotransmission, particularly on glutamate and GABA neurotransmission, are also conserved across species [69, 71, 215]. Alcohol affects GABA neurotransmission through binding to $GABA_A$ and $GABA_B$ receptors [215]. In *Drosophila*, $GABA_B$ receptor activity mediates alcohol sensitivity and upregulation inhibits rapid tolerance to alcohol exposure [228]. Flies with $GABA_BR1$ downregulation through RNAi expression have decreased $GABA_B$ receptor function and exhibit decreased alcohol-induced motor impairments [228]. Pharmacological downregulation of $GABA_B$ also decreases alcohol sensitivity whereas flies treated with a $GABA_B$ agonist (3-APMPA) fail to develop rapid alcohol tolerance [228]. Similarly in mice, the $GABA_B$ agonist baclofen blocks the development of rapid tolerance [229] and $GABA_B$ antagonists attenuate the acute sensitivity to alcohol [230]. However, the observed effect of baclofen on self-administration of alcohol has varied with some studies indicating that baclofen decreases voluntary alcohol consumption [231, 232] while others demonstrate increased alcohol consumption [233, 234]. This confusion has recently been answered, at least in part, as enantiomer specificity was found to be a critical factor in the directionality of baclofen on alcohol consumption [235]. In alcoholic patients, baclofen has also been shown to reduce alcohol craving [236–240].

5.2.4. Glutamate Signaling. The protein Homer functions as an adaptor protein in the postsynaptic density coupling membrane proteins with downstream signaling, including glutamate receptors. Transcript levels of *homer* decrease in wild-type flies following alcohol exposure, and *homer*[R102] mutant flies demonstrate increased sensitivity and decreased tolerance to alcohol exposure [241]. *Homer2*-KO mice demonstrate reduced voluntary drinking, reduced preference for alcohol, and increased sensitivity to alcohol confirming a conserved role of Homer function in the regulation of alcohol-induced behaviors [242]. More recently, chronic alcohol exposure has been shown to increase *Homer2a/b* and *mGluR1* expression in the nucleus accumbens core (NaCc) and central amygdala (CeA) of rats reinforcing previous research that chronic alcohol induces glutamatergic plasticity in the brain [243, 244].

5.2.5. Potassium Channels. Further evidence for the high degree of conservation in alcohol tolerance arises from the studies of the gene *slowpoke* (*slo*) that encodes the *Big Potassium* (BK) channel-forming subunits. SLO is necessary for the acquisition of rapid tolerance with reduced *slo* expression in flies eliminating the ability to acquire tolerance [245–247]. Increasing *slo* expression in the *Drosophila* brain mimics functional alcohol tolerance [245, 248]. Mammalian BK channels encoded by *slo* are inhibited and potentiated by alcohol [249–251]. Stimulation of BK channels in the rat supraoptic nucleus and striatum increases the response to alcohol-induced tolerance [252]. The actions of alcohol on BK channels are dependent upon the ?1–?4 subunits shown to reduce the potentiation of BK channels following acute alcohol exposure [250, 253–255].

5.2.6. Reward Signaling: Dopamine and NPY. Reward pathways mediating alcohol addiction and abuse are also conserved between flies and mammals [69, 139]. Dopamine is a pleiotropic modulator of behavior strongly implicated in the development of reward and addiction in mammals and flies [256–260]. In flies, dopamine signaling via D_1 receptors is necessary for alcohol-induced hyperactivity and preference [200, 257, 261] with dopaminergic neurons in the ellipsoid body of the central complex critical for the regulation of alcohol-induced hyperactivity [257]. Similarly, fast and steep increases in dopamine activate low-affinity D_1 dopamine receptors necessary for the rewarding effects of alcohol and triggering alcohol-induced conditioned responses in mammals [262].

Another neuropeptide, neuropeptide Y (NPY), plays a prominent role in the negative affective behaviors associated with stress and alcohol [263, 264] with a conserved role in reward pathways across species. In mammalian studies, rats selectively bred for high alcohol preferences have low levels of NPY expression in the striatum and increased anxiety-like behaviors [265]. Mice selected for high alcohol preference also show blunted NPY in the nucleus accumbens core and shell in response to acute alcohol exposure compared to control mice [266]. Manipulations of NPF signaling, the *Drosophila* homolog of NPY, affect alcohol preference with inhibition of the NPF pathway enhancing alcohol preference while NPF activation reduces alcohol preference [267]. Flies with loss-of-function mutations in NPF/NPFR1 signaling also exhibit decreased sensitivity to alcohol sedation whereas flies in which NPF is overexpressed show increased sensitivity to alcohol sedation [268].

5.2.7. Cellular Stress Pathways. Genes involved in cellular stress responses may also have a conserved role in the development of alcohol tolerance including heat shock proteins, cytochrome P450 proteins, and glutathione transferases [269]. The *hangover* gene is a Zn-finger transcription factor necessary for cellular oxidative stress responses [270]. Flies with a mutation in *hangover* exhibit decreased rapid alcohol tolerance, although no differences are observed in alcohol-induced sedation [247]. The human ortholog of *hangover* is *ZNF699*, and human studies have identified polymorphisms in this gene associated with alcohol dependence [271, 272].

Another stress-related gene involved in alcohol tolerance is the microtubule-associated protein *jwa* (alias *ARL6IP5*, *addicsin*), which increases in response to oxidative stress and heat shock in mammals [273, 274]. In flies, RNAi-mediated knockdown of *djwa* decreases the development of alcohol tolerance [275]. In mammals, the homologous *addicsin* has been implicated in the development of morphine tolerance [276]. While considerably more research needs to be done, there appears to be a conserved role for proteins involved in cellular stress responses in alcohol and drug tolerance across species.

5.2.8. Regulation of Cytoskeletal Elements. Regulation of actin dynamics also has been implicated in alcohol-induced behavioral responses. The Rho family of GTPases, including Rho1, Rac1, and Cdc42, regulates actin dynamics. In flies, *Ras suppressor1* (*Rsu1*) regulates alcohol sensitivity functioning through the regulation of actin dynamics upstream of Rac1 GTPase [277]. Flies with mutations in *Rsu1* exhibit reduced sensitivity to alcohol and a naïve preference for higher alcohol consumption that remains unchanged with experience [277]. Furthermore, the Rho GTPase activator protein 18B (RhoGAP18B) with three protein isoforms affect actin dynamics of which the RhoGAP18B PC isoform also affects the sensitivity to alcohol-induced sedation and hyperactivity [278, 279]. The loss of the full-length RhoGAP18B PC protein decreases alcohol sensitivity [278, 280]. Human genome-wide association studies have found correlations between *Rsu1* SNP and ventral striatum activity, and a mutation in *Rsu1* is associated with alcohol dependence [277]. Further, activation of the *Arf6* small GTPase results in increased resistance to alcohol-induced sedation, and flies with reduced expression are more sensitive to alcohol [281, 282]. The Efa6 activation of Arf6 is required for normal responses to alcohol-induced sedation as Arf6 and Efa6 mutant flies show reduced sensitivity to alcohol-induced sedation and no rapid tolerance to alcohol exposure [283]. Human genome-wide association studies show correlations between SNPs of Arf6 and Efa6 and increased alcohol drinking behavior [283].

The strikingly similar molecular and cellular mechanisms underlying alcohol-responsive behaviors in flies and mammals validate *Drosophila* as a model for alcohol research. Although obvious neuroanatomical differences exist between mammals and flies, alcohol affects brain regions in flies for which functionally similar parallels can be drawn to specific mammalian brain regions [139, 199]. The brain regions involved in *Drosophila* alcohol neurobiology and detailed description of genes and molecular pathways have been the subject of several recent reviews [71, 139, 199, 200, 284].

6. *Drosophila* Links Circadian and Alcohol Neurobiology

The interaction between time of day and the sensitivity to alcohol was described more than a half-century ago with studies in mice detailing time-of-day differences in alcohol toxicity [285]. Since that time, numerous behavioral studies have documented the circadian regulation of alcohol sensitivity and the bidirectional influence of alcohol on the functioning of the circadian clock [286–289]. The emergence of *Drosophila* as a model for alcohol research has expanded the opportunities for defining the bidirectional interactions between alcohol and the circadian clock using behavioral and genetic studies.

6.1. Circadian Regulation of Alcohol Behavioral Sensitivity. As the neural circuitry and molecular signaling pathways may differ between alcohol-induced behaviors, the potential for circadian regulation of multiple behaviors has been examined in *Drosophila* including the loss of righting reflex which reflects the loss of postural motor control after alcohol exposure, alcohol-induced sedation, the recovery from sedation, and functional tolerance. In *Drosophila*, the circadian clock differentially regulates acute behavioral sensitivity to alcohol dependent upon time of day with circadian rhythms in alcohol-induced loss of righting reflex and sedation occurring in both light-dark cycles and constant darkness [202, 290]. Flies exhibit the greatest sensitivity to alcohol during the mid-to-late subjective night in correspondence to the flies' inactive phase [202, 290]. The time to recover from the sedative effects of alcohol is also significantly greater at night [202]. Phase-dependent correlation of alcohol sensitivity with activity may be a conserved feature of circadian regulation as mice also exhibit rhythms in alcohol sensitivity with increased sensitivity during the day (inactive period) and decreased sensitivity at night (active period) [291]. Humans show time-of-day rhythms in the consumption of alcohol and alcohol sensitivity [292, 293]. However, not all alcohol-induced behaviors are directly regulated by the circadian clock. In *Drosophila*, the degree of rapid tolerance assessed at four hours does not show dependence upon the time of alcohol exposure, although rhythms are observed in the loss of righting reflex in both the initial alcohol exposure and the test exposure [290]. Alcohol absorbance also does not vary based upon time of exposure [290] or between circadian clock mutants and wild-type flies [294].

6.2. Circadian Dysfunction Increases Alcohol Sensitivity. When the circadian clock is rendered nonfunctional through either genetic or environmental manipulations, *Drosophila* exhibits significantly increased behavioral sensitivity to alcohol [202]. *per^{01}* mutant flies are more susceptible to alcohol-induced sedation with significantly shorter alcohol exposure required for sedation and longer recovery times to regain postural control compared to wild-type flies [202]. Constant light is frequently used in *Drosophila* as an environmental method to ablate molecular and behavioral circadian rhythmicity without the need for genetic manipulations [150, 290, 295–297] as genetic mutations or constitutive knockouts present during development may affect neural circuitry thus influencing adult behavior. Flies housed in constant light exhibit increased sensitivity to alcohol and longer recovery times [202, 290]. Circadian arrhythmicity arising from the *per^{01}* mutation or constant light exposure also appears associated with increased alcohol-induced mortality in *Drosophila* [298].

Disruption of the circadian oscillator affects alcohol behaviors and toxicity across species. *mPer2* mutant mice display increased voluntary alcohol intake and fail to exhibit diurnal rhythms in the behavioral response to alcohol [291, 299]. In humans, the regulation of alcohol consumption appears altered with gene variations in *hper2* determined by single-nucleotide polymorphism analysis correlated with higher or lower alcohol consumption [299, 300]. The Per2 gene and the circadian clock have also been postulated to play a role in regulating developmental changes following alcohol exposure as *mper2* mutant mice fail to exhibit the persistent hypothalamic changes associated with early-life alcohol exposure in wild-type mice [301]. In mice, genetic or environmental disruption of the circadian clock increases alcohol-induced pathologies including intestinal permeability and hepatic inflammation [302] and significantly alters gene expression for many genes involved in inflammation or metabolic responses [303]. Alcohol-induced colorectal cancer in mice is also increased with circadian desynchronization from shifting light-dark cycles [304]. In humans, circadian misalignment in night-shift workers is postulated to be a contributing factor to the development of liver injury with alcohol consumption [30]. Thus, circadian desynchronization appears to be a key factor in alcohol sensitivity and alcohol-induced pathologies across species.

6.3. Circadian Clock and Alcohol Tolerance. The development of alcohol tolerance and associated changes in neural plasticity also appears to require a functional circadian clock, even though the degree of rapid tolerance following alcohol exposure does not vary with time of day [290]. Flies with mutations in core oscillator genes including *per^{01}* and *tim^{01}* fail to develop functional tolerance following alcohol exposure while *cyc^{01}* flies only acquire weak tolerance [294]. Flies with the circadian clock rendered nonfunctional by constant light also fail to develop tolerance [294]. However, mutant *Clk^{Jrk}* flies develop tolerance similar to that of wild-type flies raising the possibility that PER and other core clock components regulate alcohol-induced behaviors independent of the circadian clock [294].

6.4. Effect of Alcohol on the Circadian Clock. The interactions between the circadian clock and alcohol are bidirectional. In rodent models, acute and chronic alcohol exposure results in phase shifts in locomotor activity rhythms and alters the ability of the circadian system to respond to perturbations [305–308]. Furthermore, chronic alcohol administration alters SCN function by disrupting the SCN responsiveness to light and nonphotic resetting as shown through *in vivo* and *in vitro* studies [305, 309]. Chronic alcohol exposure also affects neuropeptide signaling in the SCN decreasing the amount of vasopressin and VIP in SCN neurons [286]. In humans, chronic alcohol use or acute binge alcohol consumption appear to be strongly linked to sleep and circadian disorders [3, 310, 311]. The mRNA expression of *clk1*, *bmal1*, *per2*, *cry1*, and *cry2* is significantly reduced in alcoholic patients [312]. However, unlike rodent models, a single acute alcohol exposure in humans does not appear

sufficient to affect the phase-shifting ability of the circadian system [313].

Alcohol differentially affects central and peripheral oscillators. Studies in mice and rats demonstrate that repeated alcohol exposure results in major alterations in peripheral rhythms reducing the correlation in the phase relationships between body temperature and activity rhythms as well as altering and blunting the rhythms in plasma corticosterone, glucose, lactic acid, triglycerides, and cholesterol [287, 314, 315]. Distinct tissue-specific interactions and changes in gene expression have also been observed following chronic alcohol use in *clock* mutant mice for the hippocampus, liver, and colon [303]. Alcohol administration increases CLOCK and PER2 protein levels in intestinal epithelial cell cultures and increases measures of alcohol-induced permeability [316]. At the molecular level, chronic alcohol exposure appears to have the greatest effect on phase shifts or disruptions of core clock and clock-controlled genes in the liver rather than in the SCN [315, 317]. Chronic alcohol phase advances the rhythms in *Per1* expression in the adrenal and pituitary clocks and *Per2* expression in the liver clocks, without affecting the molecular clock in the SCN resulting in discord in the phase relationships between the SCN and peripheral oscillators [314, 317]. However, earlier research suggested that chronic alcohol administration affected the rhythmic expression of proopiomelanocortin, Per2, and Per3 in the SCN [318].

Bidirectional interactions between alcohol and the circadian clock are also conserved in *Drosophila*. For example, developmental alcohol exposure during the third larval instar affects period length in adult flies [319, 320]. With substantial evidence attesting to the value of *Drosophila* as a model for alcohol research and the parallels between the interactions of the circadian system with alcohol neurobiology across species (see Table 2), *Drosophila* appears poised for future studies probing the mechanism through which the circadian clock modulates these behaviors.

7. Interactions of the Circadian System with Cocaine

7.1. Circadian Modulation of Cocaine Behaviors. One of the earliest hints of an interaction between cocaine and the circadian system arose from studies of patients with seasonal affective disorder and seasonal variations in cocaine abuse [321, 322]. Subsequent research in rodent models found that the effects of acute cocaine exposure on locomotor activity were dependent upon the time of day [323] as was cocaine-induced behavioral sensitization [324–326]. Similar to alcohol behaviors, cocaine sensitization appears lowest during the night [324–326] correlated with the animal's activity period. Cocaine self-administration also varies with the circadian cycle [327] suggesting strong interactions between cocaine and the circadian system.

7.2. Cocaine's Effects on the Circadian Clock. Similar to alcohol, cocaine also bidirectionally interacts with the circadian clock. Cocaine administration disrupts light-induced phase shifts of the SCN during the night while cocaine

TABLE 2: Genes that mediate circadian and alcohol interactions.

Fly ortholog	Encoded protein	Genetic manipulation	*Drosophila* alcohol-related phenotypes	Mammalian homolog	References
per^{01}	PER	↓ expression	↑ alcohol sensitivity ↓ rapid tolerance ↑ recovery time	mPer1; mPer2	[202, 290, 291, 294, 299, 301, 318]
tim^{01}	TIM	↓ expression	↑ alcohol sensitivity ↓ rapid tolerance	—	[294]
cyc^{01}	CYCLE	↓ expression	↑ alcohol sensitivity ↓ rapid tolerance	BMAL	[30, 294]
Clk^{JRK}	CLOCK	↓ expression	No change	CLOCK	[294, 434]

TABLE 3: Genes mediating circadian and drug interactions in flies and mammals.

Gene/manipulation	Mechanism of action	Drug-related phenotypes in *Drosophila*	Reference	Drug studied in mammals	Reference
per^{01}	Regulation of circadian rhythms	↓ behavioral sensitization to cocaine	[334]	*mPer1* and *mPer2*: cocaine, morphine, and amphetamines	[324, 326, 336, 435, 436]
clk	Regulation of circadian rhythms	↓ behavioral sensitization to cocaine	[334]	*Clk*: cocaine, morphine, and amphetamines	[324, 336, 437, 438]
cyc^{01}	Regulation of circadian rhythms	↓ behavioral sensitization to cocaine	[334]	*Bmal*: cocaine and amphetamine	[324, 336, 436]
tim^{01}	Regulation of circadian rhythms	No change in response to cocaine	[334]	—	—
dbt	Regulation of circadian rhythms	↓ behavioral sensitization to cocaine	[334]	*Csnk1?*: cocaine, amphetamines, and opiods	[439–442]
dLmo	Regulation of dopamine receptor expression	↑ sensitivity to cocaine and nicotine and weak circadian rhythms in locomotor activity	[333]	*Lmo4*: cocaine	[338, 443]

administration during the day induces phase advances as shown through *in vivo* studies in mice and *in vitro* studies using SCN slices [328, 329]. The effects of cocaine on phase shifting of the circadian clock appear mediated through serotonin transporter antagonism and Per2 [329]. Repeated cocaine exposure has also been shown to differentially affect *per2* gene expression in the caudate putamen in rats [330].

7.3. Genes Mediating Circadian Cocaine Responses. At the first glance, *Drosophila* may seem an unusual model to forward the studies of drug abuse, but the extent of readily available mutants and the ease of behavioral screens accelerated the identification of genes involved in circadian-cocaine interactions (Table 3). In response to cocaine, *Drosophila* exhibits motor and reflexive behaviors including grooming and locomotor circling similar to those of mammals [331–333]. One of the first studies demonstrating the interplay between circadian genes and the drugs of abuse showed that flies with mutations in the circadian gene *per* failed to sensitize to cocaine (indicated by erratic jumping, twirling, and paralysis) even after repeated exposures to cocaine compared to wild-type Canton-S flies [334]. However, *per* mutants with altered period length rather than arrhythmicity display differential responses to cocaine; *per^S* mutants exhibit increased responsiveness followed by a weak sensitization to

cocaine exposure while *per^L* mutants show normal initial behavioral responses to cocaine but no sensitization [334].

This research spurred subsequent studies in mice examining the relationship between *per* and cocaine responsiveness. In mice, the *period* gene also appears strongly linked to cocaine behaviors. Mice with a mutation in *mPer1* do not sensitize to cocaine [324], and circadian rhythms in Per1 expression in the striatum appear necessary for rhythms in cocaine sensitization [326]. Recently, a variable repeat polymorphism in hPer2 was correlated with higher expression in cocaine-addicted individuals and cocaine users [335]. *mPer2* mutant mice display hypersensitization to cocaine, although they exhibit normal levels of conditioned place preference (CPP) with cocaine reward [324].

Additional evidence for the role of PER in cocaine responses comes from studies of flies with mutations in proteins that interact with PER. Flies with a mutation in *doubletime (homolog of casein kinase 1-epsilon)* require a higher dosage of cocaine to exhibit cocaine-induced behaviors with the first cocaine exposure but do not show significant sensitization with multiple exposures [334]. CLK and CYC mutant flies display increased initial sensitivity to cocaine compared to wild-type flies but fail to develop sensitization following the second exposure [334]. In mammals, additional circadian genes have also been implicated in cocaine responses. $Clock^{\Delta 19}$ mutant mice exhibit increased cocaine self-administration and conditioned place preference in response to cocaine compared to wild-type mice [336, 337].

While the above studies highlight the role of multiple circadian genes, particularly *per*, in mediating drug-induced behaviors, the function of these genes in drug behaviors may be distinct from their function in the regulation of the circadian clock. For example, tim^0 flies exhibit behavioral responses to cocaine similar to wild-type flies suggesting a divergence between the regulation of circadian function and that of cocaine behavior [334]. Intriguingly, regulation of cocaine behaviors appears to involve the small ventral lateral neurons in *Drosophila*, considered circadian pacemaker neurons, although neurotransmission through the primary circadian neuropeptide PDF is not required for cocaine behavioral responses [333]. Within the small ventral lateral neurons, the Lim-only gene *lmo* appears involved in both cocaine sensitization and circadian locomotor activity rhythms. *lmo* expression/function is inversely correlated with cocaine sensitivity as mutants with low levels of LMO exhibit increased cocaine sensitivity while flies in which overexpression of LMO occurs demonstrate increased resistance to the acute effects of cocaine [333]. *lmo* mutant flies display poor locomotor activity rhythms. In mice, *lmo4* also regulates cocaine sensitization [221] and the expression of *lmo4* is regulated by the circadian clock [338] reinforcing the relationship between the circadian clock and cocaine behaviors.

7.4. Circadian Regulation of the Reward System. A conserved feature of circadian influence on drug abuse and addiction arises from circadian regulation of the reward system. Biogenic amines produced in both the central and peripheral nervous system control motor behaviors in vertebrates and invertebrates [339–342]. Cocaine and other drugs of abuse act directly on the mesolimbic dopamine system and other pathways to promote drug-seeking behavior. In mammals and flies during reward learning, the valence and reward properties of a stimulus involve dopamine signaling, glutamate, and GABA in a complex feedback and feedforward network [343, 344]. In *Drosophila*, reward learning requires dopaminergic projections to the mushroom body neurons [125, 345] whereas in mammals, dopaminergic innervation from the ventral tegmental area to the striatum, the bed nucleus of the stria terminalis, and the nucleus accumbens is required for reward preference [346].

In *Drosophila* and mammals, the responsiveness of dopamine receptors is regulated by the circadian clock and dependent on functional expression of the *per* gene [347–349]. Using direct application of a D2 agonist, quinpirole, to the D2 receptors of the ventral nerve cord, Andretic and colleagues found that functional circadian genes are necessary for behavioral responses to cocaine in behaviorally active decapitated flies [334]. Furthermore, flies with mutations in *per*, *clock*, or *cycle* show no induction of tyrosine decarboxylase activity (TDC) which is necessary for the synthesis of tyramine, an important element for cocaine sensitization in *Drosophila* [332, 334]. Similarly in mammals, mice mutant in *Clock* show increased tyrosine hydroxylase (TH), the

rate-limiting enzyme for dopamine synthesis as well as other dopamine-related genes, and increased cocaine CPP [336]. Furthermore, many of the diurnal differences in cocaine self-administration may be due to the regulation of dopaminergic transmission. Andretic and Hirsh [347] identified diurnal regulation of dopamine receptor responsiveness in *Drosophila*. Likewise in mammals, most of the components of dopaminergic transmission including the dopamine receptor, dopamine transporter, and tyrosine hydroxylase exhibit diurnal rhythms [350–352]. More detailed discussions of the interactions of the circadian system with drug neurobiology in mammals may be found in recent reviews [348, 353–355].

Per1-knockout mice fail to display conditioned place preference (CPP) with cocaine reward [324] which is regulated by the circadian clock through the pineal gland and melatonin [356]. Recently, melatonin also was shown to significantly reduce motivation for cocaine and cocaine-seeking behavior in rats [357]. In summary, these studies suggest that a functional core circadian oscillator is necessary to drive pineal gland/melatonin outputs that regulate striatal *per1* gene expression to affect cocaine behaviors. However, the relationship between *per1* regulation and cocaine behavior is complicated as *Per1* mutant mice self-administer cocaine and display reinstatement of cocaine administration following extinction similar to wild-type counterparts [358]. This is reminiscent of the differential circadian modulation of alcohol-induced behaviors and suggests different neurobiological mechanisms underlying various drug behaviors.

7.5. Impact of Drosophila Circadian Cocaine Research. Despite the successes with the use of *Drosophila* as a model for investigations of drug abuse, surprisingly little research in *Drosophila* has been performed in the past few years delineating additional circadian-drug interactions outside of alcohol neurobiology. However, the research in *Drosophila* identifying links between PER and cocaine sensitization directly fostered research in mammals investigating circadian interactions with morphine [359–361] and methamphetamine [362]. Thus, research in *Drosophila* has provided impetus and conceptual advances in our understanding of the influence of the circadian clock on behavioral responses to drugs as well outlining roles circadian genes and neurons can play outside of the circadian clock in drug responses.

8. Potential Avenues for Future *Drosophila* Research

Despite the progress in research outlining connections between the circadian system, substance abuse, and the reward system, our understanding of the scope of these interactions and the underlying mechanisms through which these connections occur remains limited in both *Drosophila* and mammalian models directly impacting the prevention and treatment of drug-induced pathologies and addiction disorders. Techniques in rodent models have rapidly advanced over the past decade with sophisticated innovations permitting tissue-specific manipulations in gene expression and neuronal activity. Despite these advances, research in rodent models remains expensive and time consuming, reinforcing a need for the continued use of alternative model systems. The ease of maintenance, relatively short lifespan, and the neurogenetic approaches possibly have permitted *Drosophila* to remain at the forefront of neuroscience and disease research facilitating more targeted research in mammalian models. Primary areas of circadian-drug research in which *Drosophila* could provide advancement can be grouped into three strategic classifications: (1) system-level research (behavioral sensitivity and pathology) for defining the interactions between the circadian clock, sleep, and substance abuse; (2) identification of molecular networks for identifying the connections between the circadian system and substance neurobiology; and (3) drug discovery and small-molecule screening for therapy development.

8.1. System-Level Research. Behavioral research has exposed bidirectional interactions between the circadian system and substance abuse; however, the scope of these interactions remains undefined. Alcohol and cocaine represent the only drugs of abuse for which circadian interactions have been studied in *Drosophila*. Yet, considerable research has been done on dopaminergic signaling and reward pathways in *Drosophila* with significant parallels shown to mammals making *Drosophila* a suitable choice for studies of additional drugs of abuse. For example, dopamine and octopamine modulate the acute activating effects of nicotine on locomotion and the startle response [261, 363]. As substance abuse is often comorbid with additional substance abuse, poor nutrition, or sleep disorders, the ease of large-scale behavioral studies in *Drosophila* facilitates combinatorial studies.

The effects of other drugs of abuse including nicotine, morphine, amphetamine, and cannabinoids have been studied in *Drosophila* [364–366], expanding the possibilities for further investigation of the bidirectional interactions between the circadian clock and drug neurobiology using *Drosophila*. Comparatively little research has been done to dissect the relationship between endocannabinoid or cannabinoid use and circadian clock function in humans or rodent models [367–369]. However, research has shown that cannabinoids can excite circadian clock neurons, and this may be linked to the behavioral effects of time dissociation experienced by marijuana users [370, 371]. Given the increasing prevalence of marijuana use with the number of users in the United States more than doubling since 2002 to 9.5% of the adult population and approximately 30% of those individuals meeting the criteria for addiction [372], more research is needed on the interactions of marijuana with the circadian clock. The physiological activities of endocannabinoids on cell signaling appear conserved between *Drosophila* and mammalian systems [373], and *Drosophila* has been used to investigate the role of cannabinoids as therapeutics [374, 375]. As concurrent use of marijuana and alcohol increases the effects of the individual drugs [376–378], combinatorial studies are needed. Thus, *Drosophila* may be a practical model for fast high-throughput studies translatable to mammalian models.

Considerably more behavioral research is needed to identify circadian modulation of sensitivity or toxicity

encompassing multiple exposure paradigms across age groups. The circadian system weakens with age across species resulting in damped molecular rhythms and altered behavioral and metabolic rhythms [89, 379, 380]. In both humans and animal models, older subjects demonstrate greater difficulty in phase shifting after perturbations to the circadian system [381, 382]. The weakening of the circadian system with age may contribute to the increased sensitivity to or toxicity of drugs of abuse observed in older individuals. In rodent models, aged animals appear more sensitive to the effects of alcohol and alcohol withdrawal [383, 384], although little research has been done examining circadian interactions with alcohol or drugs of abuse in aged animals. With its relatively short lifespan, *Drosophila* is an excellent system for the aging system with analogous age-related changes to those observed in rodent models and humans.

8.2. Molecular Networks. With approximately 20,000 estimated human genes and an untold number of regulatory elements [385], identifying the underlying molecular or genetic mechanisms for complex behavioral and physiological issues remains an enormous challenge without potential candidates identified from animal models. This is particularly true for substance abuse disorders affecting the central nervous system that also result in widespread damage across tissues. Despite the neuroanatomical and morphological differences separating flies from humans, parallels exist for disease research affecting the central nervous system, heart, liver, kidneys, and gut [386], crucial organs for understanding the addictive and pathophysiological impacts of drug abuse.

Drosophila orthologs have been identified for approximately 75% of known human disease genes [105, 386–390]. The rapid cross-species translational value of *Drosophila* research has been demonstrated in alcohol neurobiology through the identification of the epidermal growth factor signaling pathway [195] and the role of a tyrosine kinase receptor, anaplastic lymphoma kinase [223], and the transcriptional regulator *Lmo* in alcohol behaviors [221]. Likewise, *Drosophila* has provided a model for the identification of candidate genes involved in addiction and reward behaviors [71, 139, 391]. The wide repertoire of tools in *Drosophila* to permit cost-effective large-scale genetic screens includes genome-wide RNAi screens with available collections of RNAi transgenic lines against every *Drosophila* gene [392], complete sets of micro RNA sponges with conditional expression possible [124, 393], and CRISPR-mediated mutations [394, 395].

8.3. Drug Discovery. The identification of new drugs for pharmaceutical use starting with target identification or small-molecule screening is a lengthy and expensive process often lasting more than a decade with costs up to $1 billion [396]. To streamline this process, high-throughput screens in *Drosophila* and other invertebrate models such as *C. elegans* have been employed more frequently in the past few years as a platform for target identification, drug discovery, and small-molecule screening. Previous research has demonstrated the predictive validity of *Drosophila* in preclinical research. *Drosophila* has proven beneficial for the validation and development of cancer drugs as well as for screening previously approved drugs for alternate purposes [397]. The tractability of *Drosophila* for large-scale screens include (1) viability and development assays for embryos, larvae, pupae, and adults; (2) whole-organism drug screens for absorption, metabolism, or toxicity; and (3) reporter assays including luciferase or GFP expression assays [397]. With the high degree of phylogenetic conservation in cellular signaling pathways, mechanistically the similarities between the *Drosophila* and mammalian circadian system make *Drosophila* an ideal platform for drug discovery for the identification of potential targets or therapeutics impacting the circadian system.

Through the ages, technological innovations have engineered societal changes transforming cultural norms and causing the urbanization of societies. Rapid advances in communication, networking, and information dissemination in the past two decades have solidified the establishment of a 24/7 global society further contributing to the rise of individual circadian and sleep disorders. The swiftness with which these technology-driven societal and cultural changes have become entrenched in children, adolescents, and adults makes it unlikely that the physical and mental health problems arising from circadian and sleep disorders will vanish. Thus, there is a critical need for continued research to delineate the mechanisms through which the circadian clock or circadian dysfunction affects substance abuse and conversely how substance abuse contributes to alterations in the functioning of the circadian system. Renewed research emphasis on invertebrate models as a practical and economical model to tackle these problems will provide basic biological insights into molecular pathways and cellular interactions associated with defined behaviors that can subsequently be investigated in more complex model systems with rapid translational impacts. Research in *Drosophila* has the capability to advance the understanding of the molecular changes or the genetic risk factors that transform substance use to abuse and addiction potentially providing new avenues for the identification of therapeutic interventions to minimize the risk of drug abuse and drug toxicity.

Acknowledgments

This work was supported by the National Institute on Alcohol Abuse and Alcoholism Grant R21AA021233.

References

[1] J. J. Sacks, K. R. Gonzales, E. E. Bouchery, L. E. Tomedi, and R. D. Brewer, "2010 national and state costs of excessive alcohol consumption," *American Journal of Preventive Medicine*, vol. 49, no. 5, pp. e73–e79, 2015.

[2] J. M. McGinnis and W. H. Foege, "Mortality and morbidity attributable to use of addictive substances in the United States," *Proceedings of the Association of American Physicians*, vol. 111, no. 2, pp. 109–118, 1999.

[3] D. A. Conroy and J. T. Arnedt, "Sleep and substance use disorders: an update," *Current Psychiatry Reports*, vol. 16, no. 10, p. 487, 2014.

[4] SAMSHA, *Results from the 2013 National Survey on Drug Use and Health. Summary of National Findings*, NSDUH Series H-48, HHS Publication No. (SMA) 14-4863(Substance Abuse and Mental Health Services Administration), Rockville, MD, USA, 2014.

[5] J. Rehm, C. Mathers, S. Popova, M. Thavorncharoensap, Y. Teerawattananon, and J. Patra, "Global burden of disease and injury and economic cost attributable to alcohol use and alcohol-use disorders," *The Lancet*, vol. 373, no. 9682, pp. 2223–2233, 2009.

[6] A. H. Mokdad, J. S. Marks, D. F. Stroup, and J. L. Gerberding, "Actual causes of death in the United States, 2000," *JAMA*, vol. 291, no. 10, pp. 1238–1245, 2004.

[7] D. Kanny, R. D. Brewer, J. B. Mesnick, L. J. Paulozzi, T. S. Naimi, and H. Lu, "Vital signs: alcohol poisoning deaths – United States, 2010-2012," *Morbidity and Mortality Weekly Report*, vol. 63, no. 53, pp. 1238–1242, 2015.

[8] H. G. Birnbaum, A. G. White, M. Schiller, T. Waldman, J. M. Cleveland, and C. L. Roland, "Societal costs of prescription opioid abuse, dependence, and misuse in the United States," *Pain Medicine*, vol. 12, no. 4, pp. 657–667, 2011.

[9] X. Xu, E. E. Bishop, S. M. Kennedy, S. A. Simpson, and T. F. Pechacek, "Annual healthcare spending attributable to cigarette smoking: an update," *American Journal of Preventive Medicine*, vol. 48, no. 3, pp. 326–333, 2015.

[10] C. S. Florence, C. Zhou, F. Luo, and L. Xu, "The economic burden of prescription opioid overdose, abuse, and dependence in the United States, 2013," *Medical Care*, vol. 54, no. 10, pp. 901–906, 2016.

[11] A. Hughes, M. R. Williams, R. N. Lipari, and S. Van Horn, "State estimates of past year cocaine use among young adults: 2014 and 2015," *The CBHSQ Report*, Center for Behavioral Health Statistics and Quality, Substance Abuse and Mental Health Services Administration, Rockville, MD, USA, 2016.

[12] R. E. Mistlberger and D. J. Skene, "Social influences on mammalian circadian rhythms: animal and human studies," *Biological Reviews of the Cambridge Philosophical Society*, vol. 79, no. 3, pp. 533–556, 2004.

[13] T. Roenneberg and M. Merrow, "The circadian clock and human health," *Current Biology*, vol. 26, no. 10, pp. R432–R443, 2016.

[14] U. Schibler, I. Gotic, C. Saini et al., "Clock-talk: interactions between central and peripheral circadian oscillators in mammals," *Cold Spring Harbor Symposia on Quantitative Biology*, vol. 80, pp. 223–232, 2015.

[15] J. Bass and J. S. Takahashi, "Circadian integration of metabolism and energetics," *Science*, vol. 330, no. 6009, pp. 1349–1354, 2010.

[16] W. Huang, K. M. Ramsey, B. Marcheva, and J. Bass, "Circadian rhythms, sleep, and metabolism," *Journal of Clinical Investigation*, vol. 121, no. 6, pp. 2133–2141, 2011.

[17] M. V. Plikus, E. N. Van Spyk, K. Pham et al., "The circadian clock in skin: implications for adult stem cells, tissue regeneration, cancer, aging, and immunity," *Journal of Biological Rhythms*, vol. 30, no. 3, pp. 163–182, 2015.

[18] M. Wittmann, M. Paulus, and T. Roenneberg, "Decreased psychological well-being in late 'chronotypes' is mediated by smoking and alcohol consumption," *Substance Use & Misuse*, vol. 45, no. 1-2, pp. 15–30, 2010.

[19] B. P. Hasler, S. L. Sitnick, D. S. Shaw, and E. E. Forbes, "An altered neural response to reward may contribute to alcohol problems among late adolescents with an evening chronotype," *Psychiatry Research*, vol. 214, no. 3, pp. 357–364, 2013.

[20] U. Broms, J. Kaprio, C. Hublin, M. Partinen, P. A. Madden, and M. Koskenvuo, "Evening types are more often current smokers and nicotine-dependent—a study of Finnish adult twins," *Addiction*, vol. 106, no. 1, pp. 170–177, 2011.

[21] S. S. Gau, C. Y. Shang, K. R. Merikangas, Y. N. Chiu, W. T. Soong, and A. T. Cheng, "Association between morningness-eveningness and behavioral/emotional problems among adolescents," *Journal of Biological Rhythms*, vol. 22, no. 3, pp. 268–274, 2007.

[22] B. P. Hasler and D. B. Clark, "Circadian misalignment, reward-related brain function, and adolescent alcohol involvement," *Alcoholism, Clinical and Experimental Research*, vol. 37, no. 4, pp. 558–565, 2013.

[23] T. Bogg, P. R. Finn, and K. E. Monsey, "A year in the college life: evidence for the social investment hypothesis via trait self-control and alcohol consumption," *Journal of Research in Personality*, vol. 46, no. 6, pp. 694–699, 2012.

[24] U. Albrecht, "The circadian clock, metabolism and obesity," *Obesity Reviews*, vol. 18, Supplement 1, pp. 25–33, 2017.

[25] G. R. Sridhar and N. S. Sanjana, "Sleep, circadian dysrhythmia, obesity and diabetes," *World Journal of Diabetes*, vol. 7, no. 19, pp. 515–522, 2016.

[26] F. A. Scheer, M. F. Hilton, C. S. Mantzoros, and S. A. Shea, "Adverse metabolic and cardiovascular consequences of circadian misalignment," *Proceedings of the National Academy of Sciences of the United States of America*, vol. 106, no. 11, pp. 4453–4458, 2009.

[27] D. M. Arble, K. M. Ramsey, J. Bass, and F. W. Turek, "Circadian disruption and metabolic disease: findings from animal models," *Best Practice & Research Clinical Endocrinology & Metabolism*, vol. 24, no. 5, pp. 785–800, 2010.

[28] A. W. McHill and K. P. Wright, "Role of sleep and circadian disruption on energy expenditure and in metabolic predisposition to human obesity and metabolic disease," *Obesity Reviews*, vol. 18, Supplement 1, pp. 15–24, 2017.

[29] B. P. Hasler, L. J. Smith, J. C. Cousins, and R. R. Bootzin, "Circadian rhythms, sleep, and substance abuse," *Sleep Medicine Reviews*, vol. 16, no. 1, pp. 67–81, 2012.

[30] G. R. Swanson, A. Gorenz, M. Shaikh et al., "Night workers with circadian misalignment are susceptible to alcohol-induced intestinal hyperpermeability with social drinking," *American Journal of Physiology - Gastrointestinal and Liver Physiology*, vol. 311, no. 1, pp. G192–G201, 2016.

[31] A. R. Meyers and M. W. Perrine, "Drinking by police officers, general drivers and late-night drivers," *Journal of Studies on Alcohol*, vol. 57, no. 2, pp. 187–192, 1996.

[32] A. S. Keuroghlian, A. S. Barry, and R. D. Weiss, "Circadian dysregulation, zolpidem dependence, and withdrawal seizure in a resident physician performing shift work," *The American Journal on Addictions*, vol. 21, no. 6, pp. 576-577, 2012.

[33] K. S. Kendler, H. Ohlsson, J. Sundquist, and K. Sundquist, "Alcohol use disorder and mortality across the lifespan: a longitudinal cohort and co-relative analysis," *JAMA Psychiatry*, vol. 73, no. 6, pp. 575–581, 2016.

[34] H. Wan, D. Goodkind, and P. Kowal, *An Aging World: 2015*, U.S. Census Bureau, International Population Reports, Washington, DC, USA, 2015, P95(16-1).

[35] C. C. Caruso, E. M. Hitchcock, R. B. Dick, J. M. Russo, and J. M. Schmit, *Overtime and Extended Work Shifts: Recent Findings on Illnesses, Injuries and Health Behavior*, U.S. Department of Health and Human Services, Centers for Disease control and Prevention, Cincinatti, OH, USA, 2004.

[36] T. Alterman, S. E. Luckhaupt, J. M. Dahlhamer, B. W. Ward, and G. M. Calvert, "Prevalence rates of work organization characteristics among workers in the U.S.: data from the 2010 National Health Interview Survey," *American Journal of Industrial Medicine*, vol. 56, no. 6, pp. 647–659, 2013.

[37] Institute of Medicine (US) Committee on Sleep Medicine and Research, H. R. Colten, and B. M. Altevogt, *Sleep Disorders and Sleep Deprivation: An Unmet Public Health Problem*, National Academies Press, Washington, DC, USA, 2006.

[38] A. D. Laposky, E. Van Cauter, and A. V. Diez-Roux, "Reducing health disparities: the role of sleep deficiency and sleep disorders," *Sleep Medicine*, vol. 18, pp. 3–6, 2016.

[39] K. G. Lambert, R. J. Nelson, T. Jovanovic, and M. Cerdá, "Brains in the city: neurobiological effects of urbanization," *Neuroscience & Biobehavioral Reviews*, vol. 58, pp. 107–122, 2015.

[40] C. J. Matz, D. M. Stieb, K. Davis et al., "Effects of age, season, gender and urban-rural status on time-activity: Canadian Human Activity Pattern Survey 2 (CHAPS 2)," *International Journal of Environmental Research and Public Health*, vol. 11, no. 2, pp. 2108–2124, 2014.

[41] R. C. Espiritu, D. F. Kripke, S. Ancoli-Israel et al., "Low illumination experienced by San Diego adults: association with atypical depressive symptoms," *Biological Psychiatry*, vol. 35, no. 6, pp. 403–407, 1994.

[42] B. L. Diffey, "An overview analysis of the time people spend outdoors," *British Journal of Dermatology*, vol. 164, no. 4, pp. 848–854, 2011.

[43] M. H. Smolensky, L. L. Sackett-Lundeen, and F. Portaluppi, "Nocturnal light pollution and underexposure to daytime sunlight: complementary mechanisms of circadian disruption and related diseases," *Chronobiology International*, vol. 32, no. 8, pp. 1029–1048, 2015.

[44] R. M. Lunn, D. E. Blask, A. N. Coogan et al., "Health consequences of electric lighting practices in the modern world: a report on the National Toxicology Program's workshop on shift work at night, artificial light at night, and circadian disruption," *Science of The Total Environment*, vol. 607-608, pp. 1073–1084, 2017.

[45] T. A. Bedrosian and R. J. Nelson, "Timing of light exposure affects mood and brain circuits," *Translational Psychiatry*, vol. 7, no. 1, article e1017, 2017.

[46] F. Falchi, P. Cinzano, D. Duriscoe et al., "The new world atlas of artificial night sky brightness," *Science Advances*, vol. 2, no. 6, article e1600377, 2016.

[47] S. Hattar, H. W. Liao, M. Takao, D. M. Berson, and K. W. Yau, "Melanopsin-containing retinal ganglion cells: architecture, projections, and intrinsic photosensitivity," *Science*, vol. 295, no. 5557, pp. 1065–1070, 2002.

[48] S. Hattar, R. J. Lucas, N. Mrosovsky et al., "Melanopsin and rod-cone photoreceptive systems account for all major

accessory visual functions in mice," *Nature*, vol. 424, no. 6944, pp. 76–81, 2003.

[49] K. J. Navara and R. J. Nelson, "The dark side of light at night: physiological, epidemiological, and ecological consequences," *Journal of Pineal Research*, vol. 43, no. 3, pp. 215–224, 2007.

[50] L. K. Fonken, J. L. Workman, J. C. Walton et al., "Light at night increases body mass by shifting the time of food intake," *Proceedings of the National Academy of Sciences of the United States of America*, vol. 107, no. 43, pp. 18664–18669, 2010.

[51] I. Kloog, A. Haim, R. G. Stevens, M. Barchana, and B. A. Portnov, "Light at night co-distributes with incident breast but not lung cancer in the female population of Israel," *Chronobiology International*, vol. 25, no. 1, pp. 65–81, 2008.

[52] C. C. Kyba, K. P. Tong, J. Bennie et al., "Worldwide variations in artificial skyglow," *Scientific Reports*, vol. 5, p. 8409, 2015.

[53] K. P. Wright, A. W. McHill, B. R. Birks, B. R. Griffin, T. Rusterholz, and E. D. Chinoy, "Entrainment of the human circadian clock to the natural light-dark cycle," *Current Biology*, vol. 23, no. 16, pp. 1554–1558, 2013.

[54] M. H. Hagenauer and T. M. Lee, "The neuroendocrine control of the circadian system: adolescent chronotype," *Frontiers in Neuroendocrinology*, vol. 33, no. 3, pp. 211–229, 2012.

[55] T. Roenneberg, T. Kuehnle, P. P. Pramstaller et al., "A marker for the end of adolescence," *Current Biology*, vol. 14, no. 24, pp. R1038–R1039, 2004.

[56] S. J. Crowley, C. Acebo, and M. A. Carskadon, "Sleep, circadian rhythms, and delayed phase in adolescence," *Sleep Medicine*, vol. 8, no. 6, pp. 602–612, 2007.

[57] C. Cajochen, S. Frey, D. Anders et al., "Evening exposure to a light-emitting diodes (LED)-backlit computer screen affects circadian physiology and cognitive performance," *Journal of Applied Physiology*, vol. 110, no. 5, pp. 1432–1438, 2011.

[58] J. H. Oh, H. Yoo, H. K. Park, and Y. R. Do, "Analysis of circadian properties and healthy levels of blue light from smartphones at night," *Scientific Reports*, vol. 5, article 11325, 2015.

[59] A. L. Gamble, A. L. D'Rozario, D. J. Bartlett et al., "Adolescent sleep patterns and night-time technology use: results of the Australian Broadcasting Corporation's Big Sleep Survey," *PLoS One*, vol. 9, no. 11, article e111700, 2014.

[60] C. S. Nikhita, P. R. Jadhav, and S. A. Ajinkya, "Prevalence of mobile phone dependence in secondary school adolescents," *Journal of Clinical and Diagnostic Research*, vol. 9, no. 11, pp. VC06–VC09, 2015.

[61] N. L. Bragazzi and G. Del Puente, "A proposal for including nomophobia in the new DSM-V," *Psychology Research and Behavior Management*, vol. 7, pp. 155–160, 2014.

[62] N. Nathan and J. Zeitzer, "A survey study of the association between mobile phone use and daytime sleepiness in California high school students," *BMC Public Health*, vol. 13, p. 840, 2013.

[63] S. Sahin, K. Ozdemir, A. Unsal, and N. Temiz, "Evaluation of mobile phone addiction level and sleep quality in university students," *Pakistan Journal of Medical Sciences*, vol. 29, no. 4, pp. 913–918, 2013.

[64] B. Tassino, S. Horta, N. Santana, R. Levandovski, and A. Silva, "Extreme late chronotypes and social jetlag challenged by Antarctic conditions in a population of university students from Uruguay," *Sleep Science*, vol. 9, no. 1, pp. 20–28, 2016.

[65] T. Roenneberg, K. V. Allebrandt, M. Merrow, and C. Vetter, "Social jetlag and obesity," *Current Biology*, vol. 22, no. 10, pp. 939–943, 2012.

[66] F. Rutters, S. G. Lemmens, T. C. Adam et al., "Is social jetlag associated with an adverse endocrine, behavioral, and cardiovascular risk profile?," *Journal of Biological Rhythms*, vol. 29, no. 5, pp. 377–383, 2014.

[67] P. M. Wong, B. P. Hasler, T. W. Kamarck, M. F. Muldoon, and S. B. Manuck, "Social jetlag, chronotype, and cardiometabolic risk," *The Journal of Clinical Endocrinology & Metabolism*, vol. 100, no. 12, pp. 4612–4620, 2015.

[68] R. Levandovski, G. Dantas, L. C. Fernandes et al., "Depression scores associate with chronotype and social jetlag in a rural population," *Chronobiology International*, vol. 28, no. 9, pp. 771–778, 2011.

[69] D. Landayan and F. W. Wolf, "Shared neurocircuitry underlying feeding and drugs of abuse in *Drosophila*," *Biomedical Journal*, vol. 38, no. 6, pp. 496–509, 2015.

[70] A. S. Narayanan and A. Rothenfluh, "I believe I can fly!: use of drosophila as a model organism in neuropsychopharmacology research," *Neuropsychopharmacology*, vol. 41, no. 6, pp. 1439–1446, 2016.

[71] A. Park, A. Ghezzi, T. P. Wijesekera, and N. S. Atkinson, "Genetics and genomics of alcohol responses in Drosophila," *Neuropharmacology*, vol. 122, 2017.

[72] S. Fujii, P. Krishnan, P. Hardin, and H. Amrein, "Nocturnal male sex drive in *Drosophila*," *Current Biology*, vol. 17, no. 3, pp. 244–251, 2007.

[73] Y. Zhang, Y. Liu, D. Bilodeau-Wentworth, P. E. Hardin, and P. Emery, "Light and temperature control the contribution of specific DN1 neurons to *Drosophila* circadian behavior," *Current Biology*, vol. 20, no. 7, pp. 600–605, 2010.

[74] A. V. Devineni and U. Heberlein, "The evolution of *Drosophila melanogaster* as a model for alcohol research," *Annual Review of Neuroscience*, vol. 36, pp. 121–138, 2013.

[75] J. H. Jennings, D. Mazzi, M. G. Ritchie, and A. Hoikkala, "Sexual and postmating reproductive isolation between allopatric *Drosophila montana* populations suggest speciation potential," *BMC Evolutionary Biology*, vol. 11, p. 68, 2011.

[76] E. Bier, "*Drosophila*, the golden bug, emerges as a tool for human genetics," *Nature Reviews Genetics*, vol. 6, no. 1, pp. 9–23, 2005.

[77] R. J. Greenspan and H. A. Dierick, "'Am not I a fly like thee?' from genes in fruit flies to behavior in humans," *Human Molecular Genetics*, vol. 13, Spec No 2, pp. R267–R273, 2004.

[78] K. G. Hales, C. A. Korey, A. M. Larracuente, and D. M. Roberts, "Genetics on the fly: a primer on the *Drosophila* model system," *Genetics*, vol. 201, no. 3, pp. 815–842, 2015.

[79] D. B. Sattelle and S. D. Buckingham, "Invertebrate studies and their ongoing contributions to neuroscience," *Invertebrate Neuroscience*, vol. 6, no. 1, pp. 1–3, 2006.

[80] K. J. Venken, K. L. Schulze, N. A. Haelterman et al., "MiMIC: a highly versatile transposon insertion resource for engineering *Drosophila melanogaster* genes," *Nature Methods*, vol. 8, no. 9, pp. 737–743, 2011.

[81] K. J. Venken, J. H. Simpson, and H. J. Bellen, "Genetic manipulation of genes and cells in the nervous system of the fruit fly," *Neuron*, vol. 72, no. 2, pp. 202–230, 2011.

[82] Y. He and H. Jasper, "Studying aging in *Drosophila*," *Methods*, vol. 68, no. 1, pp. 129–133, 2014.

[83] A. Bitto, A. M. Wang, C. F. Bennett, and M. Kaeberlein, "Biochemical genetic pathways that modulate aging in multiple species," *Cold Spring Harbor Perspectives in Medicine*, vol. 5, no. 11, 2015.

[84] Y. Sun, J. Yolitz, C. Wang, E. Spangler, M. Zhan, and S. Zou, "Aging studies in Drosophila melanogaster," *Methods in Molecular Biology*, vol. 1048, pp. 77–93, 2013.

[85] M. S. Grotewiel, I. Martin, P. Bhandari, and E. Cook-Wiens, "Functional senescence in *Drosophila melanogaster*," *Ageing Research Reviews*, vol. 4, no. 3, pp. 372–397, 2005.

[86] E. P. Ratliff, R. E. Mauntz, R. W. Kotzebue et al., "Aging and autophagic function influences the progressive decline of adult Drosophila behaviors," *PLoS One*, vol. 10, no. 7, article e0132768, 2015.

[87] S. Poddighe, K. M. Bhat, M. D. Setzu et al., "Impaired sense of smell in a Drosophila Parkinson's model," *PLoS One*, vol. 8, no. 8, article e73156, 2013.

[88] C. Cirelli, "Brain plasticity, sleep and aging," *Gerontology*, vol. 58, no. 5, pp. 441–5, 2012.

[89] G. Cornelissen and K. Otsuka, "Chronobiology of aging: a mini-review," *Gerontology*, vol. 63, no. 2, pp. 118–128, 2017.

[90] K. Rakshit, N. Krishnan, E. M. Guzik, E. Pyza, and J. M. Giebultowicz, "Effects of aging on the molecular circadian oscillations in *Drosophila*," *Chronobiology International*, vol. 29, no. 1, pp. 5–14, 2012.

[91] M. Robertson and A. C. Keene, "Molecular mechanisms of age-related sleep loss in the fruit fly - a mini-review," *Gerontology*, vol. 59, no. 4, pp. 334–339, 2013.

[92] A. Vaccaro, S. Birman, and A. Klarsfeld, "Chronic jet lag impairs startle-induced locomotion in *Drosophila*," *Experimental Gerontology*, vol. 85, pp. 24–27, 2016.

[93] M. Saitoe, J. Horiuchi, T. Tamura, and N. Ito, "*Drosophila* as a novel animal model for studying the genetics of age-related memory impairment," *Reviews in the Neurosciences*, vol. 16, no. 2, pp. 137–149, 2005.

[94] D. Yamazaki and M. Saitoe, "cAMP/PKA signaling underlies age-related memory impairment," *Brain and Nerve*, vol. 60, no. 7, pp. 717–724, 2008.

[95] T. Kudo, M. Uchigashima, T. Miyazaki et al., "Three types of neurochemical projection from the bed nucleus of the stria terminalis to the ventral tegmental area in adult mice," *Journal of Neuroscience*, vol. 32, no. 50, pp. 18035–18046, 2012.

[96] A. Beramendi, S. Peron, G. Casanova, C. Reggiani, and R. Cantera, "Neuromuscular junction in abdominal muscles of *Drosophila melanogaster* during adulthood and aging," *The Journal of Comparative Neurology*, vol. 501, no. 4, pp. 498–508, 2007.

[97] N. Krishnan, K. Rakshit, E. S. Chow, J. S. Wentzell, D. Kretzschmar, and J. M. Giebultowicz, "Loss of circadian clock accelerates aging in neurodegeneration-prone mutants," *Neurobiology of Disease*, vol. 45, no. 3, pp. 1129–1135, 2012.

[98] M. S. Miller, P. Lekkas, J. M. Braddock et al., "Aging enhances indirect flight muscle fiber performance yet decreases flight ability in *Drosophila*," *Biophysical Journal*, vol. 95, no. 5, pp. 2391–2401, 2008.

[99] S. M. Egenriether, E. S. Chow, N. Krauth, and J. M. Giebultowicz, "Accelerated food source location in aging *Drosophila*," *Aging Cell*, vol. 14, no. 5, pp. 916–918, 2015.

[100] I. Eleftherianos and J. C. Castillo, "Molecular mechanisms of aging and immune system regulation in *Drosophila*," *International Journal of Molecular Sciences*, vol. 13, no. 8, pp. 9826–9844, 2012.

[101] K. Ocorr, L. Perrin, H. Y. Lim, L. Qian, X. Wu, and R. Bodmer, "Genetic control of heart function and aging in *Drosophila*," *Trends in Cardiovascular Medicine*, vol. 17, no. 5, pp. 177–182, 2007.

[102] S. C. Pandey, "Neuronal signaling systems and ethanol dependence," *Molecular Neurobiology*, vol. 17, no. 1–3, pp. 1–15, 1998.

[103] U. B. Pandey and C. D. Nichols, "Human disease models in *Drosophila melanogaster* and the role of the fly in therapeutic drug discovery," *Pharmacological Reviews*, vol. 63, no. 2, pp. 411–436, 2011.

[104] M. D. Adams, S. E. Celniker, R. A. Holt et al., "The genome sequence of *Drosophila melanogaster*," *Science*, vol. 287, no. 5461, pp. 2185–2195, 2000.

[105] T. E. Lloyd and J. P. Taylor, "Flightless flies: *Drosophila* models of neuromuscular disease," *Annals of the New York Academy of Sciences*, vol. 1184, pp. e1–20, 2010.

[106] L. T. Reiter, L. Potocki, S. Chien, M. Gribskov, and E. Bier, "A systematic analysis of human disease-associated gene sequences in *Drosophila melanogaster*," *Genome Research*, vol. 11, no. 6, pp. 1114–1125, 2001.

[107] R. Brandt and A. Paululat, "Microcompartments in the *Drosophila* heart and the mammalian brain: general features and common principles," *Biological Chemistry*, vol. 394, no. 2, pp. 217–230, 2013.

[108] L. Ma, "Can the *Drosophila* model help in paving the way for translational medicine in heart failure?," *Biochemical Society Transactions*, vol. 44, no. 5, pp. 1549–1560, 2016.

[109] D. Seyres, L. Röder, and L. Perrin, "Genes and networks regulating cardiac development and function in flies: genetic and functional genomic approaches," *Briefings in Functional Genomics*, vol. 11, no. 5, pp. 366–374, 2012.

[110] T. Roeder, K. Isermann, K. Kallsen, K. Uliczka, and C. Wagner, "A *Drosophila* asthma model – what the fly tells us about inflammatory diseases of the lung," *Advances in Experimental Medicine and Biology*, vol. 710, pp. 37–47, 2012.

[111] L. Zuo, E. Iordanou, R. R. Chandran, and L. Jiang, "Novel mechanisms of tube-size regulation revealed by the *Drosophila* trachea," *Cell and Tissue Research*, vol. 354, no. 2, pp. 343–354, 2013.

[112] J. A. Dow and M. F. Romero, "*Drosophila* provides rapid modeling of renal development, function, and disease," *American Journal of Physiology - Renal Physiology*, vol. 299, no. 6, pp. F1237–F1244, 2010.

[113] J. Miller, T. Chi, P. Kapahi et al., "Drosophila melanogaster as an emerging translational model of human nephrolithiasis," *The Journal of Urology*, vol. 190, no. 5, pp. 1648–1656, 2013.

[114] B. Erkosar and F. Leulier, "Transient adult microbiota, gut homeostasis and longevity: novel insights from the *Drosophila* model," *FEBS Letters*, vol. 588, no. 22, pp. 4250–4257, 2014.

[115] R. J. Katzenberger, B. Ganetzky, and D. A. Wassarman, "The gut reaction to traumatic brain injury," *Fly*, vol. 9, no. 2, pp. 68–74, 2015.

[116] M. Y. Pasco, R. Loudhaief, and A. Gallet, "The cellular homeostasis of the gut: what the *Drosophila* model points out," *Histology and Histopathology*, vol. 30, no. 3, pp. 277–292, 2015.

[117] J. M. McLaughlin and D. P. Bratu, "*Drosophila melanogaster* oogenesis: an overview," *Methods in Molecular Biology*, vol. 1328, pp. 1–20, 2015.

[118] N. A. Siddall and G. R. Hime, "A *Drosophila* toolkit for defining gene function in spermatogenesis," *Reproduction*, vol. 153, no. 4, pp. R121–R132, 2017.

[119] H. Kazama, "Systems neuroscience in *Drosophila*: conceptual and technical advantages," *Neuroscience*, vol. 296, pp. 3–14, 2015.

[120] C. Maximino, R. X. Silva, N. da Silva Sde et al., "Non-mammalian models in behavioral neuroscience: consequences for biological psychiatry," *Frontiers in Behavioral Neuroscience*, vol. 9, p. 233, 2015.

[121] G. Artiushin and A. Sehgal, "The *Drosophila* circuitry of sleep-wake regulation," *Current Opinion in Neurobiology*, vol. 44, pp. 243–250, 2017.

[122] K. M. Parisky, J. L. Agosto Rivera, N. C. Donelson, S. Kotecha, and L. C. Griffith, "Reorganization of sleep by temperature in drosophila requires light, the homeostat, and the circadian clock," *Current Biology*, vol. 26, no. 7, pp. 882–892, 2016.

[123] S. Potdar and V. Sheeba, "Lessons from sleeping flies: insights from *Drosophila melanogaster* on the neuronal circuitry and importance of sleep," *Journal of Neurogenetics*, vol. 27, no. 1-2, pp. 23–42, 2013.

[124] G. U. Busto, T. Guven-Ozkan, and R. L. Davis, "MicroRNA function in *Drosophila* memory formation," *Current Opinion in Neurobiology*, vol. 43, pp. 15–24, 2016.

[125] K. R. Kaun and A. Rothenfluh, "Dopaminergic rules of engagement for memory in *Drosophila*," *Current Opinion in Neurobiology*, vol. 43, pp. 56–62, 2017.

[126] A. French, M. Ali Agha, A. Mitra, A. Yanagawa, M. J. Sellier, and F. Marion-Poll, "*Drosophila* bitter taste(s)," *Frontiers in Integrative Neuroscience*, vol. 9, p. 58, 2015.

[127] A. S. French, M. J. Sellier, M. Ali Agha et al., "Dual mechanism for bitter avoidance in *Drosophila*," *Journal of Neuroscience*, vol. 35, no. 9, pp. 3990–4004, 2015.

[128] R. M. Joseph and J. R. Carlson, "*Drosophila* chemoreceptors: a molecular interface between the chemical world and the brain," *Trends in Genetics*, vol. 31, no. 12, pp. 683–695, 2015.

[129] C. Melcher, R. Bader, and M. J. Pankratz, "Amino acids, taste circuits, and feeding behavior in *Drosophila*: towards understanding the psychology of feeding in flies and man," *Journal of Endocrinology*, vol. 192, no. 3, pp. 467–472, 2007.

[130] E. J. Beckwith and M. F. Ceriani, "Communication between circadian clusters: the key to a plastic network," *FEBS Letters*, vol. 589, no. 22, pp. 3336–3342, 2015.

[131] E. J. Beckwith and M. F. Ceriani, "Experimental assessment of the network properties of the *Drosophila* circadian clock," *Journal of Comparative Neurology*, vol. 523, no. 6, pp. 982–996, 2015.

[132] C. Helfrich-Förster, "From neurogenetic studies in the fly brain to a concept in circadian biology," *Journal of Neurogenetics*, vol. 28, no. 3-4, pp. 329–347, 2014.

[133] C. Helfrich-Förster, M. Stengl, and U. Homberg, "Organization of the circadian system in insects," *Chronobiology International*, vol. 15, no. 6, pp. 567–594, 1998.

[134] O. Tataroglu and P. Emery, "Studying circadian rhythms in *Drosophila melanogaster*," *Methods*, vol. 68, no. 1, pp. 140–150, 2014.

[135] E. D. Hoopfer, "Neural control of aggression in *Drosophila*," *Current Opinion in Neurobiology*, vol. 38, pp. 109–118, 2016.

[136] E. A. Kravitz and L. Fernandez Mde, "Aggression in *Drosophila*," *Behavioral Neuroscience*, vol. 129, no. 5, pp. 549–563, 2015.

[137] D. Yamamoto and K. Sato, "The female brain and the male brain," *Brain and Nerve*, vol. 65, no. 10, pp. 1147–1158, 2013.

[138] D. Yamamoto, K. Sato, and M. Koganezawa, "Neuroethology of male courtship in *Drosophila*: from the gene to behavior," *Journal of Comparative Physiology A*, vol. 200, no. 4, pp. 251–264, 2014.

[139] K. R. Kaun, A. V. Devineni, and U. Heberlein, "*Drosophila melanogaster* as a model to study drug addiction," *Human Genetics*, vol. 131, no. 6, pp. 959–975, 2012.

[140] J. T. Littleton and B. Ganetzky, "Ion channels and synaptic organization: analysis of the *Drosophila* genome," *Neuron*, vol. 26, no. 1, pp. 35–43, 2000.

[141] C. A. Martin and D. E. Krantz, "*Drosophila melanogaster* as a genetic model system to study neurotransmitter transporters," *Neurochemistry International*, vol. 73, pp. 71–88, 2014.

[142] D. R. Nässel and A. M. Winther, "*Drosophila* neuropeptides in regulation of physiology and behavior," *Progress in Neurobiology*, vol. 92, no. 1, pp. 42–104, 2010.

[143] R. J. Konopka, C. Pittendrigh, and D. Orr, "Reciprocal behaviour associated with altered homeostasis and photosensitivity of *Drosophila* clock mutants," *Journal of Neurogenetics*, vol. 6, no. 1, pp. 1–10, 1989.

[144] C. S. Pittendrigh, P. C. Caldarola, and E. S. Cosbey, "A differential effect of heavy water on temperature-dependent and temperature-compensated aspects of circadian system of *Drosophila pseudoobscura*," *Proceedings of the National Academy of Sciences of the United States of America*, vol. 70, no. 7, pp. 2037–2041, 1973.

[145] C. S. Pittendrigh, W. T. Kyner, and T. Takamura, "The amplitude of circadian oscillations: temperature dependence, latitudinal clines, and the photoperiodic time measurement," *Journal of Biological Rhythms*, vol. 6, no. 4, pp. 299–313, 1991.

[146] C. S. Pittendrigh and D. H. Minis, "Circadian systems: longevity as a function of circadian resonance in *Drosophila melanogaster*," *Proceedings of the National Academy of Sciences of the United States of America*, vol. 69, no. 6, pp. 1537–1539, 1972.

[147] C. S. Pittendrigh and T. Takamura, "Latitudinal clines in the properties of a circadian pacemaker," *Journal of Biological Rhythms*, vol. 4, no. 2, pp. 217–235, 1989.

[148] Y. Zhang, J. Ling, C. Yuan, R. Dubruille, and P. Emery, "A role for *Drosophila* ATX2 in activation of PER translation and circadian behavior," *Science*, vol. 340, no. 6134, pp. 879–882, 2013.

[149] Y. Zhang and P. Emery, "GW182 controls *Drosophila* circadian behavior and PDF-receptor signaling," *Neuron*, vol. 78, no. 1, pp. 152–165, 2013.

[150] L. C. Lyons and G. Roman, "Circadian modulation of short-term memory in *Drosophila*," *Learning & Memory*, vol. 16, no. 1, pp. 19–27, 2009.

[151] F. Guo, J. Yu, H. J. Jung et al., "Circadian neuron feedback controls the *Drosophila* sleep–activity profile," *Nature*, vol. 536, no. 7616, pp. 292–297, 2016.

[152] R. Allada and B. Y. Chung, "Circadian organization of behavior and physiology in *Drosophila*," *Annual Review of Physiology*, vol. 72, pp. 605–624, 2010.

[153] J. Tomita, G. Ban, and K. Kume, "Genes and neural circuits for sleep of the fruit fly," *Neuroscience Research*, vol. 118, pp. 82–91, 2017.

[154] Y. Hamasaka, T. Suzuki, S. Hanai, and N. Ishida, "Evening circadian oscillator as the primary determinant of rhythmic motivation for *Drosophila* courtship behavior," *Genes to Cells*, vol. 15, no. 12, pp. 1240–1248, 2010.

[155] I. Medina, J. Casal, and C. C. Fabre, "Do circadian genes and ambient temperature affect substrate-borne signalling during *Drosophila* courtship?," *Biology Open*, vol. 4, no. 11, pp. 1549–1557, 2015.

[156] H. C. Krishnan and L. C. Lyons, "Synchrony and desynchrony in circadian clocks: impacts on learning and memory," *Learning & Memory*, vol. 22, no. 9, pp. 426–437, 2015.

[157] J. E. Lee and I. Edery, "Circadian regulation in the ability of *Drosophila* to combat pathogenic infections," *Current Biology*, vol. 18, no. 3, pp. 195–199, 2008.

[158] A. Chatterjee and P. E. Hardin, "Time to taste: circadian clock function in the *Drosophila* gustatory system," *Fly*, vol. 4, no. 4, pp. 283–287, 2010.

[159] A. Chatterjee, S. Tanoue, J. H. Houl, and P. E. Hardin, "Regulation of gustatory physiology and appetitive behavior by the *Drosophila* circadian clock," *Current Biology*, vol. 20, no. 4, pp. 300–309, 2010.

[160] N. Krishnan, D. Kretzschmar, K. Rakshit, E. Chow, and J. M. Giebultowicz, "The circadian clock gene period extends healthspan in aging *Drosophila melanogaster*," *Aging*, vol. 1, no. 11, pp. 937–948, 2009.

[161] P. Karpowicz, Y. Zhang, J. B. Hogenesch, P. Emery, and N. Perrimon, "The circadian clock gates the intestinal stem cell regenerative state," *Cell Reports*, vol. 3, no. 4, pp. 996–1004, 2013.

[162] R. J. Konopka and S. Benzer, "Clock mutants of *Drosophila melanogaster*," *Proceedings of the National Academy of Sciences of the United States of America*, vol. 68, no. 9, pp. 2112–2116, 1971.

[163] J. Y. Fan, B. Agyekum, A. Venkatesan et al., "Noncanonical FK506-binding protein BDBT binds DBT to enhance its circadian function and forms foci at night," *Neuron*, vol. 80, no. 4, pp. 984–996, 2013.

[164] J. M. Lin, V. L. Kilman, K. Keegan et al., "A role for casein kinase 2α in the *Drosophila* circadian clock," *Nature*, vol. 420, no. 6917, pp. 816–820, 2002.

[165] J. L. Price, J. Blau, A. Rothenfluh, M. Abodeely, B. Kloss, and M. W. Young, "*double-time* is a novel *Drosophila* clock gene that regulates PERIOD protein accumulation," *Cell*, vol. 94, no. 1, pp. 83–95, 1998.

[166] S. M. Reppert and I. Sauman, "*period* and *timeless* tango: a dance of two clock genes," *Neuron*, vol. 15, no. 5, pp. 983–986, 1995.

[167] A. Sehgal, J. L. Price, B. Man, and M. W. Young, "Loss of circadian behavioral rhythms and per RNA oscillations in the Drosophila mutant timeless," *Science*, vol. 263, no. 5153, pp. 1603–1606, 1994.

[168] R. Allada, N. E. White, W. V. So, J. C. Hall, and M. Rosbash, "A mutant *Drosophila* homolog of mammalian *Clock* disrupts circadian rhythms and transcription of *period* and *timeless*," *Cell*, vol. 93, no. 5, pp. 791–804, 1998.

[169] B. Akten, E. Jauch, G. K. Genova et al., "A role for CK2 in the *Drosophila* circadian oscillator," *Nature Neuroscience*, vol. 6, no. 3, pp. 251–257, 2003.

[170] S. Martinek, S. Inonog, A. S. Manoukian, and M. W. Young, "A role for the segment polarity gene *shaggy*/GSK-3 in the *Drosophila* circadian clock," *Cell*, vol. 105, no. 6, pp. 769–779, 2001.

[171] J. E. Rutila, V. Suri, M. Le, W. V. So, M. Rosbash, and J. C. Hall, "CYCLE is a second bHLH-PAS clock protein essential for circadian rhythmicity and transcription of *Drosophila period* and *timeless*," *Cell*, vol. 93, no. 5, pp. 805–814, 1998.

[172] B. Kloss, J. L. Price, L. Saez et al., "The *Drosophila* clock gene *double-time* encodes a protein closely related to human casein kinase Iε," *Cell*, vol. 94, no. 1, pp. 97–107, 1998.

[173] H. Tei, H. Okamura, Y. Shigeyoshi et al., "Circadian oscillation of a mammalian homologue of the *Drosophila* period gene," *Nature*, vol. 389, no. 6650, pp. 512–516, 1997.

[174] D. P. King, Y. Zhao, A. M. Sangoram et al., "Positional cloning of the mouse circadian clock gene," *Cell*, vol. 89, no. 4, pp. 641–653, 1997.

[175] M. P. Antoch, E. J. Song, A. M. Chang et al., "Functional identification of the mouse circadian *Clock* gene by transgenic BAC rescue," *Cell*, vol. 89, no. 4, pp. 655–667, 1997.

[176] T. Yoshii, C. Hermann-Luibl, and C. Helfrich-Förster, "Circadian light-input pathways in *Drosophila*," *Communicative & Integrative Biology*, vol. 9, no. 1, article e1102805, 2016.

[177] Z. Yao and O. T. Shafer, "The *Drosophila* circadian clock is a variably coupled network of multiple peptidergic units," *Science*, vol. 343, no. 6178, pp. 1516–1520, 2014.

[178] P. E. Hardin and S. Panda, "Circadian timekeeping and output mechanisms in animals," *Current Opinion in Neurobiology*, vol. 23, no. 5, pp. 724–731, 2013.

[179] O. Ozkaya and E. Rosato, "Chapter 4 - the circadian clock of the fly: a neurogenetics journey through time," *Advances in Genetics*, vol. 77, pp. 79–123, 2012.

[180] C. Dibner, U. Schibler, and U. Albrecht, "The mammalian circadian timing system: organization and coordination of central and peripheral clocks," *Annual Review of Physiology*, vol. 72, pp. 517–549, 2010.

[181] C. H. Ko and J. S. Takahashi, "Molecular components of the mammalian circadian clock," *Human Molecular Genetics*, vol. 15, Spec No 2, pp. R271–R277, 2006.

[182] N. R. Glossop, L. C. Lyons, and P. E. Hardin, "Interlocked feedback loops within the *Drosophila* circadian oscillator," *Science*, vol. 286, no. 5440, pp. 766–768, 1999.

[183] P. E. Hardin, J. C. Hall, and M. Rosbash, "Circadian oscillations in period gene mRNA levels are transcriptionally regulated," *Proceedings of the National Academy of Sciences of the United States of America*, vol. 89, no. 24, pp. 11711–11715, 1992.

[184] C. Dubowy and A. Sehgal, "Circadian rhythms and sleep in *Drosophila melanogaster*," *Genetics*, vol. 205, no. 4, pp. 1373–1397, 2017.

[185] S. Panda, "Circadian physiology of metabolism," *Science*, vol. 354, no. 6315, pp. 1008–1015, 2016.

[186] J. S. Takahashi, "Transcriptional architecture of the mammalian circadian clock," *Nature Reviews Genetics*, vol. 18, no. 3, pp. 164–179, 2017.

[187] J. S. Menet, K. C. Abruzzi, J. Desrochers, J. Rodriguez, and M. Rosbash, "Dynamic PER repression mechanisms in the *Drosophila* circadian clock: from on-DNA to off-DNA," *Genes & Development*, vol. 24, no. 4, pp. 358–367, 2010.

[188] K. C. Abruzzi, J. Rodriguez, J. S. Menet et al., "*Drosophila* CLOCK target gene characterization: implications for

circadian tissue-specific gene expression," *Genes & Development*, vol. 25, no. 22, pp. 2374–2386, 2011.

[189] Q. He, B. Wu, J. L. Price, and Z. Zhao, "Circadian rhythm neuropeptides in *Drosophila*: signals for normal circadian function and circadian neurodegenerative disease," *International Journal of Molecular Sciences*, vol. 18, no. 4, 2017.

[190] N. Huang, Y. Chelliah, Y. Shan et al., "Crystal structure of the heterodimeric CLOCK:BMAL1 transcriptional activator complex," *Science*, vol. 337, no. 6091, pp. 189–194, 2012.

[191] C. L. Partch, C. B. Green, and J. S. Takahashi, "Molecular architecture of the mammalian circadian clock," *Trends in Cell Biology*, vol. 24, no. 2, pp. 90–99, 2014.

[192] H. W. Ko, E. Y. Kim, J. Chiu, J. T. Vanselow, A. Kramer, and I. Edery, "A hierarchical phosphorylation cascade that regulates the timing of PERIOD nuclear entry reveals novel roles for proline-directed kinases and GSK-3β/SGG in circadian clocks," *Journal of Neuroscience*, vol. 30, no. 38, pp. 12664–12675, 2010.

[193] C. Iitaka, K. Miyazaki, T. Akaike, and N. Ishida, "A role for glycogen synthase kinase-3β in the mammalian circadian clock," *Journal of Biological Chemistry*, vol. 280, no. 33, pp. 29397–29402, 2005.

[194] O. Tataroglu and P. Emery, "The molecular ticks of the *Drosophila* circadian clock," *Current Opinion in Insect Science*, vol. 7, pp. 51–57, 2015.

[195] A. B. Corl, K. H. Berger, G. Ophir-Shohat et al., "Happyhour, a Ste20 family kinase, implicates EGFR signaling in ethanol-induced behaviors," *Cell*, vol. 137, no. 5, pp. 949–960, 2009.

[196] D. Kapfhamer, S. Taylor, M. E. Zou, J. P. Lim, V. Kharazia, and U. Heberlein, "Taok2 controls behavioral response to ethanol in mice," *Genes, Brain, and Behavior*, vol. 12, no. 1, pp. 87–97, 2013.

[197] H. Scholz and J. A. Mustard, "Invertebrate models of alcoholism," *Current Topics in Behavioral Neurosciences*, vol. 13, pp. 433–457, 2013.

[198] A. V. Devineni and U. Heberlein, "Preferential ethanol consumption in *Drosophila* models features of addiction," *Current Biology*, vol. 19, no. 24, pp. 2126–2132, 2009.

[199] A. R. Rodan and A. Rothenfluh, "The genetics of behavioral alcohol responses in *Drosophila*," *International Review of Neurobiology*, vol. 91, pp. 25–51, 2010.

[200] K. R. Kaun, R. Azanchi, Z. Maung, J. Hirsh, and U. Heberlein, "A *Drosophila* model for alcohol reward," *Nature Neuroscience*, vol. 14, no. 5, pp. 612–619, 2011.

[201] A. V. Devineni and U. Heberlein, "Acute ethanol responses in *Drosophila* are sexually dimorphic," *Proceedings of the National Academy of Sciences of the United States of America*, vol. 109, no. 51, pp. 21087–21092, 2012.

[202] A. K. De Nobrega and L. C. Lyons, "Circadian modulation of alcohol-induced sedation and recovery in male and female *Drosophila*," *Journal of Biological Rhythms*, vol. 31, no. 2, pp. 142–160, 2016.

[203] A. V. Devineni, K. D. McClure, D. J. Guarnieri et al., "The genetic relationships between ethanol preference, acute ethanol sensitivity, and ethanol tolerance in *Drosophila melanogaster*," *Fly*, vol. 5, no. 3, pp. 191–199, 2011.

[204] K. H. Berger, U. Heberlein, and M. S. Moore, "Rapid and chronic: two distinct forms of ethanol tolerance in Drosophila," *Alcoholism, Clinical and Experimental Research*, vol. 28, no. 10, pp. 1469–1480, 2004.

[205] H. Scholz, J. Ramond, C. M. Singh, and U. Heberlein, "Functional ethanol tolerance in *Drosophila*," *Neuron*, vol. 28, no. 1, pp. 261–271, 2000.

[206] H. R. Krishnan, X. Li, A. Ghezzi, and N. S. Atkinson, "A DNA element in the *slo* gene modulates ethanol tolerance," *Alcohol*, vol. 51, pp. 37–42, 2016.

[207] W. W. Ja, G. B. Carvalho, E. M. Mak et al., "Prandiology of *Drosophila* and the CAFE assay," *Proceedings of the National Academy of Sciences of the United States of America*, vol. 104, no. 20, pp. 8253–8256, 2007.

[208] A. V. Devineni and U. Heberlein, "Addiction-like behavior in Drosophila," *Communicative & Integrative Biology*, vol. 3, no. 4, pp. 357–359, 2010.

[209] S. Xu, T. Chan, V. Shah, S. Zhang, S. D. Pletcher, and G. Roman, "The propensity for consuming ethanol in *Drosophila* requires *rutabaga* adenylyl cyclase expression within mushroom body neurons," *Genes, Brain, and Behavior*, vol. 11, no. 6, pp. 727–739, 2012.

[210] J. B. Pohl, B. A. Baldwin, B. L. Dinh et al., "Ethanol preference in *Drosophila melanogaster* is driven by its caloric value," *Alcoholism, Clinical and Experimental Research*, vol. 36, no. 11, pp. 1903–1912, 2012.

[211] R. L. Peru Y Colón de Portugal, S. A. Ojelade, P. S. Penninti et al., "Long-lasting, experience-dependent alcohol preference in *Drosophila*," *Addiction Biology*, vol. 19, no. 3, pp. 392–401, 2014.

[212] D. J. Guarnieri and U. Heberlein, "*Drosophila melanogaster*, a genetic model system for alcohol research," *International Review of Neurobiology*, vol. 54, pp. 199–228, 2003.

[213] L. Sivanantharajah and B. Zhang, "Current techniques for high-resolution mapping of behavioral circuits in *Drosophila*," *Journal of Comparative Physiology A*, vol. 201, no. 9, pp. 895–909, 2015.

[214] D. M. Lovinger, G. White, and F. F. Weight, "Ethanol inhibits NMDA-activated ion current in hippocampal neurons," *Science*, vol. 243, no. 4899, pp. 1721–1724, 1989.

[215] M. Roberto and F. P. Varodayan, "Synaptic targets: chronic alcohol actions," *Neuropharmacology*, vol. 122, pp. 85–99, 2017.

[216] M. S. Moore, J. DeZazzo, A. Y. Luk, T. Tully, C. M. Singh, and U. Heberlein, "Ethanol intoxication in *Drosophila*: genetic and pharmacological evidence for regulation by the cAMP signaling pathway," *Cell*, vol. 93, no. 6, pp. 997–1007, 1998.

[217] S. K. Park, S. A. Sedore, C. Cronmiller, and J. Hirsh, "Type II cAMP-dependent protein kinase-deficient *Drosophila* are viable but show developmental, circadian, and drug response phenotypes," *Journal of Biological Chemistry*, vol. 275, no. 27, pp. 20588–20596, 2000.

[218] G. Wand, M. Levine, L. Zweifel, W. Schwindinger, and T. Abel, "The cAMP-protein kinase A signal transduction pathway modulates ethanol consumption and sedative effects of ethanol," *Journal of Neuroscience*, vol. 21, no. 14, pp. 5297–5303, 2001.

[219] T. E. Thiele, B. Willis, J. Stadler, J. G. Reynolds, I. L. Bernstein, and G. S. McKnight, "High ethanol consumption and low sensitivity to ethanol-induced sedation in protein kinase A-mutant mice," *Journal of Neuroscience*, vol. 20, no. 10, article RC75, 2000.

[220] M. B. Feany and W. G. Quinn, "A neuropeptide gene defined by the Drosophila memory mutant amnesiac," *Science*, vol. 268, no. 5212, pp. 869–873, 1995.

[221] A. W. Lasek, F. Giorgetti, K. H. Berger, S. Tayor, and U. Heberlein, "*Lmo* genes regulate behavioral responses to ethanol in *Drosophila melanogaster* and the mouse," *Alcoholism, Clinical and Experimental Research*, vol. 35, no. 9, pp. 1600–1606, 2011.

[222] A. Savarese, M. E. Zou, V. Kharazia, R. Maiya, and A. W. Lasek, "Increased behavioral responses to ethanol in *Lmo3* knockout mice," *Genes, Brain, and Behavior*, vol. 13, no. 8, pp. 777–783, 2014.

[223] A. W. Lasek, J. Lim, C. L. Kliethermes et al., "An evolutionary conserved role for anaplastic lymphoma kinase in behavioral responses to ethanol," *PLoS One*, vol. 6, no. 7, article e22636, 2011.

[224] J. Y. Gouzi, A. Moressis, J. A. Walker et al., "The receptor tyrosine kinase Alk controls neurofibromin functions in Drosophila growth and learning," *PLoS Genetics*, vol. 7, no. 9, article e1002281, 2011.

[225] J. W. Dutton, H. Chen, C. You, M. S. Brodie, and A. W. Lasek, "Anaplastic lymphoma kinase regulates binge-like drinking and dopamine receptor sensitivity in the ventral tegmental area," *Addiction Biology*, vol. 22, no. 3, pp. 665–678, 2017.

[226] P. Schweitzer, C. Cates-Gatto, F. P. Varodayan et al., "Dependence-induced ethanol drinking and GABA neurotransmission are altered in *Alk* deficient mice," *Neuropharmacology*, vol. 107, pp. 1–8, 2016.

[227] J. Wang, W. Yuan, and M. D. Li, "Genes and pathways co-associated with the exposure to multiple drugs of abuse, including alcohol, amphetamine/methamphetamine, cocaine, marijuana, morphine, and/or nicotine: a review of proteomics analyses," *Molecular Neurobiology*, vol. 44, no. 3, pp. 269–286, 2011.

[228] S. Dzitoyeva, N. Dimitrijevic, and H. Manev, "γ-Aminobutyric acid B receptor 1 mediates behavior-impairing actions of alcohol in *Drosophila*: adult RNA interference and pharmacological evidence," *Proceedings of the National Academy of Sciences of the United States of America*, vol. 100, no. 9, pp. 5485–5490, 2003.

[229] M. J. Zaleski, J. R. Nunes Filho, T. Lemos, and G. S. Morato, "GABA_B receptors play a role in the development of tolerance to ethanol in mice," *Psychopharmacology*, vol. 153, no. 4, pp. 415–424, 2001.

[230] M. S. Dar, "Mouse cerebellar GABA_B participation in the expression of acute ethanol-induced ataxia and in its modulation by the cerebellar adenosinergic A_1 system," *Brain Research Bulletin*, vol. 41, no. 1, pp. 53–59, 1996.

[231] B. M. Walker and G. F. Koob, "The γ-aminobutyric acid-B receptor agonist baclofen attenuates responding for ethanol in ethanol-dependent rats," *Alcoholism, Clinical and Experimental Research*, vol. 31, no. 1, pp. 11–18, 2007.

[232] J. Besheer, V. Lepoutre, and C. W. Hodge, "GABA_B receptor agonists reduce operant ethanol self-administration and enhance ethanol sedation in C57BL/6J mice," *Psychopharmacology*, vol. 174, no. 3, pp. 358–366, 2004.

[233] E. M. Moore, K. M. Serio, K. J. Goldfarb, S. Stepanovska, D. N. Linsenbardt, and S. L. Boehm, "GABAergic modulation of binge-like ethanol intake in C57BL/6J mice," *Pharmacology, Biochemistry, and Behavior*, vol. 88, no. 1, pp. 105–113, 2007.

[234] C. L. Czachowski, B. H. Legg, and K. H. Stansfield, "Ethanol and sucrose seeking and consumption following repeated administration of the GABA_B agonist baclofen in rats," *Alcoholism, Clinical and Experimental Research*, vol. 30, no. 5, pp. 812–818, 2006.

[235] C. R. Kasten, S. N. Blasingame, and S. L. Boehm, "Bidirectional enantioselective effects of the GABA_B receptor agonist baclofen in two mouse models of excessive ethanol consumption," *Alcohol*, vol. 49, no. 1, pp. 37–46, 2015.

[236] G. Addolorato, F. Caputo, E. Capristo et al., "Baclofen efficacy in reducing alcohol craving and intake: a preliminary double-blind randomized controlled study," *Alcohol and Alcoholism*, vol. 37, no. 5, pp. 504–508, 2002.

[237] G. Addolorato, F. Caputo, E. Capristo et al., "Rapid suppression of alcohol withdrawal syndrome by baclofen," *The American Journal of Medicine*, vol. 112, no. 3, pp. 226–229, 2002.

[238] A. Mirijello, F. Caputo, G. Vassallo et al., "GABAB agonists for the treatment of alcohol use disorder," *Current Pharmaceutical Design*, vol. 21, no. 23, pp. 3367–3372, 2015.

[239] A. Mirijello, C. D'Angelo, A. Ferrulli et al., "Identification and management of alcohol withdrawal syndrome," *Drugs*, vol. 75, no. 4, pp. 353–365, 2015.

[240] L. Leggio, W. H. Zywiak, J. E. McGeary et al., "A human laboratory pilot study with baclofen in alcoholic individuals," *Pharmacology, Biochemistry, and Behavior*, vol. 103, no. 4, pp. 784–791, 2013.

[241] N. L. Urizar, Z. Yang, H. J. Edenberg, and R. L. Davis, "*Drosophila* homer is required in a small set of neurons including the ellipsoid body for normal ethanol sensitivity and tolerance," *Journal of Neuroscience*, vol. 27, no. 17, pp. 4541–4551, 2007.

[242] K. K. Szumlinski, K. D. Lominac, E. B. Oleson et al., "Homer2 is necessary for EtOH-induced neuroplasticity," *Journal of Neuroscience*, vol. 25, no. 30, pp. 7054–7061, 2005.

[243] A. Haider, N. C. Woodward, K. D. Lominac et al., "Homer2 within the nucleus accumbens core bidirectionally regulates alcohol intake by both P and Wistar rats," *Alcohol*, vol. 49, no. 6, pp. 533–542, 2015.

[244] I. Obara, R. L. Bell, S. P. Goulding et al., "Differential effects of chronic ethanol consumption and withdrawal on homer/glutamate receptor expression in subregions of the accumbens and amygdala of P rats," *Alcoholism, Clinical and Experimental Research*, vol. 33, no. 11, pp. 1924–1934, 2009.

[245] R. B. Cowmeadow, H. R. Krishnan, A. Ghezzi, Y. M. Al'Hasan, Y. Z. Wang, and N. S. Atkinson, "Ethanol tolerance caused by *slowpoke* induction in Drosophila," *Alcoholism, Clinical and Experimental Research*, vol. 30, no. 5, pp. 745–753, 2006.

[246] A. Ghezzi, Y. M. Al-Hasan, L. E. Larios, R. A. Bohm, and N. S. Atkinson, "*slo* K^+ channel gene regulation mediates rapid drug tolerance," *Proceedings of the National Academy of Sciences of the United States of America*, vol. 101, no. 49, pp. 17276–17281, 2004.

[247] N. S. Atkinson, "Tolerance in *Drosophila*," *Journal of Neurogenetics*, vol. 23, no. 3, pp. 293–302, 2009.

[248] R. B. Cowmeadow, H. R. Krishnan, and N. S. Atkinson, "The *slowpoke* gene is necessary for rapid ethanol tolerance in *Drosophila*," *Alcoholism, Clinical and Experimental Research*, vol. 29, no. 10, pp. 1777–1786, 2005.

[249] S. N. Treistman and G. E. Martin, "BK channels: mediators and models for alcohol tolerance," *Trends in Neurosciences*, vol. 32, no. 12, pp. 629–637, 2009.

[250] P. M. Wynne, S. I. Puig, G. E. Martin, and S. N. Treistman, "Compartmentalized β subunit distribution determines

characteristics and ethanol sensitivity of somatic, dendritic, and terminal large-conductance calcium-activated potassium channels in the rat central nervous system," *Journal of Pharmacology and Experimental Therapeutics*, vol. 329, no. 3, pp. 978–986, 2009.

[251] B. D. Kyle and A. P. Braun, "The regulation of BK channel activity by pre- and post-translational modifications," *Frontiers in Physiology*, vol. 5, p. 316, 2014.

[252] A. Z. Pietrzykowski, R. M. Friesen, G. E. Martin et al., "Posttranscriptional regulation of BK channel splice variant stability by miR-9 underlies neuroadaptation to alcohol," *Neuron*, vol. 59, no. 2, pp. 274–287, 2008.

[253] P. Orio and R. Latorre, "Differential effects of β1 and β2 subunits on BK channel activity," *The Journal of General Physiology*, vol. 125, no. 4, pp. 395–411, 2005.

[254] P. Orio, P. Rojas, G. Ferreira, and R. Latorre, "New disguises for an old channel: MaxiK channel β subunits," *News in Physiological Sciences*, vol. 17, pp. 156–161, 2002.

[255] P. L. Feinberg-Zadek and S. N. Treistman, "Beta-subunits are important modulators of the acute response to alcohol in human BK channels," *Alcoholism, Clinical and Experimental Research*, vol. 31, no. 5, pp. 737–744, 2007.

[256] K. Keleman, E. Vrontou, S. Krüttner, J. Y. Yu, A. Kurtovic-Kozaric, and B. J. Dickson, "Dopamine neurons modulate pheromone responses in *Drosophila* courtship learning," *Nature*, vol. 489, no. 7414, pp. 145–149, 2012.

[257] E. C. Kong, K. Woo, H. Li et al., "A pair of dopamine neurons target the D1-like dopamine receptor DopR in the central complex to promote ethanol-stimulated locomotion in *Drosophila*," *PLoS One*, vol. 5, no. 4, article e9954, 2010.

[258] D. Ron and R. O. Messing, "Signaling pathways mediating alcohol effects," *Current Topics in Behavioral Neurosciences*, vol. 13, pp. 87–126, 2013.

[259] N. D. Volkow, G. J. Wang, F. Telang et al., "Profound decreases in dopamine release in striatum in detoxified alcoholics: possible orbitofrontal involvement," *Journal of Neuroscience*, vol. 27, no. 46, pp. 12700–12706, 2007.

[260] S. Waddell, "Reinforcement signalling in *Drosophila*; dopamine does it all after all," *Current Opinion in Neurobiology*, vol. 23, no. 3, pp. 324–329, 2013.

[261] R. J. Bainton, L. T. Tsai, C. M. Singh, M. S. Moore, W. S. Neckameyer, and U. Heberlein, "Dopamine modulates acute responses to cocaine, nicotine and ethanol in *Drosophila*," *Current Biology*, vol. 10, no. 4, pp. 187–194, 2000.

[262] O. Neznanova, K. Björk, R. Rimondini et al., "Acute ethanol challenge inhibits glycogen synthase kinase-3β in the rat prefrontal cortex," *The International Journal of Neuropsychopharmacology*, vol. 12, no. 2, pp. 275–280, 2009.

[263] K. E. Pleil, A. Lopez, N. McCall, A. M. Jijon, J. P. Bravo, and T. L. Kash, "Chronic stress alters neuropeptide Y signaling in the bed nucleus of the stria terminalis in DBA/2J but not C57BL/6J mice," *Neuropharmacology*, vol. 62, no. 4, pp. 1777–1786, 2012.

[264] K. E. Pleil, J. A. Rinker, E. G. Lowery-Gionta et al., "NPY signaling inhibits extended amygdala CRF neurons to suppress binge alcohol drinking," *Nature Neuroscience*, vol. 18, no. 4, pp. 545–552, 2015.

[265] N. W. Gilpin and M. Roberto, "Neuropeptide modulation of central amygdala neuroplasticity is a key mediator of alcohol dependence," *Neuroscience and Biobehavioral Reviews*, vol. 36, no. 2, pp. 873–888, 2012.

[266] A. M. Barkley-Levenson, A. E. Ryabinin, and J. C. Crabbe, "Neuropeptide Y response to alcohol is altered in nucleus accumbens of mice selectively bred for drinking to intoxication," *Behavioural Brain Research*, vol. 302, pp. 160–170, 2016.

[267] G. Shohat-Ophir, K. R. Kaun, R. Azanchi, H. Mohammed, and U. Heberlein, "Sexual deprivation increases ethanol intake in *Drosophila*," *Science*, vol. 335, no. 6074, pp. 1351–1355, 2012.

[268] T. Wen, C. A. Parrish, D. Xu, Q. Wu, and P. Shen, "*Drosophila* neuropeptide F and its receptor, NPFR1, define a signaling pathway that acutely modulates alcohol sensitivity," *Proceedings of the National Academy of Sciences of the United States of America*, vol. 102, no. 6, pp. 2141–6, 2005.

[269] H. Scholz, M. Franz, and U. Heberlein, "The hangover gene defines a stress pathway required for ethanol tolerance development," *Nature*, vol. 436, no. 7052, pp. 845–847, 2005.

[270] I. Schwenkert, R. Eltrop, N. Funk, J. R. Steinert, C. M. Schuster, and H. Scholz, "The *hangover* gene negatively regulates bouton addition at the *Drosophila* neuromuscular junction," *Mechanisms of Development*, vol. 125, no. 8, pp. 700–711, 2008.

[271] X. Ma, Q. Wang, G. Qin et al., "Predictive value of liver enzymes and alcohol consumption for risk of type 2 diabetes," *Zhonghua Gan Zang Bing Za Zhi*, vol. 23, no. 1, pp. 55–58, 2015.

[272] B. P. Riley, G. Kalsi, P. H. Kuo et al., "Alcohol dependence is associated with the ZNF699 gene, a human locus related to *Drosophila hangover*, in the Irish affected sib pair study of alcohol dependence (IASPSAD) sample," *Molecular Psychiatry*, vol. 11, no. 11, pp. 1025–1031, 2006.

[273] Z. W. Chen and R. W. Olsen, "GABA_A receptor associated proteins: a key factor regulating GABA_A receptor function," *Journal of Neurochemistry*, vol. 100, no. 2, pp. 279–294, 2007.

[274] J. Zhou, J. Ye, X. Zhao, and A. Li, "JWA is required for arsenic trioxide induced apoptosis in HeLa and MCF-7 cells via reactive oxygen species and mitochondria linked signal pathway," *Toxicology and Applied Pharmacology*, vol. 230, no. 1, pp. 33–40, 2008.

[275] C. Li, X. Zhao, X. Cao, D. Chu, J. Chen, and J. Zhou, "The *Drosophila* homolog of *jwa* is required for ethanol tolerance," *Alcohol and Alcoholism*, vol. 43, no. 5, pp. 529–536, 2008.

[276] M. J. Ikemoto, K. Inoue, S. Akiduki et al., "Identification of addicsin/GTRAP3-18 as a chronic morphine-augmented gene in amygdala," *Neuroreport*, vol. 13, no. 16, pp. 2079–2084, 2002.

[277] S. A. Ojelade, T. Jia, A. R. Rodan et al., "Rsu1 regulates ethanol consumption in *Drosophila* and humans," *Proceedings of the National Academy of Sciences of the United States of America*, vol. 112, no. 30, pp. E4085–E4093, 2015.

[278] S. A. Ojelade, S. F. Acevedo, G. Kalahasti, A. R. Rodan, and A. Rothenfluh, "RhoGAP18B isoforms act on distinct rho-family GTPases and regulate behavioral responses to alcohol via cofilin," *PLoS One*, vol. 10, no. 9, article e0137465, 2015.

[279] A. Rothenfluh, R. J. Threlkeld, R. J. Bainton, L. T. Tsai, A. W. Lasek, and U. Heberlein, "Distinct behavioral responses to ethanol are regulated by alternate RhoGAP18B isoforms," *Cell*, vol. 127, no. 1, pp. 199–211, 2006.

[280] P. Bhandari, K. S. Kendler, J. C. Bettinger, A. G. Davies, and M. Grotewiel, "An assay for evoked locomotor behavior in *Drosophila* reveals a role for integrins in ethanol sensitivity

and rapid ethanol tolerance," *Alcoholism, Clinical and Experimental Research*, vol. 33, no. 10, pp. 1794–1805, 2009.

[281] S. F. Acevedo, R. L. Peru, R. L. Peru y Colón de Portugal, D. A. Gonzalez, A. R. Rodan, and A. Rothenfluh, "S6 kinase reflects and regulates ethanol-induced sedation," *Journal of Neuroscience*, vol. 35, no. 46, pp. 15396–15402, 2015.

[282] R. L. Peru y Colón de Portugal, S. F. Acevedo, A. R. Rodan, L. Y. Chang, B. A. Eaton, and A. Rothenfluh, "Adult neuronal Arf6 controls ethanol-induced behavior with arfaptin downstream of Rac1 and RhoGAP18B," *Journal of Neuroscience*, vol. 32, no. 49, pp. 17706–17713, 2012.

[283] D. A. Gonzalez, T. Jia, J. H. Pinzón et al., "The Arf6 activator Efa6/PSD3 confers regional specificity and modulates ethanol consumption in *Drosophila* and humans," *Molecular Psychiatry*, 2017.

[284] M. Grotewiel and J. C. Bettinger, "*Drosophila* and *Caenorhabditis elegans* as discovery platforms for genes involved in human alcohol use disorder," *Alcoholism, Clinical and Experimental Research*, vol. 39, no. 8, pp. 1292–1311, 2015.

[285] E. Haus and F. Halberg, "24-hour rhythm in susceptibility of C mice to a toxic dose of ethanol," *Journal of Applied Physiology*, vol. 14, pp. 878–880, 1959.

[286] M. D. Madeira, J. P. Andrade, A. R. Lieberman, N. Sousa, O. F. Almeida, and M. M. Paula-Barbosa, "Chronic alcohol consumption and withdrawal do not induce cell death in the suprachiasmatic nucleus, but lead to irreversible depression of peptide immunoreactivity and mRNA levels," *Journal of Neuroscience*, vol. 17, no. 4, pp. 1302–1319, 1997.

[287] V. Rajakrishnan, P. Subramanian, P. Viswanathan, and V. P. Menon, "Effect of chronic ethanol ingestion on biochemical circadian rhythms in Wistar rats," *Alcohol*, vol. 18, no. 2-3, pp. 147–152, 1999.

[288] R. Spanagel, A. M. Rosenwasser, G. Schumann, and D. K. Sarkar, "Alcohol consumption and the body's biological clock," *Alcoholism, Clinical and Experimental Research*, vol. 29, no. 8, pp. 1550–1557, 2005.

[289] E. Van Reen, T. L. Rupp, C. Acebo, R. Seifer, and M. A. Carskadon, "Biphasic effects of alcohol as a function of circadian phase," *Sleep*, vol. 36, no. 1, pp. 137–145, 2013.

[290] K. van der Linde and L. C. Lyons, "Circadian modulation of acute alcohol sensitivity but not acute tolerance in *Drosophila*," *Chronobiology International*, vol. 28, no. 5, pp. 397–406, 2011.

[291] S. Perreau-Lenz, T. Zghoul, F. R. de Fonseca, R. Spanagel, and A. Bilbao, "Circadian regulation of central ethanol sensitivity by the mPer2 gene," *Addiction Biology*, vol. 14, no. 3, pp. 253–259, 2009.

[292] T. Danel, R. Jeanson, and Y. Touitou, "Temporal pattern in consumption of the first drink of the day in alcohol-dependent persons," *Chronobiology International*, vol. 20, no. 6, pp. 1093–1102, 2003.

[293] T. Danel and Y. Touitou, "Chronobiology of alcohol: from chronokinetics to alcohol-related alterations of the circadian system," *Chronobiology International*, vol. 21, no. 6, pp. 923–935, 2004.

[294] J. B. Pohl, A. Ghezzi, L. K. Lew, R. B. Robles, L. Cormack, and N. S. Atkinson, "Circadian genes differentially affect tolerance to ethanol in Drosophila," *Alcoholism, Clinical and Experimental Research*, vol. 37, no. 11, pp. 1862–1871, 2013.

[295] J. Ewer, B. Frisch, M. J. Hamblen-Coyle, M. Rosbash, and J. C. Hall, "Expression of the period clock gene within different cell types in the brain of Drosophila adults and mosaic analysis of these cells' influence on circadian behavioral rhythms," *Journal of Neuroscience*, vol. 12, no. 9, pp. 3321–3349, 1992.

[296] J. L. Price, M. E. Dembinska, M. W. Young, and M. Rosbash, "Suppression of PERIOD protein abundance and circadian cycling by the *Drosophila* clock mutation *timeless*," *The EMBO Journal*, vol. 14, no. 16, pp. 4044–4049, 1995.

[297] T. Yoshii, Y. Heshiki, T. Ibuki-Ishibashi, A. Matsumoto, T. Tanimura, and K. Tomioka, "Temperature cycles drive *Drosophila* circadian oscillation in constant light that otherwise induces behavioural arrhythmicity," *European Journal of Neuroscience*, vol. 22, no. 5, pp. 1176–1184, 2005.

[298] A. K. De Nobrega, A. P. Mellers, and L. C. Lyons, "Aging and circadian dysfunction increase alcohol sensitivity and exacerbate mortality in *Drosophila melanogaster*," *Experimental Gerontology*, vol. 97, pp. 49–59, 2017.

[299] R. Spanagel, G. Pendyala, C. Abarca et al., "The clock gene Per2 influences the glutamatergic system and modulates alcohol consumption," *Nature Medicine*, vol. 11, no. 1, pp. 35–42, 2005.

[300] E. Comasco, N. Nordquist, C. Göktürk et al., "The clock gene PER2 and sleep problems: association with alcohol consumption among Swedish adolescents," *Upsala Journal of Medical Sciences*, vol. 115, no. 1, pp. 41–48, 2010.

[301] M. A. Agapito, J. C. Barreira, R. W. Logan, and D. K. Sarkar, "Evidence for possible period 2 gene mediation of the effects of alcohol exposure during the postnatal period on genes associated with maintaining metabolic signaling in the mouse hypothalamus," *Alcoholism, Clinical and Experimental Research*, vol. 37, no. 2, pp. 263–269, 2013.

[302] K. C. Summa, R. M. Voigt, C. B. Forsyth et al., "Disruption of the circadian clock in mice increases intestinal permeability and promotes alcohol-induced hepatic pathology and inflammation," *PLoS One*, vol. 8, no. 6, article e67102, 2013.

[303] K. C. Summa, P. Jiang, K. Fitzpatrick et al., "Chronic alcohol exposure and the circadian clock mutation exert tissue-specific effects on gene expression in mouse hippocampus, liver, and proximal colon," *Alcoholism, Clinical and Experimental Research*, vol. 39, no. 10, pp. 1917–1929, 2015.

[304] F. Bishehsari, A. Saadalla, K. Khazaie et al., "Light/dark shifting promotes alcohol-induced colon carcinogenesis: possible role of intestinal inflammatory milieu and microbiota," *International Journal of Molecular Sciences*, vol. 17, no. 12, 2016.

[305] J. A. Seggio, R. W. Logan, and A. M. Rosenwasser, "Chronic ethanol intake modulates photic and non-photic circadian phase responses in the Syrian hamster," *Pharmacology, Biochemistry, and Behavior*, vol. 87, no. 3, pp. 297–305, 2007.

[306] A. J. Brager, C. L. Ruby, R. A. Prosser, and J. D. Glass, "Acute ethanol disrupts photic and serotonergic circadian clock phase-resetting in the mouse," *Alcoholism, Clinical and Experimental Research*, vol. 35, no. 8, pp. 1467–1474, 2011.

[307] C. L. Ruby, A. J. Brager, M. A. DePaul, R. A. Prosser, and J. D. Glass, "Chronic ethanol attenuates circadian photic phase resetting and alters nocturnal activity patterns in the hamster," *American Journal of Physiology - Regulatory, Integrative and Comparative Physiology*, vol. 297, no. 3, pp. R729–R737, 2009.

[308] C. L. Ruby, R. A. Prosser, M. A. DePaul, R. J. Roberts, and J. D. Glass, "Acute ethanol impairs photic and nonphotic circadian phase resetting in the Syrian hamster," *American*

Journal of Physiology - Regulatory, Integrative and Comparative Physiology, vol. 296, no. 2, pp. R411–R418, 2009.

[309] R. A. Prosser and J. D. Glass, "Assessing ethanol's actions in the suprachiasmatic circadian clock using *in vivo* and *in vitro* approaches," *Alcohol*, vol. 49, no. 4, pp. 321–339, 2015.

[310] T. Partonen, "Clock genes in human alcohol abuse and comorbid conditions," *Alcohol*, vol. 49, no. 4, pp. 359–365, 2015.

[311] S. Perreau-Lenz and R. Spanagel, "Clock genes × stress × reward interactions in alcohol and substance use disorders," *Alcohol*, vol. 49, no. 4, pp. 351–357, 2015.

[312] M. C. Huang, C. W. Ho, C. H. Chen, S. C. Liu, C. C. Chen, and S. J. Leu, "Reduced expression of circadian clock genes in male alcoholic patients," *Alcoholism, Clinical and Experimental Research*, vol. 34, no. 11, pp. 1899–1904, 2010.

[313] H. J. Burgess, M. Rizvydeen, L. F. Fogg, and A. Keshavarzian, "A single dose of alcohol does not meaningfully alter circadian phase advances and phase delays to light in humans," *American Journal of Physiology - Regulatory, Integrative and Comparative Physiology*, vol. 310, no. 8, pp. R759–R765, 2016.

[314] R. Guo, S. M. Simasko, and H. T. Jansen, "Chronic alcohol consumption in rats leads to desynchrony in diurnal rhythms and molecular clocks," *Alcoholism, Clinical and Experimental Research*, vol. 40, no. 2, pp. 291–300, 2016.

[315] P. Zhou, R. A. Ross, C. M. Pywell, S. Liangpunsakul, and G. E. Duffield, "Disturbances in the murine hepatic circadian clock in alcohol-induced hepatic steatosis," *Scientific Reports*, vol. 4, p. 3725, 2014.

[316] G. Swanson, C. B. Forsyth, Y. Tang et al., "Role of intestinal circadian genes in alcohol-induced gut leakiness," *Alcoholism, Clinical and Experimental Research*, vol. 35, no. 7, pp. 1305–1314, 2011.

[317] A. N. Filiano, T. Millender-Swain, R. Johnson, M. E. Young, K. L. Gamble, and S. M. Bailey, "Chronic ethanol consumption disrupts the core molecular clock and diurnal rhythms of metabolic genes in the liver without affecting the suprachiasmatic nucleus," *PLoS One*, vol. 8, no. 8, article e71684, 2013.

[318] C. P. Chen, P. Kuhn, J. P. Advis, and D. K. Sarkar, "6," *Journal of Neurochemistry*, vol. 88, no. 6, pp. 1547–1554, 2004.

[319] J. A. Seggio, B. Possidente, and S. T. Ahmad, "Larval ethanol exposure alters adult circadian free-running locomotor activity rhythm in *Drosophila melanogaster*," *Chronobiology International*, vol. 29, no. 1, pp. 75–81, 2012.

[320] S. T. Ahmad, S. B. Steinmetz, H. M. Bussey, B. Possidente, and J. A. Seggio, "Larval ethanol exposure alters free-running circadian rhythm and *per Locus* transcription in adult *D. melanogaster period* mutants," *Behavioural Brain Research*, vol. 241, pp. 50–55, 2013.

[321] R. Sandyk and J. D. Kanofsky, "Cocaine addiction: relationship to seasonal affective disorder," *International Journal of Neuroscience*, vol. 64, no. 1–4, pp. 195–201, 1992.

[322] S. L. Satel and F. H. Gawin, "Seasonal cocaine abuse," *American Journal of Psychiatry*, vol. 146, no. 4, pp. 534–535, 1989.

[323] Y. Iijima, M. Shinoda, H. Kuribara, T. Asami, and Y. Uchihashi, "Evaluation of acute and sub-acute effects of cocaine by means of circadian variation in wheel-running and drinking in mice," *Nihon Shinkei Seishin Yakurigaku Zasshi*, vol. 15, no. 4, pp. 315–321, 1995.

[324] C. Abarca, U. Albrecht, and R. Spanagel, "Cocaine sensitization and reward are under the influence of circadian genes and rhythm," *Proceedings of the National Academy of Sciences of the United States of America*, vol. 99, no. 13, pp. 9026–9030, 2002.

[325] M. Akhisaroglu, R. Ahmed, M. Kurtuncu, H. Manev, and T. Uz, "Diurnal rhythms in cocaine sensitization and in Period1 levels are common across rodent species," *Pharmacology, Biochemistry, and Behavior*, vol. 79, no. 1, pp. 37–42, 2004.

[326] T. Uz, M. Akhisaroglu, R. Ahmed, and H. Manev, "The pineal gland is critical for circadian Period1 expression in the striatum and for circadian cocaine sensitization in mice," *Neuropsychopharmacology*, vol. 28, no. 12, pp. 2117–2123, 2003.

[327] T. J. Baird and D. Gauvin, "Characterization of cocaine self-administration and pharmacokinetics as a function of time of day in the rat," *Pharmacology, Biochemistry, and Behavior*, vol. 65, no. 2, pp. 289–299, 2000.

[328] J. D. Glass, A. J. Brager, A. C. Stowie, and R. A. Prosser, "Cocaine modulates pathways for photic and nonphotic entrainment of the mammalian SCN circadian clock," *American Journal of Physiology - Regulatory, Integrative and Comparative Physiology*, vol. 302, no. 6, pp. R740–R750, 2012.

[329] R. A. Prosser, A. Stowie, M. Amicarelli, A. G. Nackenoff, R. D. Blakely, and J. D. Glass, "Cocaine modulates mammalian circadian clock timing by decreasing serotonin transport in the SCN," *Neuroscience*, vol. 275, pp. 184–193, 2014.

[330] V. Yuferov, T. Kroslak, K. S. Laforge, Y. Zhou, A. Ho, and M. J. Kreek, "Differential gene expression in the rat caudate putamen after "binge" cocaine administration: advantage of triplicate microarray analysis," *Synapse*, vol. 48, no. 4, pp. 157–169, 2003.

[331] R. George, K. Lease, J. Burnette, and J. Hirsh, "A "bottom-counting" video system for measuring cocaine-induced behaviors in *Drosophila*," *Methods in Enzymology*, vol. 393, pp. 841–851, 2005.

[332] C. McClung and J. Hirsh, "Stereotypic behavioral responses to free-base cocaine and the development of behavioral sensitization in *Drosophila*," *Current Biology*, vol. 8, no. 2, pp. 109–112, 1998.

[333] L. T. Tsai, R. J. Bainton, J. Blau, and U. Heberlein, "*Lmo* mutants reveal a novel role for circadian pacemaker neurons in cocaine-induced behaviors," *PLoS Biology*, vol. 2, no. 12, article e408, 2004.

[334] R. Andretic, S. Chaney, and J. Hirsh, "Requirement of circadian genes for cocaine sensitization in *Drosophila*," *Science*, vol. 285, no. 5430, pp. 1066–1068, 1999.

[335] E. Shumay, J. S. Fowler, G. J. Wang et al., "Repeat variation in the human PER2 gene as a new genetic marker associated with cocaine addiction and brain dopamine D2 receptor availability," *Translational Psychiatry*, vol. 2, article e86, 2012.

[336] C. A. McClung, K. Sidiropoulou, M. Vitaterna et al., "Regulation of dopaminergic transmission and cocaine reward by the *Clock* gene," *Proceedings of the National Academy of Sciences of the United States of America*, vol. 102, no. 26, pp. 9377–9381, 2005.

[337] A. R. Ozburn, E. B. Larson, D. W. Self, and C. A. McClung, "Cocaine self-administration behaviors in *Clock*Δ19 mice," *Psychopharmacology*, vol. 223, no. 2, pp. 169–177, 2012.

[338] U. Heberlein, L. T. Tsai, D. Kapfhamer, and A. W. Lasek, "*Drosophila*, a genetic model system to study cocaine-

related behaviors: a review with focus on LIM-only proteins," *Neuropharmacology*, vol. 56, Supplement 1, pp. 97–106, 2009.

[339] R. M. Harris-Warrick and E. A. Kravitz, "Cellular mechanisms for modulation of posture by octopamine and serotonin in the lobster," *Journal of Neuroscience*, vol. 4, no. 8, pp. 1976–1993, 1984.

[340] E. A. Kravitz, S. Glusman, R. M. Harris-Warrick, M. S. Livingstone, T. Schwarz, and M. F. Goy, "Amines and a peptide as neurohormones in lobsters: actions on neuromuscular preparations and preliminary behavioural studies," *Journal of Experimental Biology*, vol. 89, pp. 159–175, 1980.

[341] B. D. Sloley and A. V. Juorio, "Monoamine neurotransmitters in invertebrates and vertebrates: an examination of the diverse enzymatic pathways utilized to synthesize and inactivate biogenic amines," *International Review of Neurobiology*, vol. 38, pp. 253–303, 1995.

[342] J. R. Cazalets, P. Grillner, I. Menard, J. Cremieux, and F. Clarac, "Two types of motor rhythm induced by NMDA and amines in an in vitro spinal cord preparation of neonatal rat," *Neuroscience Letters*, vol. 111, no. 1-2, pp. 116–121, 1990.

[343] M. Matsumoto and O. Hikosaka, "Two types of dopamine neuron distinctly convey positive and negative motivational signals," *Nature*, vol. 459, no. 7248, pp. 837–841, 2009.

[344] H. M. Nasser, D. J. Calu, G. Schoenbaum, and M. J. Sharpe, "The dopamine prediction error: contributions to associative models of reward learning," *Frontiers in Psychology*, vol. 8, p. 244, 2017.

[345] C. J. Perry and A. B. Barron, "Neural mechanisms of reward in insects," *Annual Review of Entomology*, vol. 58, pp. 543–562, 2013.

[346] G. F. Koob and N. D. Volkow, "Neurobiology of addiction: a neurocircuitry analysis," *Lancet Psychiatry*, vol. 3, no. 8, pp. 760–773, 2016.

[347] R. Andretic and J. Hirsh, "Circadian modulation of dopamine receptor responsiveness in *Drosophila melanogaster*," *Proceedings of the National Academy of Sciences of the United States of America*, vol. 97, no. 4, pp. 1873–1878, 2000.

[348] C. A. McClung, "Circadian rhythms, the mesolimbic dopaminergic circuit, and drug addiction," *Scientific World Journal*, vol. 7, pp. 194–202, 2007.

[349] M. J. Lee, K. D. Burau, and N. Dafny, "Behavioral daily rhythmic activity pattern of adolescent female rat is modulated by acute and chronic cocaine," *Journal of Neural Transmission*, vol. 120, no. 5, pp. 733–744, 2013.

[350] M. Weber, T. Lauterburg, I. Tobler, and J. M. Burgunder, "Circadian patterns of neurotransmitter related gene expression in motor regions of the rat brain," *Neuroscience Letters*, vol. 358, no. 1, pp. 17–20, 2004.

[351] K. R. Shieh, Y. S. Chu, and J. T. Pan, "Circadian change of dopaminergic neuron activity: effects of constant light and melatonin," *Neuroreport*, vol. 8, no. 9-10, pp. 2283–2287, 1997.

[352] R. Schade, K. Vick, T. Ott et al., "Circadian rhythms of dopamine and cholecystokinin in nucleus accumbens and striatum of rats—influence on dopaminergic stimulation," *Chronobiology International*, vol. 12, no. 2, pp. 87–99, 1995.

[353] P. K. Parekh, A. R. Ozburn, and C. A. McClung, "Circadian clock genes: effects on dopamine, reward and addiction," *Alcohol*, vol. 49, no. 4, pp. 341–349, 2015.

[354] I. C. Webb, "Circadian rhythms and substance abuse: chronobiological considerations for the treatment of addiction," *Current Psychiatry Reports*, vol. 19, no. 2, p. 12, 2017.

[355] R. W. Logan, W. P. Williams, and C. A. McClung, "Circadian rhythms and addiction: mechanistic insights and future directions," *Behavioral Neuroscience*, vol. 128, no. 3, pp. 387–412, 2014.

[356] M. Kurtuncu, A. D. Arslan, M. Akhisaroglu, H. Manev, and T. Uz, "Involvement of the pineal gland in diurnal cocaine reward in mice," *European Journal of Pharmacology*, vol. 489, no. 3, pp. 203–205, 2004.

[357] T. T. Takahashi, V. Vengeliene, and R. Spanagel, "Melatonin reduces motivation for cocaine self-administration and prevents relapse-like behavior in rats," *Psychopharmacology*, vol. 234, no. 11, pp. 1741–1748, 2017.

[358] B. Halbout, S. Perreau-Lenz, C. I. Dixon, D. N. Stephens, and R. Spanagel, "Per1Brdm1 mice self-administer cocaine and reinstate cocaine-seeking behaviour following extinction," *Behavioural Pharmacology*, vol. 22, no. 1, pp. 76–80, 2011.

[359] Y. Liu, Y. Wang, Z. Jiang, C. Wan, W. Zhou, and Z. Wang, "The extracellular signal-regulated kinase signaling pathway is involved in the modulation of morphine-induced reward by mPer1," *Neuroscience*, vol. 146, no. 1, pp. 265–271, 2007.

[360] Y. Liu, Y. Wang, C. Wan et al., "The role of mPer1 in morphine dependence in mice," *Neuroscience*, vol. 130, no. 2, pp. 383–388, 2005.

[361] X. Wang, Y. Wang, H. Xin et al., "Altered expression of circadian clock gene, mPer1, in mouse brain and kidney under morphine dependence and withdrawal," *Journal of Circadian Rhythms*, vol. 4, p. 9, 2006.

[362] T. Nikaido, M. Akiyama, T. Moriya, and S. Shibata, "Sensitized increase of period gene expression in the mouse caudate/putamen caused by repeated injection of methamphetamine," *Molecular Pharmacology*, vol. 59, no. 4, pp. 894–900, 2001.

[363] N. Fuenzalida-Uribe, R. C. Meza, H. A. Hoffmann, R. Varas, and J. M. Campusano, "nAChR-induced octopamine release mediates the effect of nicotine on a startle response in *Drosophila melanogaster*," *Journal of Neurochemistry*, vol. 125, no. 2, pp. 281–290, 2013.

[364] R. Andretic, B. van Swinderen, and R. J. Greenspan, "Dopaminergic modulation of arousal in *Drosophila*," *Current Biology*, vol. 15, no. 13, pp. 1165–1175, 2005.

[365] E. Tekieh, M. Kazemi, L. Dehghani et al., "Effects of oral morphine on the larvae, pupae and imago development in *Drosophila melanogaster*," *Cell Journal*, vol. 13, no. 3, pp. 149–154, 2011.

[366] N. A. Velazquez-Ulloa, "A *Drosophila* model for developmental nicotine exposure," *PLoS One*, vol. 12, no. 5, article e0177710, 2017.

[367] E. S. Barratt and P. M. Adams, "Chronic marijuana usage and sleep-wakefulness cycles in cats," *Biological Psychiatry*, vol. 6, no. 3, pp. 207–214, 1973.

[368] A. E. Sanford, E. Castillo, and R. L. Gannon, "Cannabinoids and hamster circadian activity rhythms," *Brain Research*, vol. 1222, pp. 141–148, 2008.

[369] L. N. Whitehurst, K. Fogler, K. Hall, M. Hartmann, and J. Dyche, "The effects of chronic marijuana use on circadian entrainment," *Chronobiology International*, vol. 32, no. 4, pp. 561–567, 2015.

[370] C. Acuna-Goycolea, K. Obrietan, and A. N. van den Pol, "Cannabinoids excite circadian clock neurons," *Journal of Neuroscience*, vol. 30, no. 30, pp. 10061–10066, 2010.

[371] J. R. Tinklenberg, W. T. Roth, and B. S. Kopell, "Marijuana and ethanol: differential effects on time perception, heart rate, and subjective response," *Psychopharmacology*, vol. 49, no. 3, pp. 275–279, 1976.

[372] D. S. Hasin, T. D. Saha, B. T. Kerridge et al., "Prevalence of marijuana use disorders in the United States between 2001-2002 and 2012-2013," *JAMA Psychiatry*, vol. 72, no. 12, pp. 1235–1242, 2015.

[373] H. Khaliullina, M. Bilgin, J. L. Sampaio, A. Shevchenko, and S. Eaton, "Endocannabinoids are conserved inhibitors of the Hedgehog pathway," *Proceedings of the National Academy of Sciences of the United States of America*, vol. 112, no. 11, pp. 3415–3420, 2015.

[374] M. Jimenez-Del-Rio, A. Daza-Restrepo, and C. Velez-Pardo, "The cannabinoid CP55,940 prolongs survival and improves locomotor activity in *Drosophila melanogaster* against paraquat: implications in Parkinson's disease," *Neuroscience Research*, vol. 61, no. 4, pp. 404–411, 2008.

[375] M. J. Lee, M. S. Park, S. Hwang et al., "Dietary hempseed meal intake increases body growth and shortens the larval stage via the upregulation of cell growth and sterol levels in *Drosophila melanogaster*," *Molecules and Cells*, vol. 30, no. 1, pp. 29–36, 2010.

[376] R. L. Hartman, T. L. Brown, G. Milavetz et al., "Controlled vaporized cannabis, with and without alcohol: subjective effects and oral fluid-blood cannabinoid relationships," *Drug Testing and Analysis*, vol. 8, no. 7, pp. 690–701, 2016.

[377] R. L. Hartman, T. L. Brown, G. Milavetz et al., "Cannabis effects on driving lateral control with and without alcohol," *Drug and Alcohol Dependence*, vol. 154, pp. 25–37, 2015.

[378] J. Hayaki, B. J. Anderson, and M. D. Stein, "Dual cannabis and alcohol use disorders in young adults: problems magnified," *Substance Abuse*, vol. 37, no. 4, pp. 579–583, 2016.

[379] J. F. Duffy, K. M. Zitting, and E. D. Chinoy, "Aging and circadian rhythms," *Sleep Medicine Clinics*, vol. 10, no. 4, pp. 423–434, 2015.

[380] J. Mattis and A. Sehgal, "Circadian rhythms, sleep, and disorders of aging," *Trends in Endocrinology and Metabolism*, vol. 27, no. 4, pp. 192–203, 2016.

[381] S. Benloucif, M. I. Masana, and M. L. Dubocovich, "Light-induced phase shifts of circadian activity rhythms and immediate early gene expression in the suprachiasmatic nucleus are attenuated in old C3H/HeN mice," *Brain Research*, vol. 747, no. 1, pp. 34–42, 1997.

[382] C. Y. Chen, R. W. Logan, T. Ma et al., "Effects of aging on circadian patterns of gene expression in the human prefrontal cortex," *Proceedings of the National Academy of Sciences of the United States of America*, vol. 113, no. 1, pp. 206–211, 2016.

[383] A. Novier, L. C. Ornelas, J. L. Diaz-Granados, and D. B. Matthews, "Differences in behavioral responding in adult and aged rats following chronic ethanol exposure," *Alcoholism, Clinical and Experimental Research*, vol. 40, no. 7, pp. 1462–1472, 2016.

[384] A. Novier, C. E. Van Skike, J. L. Diaz-Granados, G. Mittleman, and D. B. Matthews, "Acute alcohol produces ataxia and cognitive impairments in aged animals: a comparison between young adult and aged rats," *Alcoholism, Clinical and Experimental Research*, vol. 37, no. 8, pp. 1317–1324, 2013.

[385] International Human Genome Sequencing Consortium, "Finishing the euchromatic sequence of the human genome," *Nature*, vol. 431, no. 7011, pp. 931–945, 2004.

[386] B. Ugur, K. Chen, and H. J. Bellen, "*Drosophila* tools and assays for the study of human diseases," *Disease Models & Mechanisms*, vol. 9, no. 3, pp. 235–244, 2016.

[387] N. Perrimon, N. M. Bonini, and P. Dhillon, "Fruit flies on the front line: the translational impact of *Drosophila*," *Disease Models & Mechanisms*, vol. 9, no. 3, pp. 229–231, 2016.

[388] N. Perrimon, C. Pitsouli, and B. Z. Shilo, "Signaling mechanisms controlling cell fate and embryonic patterning," *Cold Spring Harbor Perspectives in Biology*, vol. 4, no. 8, article a005975, 2012.

[389] S. Chien, L. T. Reiter, E. Bier, and M. Gribskov, "Homophila: human disease gene cognates in *Drosophila*," *Nucleic Acids Research*, vol. 30, no. 1, pp. 149–151, 2002.

[390] S. Yamamoto, M. Jaiswal, W. L. Charng et al., "A *Drosophila* genetic resource of mutants to study mechanisms underlying human genetic diseases," *Cell*, vol. 159, no. 1, pp. 200–214, 2014.

[391] K. H. Berger, E. C. Kong, J. Dubnau, T. Tully, M. S. Moore, and U. Heberlein, "Ethanol sensitivity and tolerance in long-term memory mutants of *Drosophila melanogaster*," *Alcoholism, Clinical and Experimental Research*, vol. 32, no. 5, pp. 895–908, 2008.

[392] G. Dietzl, D. Chen, F. Schnorrer et al., "A genome-wide transgenic RNAi library for conditional gene inactivation in *Drosophila*," *Nature*, vol. 448, no. 7150, pp. 151–156, 2007.

[393] T. A. Fulga, E. M. McNeill, R. Binari et al., "A transgenic resource for conditional competitive inhibition of conserved *Drosophila* microRNAs," *Nature Communications*, vol. 6, p. 7279, 2015.

[394] A. R. Bassett and J. L. Liu, "CRISPR/Cas9 and genome editing in *Drosophila*," *Journal of Genetics and Genomics*, vol. 41, no. 1, pp. 7–19, 2014.

[395] J. Xu, X. Ren, J. Sun et al., "A toolkit of CRISPR-based genome editing systems in *Drosophila*," *Journal of Genetics and Genomics*, vol. 42, no. 4, pp. 141–149, 2015.

[396] R. Ghaemi and P. R. Selvaganapathy, "Microfluidic devices for automation of assays on Drosophila melanogaster for applications in drug discovery and biological studies," *Current Pharmaceutical Biotechnology*, vol. 17, no. 9, pp. 822–836, 2016.

[397] A. K. Yadav, S. Srikrishna, and S. C. Gupta, "Cancer drug development using *Drosophila* as an *in vivo* tool: from bedside to bench and back," *Trends in Pharmacological Sciences*, vol. 37, no. 9, pp. 789–806, 2016.

[398] N. Cadieu, J. Cadieu, L. El Ghadraoui, A. Grimal, and Y. Lamboeuf, "Conditioning to ethanol in the fruit fly—a study using an inhibitor of ADH," *Journal of Insect Physiology*, vol. 45, no. 6, pp. 579–586, 1999.

[399] M. B. Acevedo, M. E. Nizhnikov, N. E. Spear, J. C. Molina, and R. M. Pautassi, "Ethanol-induced locomotor activity in adolescent rats and the relationship with ethanol-induced conditioned place preference and conditioned taste aversion," *Developmental Psychobiology*, vol. 55, no. 4, pp. 429–442, 2013.

[400] N. A. Holtz, A. K. Radke, N. E. Zlebnik, A. C. Harris, and M. E. Carroll, "Intracranial self-stimulation reward

thresholds during morphine withdrawal in rats bred for high (HiS) and low (LoS) saccharin intake," *Brain Research*, vol. 1602, pp. 119–126, 2015.

[401] F. D. Zeeb, G. A. Higgins, and P. J. Fletcher, "The serotonin 2C receptor agonist lorcaserin attenuates intracranial self-stimulation and blocks the reward-enhancing effects of nicotine," *ACS Chemical Neuroscience*, vol. 6, no. 7, pp. 1231–1240, 2015.

[402] B. T. Lett and V. L. Grant, "Conditioned taste preference produced by pairing a taste with a low dose of morphine or sufentanil," *Psychopharmacology*, vol. 98, no. 2, pp. 236–239, 1989.

[403] Z. I. Su, J. Wenzel, A. Ettenberg, and O. Ben-Shahar, "Prior extended daily access to cocaine elevates the reward threshold in a conditioned place preference test," *Addiction Biology*, vol. 19, no. 5, pp. 826–837, 2014.

[404] H. B. Madsen and S. H. Ahmed, "Drug versus sweet reward: greater attraction to and preference for sweet versus drug cues," *Addiction Biology*, vol. 20, no. 3, pp. 433–444, 2015.

[405] C. M. Davis, I. de Brugada, and A. L. Riley, "The role of injection cues in the production of the morphine preexposure effect in taste aversion learning," *Learning & Behavior*, vol. 38, no. 2, pp. 103–110, 2010.

[406] H. E. King and A. L. Riley, "A history of morphine-induced taste aversion learning fails to affect morphine-induced place preference conditioning in rats," *Learning & Behavior*, vol. 41, no. 4, pp. 433–442, 2013.

[407] D. J. Fachin-Scheit, A. Frozino Ribeiro, G. Pigatto, F. Oliveira Goeldner, and R. Boerngen de Lacerda, "Development of a mouse model of ethanol addiction: naltrexone efficacy in reducing consumption but not craving," *Journal of Neural Transmission*, vol. 113, no. 9, pp. 1305–1321, 2006.

[408] B. R. Lee, Y. Y. Ma, Y. H. Huang et al., "Maturation of silent synapses in amygdala-accumbens projection contributes to incubation of cocaine craving," *Nature Neuroscience*, vol. 16, no. 11, pp. 1644–1651, 2013.

[409] A. Shahbabaie, M. Golesorkhi, B. Zamanian et al., "State dependent effect of transcranial direct current stimulation (tDCS) on methamphetamine craving," *The International Journal of Neuropsychopharmacology*, vol. 17, no. 10, pp. 1591–1598, 2014.

[410] B. Wang, B. Zhang, X. Ge, F. Luo, and J. Han, "Inhibition by peripheral electric stimulation of the reinstatement of morphine-induced place preference in rats and drug-craving in heroin addicts," *Beijing Da Xue Xue Bao Yi Xue Ban*, vol. 35, no. 3, pp. 241–247, 2003.

[411] C. Quoilin, V. Didone, E. Tirelli, and E. Quertemont, "Chronic tolerance to ethanol-induced sedation: implication for age-related differences in locomotor sensitization," *Alcohol*, vol. 47, no. 4, pp. 317–322, 2013.

[412] P. Maccioni, D. Vargiolu, A. W. Thomas et al., "Inhibition of alcohol self-administration by positive allosteric modulators of the GABA$_B$ receptor in rats: lack of tolerance and potentiation of baclofen," *Psychopharmacology*, vol. 232, no. 10, pp. 1831–1841, 2015.

[413] C. Arias, D. A. Revillo, and N. E. Spear, "Chronic tolerance to the locomotor stimulating effect of ethanol in preweanling rats as a function of social stress," *Alcohol*, vol. 46, no. 3, pp. 245–252, 2012.

[414] S. Talarek, J. Orzelska, J. Listos, and S. Fidecka, "Effects of sildenafil treatment on the development of tolerance to diazepam-induced motor impairment and sedation in mice," *Pharmacological Reports*, vol. 62, no. 4, pp. 627–634, 2010.

[415] H. Li, S. Chaney, I. J. Roberts, M. Forte, and J. Hirsh, "Ectopic G-protein expression in dopamine and serotonin neurons blocks cocaine sensitization in *Drosophila melanogaster*," *Current Biology*, vol. 10, no. 4, pp. 211–4, 2000.

[416] C. McClung and J. Hirsh, "The trace amine tyramine is essential for sensitization to cocaine in *Drosophila*," *Current Biology*, vol. 9, no. 16, pp. 853–860, 1999.

[417] E. S. Calipari, M. J. Ferris, C. A. Siciliano, B. A. Zimmer, and S. R. Jones, "Intermittent cocaine self-administration produces sensitization of stimulant effects at the dopamine transporter," *Journal of Pharmacology and Experimental Therapeutics*, vol. 349, no. 2, pp. 192–198, 2014.

[418] N. R. Gubner and T. J. Phillips, "Effects of nicotine on ethanol-induced locomotor sensitization: a model of neuroadaptation," *Behavioural Brain Research*, vol. 288, pp. 26–32, 2015.

[419] E. Valjent, J. Bertran-Gonzalez, B. Aubier, P. Greengard, D. Hervé, and J. A. Girault, "Mechanisms of locomotor sensitization to drugs of abuse in a two-injection protocol," *Neuropsychopharmacology*, vol. 35, no. 2, pp. 401–415, 2010.

[420] J. Zhu, N. M. Midde, A. M. Gomez, W. L. Sun, and S. B. Harrod, "Intra-ventral tegmental area HIV-1 Tat1–86 attenuates nicotine-mediated locomotor sensitization and alters mesocorticolimbic ERK and CREB signaling in rats," *Frontiers in Microbiology*, vol. 6, p. 540, 2015.

[421] A. Ghezzi, H. R. Krishnan, and N. S. Atkinson, "Susceptibility to ethanol withdrawal seizures is produced by BK channel gene expression," *Addiction Biology*, vol. 19, no. 3, pp. 332–337, 2014.

[422] X. Li, A. Ghezzi, J. B. Pohl, A. Y. Bohm, and N. S. Atkinson, "A DNA element regulates drug tolerance and withdrawal in Drosophila," *PLoS One*, vol. 8, no. 9, article e75549, 2013.

[423] S. Perreau-Lenz, C. Sanchis-Segura, F. Leonardi-Essmann, M. Schneider, and R. Spanagel, "Development of morphine-induced tolerance and withdrawal: involvement of the clock gene mPer2," *European Neuropsychopharmacology*, vol. 20, no. 7, pp. 509–517, 2010.

[424] S. M. Bhisikar, D. M. Kokare, K. T. Nakhate, C. T. Chopde, and N. K. Subhedar, "Tolerance to ethanol sedation and withdrawal hyper-excitability is mediated via neuropeptide Y Y1 and Y5 receptors," *Life Sciences*, vol. 85, no. 21-22, pp. 765–772, 2009.

[425] M. Naassila, O. Pierrefiche, C. Ledent, and M. Daoust, "Decreased alcohol self-administration and increased alcohol sensitivity and withdrawal in CB1 receptor knockout mice," *Neuropharmacology*, vol. 46, no. 2, pp. 243–253, 2004.

[426] C. G. Jang, T. Whitfield, G. Schulteis, G. F. Koob, and S. Wee, "A dysphoric-like state during early withdrawal from extended access to methamphetamine self-administration in rats," *Psychopharmacology*, vol. 225, no. 3, pp. 753–763, 2013.

[427] J. F. McGinty, A. Zelek-Molik, and W. L. Sun, "Cocaine self-administration causes signaling deficits in corticostriatal circuitry that are reversed by BDNF in early withdrawal," *Brain Research*, vol. 1628, Part A, pp. 82–87, 2015.

[428] B. G. Robinson, S. Khurana, A. Kuperman, and N. S. Atkinson, "Neural adaptation leads to cognitive ethanol dependence," *Current Biology*, vol. 22, no. 24, pp. 2338–2341, 2012.

[429] Y. Chen, R. Song, R. F. Yang, N. Wu, and J. Li, "A novel dopamine D3 receptor antagonist YQA14 inhibits methamphetamine self-administration and relapse to drug-seeking behaviour in rats," *European Journal of Pharmacology*, vol. 743, pp. 126–132, 2014.

[430] M. L. Logrip, L. F. Vendruscolo, J. E. Schlosburg, G. F. Koob, and E. P. Zorrilla, "Phosphodiesterase 10A regulates alcohol and saccharin self-administration in rats," *Neuropsychopharmacology*, vol. 39, no. 7, pp. 1722–1731, 2014.

[431] A. Cooper, N. Barnea-Ygael, D. Levy, Y. Shaham, and A. Zangen, "A conflict rat model of cue-induced relapse to cocaine seeking," *Psychopharmacology*, vol. 194, no. 1, pp. 117–125, 2007.

[432] N. J. Marchant, T. N. Khuc, C. L. Pickens, A. Bonci, and Y. Shaham, "Context-induced relapse to alcohol seeking after punishment in a rat model," *Biological Psychiatry*, vol. 73, no. 3, pp. 256–262, 2013.

[433] Z. J. Brown, J. N. Nobrega, and S. Erb, "Central injections of noradrenaline induce reinstatement of cocaine seeking and increase c-fos mRNA expression in the extended amygdala," *Behavioural Brain Research*, vol. 217, no. 2, pp. 472–476, 2011.

[434] A. R. Ozburn, R. A. Harris, and Y. A. Blednov, "Chronic voluntary alcohol consumption results in tolerance to sedative/hypnotic and hypothermic effects of alcohol in hybrid mice," *Pharmacology, Biochemistry, and Behavior*, vol. 104, pp. 33–39, 2013.

[435] B. Garmabi, N. Vousooghi, M. Vosough, A. Yoonessi, A. Bakhtazad, and M. R. Zarrindast, "Effect of circadian rhythm disturbance on morphine preference and addiction in male rats: involvement of period genes and dopamine D1 receptor," *Neuroscience*, vol. 322, pp. 104–114, 2016.

[436] P. Wongchitrat, S. Mukda, P. Phansuwan-Pujito, and P. Govitrapong, "Effect of amphetamine on the clock gene expression in rat striatum," *Neuroscience Letters*, vol. 542, pp. 126–130, 2013.

[437] S. X. Li, L. J. Liu, W. G. Jiang, and L. Lu, "Morphine withdrawal produces circadian rhythm alterations of clock genes in mesolimbic brain areas and peripheral blood mononuclear cells in rats," *Journal of Neurochemistry*, vol. 109, no. 6, pp. 1668–1679, 2009.

[438] S. Masubuchi, S. Honma, H. Abe, W. Nakamura, and K. Honma, "Circadian activity rhythm in methamphetamine-treated *Clock* mutant mice," *European Journal of Neuroscience*, vol. 14, no. 7, pp. 1177–1180, 2001.

[439] C. D. Bryant, M. E. Graham, M. G. Distler et al., "A role for casein kinase 1 epsilon in the locomotor stimulant response to methamphetamine," *Psychopharmacology*, vol. 203, no. 4, pp. 703–711, 2009.

[440] C. D. Bryant, C. C. Parker, L. Zhou et al., "Csnk1e is a genetic regulator of sensitivity to psychostimulants and opioids," *Neuropsychopharmacology*, vol. 37, no. 4, pp. 1026–1035, 2012.

[441] D. Li, S. Herrera, N. Bubula et al., "Casein kinase 1 enables nucleus accumbens amphetamine-induced locomotion by regulating AMPA receptor phosphorylation," *Journal of Neurochemistry*, vol. 118, no. 2, pp. 237–247, 2011.

[442] Y. Zhang, P. Svenningsson, R. Picetti et al., "Cocaine self-administration in mice is inversely related to phosphorylation at Thr34 (protein kinase A site) and Ser130 (kinase CK1 site) of DARPP-32," *Journal of Neuroscience*, vol. 26, no. 10, pp. 2645–2651, 2006.

[443] A. W. Lasek, D. Kapfhamer, V. Kharazia, J. Gesch, F. Giorgetti, and U. Heberlein, "*Lmo4* in the nucleus accumbens regulates cocaine sensitivity," *Genes, Brain and Behavior*, vol. 9, no. 7, pp. 817–824, 2010.

CRMP2 and CRMP4 Are Differentially Required for Axon Guidance and Growth in Zebrafish Retinal Neurons

Zhi-Zhi Liu,[1,2,3] Jian Zhu,[1,2,3] Chang-Ling Wang,[1,2,3] Xin Wang,[1,2,3] Ying-Ying Han,[1,2,3] Ling-Yan Liu,[1,2,3] and Hong A. Xu ⓘ[1,2,3]

[1]Institute of Life Science, Nanchang University, Nanchang, China
[2]School of Life Sciences, Nanchang University, Nanchang, China
[3]Jiangxi Provincial Collaborative Innovation Center for Cardiovascular, Digestive, and Neuropsychiatric Diseases, Nanchang, China

Correspondence should be addressed to Hong A. Xu; xuhong@ncu.edu.cn

Academic Editor: Stuart C. Mangel

Axons are directed to their correct targets by guidance cues during neurodevelopment. Many axon guidance cues have been discovered; however, much less known is about how the growth cones transduce the extracellular guidance cues to intracellular responses. Collapsin response mediator proteins (CRMPs) are a family of intracellular proteins that have been found to mediate growth cone behavior *in vitro*; however, their roles *in vivo* in axon development are much less explored. In zebrafish embryos, we find that CRMP2 and CRMP4 are expressed in the retinal ganglion cell layer when retinal axons are crossing the midline. Knocking down CRMP2 causes reduced elongation and premature termination of the retinal axons, while knocking down CRMP4 results in ipsilateral misprojections of retinal axons that would normally project to the contralateral brain. Furthermore, CRMP4 synchronizes with neuropilin 1 in retinal axon guidance, suggesting that CRMP4 might mediate the semaphorin/neuropilin signaling pathway. These results demonstrate that CRMP2 and CRMP4 function differentially in axon development *in vivo*.

1. Introduction

The correct formation of neural circuits is critical for establishing a functional nervous system. Axons grow out of neurons and usually travel a long distance to reach their correct targets. The axons must navigate accurately through the brain by following a precise path and the course is regulated by guidance cues [1, 2]. Dozens of axon guidance cues, including semaphorins, have been identified in the past decades. However, the intracellular molecular response mechanisms underlying how the growth cone of axons interpret environmental guidance cues are relatively less understood.

The collapsin response mediator protein (CRMP) is an intracellular protein discovered in a screen for components of the semaphorin 3A (originally named collapsin [3]) signaling pathway that mediates the collapse response of the growth cone [4]. Concurrently, a number of CRMPs were identified independently and referred to as turned on after division (TOAD-64) [5], dihydropyrimidinase-related protein (DRP or DPYSL) [6], unc-33-like protein (Ulip) [7], or TUC (TOAD64/Ulip/CRMP) [8]. In vertebrates, five members of CRMPs, CRMP1–5, have been identified [9, 10]. CRMPs are highly expressed in the nervous system at an early developmental stage and the expression dramatically drops in adults [9, 11]. CRMPs have been shown to be critical for many neurodevelopmental processes, such as neurogenesis, neuronal migration, and dendrite development [12]. Additionally, CRMPs might also be involved in axon regeneration, neurodegenerative diseases, and neuropsychiatric diseases [9, 12, 13]. Vertebrate CRMPs are homologous with *C. elegans unc-33*, the mutation of which results in severe defects of axon growth and guidance [14, 15]. Many studies have demonstrated that CRMPs are involved in growth cone collapse and axon growth *in vitro* [8, 10, 13, 16]. However, their roles in axon development *in vivo*, particularly in the central nervous system, still remain unclear. For example, in CMRP4 knockout mice, the apical dendrites of the CA1 pyramidal neurons are found to bifurcate precociously [17]. However, no anatomical or macroscopic changes in gross brain anatomy is observed in CMRP4 knockout mice [17, 18] although a selective decrease of axon extension and reduced growth cone area are observed in the cultured hippocampus neurons of CMRP4 knockout mice [18].

In the present study, the visual system was used to study the roles of CRMPs in axon development in the central nervous system. Both CRMP2 and CRMP4 were highly expressed in the retinal ganglion cell layer when retinal axons were crossing the chiasm and approaching the tectum in zebrafish. The two CRMPs functioned differentially in axon guidance and growth. CRMP2 was critical for axon elongation while CRMP4 was important for axon guidance. We also showed that CRMP4 synergized with neuropilin 1 in retinal axon guidance, suggesting that it might mediate the semaphorin/neuropilin signaling pathway.

2. Materials and Methods

2.1. Zebrafish Maintenance. Adult zebrafish (*Danio rerio*) were maintained in our facility on a 14–10 light–dark cycle in circulating water at 26–28°C. Embryos of either sex were raised at 28.5°C in E3 embryo medium (5 mM NaCl, 0.17 mM KCl, 0.33 mM $CaCl_2$, and 0.33 mM $MgSO_4$). Embryos to be collected for imaging were treated with 0.003% phenylthiourea (Sigma-Aldrich, St. Louis, USA) in E3 to prevent pigmentation. Embryos were staged by time after fertilization. All handling procedures were approved by the local ethical review committee at Nanchang University.

2.2. Whole-Mount In Situ Hybridization. The cDNAs used as templates to make probes were prepared by RNA extraction and reverse transcription PCR (RT-PCR). The primers for RT-PCR were designed according to the Esembl genomic sequences [19]. In situ hybridization was performed as described previously [20] with minor modifications. Briefly, DIG-labeled riboprobes were incubated with the embryos to detect the expression pattern of CRMP2 and CRMP4. Anti-DIG-alkaline phosphatase Fab fragments (Roche, Mannheim, Germany) and NBT/BCIP (Sangon Biotech, Shanghai, China) were used to detect and amplify the signals.

2.3. Morpholino Microinjections. Antisense morpholinos (MOs) were obtained from Gene Tools LLC (Philomath, OR, USA). MO sequences are as follows: CRMP2, 5'-CTT CTT GCC CTG ATA GCC AGA **CAT** C-3' [21] (underlined nucleotides corresponding to the first initiation codon); CRMP4, 5'-TCT TTT TGC CTT GGT AAG A**CA T**GG T-3' [22]; and Nrp1a, 5'-GAA TCC TGG AGT TCG GAG TGC GGA A-3' [20, 23]. The knockdown effects and specificity of CRMP2 and CRMP4 MOs have been validated by rescuing the resulting phenotypes with the corresponding mRNAs [21, 22]. Nrp1a MO has also been validated in an *in vitro* transcription and translation system [23] and *in vivo* in axon guidance [20]. The sequence of the standard control MO from Gene Tools is 5'-CCT CTT ACCTCA GTT ACA ATT TAT A-3'. Approximately 1–1.5 nl of MOs at different dosages were injected into embryo yolk at the 1-2 cell stage.

2.4. Retinal Axon Labeling. Retina axons were labeled by dye injection as previously described [24]. Briefly, zebrafish larvae were fixed at 4 dpf (days post fertilization) in 4% PFA. Retinal axons were labeled by injecting lipophilic dye DiI into one eye and DiD into the other eye. The dye-labeled retinotectal axons were scanned on an Olympus FV1000 confocal microscope and all images were presented as maximum projections of the z series. The number of the eyes were counted with normal or abnormal retinal axon guidance or growth. Fisher's exact test was used to compare the effects of the combination of the morpholinos with that of the sum of the single half doses of morpholinos.

3. Results

3.1. CRMP2 and CRMP4 Were Expressed in a Retinal Ganglion Cell Layer When Retinal Axons Were Crossing the Midline. The visual system is a classical modeling system to study axon guidance of the central nervous system since retinal axons travel a long distance through the brain [25]. Retinal axons exit the eye and extend ventrally to cross the midline at the optic chiasm. They continue to extend dorsally and posteriorly to the tectum. In contrast to binocular animals, all retinal axons cross the midline and project to the contralateral brain in zebrafish.

In order to investigate the role of CRMPs in axon growth and guidance *in vivo*, we performed in situ hybridization with antisense probes for CRMPs in zebrafish embryos. Our preliminary results revealed that CRMP1–4 were all expressed in the retina at 36 hours post fertilization (hpf). We focused on CRMP2 and CRMP4 since CRMP2 is the most studied member of the CRMP family and both CRMP2 and CRMP4 have been shown to be critical for axon regeneration. CRMP2 and CRMP4 were highly expressed in the retinal ganglion cell layer surrounding the lens at 36 hpf (Figures 1(a) and 1(b)), when the first retinal axons are exiting the eye and crossing the midline. Both of the CRMPs were still highly and specifically expressed in the retina at 48 hpf, when retinal axons are approaching and starting to arborise the tectum (Figures 1(c) and 1(d)). Besides being expressed in the retina, CRMP2 and CRMP4 were also highly expressed in specific brain regions and a subpopulation of neurons in the spinal cord, consistent with previous reports [11, 26]. We confirmed the expression patterns of CRMP2 and CRMP4 by using antisense probes targeting nonoverlapping regions of the mRNA transcripts. The spatiotemporal expression patterns of CRMP2 and CRMP4 in the retinal ganglion cell layer suggested that they might be important for axon growth and guidance *in vivo*.

3.2. Knocking Down CRMP2 Resulted in Growth Defects of Retinal Axons. CRMP2 has been shown to be critical for axon specification and growth *in vitro* [8, 16]; however, its roles *in vivo* still remain unclear. We injected morpholino (MO), an antisense oligonucleotide sequence specifically targeting

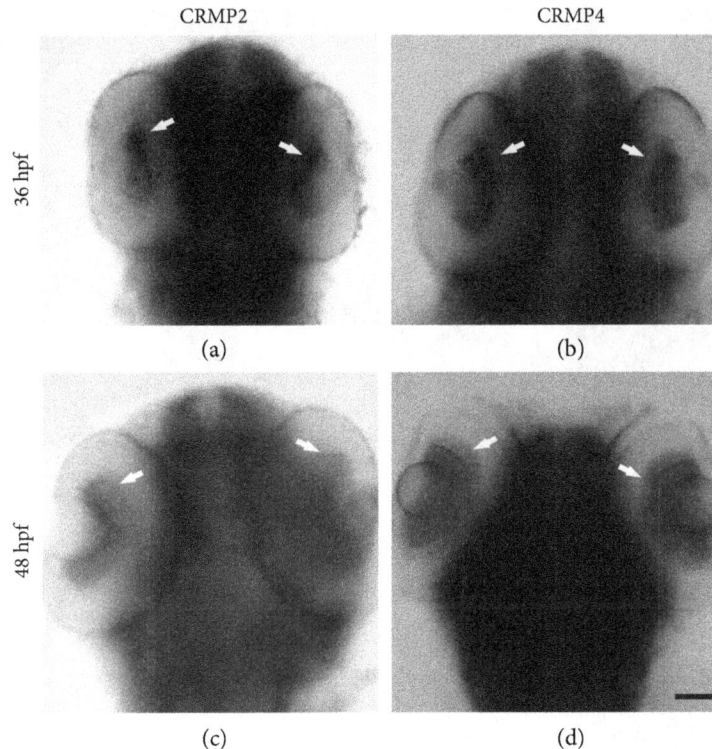

FIGURE 1: CRMP2 and CRMP4 are expressed in the retinal ganglion cell layer when retinal axons are exiting the eye and crossing the midline. Whole mount in situ hybridization was performed in zebrafish embryos using RNA probes for CRMP2. (a, b) CRMP2 and CRMP4 transcripts are detected in the retina (white arrows) at 36 hpf. (c, d) CRMP2 and CRMP4 transcripts are detected in the retina of 48 hpf embryos (white arrows). Scale bar: 50 μm.

the transcribed mRNA, into zebrafish zygotes to block the translation of CRMP2 [21]. Fluorescence lipophilic dyes were injected into the eyes of fixed embryos to label retinal axons. Normally, the first retinal axons reach and start to arborize the optic tectum at 2 dpf and a preliminary arborization of the tectum is formed at 3 dpf (data not shown). At 4 dpf, many retinal axons have arborized the whole tectum (Figure 2(a)). However, in CRMP2 MO-treated embryos (morphants), much less retinal axons arborized the tectum in morphants compared to wildtype embryos. Some retinal axons might terminate prematurely and fail to reach the tectum even at 4 dpf, although many retinal axons grew out of the eye and formed the optic tract (Figures 2(b) and 2(c)). The growth defects of retinal axons in CRMP2 morphants were dose-dependent, with much more severe defects at higher doses of morpholino (Figure 2(d)). The reduced arborization of the tectum in morphants suggested that CRMP2 might be critical for axon elongation, consistent with the reports in vitro [8, 16]. CRMP2 has long been presumed to be involved in axon guidance since its discovery. However, we only found rare axon guidance errors, such as ipsilateral misprojections (2%) and dorsal misprojections (2.6%) in CRMP2 morphants (data not shown). In most morphants, despite growth defects, the residue retinal axons still crossed the midline, followed normal optic pathways, and projected correctly into the tectum (Figures 2(b) and 2(c)). These results revealed that CRMP2 was critical for axon elongation in vivo.

3.3. Knocking Down CRMP4 Caused Retinal Axons to Misproject Ipsilaterally.
Similar to CRMP2, CRMP4 was also highly expressed in the retinal ganglion cell layer. However, different from CRMP2 morphants, only mild growth defects of retinal axons were found in CRMP4 morphants (data not shown). Unexpectedly, knocking down CRMP4 resulted in axon guidance defects. In control MO-treated larvae, nearly all retinal axons crossed the midline and projected into the contralateral tectum (Figure 3(a)). However, in CRMP4 morphants, some retinal axons failed to cross the midline and misprojected into the ipsilateral tectum (Figures 3(b) and 3(c)). The axon guidance errors caused by CRMP4 MO were dose-dependent (Figure 3(d)). The ipsilaterally misprojected retinal axons still follow the correct orbit of the normal optic tract, suggesting that CRMP4 mainly mediates axon crossing at the midline. These results demonstrated that CRMP2 and CRMP4 functioned differentially in axon guidance and growth during the development of the visual system.

3.4. CRMP4 Synergized with Neuropilin 1 in Retinal Axon Guidance.
The ipsilateral misprojection phenotypes caused by CRMP4 knockdown was reminiscent of the phenotypes induced by knocking down Sema3D, Sema3E, and their coreceptor neuropilin 1 (Nrp1) [20]. This suggested that CRMP4 might mediate the signaling transduction of Sema3/Nrp1 in axon guidance. In order to test this possibility, we knocked down Nrp1 and CRMP4 with half doses of MOs. At half doses of either the CRMP4 or Nrp1a MO,

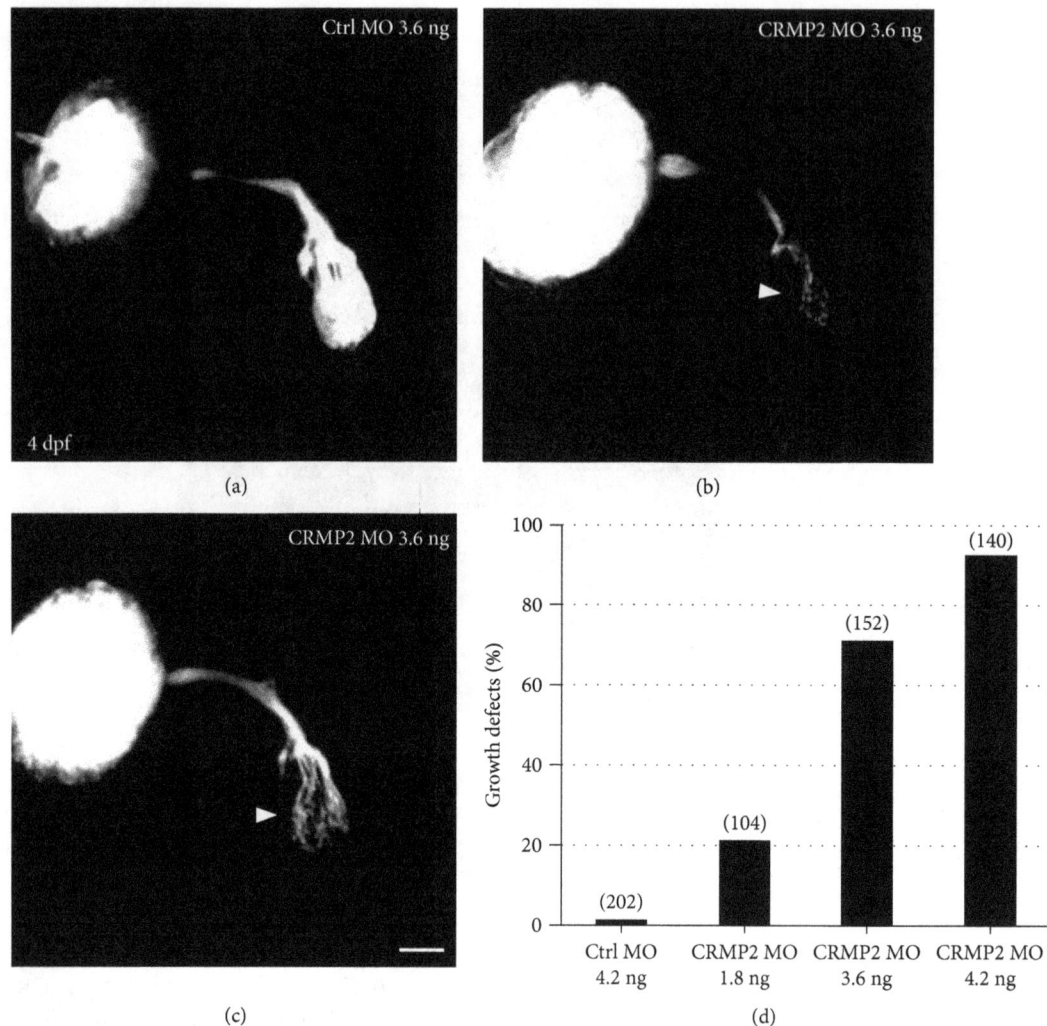

FIGURE 2: Knocking down CRMP2 induces growth defects of retinal axons. Morpholino was injected into the zygotes at the 1-2 cell stage. Embryos were allowed to grow until 4 days (4 days postfertilization, 4 dpf) and fixed with PFA. Lipophilic fluorescent dye DiI or DiD was injected into an eye of the larvae to label retinal axons. (a) An example showing that, in control MO-treated zebrafish larvae, retinal axons exit the eye, cross the midline, and grow into and arborize the whole tectum at 4 dpf. (b, c) Representative images of retinal axons of CRMP2 MO-treated embryos. Much less retinal axons grow into and arborized the tectum (white arrowheads) compared with that in control MO-treated embryos. (d) The growth defects of retinal axons induced by CRMP2 MOs are dose-dependent. The y-axis represents the percentage of eyes with growth defects of retinal axons. The doses of MOs are labeled under each column. The numbers in parentheses above each column indicate the amount of eyes. Scale bar: 50 μm.

only a low percentage of ipsilateral misprojections was observed (Figure 4(a)), much less than that caused by full doses of either corresponding MO. The combination of half doses of CRMP4 and Nrp1a induced a much higher percentage of ipsilateral misprojections than the sum by adding up that induced by single half doses of them (Figures 4(b) and 4(c)). This indicated that CRMP4 and Nrp1a synergize with each other in retinal axon guidance, suggesting that they might function in a common signaling pathway. This is consistent with the *in vitro* studies that CRMPs function downstream of semaphorin/neuropilin [27–29].

3.5. CRMP2 and CRMP4 Synergize with Each Other in Axon Growth but Not Axon Guidance. The above results suggested that CRMP2 and CRMP4 might play differential roles in

axon growth and guidance. It seemed that CRMP2 might mainly function in axon growth while CRMP4 participates in axon guidance. Since both of the two CRMPs were expressed in the retinal ganglion cell layer, we asked whether they cooperate with each other in axon development. We found that combining half doses of CRMP2 and CRMP4 MOs resulted in more axon growth defects than the sum of the defects caused by the two single half doses of morpholinos (Figure 5). The synergy between CRMP2 and CRMP4 suggested that they participate in axon growth in a common signaling pathway. However, we did not observe any synergy between the two CRMPs in retinal axon guidance (Figure 5(d)). The synergy between the two MOs in axon growth but not axon guidance suggested that the observed phenotypes could not be due to any toxic

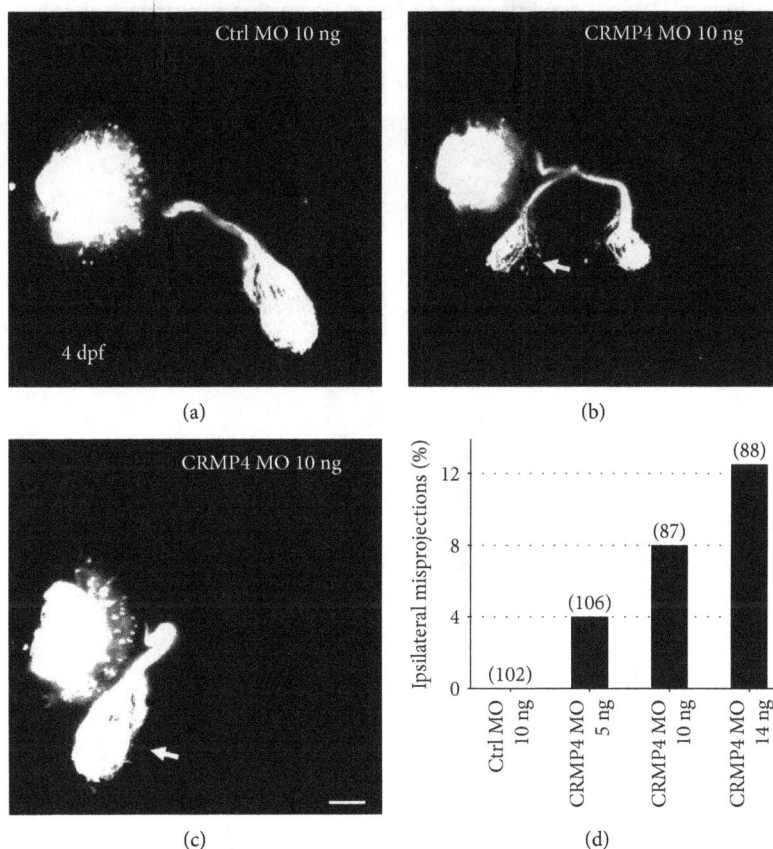

FIGURE 3: Knocking down CRMP4 causes ipsilateral misprojections of retinal axons. Morpholino was injected into 1-2 cell stage embryos and retinal axons were labeled with DiI or DiD at 4 dpf. (a) A representative image demonstrating that, in control MO-treated zebrafish larvae, all retinal axons cross the midline and project into the opposite side of the tectum. (b, c) Representative images of retinal axon guidance errors in CRMP4 MO-treated larvae. A part or all of the retinal axons fail to cross the midline and misproject into the ipsilateral tectum (arrows). Note that although the axons misproject ipsilaterally, they still follow the normal optic tract and arborize into the tectum. (d) The ipsilateral misprojections of retinal axons caused by CRMP4 MOs are dose dependent. The doses of MOs are labeled under each column. The numbers in parentheses above each column indicate the amount of eyes. Scale bar: 50 μm.

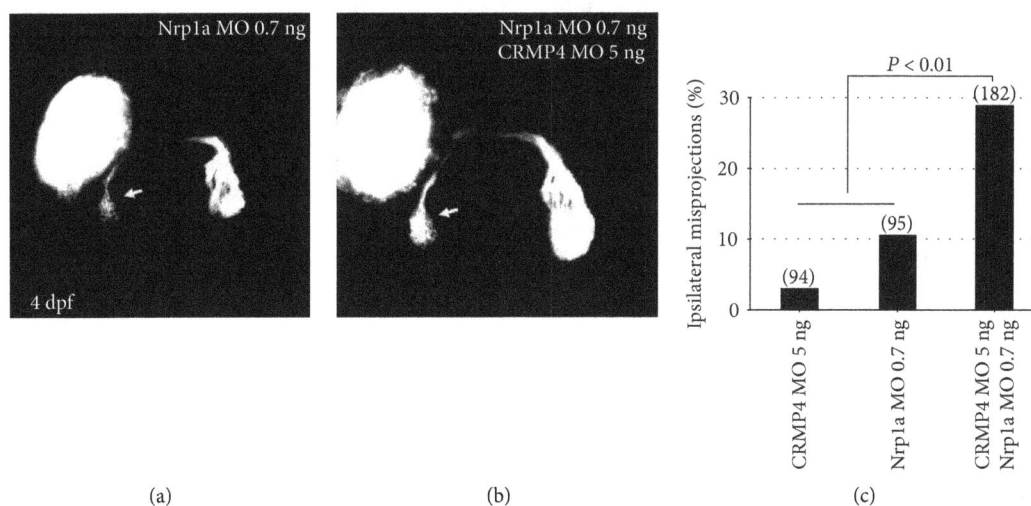

FIGURE 4: CRMP4 and Nrp1a synergize in retinal axon guidance. A low dose of either CRMP4 or Nrp1a induce a small percentage of ipsilateral misprojections. A half dose of either CRMP4 MOs or Nrp1a MOs was injected singly or in combination. (a, b) Representative images of knocking down effects by a half dose of Nrp1a MOs or Nrp1a and CRMP4 in combination. Some retinal axons fail to cross the midline and misproject ipsilaterally (arrows). (c) The combination of the two morpholinos induce a significantly higher percentage of ipsilateral misprojections than simply adding up the misprojections caused by the two half doses (Fisher's exact test, $P < 0.01$). The doses of MOs are labeled under each column. The numbers in each column indicate the amount of eyes.

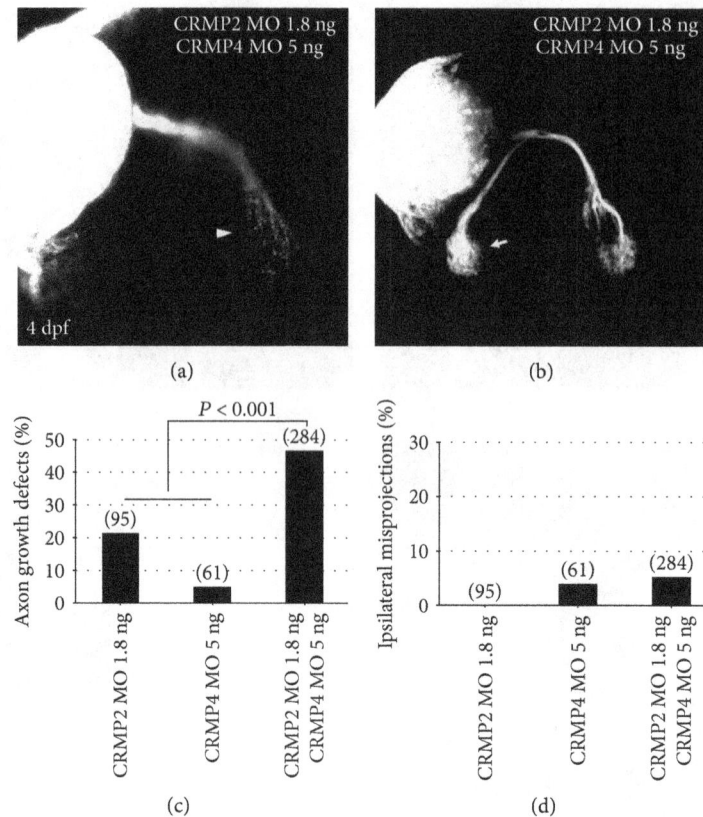

FIGURE 5: CRMP2 synergized with CRMP4 in axon growth but not axon guidance. A half dose of either CRMP2 or CRMP4 MOs was injected singly or in combination. (a, b) Representative examples of knocking down effects of CRMP2 and CRMP4 MOs in combination. (c) The combination of the two MOs causes a significantly higher percentage of axon growth defects than the sum of the defects caused by adding up the single half doses (Fisher's exact test, $P < 0.001$). (d) No obvious synergy between the two CRMPs in retinal axon guidance. The doses of MOs are labeled under each column. The numbers in parentheses above each column indicate the amount of eyes.

effect but instead due to their specific effects. These data further demonstrated that CRMP2 and CRMP4 played differential roles in axon development. CRMP2 might mainly participate in axon elongation while CRMP4 mainly function in axon guidance. Additionally, CRMP4 might coordinate with CRMP2 in axon elongation.

4. Discussion

It has long been proposed that CRMPs might play critical roles in axon development since their discovery; however, little *in vivo* evidence has been presented. In this study, we report that CRMP2 and CRMP4 are critical for retinal axon guidance and growth in zebrafish embryos. Interestingly, the two CRMPs function differentially in axon development: CRMP2 mainly participates in axon outgrowth and elongation while CRMP4 seems to play dual roles in both axon guidance and growth.

Vertebrate CRMPs share a homology with the UNC-33 protein in the nematode *C. elegans*. Mutations in the *unc-33* gene cause severe axon extension defects and guidance errors [14, 15]. Our current findings that knocking down CRMPs results in defects of axon growth and guidance suggest that the roles of vertebrate CRMPs in axon development are well conserved evolutionally between invertebrates and

vertebrates. It has been demonstrated that CRMP2 regulates axon initiation and elongation *in vitro* [16, 30]. Those findings are consistent with our results that both the number and length of retinal axons are reduced in the tectum of the CRMP2 morphants. The bundle of retinal axons in the optic nerve and optic tract seems to be thinner than that in wild type embryos, suggesting possible initiation failure of axons; however, further study is required to confirm the possibility. Some of the retinal axons terminate prematurely and fail to reach the tectum (Figures 2(b) and 2(c)), indicating the failure of axons to elongate further into the tectum in the absence of CRMP2. Besides the visual system, CRMP2 might also be broadly required for axon growth in other neural systems [31]. Furthermore, in the adult mouse hippocampal dentate gyrus, there are axonal growth and targeting defects in newborn granule neurons with CRMP2 knockdown [32]. This indicates that axon growth during embryonic development and adult newborn regeneration might share some common mechanisms related to CRMP2. CRMP4, similar to CRMP2, has been revealed to be involved in axon growth *in vitro* and *in vivo* [18, 22]. All these findings are consistent with our results, although CRMP4 seems to play only a minor role in axon growth as compared to CRMP2.

Since their discovery, CRMPs have been proposed to be involved in axon guidance by mediating the activity of semaphorins and other guidance cues. In the present study, we demonstrate that CRMP4 is critical for the proper direction of retinal axons in the chiasm. Knocking down CRMP4 causes retinal axons to misproject to the ipsilateral side of the brain. The ipsilateral misprojections of retinal axons are reminiscent of those caused by knocking down Sema3s or neuropilin 1 [20, 33]. Furthermore, the synergetic effect between CRMP4 and neuropilin 1 (Figure 4) indicates that CRMP4 might function downstream of the semaphorin/neuropilin signaling pathway in guiding axons [20]. However, the intracellular domain of neuropilin is very short (about 20 amino acids long). So it is reasonable to speculate that CRMP4, as an intracellular protein, should interact with a transmembrane receptor for semaphorin, such as plexin. Further studies are guaranteed to search for such a receptor and investigate its interaction with neuropilin and CRMP4.

It is intriguing that CRMP2 and CRMP4 cooperate in axon growth while playing differential roles in axon guidance. Continuous remodeling of the neuronal cytoskeleton is critical for axon extension and turning. Microtubules and actin filaments are central to the coordinated control of the cytoskeleton in the growth cone of the axons. It has been demonstrated that CRMP2 and CRMP4 similarly interact with tubulin while differentially involved in actin dynamics [18, 34, 35]. The cooperated and differential roles of CRMP2 and CRMP4 in axon development could partially be due to their complex interactions with tubulin and actin. The differential roles of CRMP2 and CRMP4 in axon development could also be associated with other factors, such as differential expression of CRMPs upon stimulation [36], differential response to various axon guidance cues [37], specific phosphorylation by different kinases [36, 38], and subcellular distribution [39].

Alternative splicing of CRMPs (CRMP1–4) has been shown to result in two isoforms that differ in the first exons and consequently different N-termini: the short isoforms (CRMP1–4S (Small or short)) and the isoforms that are longer by ~100 amino acids (CRMP1–4L (Large or long)) [40, 41]. It has been shown that the alternatively spliced isoforms of CRMP2 are differentially involved in axon guidance and growth [42]. Our PCR results suggest that the zebrafish CRMP2 and CRMP4 also have alternatively spliced isoforms (data not shown). However, we fail to distinguish the expression pattern of the short and long isoforms. The morpholinos used in this report are translational blockers targeting the short isoforms [22], CRMP2S and CRMP4S. Further studies are required to investigate the roles of the long isoforms of CRMPs in axon growth and guidance *in vivo*.

5. Conclusion

The study has revealed the intracellular mechanisms of how the CRMPs transduce the extracellular guidance cues into behavioral responses of the growth cone *in vivo*. CRMP2 and CRMP4 are expressed in the retinal ganglion cell layer when retinal axons are growing from the eye to the brain. CRMP2 and CRMP4 differentially participate in axon development *in vivo*. CRMP2 mainly mediates axon elongation while CRMP4 mediates axon guidance. We also demonstrate that CRMP4 phenocopies neuropilin 1a in retinal axon guidance and they synergize with each other, suggesting that they might mediate the semaphorin/neuropilin signaling pathway *in vivo*. Our findings will help to understand the underlying molecular mechanisms of axon development and regeneration and CRMP-related diseases such as neurodegeneration and neuropsychiatric disorders.

Acknowledgments

This work was supported by grants from the National Natural Science Foundation of China (Grant nos. 31400988, 31171044, 81160144, and 81760216), the Young Scientist of Jiangxi Province (Grant no. 20122BCB23007), and the Natural Science Foundation of Jiangxi Province (Grant no. 20151BAB215015).

References

[1] B. J. Dickson, "Molecular mechanisms of axon guidance," *Science*, vol. 298, no. 5600, pp. 1959–1964, 2002.

[2] M. Tessier-Lavigne and C. S. Goodman, "The molecular biology of axon guidance," *Science*, vol. 274, no. 5290, pp. 1123–1133, 1996.

[3] Y. Luo, D. Raible, and J. A. Raper, "Collapsin: a protein in brain that induces the collapse and paralysis of neuronal growth cones," *Cell*, vol. 75, no. 2, pp. 217–227, 1993.

[4] Y. Goshima, F. Nakamura, P. Strittmatter, and S. M. Strittmatter, "Collapsin-induced growth cone collapse mediated by an intracellular protein related to UNC-33," *Nature*, vol. 376, no. 6540, pp. 509–514, 1995.

[5] J. E. Minturn, H. J. Fryer, D. H. Geschwind, and S. Hockfield, "TOAD-64, a gene expressed early in neuronal differentiation in the rat, is related to unc-33, a *C. elegans* gene involved in axon outgrowth," *The Journal of Neuroscience*, vol. 15, no. 10, pp. 6757–6766, 1995.

[6] N. Hamajima, K. Matsuda, S. Sakata, N. Tamaki, M. Sasaki, and M. Nonaka, "A novel gene family defined by human dihydropyrimidinase and three related proteins with differential tissue distribution," *Gene*, vol. 180, no. 1-2, pp. 157–163, 1996.

[7] T. Byk, T. Dobransky, C. Cifuentes-Diaz, and A. Sobel, "Identification and molecular characterization of Unc-33-like phosphoprotein (Ulip), a putative mammalian homolog of the axonal guidance-associated unc-33 gene product," *The Journal of Neuroscience*, vol. 16, no. 2, pp. 688–701, 1996.

[8] C. C. Quinn, G. E. Gray, and S. Hockfield, "A family of proteins implicated in axon guidance and outgrowth," *Journal of Neurobiology*, vol. 41, no. 1, pp. 158–164, 1999.

[9] E. Charrier, S. Reibel, V. Rogemond, M. Aguera, N. Thomasset, and J. Honnorat, "Collapsin response mediator proteins (CRMPs): involvement in nervous system development and adult neurodegenerative disorders," *Molecular Neurobiology*, vol. 28, no. 1, pp. 51–64, 2003.

[10] E. F. Schmidt and S. M. Strittmatter, "The CRMP family of proteins and their role in Sema3A signaling," *Advances in Experimental Medicine and Biology*, vol. 600, pp. 1–11, 2007.

[11] J. Schweitzer, C. G. Becker, M. Schachner, and T. Becker, "Expression of collapsin response mediator proteins in the nervous system of embryonic zebrafish," *Gene Expression Patterns*, vol. 5, no. 6, pp. 809–816, 2005.

[12] J. Nagai, R. Baba, and T. Ohshima, "CRMPs function in neurons and glial cells: potential therapeutic targets for neurodegenerative diseases and CNS injury," *Molecular Neurobiology*, vol. 54, no. 6, pp. 4243–4256, 2017.

[13] T. T. Quach, J. Honnorat, P. E. Kolattukudy, R. Khanna, and A. M. Duchemin, "CRMPs: critical molecules for neurite morphogenesis and neuropsychiatric diseases," *Molecular Psychiatry*, vol. 20, no. 9, pp. 1037–1045, 2015.

[14] W. Li, R. K. Herman, and J. E. Shaw, "Analysis of the *Caenorhabditis elegans* axonal guidance and outgrowth gene unc-33," *Genetics*, vol. 132, no. 3, pp. 675–689, 1992.

[15] E. M. Hedgecock, J. G. Culotti, J. N. Thomson, and L. A. Perkins, "Axonal guidance mutants of *Caenorhabditis elegans* identified by filling sensory neurons with fluorescein dyes," *Developmental Biology*, vol. 111, no. 1, pp. 158–170, 1985.

[16] N. Inagaki, K. Chihara, N. Arimura et al., "CRMP-2 induces axons in cultured hippocampal neurons," *Nature Neuroscience*, vol. 4, no. 8, pp. 781-782, 2001.

[17] E. Niisato, J. Nagai, N. Yamashita et al., "CRMP4 suppresses apical dendrite bifurcation of CA1 pyramidal neurons in the mouse hippocampus," *Developmental Neurobiology*, vol. 72, no. 11, pp. 1447–1457, 2012.

[18] M. R. Khazaei, M. P. Girouard, R. Alchini et al., "Collapsin response mediator protein 4 regulates growth cone dynamics through the actin and microtubule cytoskeleton," *Journal of Biological Chemistry*, vol. 289, no. 43, pp. 30133–43, 2014.

[19] D. R. Zerbino, P. Achuthan, W. Akanni et al., "Ensembl 2018," *Nucleic Acids Research*, vol. 46, no. D1, pp. D754–D761, 2018.

[20] A. L. Dell, E. Fried-Cassorla, H. Xu, and J. A. Raper, "cAMP-induced expression of neuropilin1 promotes retinal axon crossing in the zebrafish optic chiasm," *The Journal of Neuroscience*, vol. 33, no. 27, pp. 11076–11088, 2013.

[21] H. Tanaka, R. Morimura, and T. Ohshima, "Dpysl2 (CRMP2) and Dpysl3 (CRMP4) phosphorylation by Cdk5 and DYRK2 is required for proper positioning of Rohon-Beard neurons and neural crest cells during neurulation in zebrafish," *Developmental Biology*, vol. 370, no. 2, pp. 223–236, 2012.

[22] H. Tanaka, Y. Nojima, W. Shoji et al., "Islet1 selectively promotes peripheral axon outgrowth in Rohon-Beard primary sensory neurons," *Developmental Dynamics*, vol. 240, no. 1, pp. 9–22, 2011.

[23] P. Lee, K. Goishi, A. J. Davidson, R. Mannix, L. Zon, and M. Klagsbrun, "Neuropilin-1 is required for vascular development and is a mediator of VEGF-dependent angiogenesis in zebrafish," *Proceedings of the National Academy of Sciences of the United States of America*, vol. 99, no. 16, pp. 10470–10475, 2002.

[24] H. Xu, S. G. Leinwand, A. L. Dell, E. Fried-Cassorla, and J. A. Raper, "The calmodulin-stimulated adenylate cyclase ADCY8 sets the sensitivity of zebrafish retinal axons to midline repellents and is required for normal midline crossing," *The Journal of Neuroscience*, vol. 30, no. 21, pp. 7423–7433, 2010.

[25] R. O. Karlstrom, T. Trowe, S. Klostermann et al., "Zebrafish mutations affecting retinotectal axon pathfinding," *Development*, vol. 123, pp. 427–438, 1996.

[26] T. L. Christie, O. Starovic-Subota, and S. Childs, "Zebrafish collapsin response mediator protein (CRMP)-2 is expressed in developing neurons," *Gene Expression Patterns*, vol. 6, no. 2, pp. 193–200, 2006.

[27] E. F. Schmidt, S. O. Shim, and S. M. Strittmatter, "Release of MICAL autoinhibition by semaphorin-plexin signaling promotes interaction with collapsin response mediator protein," *The Journal of Neuroscience*, vol. 28, no. 9, pp. 2287–2297, 2008.

[28] Y. Ito, I. Oinuma, H. Katoh, K. Kaibuchi, and M. Negishi, "Sema4D/plexin-B1 activates GSK-3beta through R-Ras GAP activity, inducing growth cone collapse," *EMBO Reports*, vol. 7, no. 7, pp. 704–709, 2006.

[29] R. C. Deo, E. F. Schmidt, A. Elhabazi, H. Togashi, S. K. Burley, and S. M. Strittmatter, "Structural bases for CRMP function in plexin-dependent semaphorin3A signaling," *EMBO Journal*, vol. 23, no. 1, pp. 9–22, 2004.

[30] Y. Fukata, T. J. Itoh, T. Kimura et al., "CRMP-2 binds to tubulin heterodimers to promote microtubule assembly," *Nature Cell Biology*, vol. 4, no. 8, pp. 583–591, 2002.

[31] L. Brautigam, L. D. Schutte, J. R. Godoy et al., "Vertebrate-specific glutaredoxin is essential for brain development," *Proceedings of the National Academy of Sciences of the United States of America*, vol. 108, no. 51, pp. 20532–20537, 2011.

[32] H. Zhang, E. Kang, Y. Wang et al., "Brain-specific *Crmp2* deletion leads to neuronal development deficits and behavioural impairments in mice," *Nature Communications*, vol. 7, 2016.

[33] J. A. Sakai and M. C. Halloran, "Semaphorin 3d guides laterality of retinal ganglion cell projections in zebrafish," *Development*, vol. 133, no. 6, pp. 1035–1044, 2006.

[34] Y. Gu and Y. Ihara, "Evidence that collapsin response mediator protein-2 is involved in the dynamics of microtubules," *Journal of Biological Chemistry*, vol. 275, no. 24, pp. 17917–17920, 2000.

[35] M. Tan, C. Cha, Y. Ye et al., "CRMP4 and CRMP2 interact to coordinate cytoskeleton dynamics, regulating growth cone development and axon elongation," *Neural Plasticity*, vol. 2015, Article ID 947423, 13 pages, 2015.

[36] T. Byk, S. Ozon, and A. Sobel, "The Ulip family phosphoproteins—common and specific properties," *European Journal of Biochemistry*, vol. 254, no. 1, pp. 14–24, 1998.

[37] N. Arimura, N. Inagaki, K. Chihara et al., "Phosphorylation of collapsin response mediator protein-2 by rho-kinase: evidence for two separate signaling pathways for growth cone collapse," *Journal of Biological Chemistry*, vol. 275, no. 31, pp. 23973–23980, 2000.

[38] Y. Z. Alabed, M. Pool, S. O. Tone, and A. E. Fournier, "Identification of CRMP4 as a convergent regulator of axon outgrowth inhibition," *Journal of Neuroscience*, vol. 27, no. 7, pp. 1702–1711, 2007.

[39] V. Rosslenbroich, L. Dai, S. Franken et al., "Subcellular localization of collapsin response mediator proteins to lipid rafts," *Biochemical and Biophysical Research Communications*, vol. 305, no. 2, pp. 392–399, 2003.

[40] J. Yuasa-Kawada, R. Suzuki, F. Kano, T. Ohkawara, M. Murata, and M. Noda, "Axonal morphogenesis controlled by antagonistic roles of two CRMP subtypes in microtubule organization," *European Journal of Neuroscience*, vol. 17, no. 11, pp. 2329–2343, 2003.

[41] C. C. Quinn, E. Chen, T. G. Kinjo et al., "TUC-4b, a novel TUC family variant, regulates neurite outgrowth and associates with vesicles in the growth cone," *The Journal of Neuroscience*, vol. 23, no. 7, pp. 2815–2823, 2003.

[42] M. Balastik, X. Z. Zhou, M. Alberich-Jorda et al., "Prolyl isomerase Pin1 regulates axon guidance by stabilizing CRMP2A selectively in distal axons," *Cell Reports*, vol. 13, no. 4, pp. 812–828, 2015.

3

Cortical AAV-CNTF Gene Therapy Combined with Intraspinal Mesenchymal Precursor Cell Transplantation Promotes Functional and Morphological Outcomes after Spinal Cord Injury in Adult Rats

Stuart I. Hodgetts [1,2] Jun Han Yoon,[1] Alysia Fogliani,[1] Emmanuel A. Akinpelu,[1] Danii Baron-Heeris,[1] Imke G. J. Houwers,[1] Lachlan P. G. Wheeler,[1] Bernadette T. Majda,[3] Sreya Santhakumar,[1,2] Sarah J. Lovett,[1] Emma Duce,[1] Margaret A. Pollett,[1] Tylie M. Wiseman,[1] Brooke Fehily,[1] and Alan R. Harvey [1,2]

[1] *School of Human Sciences, The University of Western Australia (UWA), Perth, WA 6009, Australia*
[2] *Perron Institute for Neurological and Translational Science, Nedlands, WA 6009, Australia*
[3] *University of Notre Dame Australia, Fremantle, WA 6959, Australia*

Correspondence should be addressed to Stuart I. Hodgetts; stuart.hodgetts@uwa.edu.au

Academic Editor: Michele Fornaro

Ciliary neurotrophic factor (CNTF) promotes survival and enhances long-distance regeneration of injured axons in parts of the adult CNS. Here we tested whether CNTF gene therapy targeting corticospinal neurons (CSN) in motor-related regions of the cerebral cortex promotes plasticity and regrowth of axons projecting into the female adult F344 rat spinal cord after moderate thoracic (T10) contusion injury (SCI). Cortical neurons were transduced with a bicistronic adeno-associated viral vector (AAV1) expressing a secretory form of CNTF coupled to mCHERRY (AAV-CNTF^{mCherry}) or with control AAV only (AAV-GFP) two weeks prior to SCI. In some animals, viable or nonviable F344 rat mesenchymal precursor cells (rMPCs) were injected into the lesion site two weeks after SCI to modulate the inhibitory environment. Treatment with AAV-CNTF^{mCherry}, as well as with AAV-CNTF^{mCherry} combined with rMPCs, yielded functional improvements over AAV-GFP alone, as assessed by open-field and Ladderwalk analyses. Cyst size was significantly reduced in the AAV-CNTF^{mCherry} plus viable rMPC treatment group. Cortical injections of biotinylated dextran amine (BDA) revealed more BDA-stained axons rostral and alongside cysts in the AAV-CNTF^{mCherry} versus AAV-GFP groups. After AAV-CNTF^{mCherry} treatments, many sprouting mCherry-immunopositive axons were seen rostral to the SCI, and axons were also occasionally found caudal to the injury site. These data suggest that CNTF has the potential to enhance corticospinal repair by transducing parent CNS populations.

1. Introduction

Most spinal cord injury (SCI) results from contusion rather than transection injuries, and cervical injuries (~60–70% of all SCI) produce greater deficits and threaten more critical survival systems than thoracic/lumbar SCI. The corticospinal tract (CST) is important in the control of voluntary skilled movements, especially of distal limbs. Human CST projections are not completely homologous to the descending CST in rodents (which in these species projects mainly to the forelimbs and is mainly located in the dorsal rather than lateral columns) [1], nonetheless, because of the importance of CST projections in fine manipulatory motor control, this pathway has been a focus of many experimental repair strategies aimed at restoring function following SCI. Most studies in rodents have attempted this by the delivery of purified neurotrophic growth factors and/or by cell transplantation using donor cells engineered to overexpress the growth factors, the factors usually applied to the injury site itself (see [2]). In such studies, functional improvements usually reflect sprouting and some plasticity in collateral and/or intraspinal pathways ([3, 4], c.f. [5]), rather than axonal regeneration per se.

Our gene therapy approach targets corticospinal neurons (CSN) and is aimed at enhancing axonal plasticity and inducing regeneration of CST axons, leading to behavioural improvements after SCI. Gene therapy involves the transduction of neurons in the sensorimotor cortex using a bicistronic adeno-associated viral vector (AAV) that encodes and expresses a secretory form of ciliary neurotrophic factor (CNTF) coupled to mCHERRY (AAV-CNTF^{mCherry}). Injection of AAV-CNTF^{mCherry} into the cortical regions of the brain that project onto the output pathways of the CST allows expression of CNTF in neurons, including CSN, at the time of SCI.

CNTF has been selected because it is known to promote the survival of injured CSN [6], and in other systems it promotes long-distance regeneration of injured adult CNS axons [7–10], with at least some functional outcomes [11]. CNTF is a neuropoietic member of the interleukin 6 (IL-6) cytokine family, expressed primarily in glial cells of the nervous system [12–15]. Survival effects of CNTF have been demonstrated on motor, retinal ganglion, cortical and hippocampal, red nucleus, and striatal and thalamic neuron populations [14–16] (see also [17]). CNTF has demonstrated efficacy in limiting neuronal injury in several experimental disease and injury paradigms, and has been clinically evaluated as a treatment for motor neuron-specific amyotrophic lateral sclerosis (ALS) [18, 19]. CNTF protects corticospinal neurons in the sensorimotor cortex after intracortical axotomy [6], and these neurons, at least in murine neonates, are known to express CNTF receptor α [20]. Functional improvement and enhanced remyelination has also been reported after intraspinal transplantation of oligodendrocyte precursor cells expressing CNTF [21]. However, as we have argued [2], while most SCI studies have targeted the injured cord itself for therapy, in other systems—such as the visual system—targeting the injured neurons themselves yields excellent functional outcomes [11, 22]. Most importantly there is now clear evidence in human postmortem material that there is long-term survival of CSN after SCI [23], making strategies that target these neurons of genuine clinical relevance, potentially in both acute and chronic circumstances.

In an initial study, we obtained preliminary evidence that AAV2.1-CNTF^{mCherry} transduced large numbers of neurons in the sensorimotor cortex containing CSNs projecting into the spinal cord, and after moderate thoracic T10 contusion SCI there was clear and consistent sprouting of mCherry-labelled CST axons at, and rostral to, the lesion site [2]. In the present report, cortical gene therapy has been also combined with the transplantation of mesenchymal precursor cells (MPCs) into the injured thoracic cord, a method shown by us and others consistently to limit tissue loss and promote morphological sparing as well as functional improvement following SCI [24, 25]. The rationale is that a healthier local environment at the cell-transplant injury site provides a better terrain for plasticity and regeneration of CST axons after targeted CNTF expression in the motor cortex. MPC

treatment may be especially needed for contusion injuries which tend to be more unstable and prone to cyst formation—this is vital when treating cervical injuries in humans due to ongoing cavity formation (syringomyelia) and consequent progressive, sometimes catastrophic, loss of function [26].

2. Materials and Methods

2.1. Animals and Experimental Design. Adult female Fischer (F344) rats (age 10–12 wk, 120–150 g; Animal Resource Centre, Western Australia) were used in experimental procedures conforming to National Health and Medical Research Council Guidelines (Australia) and approved by the University of Western Australia Animal Ethics Committee. A total of 43 rats was used, distributed between 4 experimental SCI groups as follows; SCI + control AAV-GFP ($n = 11$), SCI + AAV-CNTF^{mCherry} ($n = 16$), SCI + AAV-CNTF^{mCherry} + nonviable rMPCs ($n = 6$), and SCI + AAV-CNTF^{mCherry} + viable rMPCs ($n = 11$). Previous experiments conducted in our lab used SCI + either nonviable or viable rMPC cell transplantation only [24, 25], and to satisfy NHMRC guidelines to address animal welfare and minimise animal use, these groups were not repeated for the present study. Viral AAV transduction was performed 2 weeks prior to SCI, and 2 weeks prior to experimental endpoint, biotinylated dextran amine BDA conjugated to horseradish peroxidase (Thermo Fisher Scientific) was spaced and injected in virtually identical positions as the earlier AAV injections in order to cover the same hindlimb projection fields in the sensorimotor cortex. Endpoint was reached and animals culled at day 56 after SCI.

2.1.1. Viral Vectors. The bicistronic adeno-associated viral vector (AAV) encoding and expressing a secretory form of CNTF coupled to mCHERRY (AAV-CNTF^{mCherry}) or vector-alone control linked to green fluorescent protein (AAV-GFP) were made by Vector Biolabs, USA. AAV vectors consisted of an AAV2 DNA backbone in an AAV1 capsid. This particular serotype has been shown to provide excellent transduction of cortical neurons [27–29]. Transgene expression was driven by a shortened CAG2 promoter based on the typical cytomegalovirus/chicken beta-actin (CAG) promoter. For bicistronic vectors, the transgene (CNTF) and reporter (mCherry) were linked by a 2A viral peptide sequence, which causes a "translational skip" and results in a 1 : 1 expression of transgene and reporter proteins. The CNTF transgene is a mouse CNTF gene preceded by the secretory signal sequence from mouse pre-pro-NGF, to allow for local secretion of CNTF [30] (a gift from Prof. M. Sendtner, University of Wurzburg, Germany).

2.1.2. Viral Transduction of Hindlimb Sensorimotor Cortex. AAV-CNTF^{mCherry} or AAV-GFP transduction of CSN in the cortical regions that project axons to the level of the spinal cord that controls the hindlimbs [2, 31] was performed 2 weeks prior to SCI via $4 \times 0.5\,\mu l$ injections of the respective virus (~4×10^{13} genomic copies/ml) using a nanojet device and a digital stereotaxic frame (Kopf) for accurate Bregma/

Lambda coordinate positioning. Injection of AAV 2 weeks prior to SCI allowed time for onset of transgene expression and production of CNTF.

2.2. Spinal Cord Injury (SCI). Rats were anesthetized with 1.5% (v/v) halothane (Rhone-Poulenc Chemicals Pty. Ltd., Australia) combined with nitrous oxide (60%) and oxygen (38.5%). Amacin ophthalmic eye ointment was applied before rats were placed on a heating pad (37°C). Partial laminectomy at vertebral level T9-T10 exposed the SC underneath without disrupting the dura [24, 25]. Using an Infinite Horizon impactor device, a 200 kDyne contusion injury was induced at the exposed spinal cord. Postsurgery care, analgesics, food, and housing were as previously described [24, 25]. Briefly, rats were treated with Benacillin (0.02 ml/100 g body wt., 300 U/ml, i.m.) and painkiller Buprenorphine (Temgesic, 0.01 ml/100 g, 300 U/ml, ip) for 5 days.

2.3. Donor rMPCs and Transplantation. Commercially available rMPCs isolated from Fischer F344 rats (Cyagen Biosciences Inc., number RAFMX-01201) were routinely maintained in Mesenchymal Stem Cell Growth Medium (number GUXMX-90011) prior to use in transplantation experiments, or for those used for routine phenotypic characterization and differentiation [24, 25] maintained for at least 24–48 hr, in order to determine any neuronal phenotype/ marker expression using the panel of antibodies described in Section 2.7.2. For transplantation experiments, MPCs (no higher than passage number 5) were washed and resuspended in PBS. Nonviable MPCs were prepared by multiple (×3) freeze/thawing steps between −80°C and 37°C and confirming loss of viability using trypan blue staining under microscopy. At day 14 after SCI, 6×10^5 cells in a total of $4 \mu l$ were injected in a single injection directly into the lesion site (rostrocaudally at 1 mm depth) through a finely drawn (80 μm tip) glass pipette connected to a 10 μl Hamilton syringe and driven by a Harvard Pump at 0.5 μl/min (total duration is 8 min). The pipette was left in place to prevent cell leakage for 1 min before withdrawal [24, 25].

2.4. BDA Injection into Sensorimotor Cortex that Projects to Low Thoracic/Lumbar Spinal Cord. Injections of biotinylated dextran amine were spaced in virtually identical positions as the earlier AAV-CNTF^{mCherry} or AAV-GFP transduction injections in order to cover the same hindlimb projection fields in the sensorimotor cortex. For each of the 4 injections, 0.5–1 μl of 10% (w/v) BDA were injected using a nanojet device (World Precision Instruments) at a depth of 1 mm. The location of these injections is based on studies showing the location of CMN that project to the hindlimbs and forelimbs in Fischer rats [2] and confirmed by the examination of the label in appropriate thalamic motor nuclei. In some rats, gelfoam soaked in the BDA solution was placed over the exposed cortex prior to the closure of the craniotomy.

2.5. Functional Behaviour. A variety of behavioural tests for injured rats were used to give a valid indication of functional recovery [24, 25, 32–35] including (i) "open-field" locomotion test (BBB scoring method [36] to assess spontaneous movements), (ii) ladder walking [37] to assess general hindlimb recovery, and (iii) our own novel computerized quantitative gait analysis method (Ratwalk® [38]) which allows objective analyses of a large number of locomotion parameters, such as interlimb coordination (step sequence), stride length, step length, and base of support (stance width) [38]. All functional (locomotor) behaviour was assessed weekly for up to day 56 after SCI. BBB scoring was analysed using at least 3 blinded raters both at the time of assessment and later *in silica* via slow motion/frame-by-frame replay of high definition (1080 p) digital recordings taken during the test. The BBB rating score is composed of 22 nonlinear operational definitions (0–21 scale) studying several aspects involved in the locomotion of quadrupedal animals such as weight support, plantar stepping, and forelimb/hindlimb coordination. Ladderwalk and Ratwalk assays were performed on animals once they had reached weight support on their hindlimbs, and involved comparison of preinjury performance with weekly assessments from day 14 post-SCI until day 56 (endpoint). Digital recordings of animals traversing 3 lengths per time point of Ladderwalk and Ratwalk (preinjury and weekly up to day 56 post-SCI) were also similarly assessed by at least 2 blinded raters *in silica* via slow motion/frame-by-frame replay of digital recordings taken during the tests for preinjury and up to day 56 post-SCI. Ladderwalk scores are an average of missteps over a 1 m horizontal ladder with unevenly spaced bars. Ratwalk data analysis involves frame by frame designation from digital recordings of left and right fore- and hindlimb placement on a 1 m glass platform in the Ratwalk apparatus in low light, using an average of 3 "runs" per time point [38].

2.6. Perfusion and Tissue Processing. At day 56 (2 weeks after the BDA cortex injections), rats were euthanized by lethal injection of sodium pentobarbitone (50 mg/100 g) and transcardially perfused in 0.9 M with 100 ml of heparinized Dulbecco's PBS followed by 4% (w/v) paraformaldehyde in PBS pH 7.4. The head and vertebral column were dissected from each animal and postfixed for 24 hours. The brain and spinal cord were extracted from the skull and vertebra and then stored intact in 0.1 M PBS (pH 7.4). The position of the injury in the SC was measured from the caudal edge of the cerebellum to confirm that all animals were lesioned at the same level. A 2 cm segment was cut from the SC, with the lesion at the midpoint of this segment, and embedded in 1% (w/v) gelatin (Sigma-Aldrich). Using a CO_2-freezing microtome (Polycut, Reichert-Jung, Australia), proximal and distal SC close to the grafts (1 cm) was cut sagitally in 40 μm frozen sections, while the brain and brainstem were cut transversely in 50 μm frozen sections. A consecutive series of sections were transferred to 24-well plates containing 0.1 M PB with 0.01% (w/v) sodium azide (Sigma-Aldrich) and stored at 4°C until processed for immunohistochemistry.

2.7. Tissue Analysis

2.7.1. Axonal Transduction and Anterograde Tracing. Frozen coronal brain sections were examined for preinjury AAV-CNTF^{mCherry} or AAV-GFP transduction in the cortex and

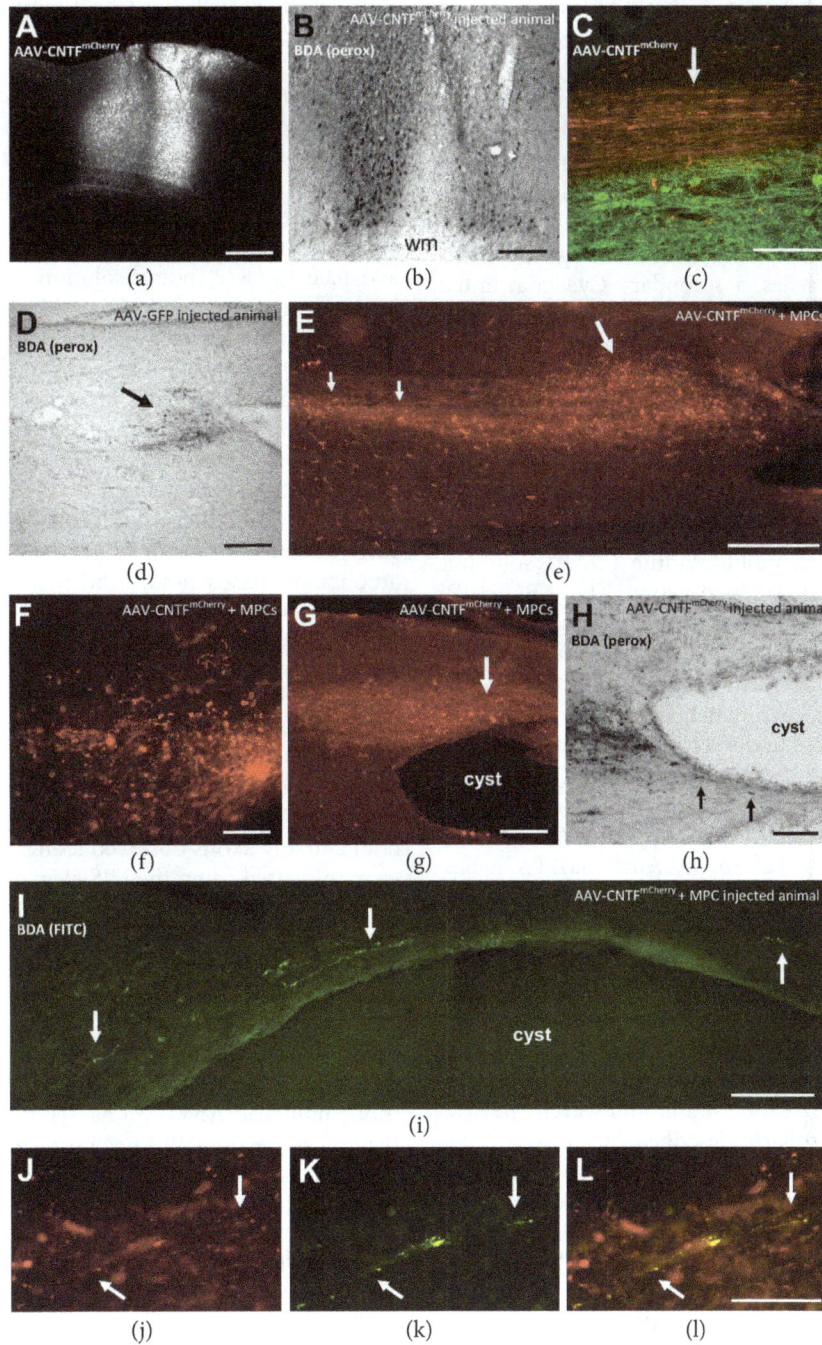

FIGURE 1: (a) Two AAV-CNTF^{mCherry} injections in the cerebral cortex. (b) BDA injections into the cortex revealed using immunoperoxidase; note the many labelled neurons in deeper layers. This animal had previously received cortical injections of AAV-CNTF^{mCherry}. (c–l) Longitudinal sections of the spinal cord—in all cases rostral is to the left of the picture. (c) Section immunostained for mCherry (red) and β-III tubulin (green) showing anterogradely labelled mCherry-positive axons (arrow) in the dorsal corticospinal tract far rostral to the lesion site. (d) Control AAV-GFP-injected rat (no MPCs injected); a small number of immunoperoxidase BDA-labelled axons and debris are visible just in front of a rostral cyst (arrow), with no axons extending beyond the injury. (e–g) Large numbers of mCherry-positive axons rostral (e, f) and running dorsally over and beyond the cyst (g); these rats received AAV-CNTF^{mCherry} cortical injections plus an intraspinal injection of viable rat mesenchymal precursor cells (rMPCs). Note in (e) the profusion of mCherry-positive profiles (large arrow) approximately 1 mm rostral to the lesion cavity, growing into regions dorsal to the corticospinal tract (small arrows). There appears to be considerable sprouting of axons in this zone (f). (h) Immunoperoxidase BDA-labelled axons and debris rostral to a cyst in a rat injected with AAV-CNTF^{mCherry}. Several axons can be seen running caudally, ventral to the cyst (arrows). (i) BDA-labelled cortical axons (arrows) visualized using a fluorescent secondary antibody (green), running over a cystic cavity. This animal also received AAV-CNTF^{mCherry} and viable MPC injections. (j–l) Cortical axons (arrows) double labelled (l) with both mCherry ((j), red) and BDA ((k), green); note, some axons are only mCherry or BDA immunoreactive. Scale bars: (a, e), 500 μm; (b, h, and i), 200 μm; (c, d, g, and j–l), 100 μm; and (f) 50 μm.

thalamus using immunofluorescence, in addition to post-SCI anterograde BDA labelling using both immunofluorescence and immunostaining with horseradish peroxidase (HRP). At the lesion site, longitudinal SC sections were similarly examined for axonal sprouting and regrowth (BDA). After blocking for 30 min in PBS containing 10% (v/v) normal goat serum and 0.02% (v/v) Triton X-100, AAV-transduced axons were immunolabelled overnight at 4°C using antibodies to mCherry (Living Colours, 1/600 in PBS). After washes, a secondary Cy3 goat anti-mouse antibody (Jackson ImmunoResearch 115613, 1/500 dilution in PBS) was applied for 30 min at room temperature, before unbound antibody was washed away and sections coverslipped. In most cases, BDA was visualized using commercial VECTASTAIN avidin-biotin (Vector Laboratories, USA, number PK-4000) kits (as per manufacturer's instructions) and horseradish peroxidase (HRP) histochemistry. Briefly, avidin-biotinylated (ABC)/HRP, followed by 3,3'-diaminobenzidine (DAB) solution was used to visualize BDA-stained axons. The ABC/HRP reagents were prepared 30 minutes before application to the sections. The sections were incubated with ABC reagents for 1.5 hours at room temperature and washed with PBS. A DAB solution (10% (v/v) DAB metal concentrate in peroxidase buffer) was then added to the sections and incubated for 5–15 minutes on a shaker. Sections were washed with PBS, allowed to air dry overnight and then counterstained with 1% (w/v) toluidine blue and coverslipped with DEPEX mounting medium (Fronine Lab Supply, Australia). To enable identification of both mCherry and BDA-labelled axons in the same longitudinal tissue sections, BDA was occasionally visualized using FITC-conjugated anti-streptavidin secondary antibodies (Thermo Fisher Scientific). In AAV-GFP-injected rats, brain and spinal cord sections were immunostained with an antibody to GFP (rabbit 1/500, Millipore, in PBS) followed by goat anti-rabbit IgG FITC-conjugated secondary antibodies (Jackson ImmunoResearch 89751, diluted 1/100 in PBS) similarly described as above.

In mCherry-, GFP-, and BDA-stained sections, the accumulation of debris and branching of CST axons were commonly seen rostral to the SCI and associated cysts. Axon sprouting was especially evident in AAV-CNTF-injected animals. In a series of sagittal sections, the rostral extent of this region was measured from the beginning of the injury site in 38 rats ($n = 6$ for AAV-GFP; $n = 15$ for AAV-CNTF^{mCherry}; $n = 6$ for AAV-CNTF^{mCherry} + nonviable rMPCs; and $n = 11$ for AAV-CNTF^{mCherry} + viable rMPCs).

2.7.2. Immunohistochemical Analyses of Glial and Neuronal Phenotypes. Brain and spinal cord tissue sections were blocked in 10% (v/v) fetal calf serum (Gibco, BRL) and 0.2% (v/v) Triton X-100 in PBS for 10 minutes at room temperature and washed in PBS. Primary antibodies (diluted at 1/500 in PBS unless otherwise stated) to confirm the expression of phenotypic markers for glial cells, GFAP in spinal cord (Millipore, AB3080), and axon populations using antibodies to β-III tubulin (Covance, PRB-435) in the brain and spinal cord were used. Detection using FITC- or Cy3-conjugated secondary goat anti-mouse or goat anti-rabbit

antibodies (diluted at 1/400 in PBS, Jackson ImmunoResearch, 115613, 89751) as described previously [24, 25].

2.7.3. Quantitative Analysis of Tissue Sparing in the Spinal Cord. At least two independent raters (blinded) also measured cyst sizes to remove bias. Tissue sparing was assessed by measuring cyst size and the amount of intact versus degenerating tissue [24, 25]. Briefly, assessment of spinal tissue sparing was carried out using 0.05% (w/v) toluidine and 0.005% (w/v) borax solution followed by dehydration in sequentially graded ethanol (v/v) of 70%, 90%, and 100%. Staining on every sixth sagittal section was used to determine the volume of spared spinal tissue. In each section, the total number of pixels in a 2.5 mm-long SC segment was determined, with the lesion epicenter in the middle, as well as the area of damaged spinal tissue around it. The border of the damaged tissue was defined by the absence of healthy cells and an obvious discontinuity in density. Measurements of each section were summed per rat and averaged to give the amount of spared tissue, and percentage was calculated as the difference between the area of damaged tissue versus the whole segment (field of view) [24, 25].

2.7.4. Microscopy. A Nikon Eclipse E800 microscope was used to visualise immunofluorescence staining as well as confirm successful BDA injection into the brain and to visualize BDA-stained axons at the SCI site. The distances between the front edge of the most rostral cyst (if there was more than one) and any axons observed alongside or caudal to the cyst were measured using the NIS elements BR 4.5 software.

2.7.5. Statistics. Using GraphPad Prism v4.03, SBSS (version 21.0) and InStat v3.06 for Windows (GraphPad Software, San Diego, USA), 1- and 2-way repeated measures using either one- or two-way analysis of variance (ANOVA) plus Tukey's post hoc analysis as required were performed, except for BBB scoring which uses Kruskal-Wallis analysis (nonparametric ANOVA) as described previously [24, 25]. In addition, Mann–Whitney post hoc testing was performed.

3. Results

3.1. Preinjury AAV Gene Therapy and Postinjury BDA Injection into the Cortex. Both GFP and mCherry expression in transduced axons following AAV-GFP control and b*icis*tronic AAV-CNTF^{mCherry} injections into the cortex prior to SCI were confirmed at day 56 post-SCI using immunofluorescence microscopy on relevant brain sections (Figure 1(a)). Note that the mCherry expression in neurons was confirmed through all the layers of cortex, including layer V containing CSN; this robust, post-2A linker expression is indicative of widespread transduction and expression of the secretable form of CNTF. BDA injection sites in the cortex were also visualized with ABC/HRP and DAB reaction (see Figure 1(b)) or immunofluorescence at day 56. BDA staining reached layer V of the cortex indicating the successful labelling of CSN and, as for mCherry expression, the label in the ventrolateral nucleus of the thalamus confirmed injection into appropriate sensorimotor cortical regions. The appearance of BDA in the same tracts in the cortex as transduced AAV-GFP control and AAV-CNTF^{mCherry} confirms that we were able to successfully label similar areas of axonal projection from the cortex that would facilitate identification within the CST regions of the spinal cord.

3.2. AAV-Transduced and BDA-Labelled Projections in the Spinal Cord.

In all treatment groups, AAV-transduced, immunostained axons and BDA-immunolabelled axons were seen in the contralateral CST rostral to the injury site. An example is shown in Figure 1(c) with AAV-CNTF^{mCherry}-labelled axons (red) in the CST adjacent to βIII tubulin-positive fibers and neurons (green). While nearly all CST fibers were well aligned in the ventral dorsal column in segments far rostral to the SCI site (Figure 1(c)), immediately in front of the injury these axons became disorganized and more broadly distributed. In this region, in addition to degenerate axon profiles and other debris, apparently intact CST axons possessed complex, irregular profiles strongly suggestive of local sprouting and regenerative responses. In AAV-GFP control rats, there were small numbers of these axons immediately rostral to the first lesion cavity; however, in this group GFP-positive or BDA-labelled CST axons were *never* seen caudal to the injury/cyst. Furthermore, compared to animals injected with AAV-CNTF^{mCherry} (Figures 1(e)–1(g)), there was greater axon dieback as well as relatively little sprouting. The best example is shown in Figure 1(f) (BDA label). By comparison, in rats with AAV-CNTF^{mCherry} cortical injections, there was consistently a much higher density of CST axons 400–1000 μm rostral to the first spinal cord cavity, as revealed in both mCherry- (Figures 1(e)–1(g)) and BDA- (Figure 1(h)) immunostained material.

In a series of mCherry- or BDA-immunostained sagittal sections, the rostral extent of the zone containing scattered, often branched, CST axons was measured from the beginning of the injury site (taken as the rostral edge of the first lesion cavity) in 38 rats. These "expanded" zones of CST label (Figures 1(e)–1(h)) were seen in 3/6 AAV-GFP-injected rats, 9/15 AAV-CNTF^{mCherry} rats, 4/6 rats with AAV-CNTF^{mCherry}+nonviable rMPCs, and 8/11 rats with AAV-CNTF^{mCherry}+viable rMPCs. The mean rostral extent of this zone was $323 \pm 125 \mu$m (S.D.), $483 \pm 226 \mu$m, $475 \pm 330 \mu$m, and $638 \pm 370 \mu$m for the four groups, respectively. There was considerable interanimal variability as shown by the large standard deviations, nonetheless the trend for increased density and greater areal extent of rostral CST sprouting in AAV-CNTF-injected animals is evident.

After AAV-CNTF but not AAV-GFP cortical injections, many labelled CST axons were located beyond the rostral edge of the cyst (Figure 1(g)). Growth of BDA-positive axons beyond the cyst was also seen (arrows, Figure 1(h)). Long-distance growth of axons was also occasionally seen as shown in Figure 1(j); again, note the irregular nature of the postinjury BDA^{FITC}-labelled axonal profiles. This animal also received a viable MHC graft. In sections immunostained for both mCherry (red) and BDA (FITC—green), we observed occasional axons that were both AAV-CNTF^{mCherry}- and anti-BDA^{FITC}-positive (arrows, Figures 1(j)–1(l)). In the example shown, the axons were located ventral to a cyst. The double labelling indicates that at last some of the

mCherry and BDA cortical injections were successfully made in overlapping regions of cortex, resulting in the dual label of the projecting layer V pyramidal neurons.

Figure 2 shows representative longitudinal spinal cord sections from three animals treated either with AAV-CNTF^{mCherry} alone (Figures 2(A)–2(H)) or AAV-CNTF^{mCherry}+viable rMPC transplantation (Figures 2(I), and 2(J)). Low power images show the size and location of cysts in two of these animals (Figures 2(A) and 2(F), resp.). The arrows in Figures 2(A) and 2(F) point to the approximate postcyst location of the mCherry-positive axons shown in Figures 2(D), 2(E), and 2(I). In the rat shown in Figures 2(A)–2(E), there were large numbers of mCherry-positive fibers dorsal to the first large cyst in regions of spared tissue midway within the lesion site (arrow, Figure 2(B), shown in higher power in Figure 2(C)). More importantly, we also observed AAV-CNTF^{mCherry}-positive fibers in the spinal cord distal to the lesion (Figures 2(D) and 2(E)). These fibers were nonlinear in orientation and, although infrequent, they were located up to 3-4 mm beyond the rostral edge of the injury site. In the animal shown in Figures 2(F)–2(H), again there were many mCherry-immunopositive axons located just in front of, and dorsal to, the rostral cavity (Figure 2(G)), and many sprouting BDA-positive axons were also seen. However, in this animal, there were only a small number of mCherry-labelled axons located caudal to the injury site (arrows, Figure 2(H)). It is worth emphasizing in Figures 2(D), 2(E), and 2(I) that the irregular course and branching of these axons are strongly suggestive of regenerative growth. One other rat, this one treated with both AAV-CNTF^{mCherry} and viable rMPCs, possessed a number of mCherry-labelled axons distal to the contusion injury and to the most caudal lesion cavity (arrows, Figures 2(I) and 2(J)).

3.3. Functional Hindlimb Recovery Is Generally Enhanced after CNTF Gene Therapy

3.3.1. Ladderwalk.

The number of missteps over the Ladderwalk apparatus showed a gradual decline for all treatment groups from day 14 through to endpoint at day 56 after SCI (Figure 3). Animals treated with control AAV-GFP after SCI had the highest misstep counts across all time points, with the average decreasing gradually from 12 at day14, to 8 at day 56, respectively. Rats with SCI followed by AAV-CNTF^{mCherry} treatment consistently displayed a lower average number of missteps than control AAV-GFP treatment, decreasing gradually from ~9 at day14 to ~6 at day 56, respectively. The combined AAV-CNTF^{mCherry} treatment with either nonviable or viable rMPC transplantation at the lesion site markedly reduced the average numbers of missteps, ranging from 3 to 6 at day 14 after SCI, with both of these groups showing very similar average missteps of 3 from day 28 until day 56 after SCI. Two-way ANOVA showed statistically significant differences (pairwise comparisons) between all groups from day 14 until day 56 after SCI ($p = 0.002$, 0.003, 0.006, 0.001, 0.013, 0.002, and 0.032 at days 14, 21, 28, 35, 42, 49, and 56, resp.). Post hoc tests revealed statistically significant differences between the AAV-GFP-treated control

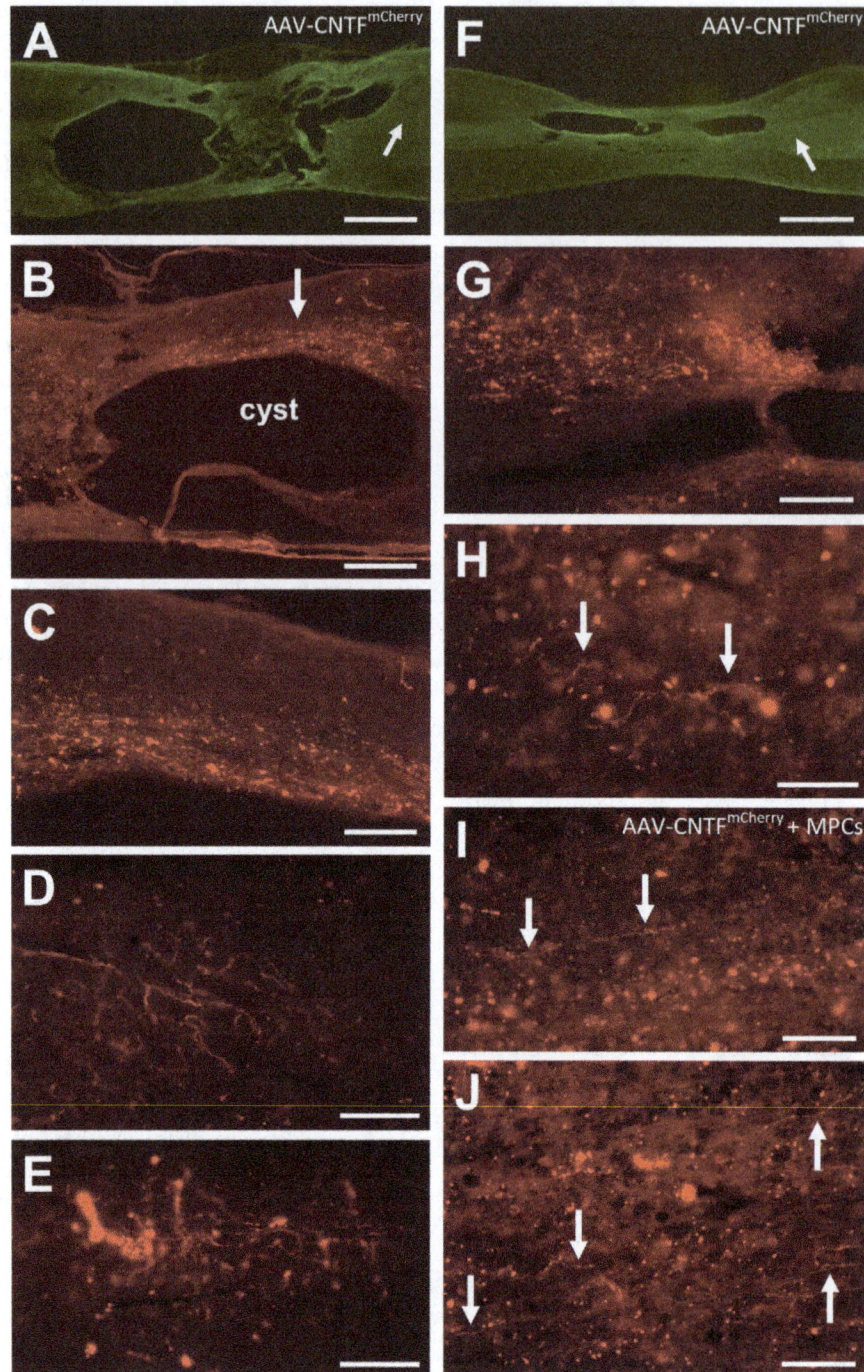

FIGURE 2: Two examples (A–E and F–H) of animals that received cortical AAV-CNTF^{mCherry} injections and with mCherry-positive corticospinal axons distal to spinal cysts (D, E, I and J), and therefore distal to the initial injury. In all images rostral is to the left. (A, F) Low power views of cysts (β-III tubulin-immunostained sections) in each rat; the arrows in (A) and (B) point to the approximate location of the axons shown in (D, E, and H), respectively. (B, C) Large numbers of mCherry-positive axons (arrow) dorsal to the large rostral cyst (see (A)), with small numbers of irregularly organized axons distal (D, E). (G) mCherry-labelled axons rostral and dorsal to the cyst, with several axons (arrows) located distal to the injury (H). In one animal injected with AAV-CNTF^{mCherry} and that received a spinal rMPC injection, numerous mCherry-positive axons (arrowed) were seen distal to the most caudal lesion cavity (I, J). Scale bars: (A, F), 1 mm; (B), 500 μm; (C, G), 200 μm; (D, E, I, and J), 100 μm; and (H) = 50 μm.

group and AAV-CNTF^{mCherry} + nonviable rMPCs at all time points as well as between the AAV-GFP-treated control group and AAV-CNTF^{mCherry} + viable rMPCs at all time points except day 14 and day 56 (Figure 3).

Because the two-way ANOVA with repeated measures described above showed a significant interaction ($p = 0.0001$), we then separated the factors and performed a one-way ANOVA on all AAV-CNTF^{mCherry}-treated animals

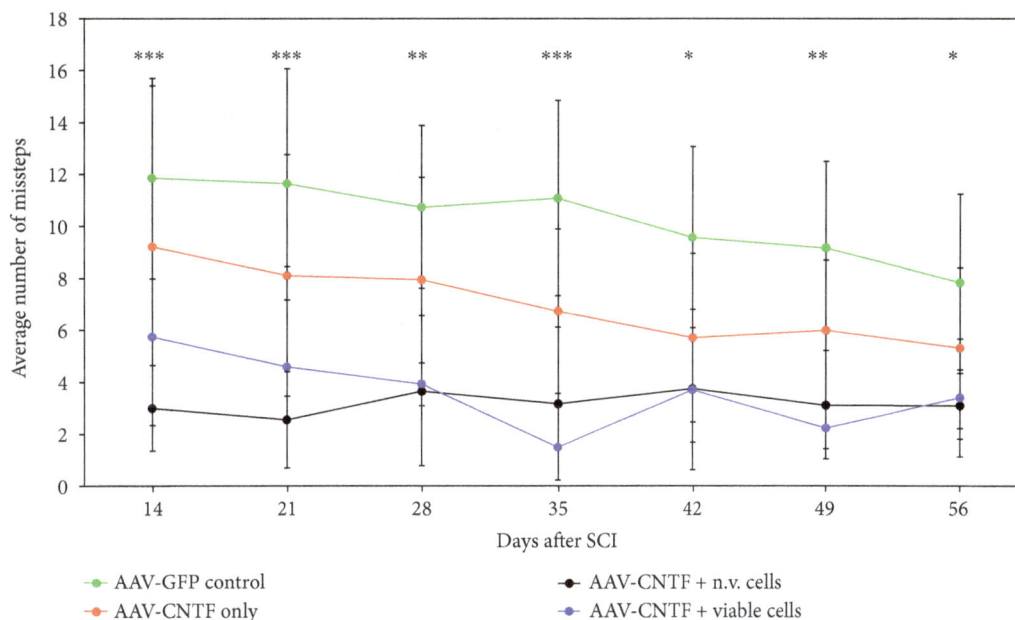

FIGURE 3: Functional hindlimb recovery promoted after AAV-CNTF gene therapy and cellular transplantation as assessed by Ladderwalk: reduced misstepping over the Ladderwalk apparatus indicates that AAV-CNTF^{mCherry} therapy (red, crosses) promoted significant functional improvement after SCI compared with control AAV-GFP treatment (green). Note that at day 14, the Ladderwalk testing was carried out prior to injection of either viable (blue) or nonviable (black) cells. Post hoc tests revealed statistically significant differences between the AAV-GFP-treated control group and AAV-CNTF^{mCherry} + nonviable rMPCs at all time points as well as between the AAV-GFP-treated control group and AAV-CNTF^{mCherry} + viable rMPCs at all time points except day 56 (*$p = 0.01 - 0.05$, **$p = 0.005 - 0.01$, and ***$p = 0.001 - 0.005$). Two-way repeated measures ANOVA was conducted using PRISM (time: $p = 0.0001$, treatment: $p = 0.0016$, and interaction: $p = 0.0001$). Standard deviation is shown.

at day 14 only. This one-way ANOVA revealed that there was no difference between the cell-type (no cell, viable, and nonviable rMPC) treatments for the AAV-CNTF^{mCherry}-treated cohort at day 14 ($p = 0.395$), to be expected given that the Ladderwalk tests were performed prior to rMPC transplantation at this time point. Note that the number of animals per group at day 14 was less than at later times because only those animals that supported their weight on their hindlimbs could be tested. Additionally, the one-way repeated measures ANOVA within the AAV-CNTF^{mCherry} animals revealed that while there was an overall effect of a reduction in missteps over time ($p = 0.001$), there was no difference between the cell-type treatment groups ($p = 0.143$). Interestingly however, in the AAV-CNTF^{mCherry}-injected rats only the AAV-CNTF^{mCherry} without rMPC group showed a significant reduction in missteps ($p = 0.05$, LSD test) across time with post hoc testing.

3.3.2. Open-Field Locomotion (BBB). BBB scores for hindlimb recovery (Figure 4) revealed significant differences between the AAV-GFP-treated control group (green) compared to the AAV-CNTF^{mCherry} (red, crosses), AAV-CNTF^{mCherry} + nonviable rMPC (black), and AAV-CNTF^{mCherry} + viable rMPC (blue) treatment groups, generally from day 21 onwards. All treatment groups followed a slow increase in average BBB scores (0-1 at day 0 following SCI) until around day 5–day 7 when average scores began to typically increase at a greater rate, with the AAV-GFP-treated control group

consistently showing the lowest average BBB scores of 5 from day 7 (which corresponds to a slight movement of two joints and an extensive movement of the third joint) until score 10 at day 56 after SCI (which corresponds to plantar stepping with occasional weight bearing and no forelimb-hindlimb coordination). AAV-CNTF^{mCherry} and AAV-CNTF^{mCherry} + nonviable rMPC groups' scores plateaued from day 21 after SCI with an average BBB score of 11 (which corresponds to plantar stepping with frequent to consistent weight bearing and NO forelimb-hindlimb coordination). Only the AAV-CNTF^{mCherry} and AAV-CNTF^{mCherry} + viable rMPC treatment group obtained higher scores from day 42 until day 56 after SCI, where average BBB scores plateaued at 12 (which corresponds to plantar stepping with frequent to consistent weight bearing and occasional forelimb-hindlimb coordination), suggesting that CNTF gene therapy alone and CNTF gene therapy + viable MPC transplantation into the lesion resulted in the best functional outcomes. Kruskal Wallis scores showed overall statistically significant differences between the AAV-GFP-treated control group and all other treatment groups at day 21 (**$p = 0.006$), day 28 (***$p = 0.0016$), and day 49 (*$p = 0.023$). Specific Mann–Whitney post hoc tests revealed statistically significant differences between the AAV-GFP-treated control group and AAV-CNTF^{mCherry} ($p = 0.001$ at day 21, $p = 0.004$ at day 28, and $p = 0.003$ at day 49), AAV-CNTF^{mCherry} + nonviable rMPCs ($p = 0.018$ at day 21, $p = 0.036$ at day 28, and $p = 0.113$ at day 49), and AAV-CNTF^{mCherry} + viable

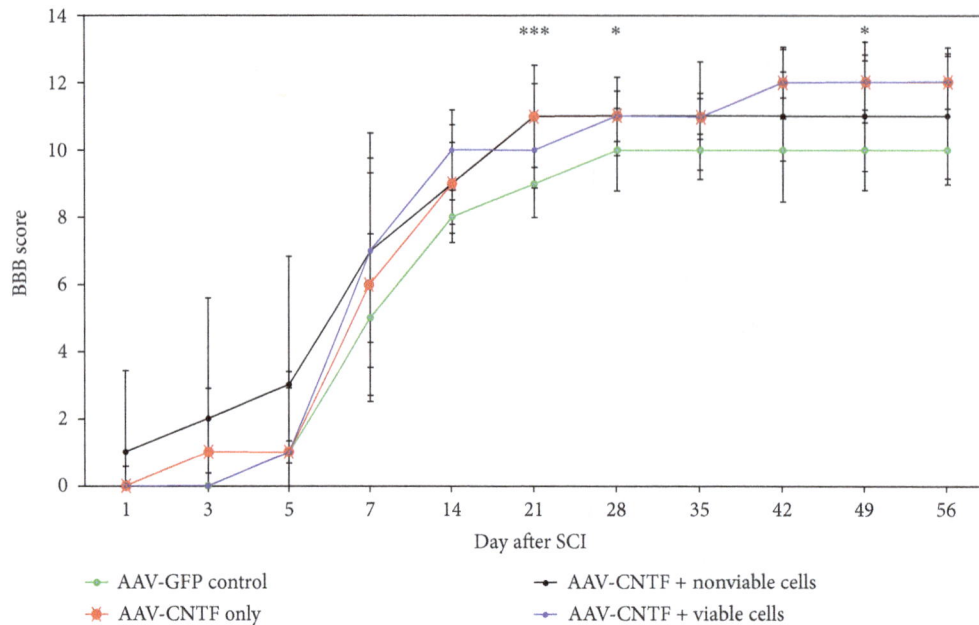

FIGURE 4: Functional hindlimb recovery promoted after AAV-CNTF gene therapy and cellular transplantation as assessed by open-field locomotion (BBB). Significant functional improvements were observed following AAV-CNTF^{mCherry} (red), AAV-CNTF^{mCherry} + nonviable rMPC (black), and AAV-CNTF^{mCherry} + viable rMPC (blue) treatment compared to AAV-GFP-treated control animals (green) generally from day 21 after SCI onwards, although statistically significant differences were not maintained at all time points ($^*p = 0.01 - 0.05$ and $^{***}p = 0.001 - 0.005$). Standard deviation is shown.

rMPCs ($p = 0.021$ at day 21, $p = 0.008$ at day 28, and $p = 0.059$ at day 49), respectively.

3.3.3. Ratwalk® Gait Analysis. Ratwalk analysis on animals showing hindlimb weight support are summarized in Figure 5, with averages of arbitrary unit values assigned by the software *in silica* for each treatment group compared to preinjury levels (dotted black lines) shown for stance width (5A), step length (5B), stride length (5C), and step sequence (5D) at day 56 after injury, by which time any differences in gait parameters should be apparent. Stance width is the average distance between each of the forelimbs (Rf/Lf), each of the hindlimbs (Rh/Lh), and each of the fore-to-hindlimb placements (Rf/Lh and Lf/Rh). There was no significant difference between any treatment group for any variable in stance width at day 56. Typically, hindlimb stance width increases slightly very early on after SCI (data not shown) and although the AAV-GFP-treated control group still showed a marginally increased average hindlimb stance width compared to all other treatment groups, there was no statistical difference between them or preinjury levels. A higher average stance width between opposing fore- and hindlimbs (Rf/Lh and Lf/Rh) was maintained at day 56 post-SCI for all treatment groups compared to preinjury levels and suggests that all animals assume a longer distance between each fore- and hindlimbs as a consequence of the injury irrespective of treatment. The stance width data suggesting these compensatory fore- and hindlimb changes in the treatment groups is confirmed by the day 56 post-SCI analyses for step length (Figure 5(b)) and stride length (Figure 5(c)), which again showed no statistically significant

differences between treatments. Step length analysis shows a higher average distance between Rf/Rh, Rf/Lh, Rh/Lf, and Lf/Lh across all groups compared to preinjury levels with no statistically significant differences between the groups (Figure 5(b)). Stride length also shows that generally forelimb strides are shorter and hindlimb strides are longer on average compared to preinjury levels (Figure 5(c)), consistent with the idea that compensatory movements to bring forelimbs closer and take shorter strides to help "pull" the animal forward correlates with longer hindlimb strides that adopt a wider stance (for more stability) and therefore longer distances. While the AAV-CNTF^{mCherry} + nonviable rMPC group of animals still showed slightly higher forelimb distances compared to preinjury levels, there were no statistically significant differences between treatments.

Step sequence analysis revealed that following SCI, there was generally a decrease in the amount of patterns of coordinated fore- and hindlimb placements designated as "cruciate," "alternate," and "rotary" using the Ratwalk software, as well as an increase in the amount of unrecognisable (non-coordinated) fore- and hindlimb placements designated as "none" (Figure 5(d)). There remained a significant decrease in the amount of cruciate patterns of sequence compared to preinjury levels, and despite some variation between treatment groups, there were no statistically significant differences between treatment groups for both alternate and rotary patterns of step sequence. The amount of uncoordinated patterns of step sequence ("none") was almost twice as high for all treatment groups at day 56 post-SCI, again with no statistically significant differences between treatment groups.

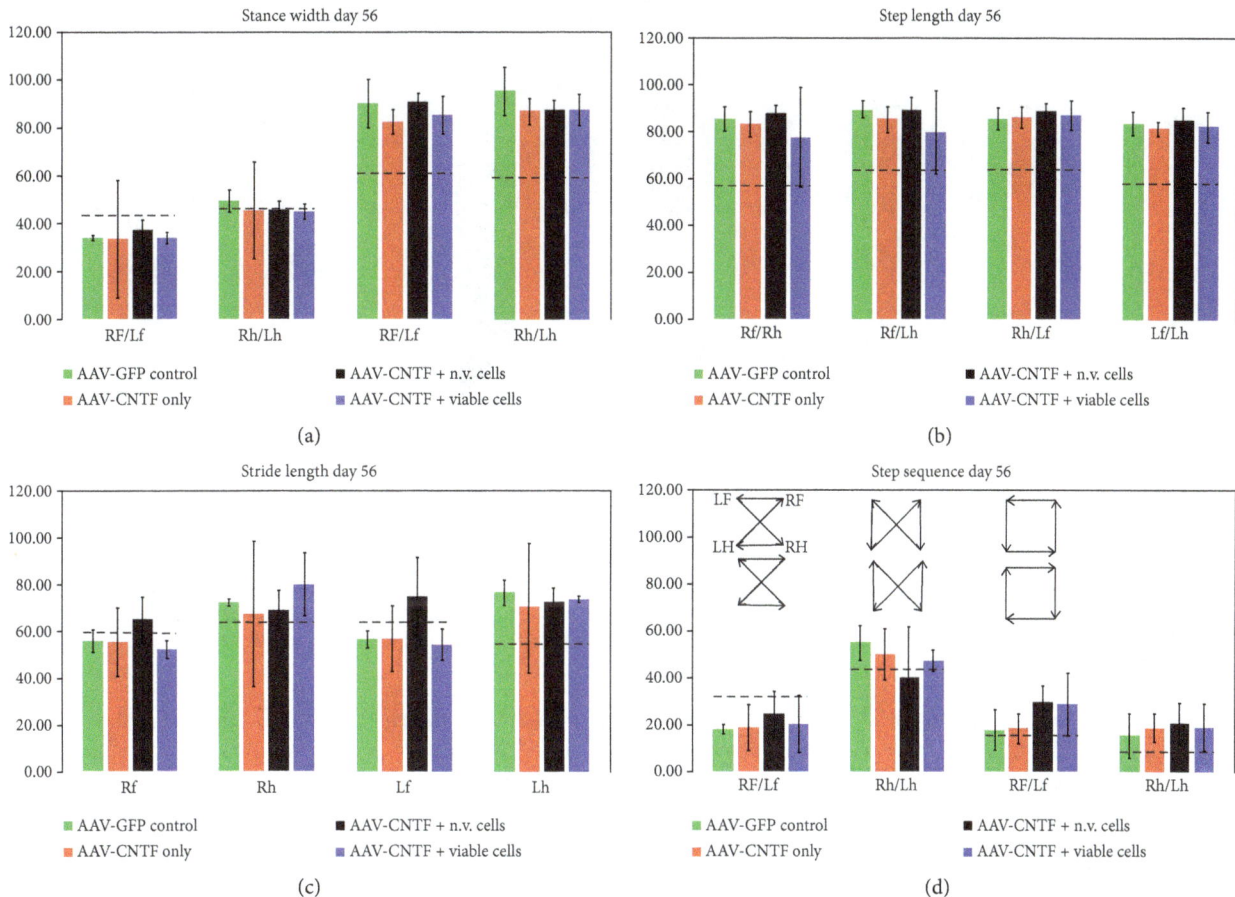

FIGURE 5: Ratwalk gait analysis at day 56 after SCI. Averages of arbitrary unit values of each treatment group compared to preinjury levels (dotted black lines) are shown for stance width (a), step length (b), stride length (c), and step sequence (d). Despite no statistically significant differences *between* any treatment group for any variable, compensatory changes such as a marked reduction in the stance width (a) of the forelimbs (Rf/Lf) between opposing fore- and hindlimbs (Rf/Lh and Lf/Rh) in all groups compared to preinjury levels were supported by data for step length (b) and stride length (c). A general decrease in the amount of patterns of coordinated fore- and hindlimb placement ("cruciate," "alternate," and "rotary" as indicated in (d)) and an increase in the amount of noncoordinated fore- and hindlimb placement ("none") was observed. Standard deviation is shown.

3.4. Transplantation of Viable rMPCs, but Not Cortical Gene Therapy, Promotes Tissue Sparing. Cysts developed at the injury site of all animals in all groups after SCI. The cyst sizes measured at day 56 after SCI are shown in Figure 6. AAV-GFP treatment and AAV-CNTF^{mCherry} treatment groups on average had a 10-11% area of field of view occupied by cysts, respectively. While AAV-CNTF^{mCherry} + nonviable rMPC-treated animals still showed slightly lower average cyst sizes of about 8%, there was no statistical difference between any of these groups. However, AAV-CNTF^{mCherry} transduction in the cortex followed by *viable* rMPC transplantation into the lesion did result in a statistically significant reduction in average cyst size, to just a 2% area of field of view, indicating that viable rMPCs are able to significantly alter the terrain of the lesion site to affect tissue sparing. Note that two of the three rats with mCherry-positive axons distal to the injury site were in the AAV-CNTF^{mCherry} + viable rMPC group. Donor rMPCs were not labelled with any marker for identification posttransplantation, and there was no evidence of individual donor rMPCs remaining in spinal cord

sections subjected to immunohistochemistry or toluidine blue staining (data not shown).

4. Discussion

In this study, we used AAV-CNTF^{mCherry} therapy to transduce neurons, including CSN, in the sensorimotor cortex of animals with a moderate thoracic (T10) contusion injury, with the aim of enhancing plasticity and promoting the regrowth of corticospinal tract axons after SCI. It is widely acknowledged that combinations of therapies are required for effective treatment of SCI, thus in some animals AAV-CNTF^{mCherry} was applied in combination with viable or nonviable rat mesenchymal precursor cells (rMPCs) grafted into the spinal lesion site two weeks after SCI to modulate the local inhibitory environment. As discussed more fully below, different types of AAV vectors have previously been injected into the cortex in SCI studies, and MPC grafts have also been tested after SCI, but to our knowledge no trials have—until now—combined these therapeutic approaches.

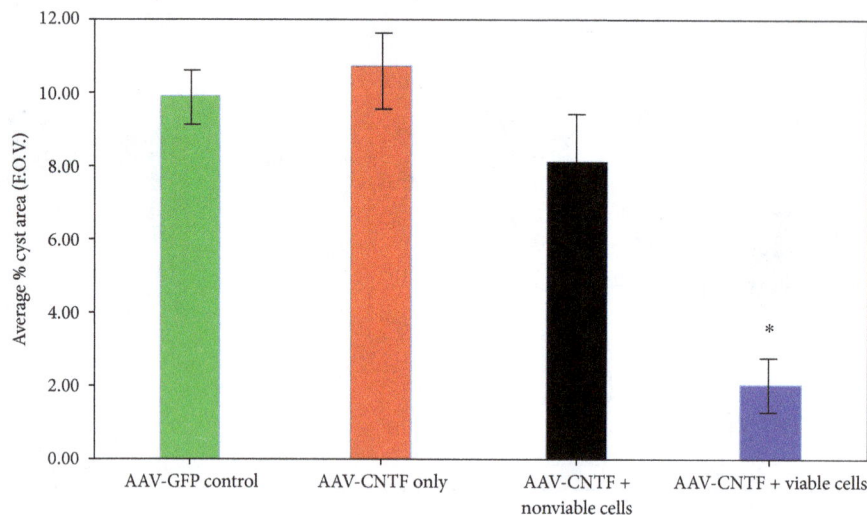

FIGURE 6: Tissue sparing promoted by combined cortical AAV-CNTF^{mCherry} therapy and local transplantation of viable rMPCs. AAV-GFP control treatment and AAV-CNTF^{mCherry} treatment groups revealed similar average areas of cyst formation in spinal cord sections stained by toluidine blue, and although AAV-CNTF^{mCherry} + nonviable rMPC treatment resulted in slightly lower average cyst sizes, only AAV-CNTF^{mCherry} + viable rMPC treatment into the lesion resulted in a statistically significant reduction in average cyst size. $^*p = 0.01 - 0.05$.

AAV-CNTF^{mCherry} therapy alone or in combination with either viable or nonviable rMPC transplantation provided a sustained improvement in functional outcome over AAV-GFP alone as measured by Ladderwalk. Note that with this behavioural test, while control and CNTF treatments differed, there was no significant difference between the different AAV-CNTF^{mCherry} groups (no cells, viable cells, and nonviable cells), thus it seems that the presence of cortical CNTF was sufficient to yield an improvement in the stepping function. AAV-CNTF^{mCherry} therapy alone and in combination with rMPC transplantation also yielded sustained improvements as assessed by open-field locomotion (BBB). Ratwalk gait analyses revealed subtle compensatory mechanisms for limb placement after injury, but it is likely that even the moderate injury used here was too severe to reveal significant statistical differences. The average cyst size was significantly reduced only in the AAV-CNTF^{mCherry} + viable rMPC group.

In addition to many degenerative profiles, the sprouting of apparently intact axons was evident in the CST immediately rostral to the injury site. Compared to AAV-GFP controls, considerably more BDA or mCherry-labelled axons with complex profiles were located just rostral to the cysts in the AAV-CNTF^{mCherry}-injected rats containing CNTF-transduced cortical neurons. Not only was the density of these axons higher, but the area of the spinal cord containing them extended further rostrally into uninjured segments. Furthermore, only in AAV-CNTF^{mCherry}-transduced treatment groups were BDA and mCherry-immunoreactive axons seen to project alongside, and sometimes several millimeters beyond, the rostral border of the lesion-induced cysts. It is important to emphasize that, compared to oriented and organized fibers in the CST far rostral to the injury site, axons were more irregularly organized immediately in front of, as well as caudal to, cysts, strongly suggestive of local sprouting and regenerative responses.

In three of the eleven animals that received cortical AAV-CNTF^{mCherry} injections, axons were seen caudal to all cysts, located up to 3-4 mm beyond the rostral edge of the injury site. These axons were seen in two non-rMPC grafted animals as well as in a rat that also received an rMPC transplant. We did not detect such axons in AAV-GFP-injected animals, again supporting the suggestion that CNTF has the potential to enhance axon regeneration in the spinal cord by transducing appropriate neuronal populations in the sensorimotor cortex. In other CNS systems, vector-mediated delivery of CNTF to parent cell bodies combined with the transplantation of an appropriate bridging substrate (peripheral nerve), promotes the long-distance regeneration of injured axons [7–10], with at least some functional outcomes [11]. Note in particular that the survival effects of CNTF have been demonstrated on numerous neuron populations [14–16], including increasing the viability of corticospinal neurons in the sensorimotor cortex after intracortical axotomy [6]. Because AAV-CNTF delivery is only to the cortex, the primary site of trophic action is at the cell bodies, and transport and release of CNTF at axon tips likely occurs at a low level (we have confirmed this previously, data not shown). Based on previous studies in the visual system, we propose that the mechanisms of protection and promotion of plasticity and regenerative capacity are mediated and amplified both by direct infection of CSN themselves but also due to bystander release of CNTF by adjacent nonprojecting cortical cells [8, 39]. Many of the biological actions of CNTF are signalled via STAT3, and it is therefore important to note that vector-mediated delivery of a hyperactivated STAT3 enhances process outgrowth in cultured cortical neurons [40], and in vivo overexpression of STAT3 enhances CSN plasticity in mice after SCI [41].

Delivery of AAV vectors to the cortex has been reported by a number of groups, some to test the optimal serotype for transduction of cortical neurons, including CSN [42, 43], others to deliver factors designed to enhance CST repair after SCI [44–49]. Such studies are nonetheless much less frequent than those involving the delivery of vectors and/or growth factors to the spinal cord injury site itself [2, 50]. In some initial studies, we tested the effect of the cortical injection of AAV1 expressing insulin-like growth factor 1 (IGF-1) on CST plasticity after SCI, but although we saw some additional sprouting rostral to the injury, this was less than that seen after the cortical delivery of AAV-CNTF vectors, and we saw no significant changes in functional recovery (unpublished data). Interestingly then, postlesion AAV-assisted coexpression of IGF1 and osteopontin in cortical neurons resulted in robust CST regrowth and the recovery of CST-dependent behavioural outcomes after SCI [50], again indicative of the therapeutic power of combined therapies.

The long-term transduction of murine cortical neurons using an AAV vector to suppress or conditionally delete expression of phosphatase and tensin homolog (PTEN), the main suppressor of the PI3K-Akt survival and growth pathway, leads to the greater regenerative growth of CST axons and some functional improvements [45]. However the resultant long-term upregulation of protein kinases such as mTOR, a key regulator of protein translation in neurons, leads to some aberrant growth [48] and progressive changes in the growth of cells, their dendrites, and their axons [46]. This is not dissimilar to the effect of long-term (up to one year) AAV-mediated expression of CNTF on retinal ganglion cells, where there are not only changes in the dendritic morphology of transduced and neighboring non-transduced cells [51], but there is also altered expression of endogenous retinal genes [52]. Whether such effects are also seen in cortical neurons transduced with AAV-CNTF is yet to be determined, but this is an important topic for future studies.

MPCs from the bone marrow stroma have the potential to differentiate into cells with many of the phenotypic characteristics of neural tissue [53–55], migrate and integrate into CNS tissues, and express markers typical of mature neurons and astrocytes [56]. MPCs have been successfully transplanted into the spinal cord and shown to (a) promote regeneration of lesioned axons into the graft, (b) differentiate into neurons, (c) remyelinate damaged myelin sheaths around CNS axons, and (d) improve functional outcomes after SCI (for extensive reviews, see [57, 58]). Our own work using purified (Stro-1+) human MPCs from the bone marrow stroma of SCI patients dramatically improved anatomical (characterized by smaller cyst sizes, as well as lower amounts of degenerative tissue) and functional recovery after both acute and subacute/chronic SCI in nude rat (T-cell immunodeficient) hosts after contusion SCI [24, 25]. Rat MPCs can be prepared to an essentially pure, minor subpopulation of adult cells [59–61] significantly lessening any potential variation in functional and morphological outcomes, often encountered in the literature when using different hMPC donor cells in transplantation experiments.

rMPC transplantation at day 14 post-SCI presumably avoids the cytotoxicity of the acute injury and presumably allows sufficient time for targeted expression of CNTF to be switched on in transduced cortical cells [2, 4, 28]. Generally, SCI studies show significant results attributable to transplantation within a few weeks of injection [24, 25, 57, 62, 63]; however, in the present study the impact of rMPCs grafted into the injury site was evident in reducing postlesion cavity dimensions, but effects were absent or inconsistent in the behavioural studies involving AAV-CNTF^{mCherry}-injected animals. It should be noted that a caveat of this study is that behavioural tests were continued after BDA was injected which could potentially obscure or increase treatment effects due to the injection-associated injury and surgery, although we did not observe any apparent reduction in functional outcomes between BDA injection and the final time points analysed. There did not appear to be greater macrophage/microglial reactivity associated with AAV transduction (either AAV-GFP-treated control or AAV-CNTF^{mCherry} treatments) beyond that typically observed in our other SCI studies [24, 25]. MPCs do produce some CNTF [64] but our experience is that, while MPCs alter the local environment to enhance axonal regrowth, few survive in the long term [24, 25]. Only viable rMPC grafts promoted statistically significant tissue sparing, yet nonviable rMPC transplantation had similar effects as viable rMPC transplantation in functional outcomes (as shown in our Ladderwalk and open-field assays). The use of (freeze-thawed) nonviable cells as appropriate controls for cell transplantation studies in SCI is by no means common. There is evidence to suggest that even fibroblasts can contribute to functional and/or morphological improvements in animal models of SCI compared to specific stem/precursor cell types [57, 63]. Indeed some studies have reported functional improvements without associated (and expected?) structural improvements, and vice versa [57, 65]. A possible scenario is that MPCs (which are known to have immunosuppressive properties [66]) may act as immune "decoys" that modulate the host immune response (e.g., [67]) and this property may still be effective even if the cells themselves are not viable. This could potentially allow the "normal" host repair mechanism to be more effective and be reflected in either functional and/or morphological outcomes.

4.1. Impact and Future Direction. The combination of AAV-targeted expression of CNTF, with or without the use of stem cell graft technology, represents a novel strategy to assess the effect of vector-mediated production of growth factors on plasticity and regeneration after SCI. A major aim of these experiments was to assess the capability of cortical gene therapy to promote potential plasticity and regrowth/regeneration of CST axons. The present behavioural and morphological data after thoracic contusion injury show the promise of using cortical AAV-CNTF gene therapy to promote repair after SCI. In future studies, we will test this approach in a model of cervical CST hemitransection, focusing on the importance of this tract in rodent forelimb function. The data presented here aid in the advancement of technologies related to the development of more effective gene therapy and begin to provide a platform for exploring the possibility of preclinical studies aimed at using gene therapy to modify cortical neurons as part of an SCI repair strategy.

Acknowledgments

The authors thank Associate Professor Peter Mark for statistical help and advice, Mary Lee for laboratory assistance and tissue processing, and Guy Ben-Ary for image analysis. Additionally, the authors thank Professor Giles Plant and Iain Sweetman (Ratwalk) for the development of the Ratwalk device and software. Professor Giles Plant is affiliated with the Stanford Partnership for Spinal Cord Injury and Repair, Stanford Institute for Neuro-Innovation and Translational Neurosciences, and Department of Neurosurgery, 265 Campus Drive, Stanford, CA 94305-5454, USA. Iain Sweetman (Ratwalk) is affiliated with the Faculty, Preventive and Social Medicine NZPhvC Health Sciences, Dunedin School of Medicine, Otago, New Zealand.

References

[1] C. Watson and A. R. Harvey, "Chapter 11. Projections from the brain to the spinal cord," in *The Spinal Cord*, pp. 168–179, Academic Press, 2009.

[2] A. R. Harvey, S. J. Lovett, B. T. Majda, J. H. Yoon, L. P. G. Wheeler, and S. I. Hodgetts, "Neurotrophic factors for spinal cord repair: which, where, how and when to apply, and for what period of time?," *Brain Research*, vol. 1619, pp. 36–71, 2015.

[3] E. J. Gonzalez-Rothi, A. M. Rombola, C. A. Rousseau et al., "Spinal interneurons and forelimb plasticity after incomplete cervical spinal cord injury in adult rats," *Journal of Neurotrauma*, vol. 32, no. 12, pp. 893–907, 2015.

[4] T. Isa and Y. Nishimura, "Plasticity for recovery after partial spinal cord injury—hierarchical organization," *Neuroscience Research*, vol. 78, pp. 3–8, 2014.

[5] C. Darian-Smith, A. Lilak, J. Garner, and K. A. Irvine, "Corticospinal sprouting differs according to spinal injury location and cortical origin in macaque monkeys," *The Journal of Neuroscience*, vol. 34, no. 37, pp. 12267–12279, 2014.

[6] S. M. Dale, R. Z. Kuang, X. Wei, and S. Varon, "Corticospinal motor neurons in the adult rat: degeneration after intracortical axotomy and protection by ciliary neurotrophic factor (CNTF)," *Experimental Neurology*, vol. 135, no. 1, pp. 67–73, 1995.

[7] A. R. Harvey, Y. Hu, S. G. Leaver et al., "Gene therapy and transplantation in CNS repair: the visual system," *Progress in Retina and Eye Research*, vol. 25, no. 5, pp. 449–489, 2006.

[8] M. Hellstrom, M. A. Pollett, and A. R. Harvey, "Post-injury delivery of rAAV2-CNTF combined with short-term pharmacotherapy is neuroprotective and promotes extensive axonal regeneration after optic nerve trauma," *Journal of Neurotrauma*, vol. 28, no. 12, pp. 2475–2483, 2011.

[9] Y. Hu, S. G. Leaver, G. W. Plant et al., "Lentiviral-mediated transfer of CNTF to Schwann cells within reconstructed peripheral nerve grafts enhances adult retinal ganglion cell survival and axonal regeneration," *Molecular Therapy*, vol. 11, no. 6, pp. 906–915, 2005.

[10] S. G. Leaver, Q. Cui, O. Bernard, and A. R. Harvey, "Cooperative effects of bcl-2 and AAV-mediated expression of CNTF on retinal ganglion cell survival and axonal regeneration in adult transgenic mice," *The European Journal of Neuroscience*, vol. 24, no. 12, pp. 3323–3332, 2006.

[11] S. W. You, M. Hellström, M. A. Pollett et al., "Large-scale reconstitution of a retina-to-brain pathway in adult rats using gene therapy and bridging grafts: an anatomical and behavioral analysis," *Experimental Neurology*, vol. 279, pp. 197–211, 2016.

[12] N. Y. Ip and G. D. Yancopoulos, "Ciliary neurotrophic factor and its receptor complex," *Progress in Growth Factor Research*, vol. 4, no. 2, pp. 139–155, 1992.

[13] N. Y. Ip and G. D. Yancopoulos, "The neurotrophins and CNTF: two families of collaborative neurotrophic factors," *Annual Review of Neuroscience*, vol. 19, no. 1, pp. 491–515, 1996.

[14] P. M. Richardson, "Ciliary neurotrophic factor: a review," *Pharmacology & Therapeutics*, vol. 63, no. 2, pp. 187–198, 1994.

[15] M. Sendtner, P. Carroll, B. Holtmann, R. A. Hughes, and H. Thoenen, "Ciliary neurotrophic factor," *Journal of Neurobiology*, vol. 25, no. 11, pp. 1436–1453, 1994.

[16] M. Sendtner, F. Dittrich, R. A. Hughes, and H. Thoenen, "Actions of CNTF and neurotrophins on degenerating motoneurons: preclinical studies and clinical implications," *Journal of the Neurological Science*, vol. 124, pp. 77–83, 1994.

[17] J. Ye, L. Cao, R. Cui et al., "The effects of ciliary neurotrophic factor on neurological function and glial activity following contusive spinal cord injury in the rats," *Brain Research*, vol. 997, no. 1, pp. 30–39, 2004.

[18] R. E. Clatterbuck, D. L. Price, and V. E. Koliatsos, "Ciliary neurotrophic factor prevents retrograde neuronal death in the adult central nervous system," *Proceedings of the National Academy of Sciences of the United States of America*, vol. 90, no. 6, pp. 2222–2226, 1993.

[19] T. Hagg and S. Varon, "Ciliary neurotrophic factor prevents degeneration of adult rat substantia nigra dopaminergic neurons in vivo," *Proceedings of the National Academy of Sciences of the United States of America*, vol. 90, no. 13, pp. 6315–6319, 1993.

[20] P. H. Ozdinler and J. D. Macklis, "IGF-I specifically enhances axon outgrowth of corticospinal motor neurons," *Nature Neuroscience*, vol. 9, no. 11, pp. 1371–1381, 2006.

[21] Q. Cao, Q. He, Y. Wang et al., "Transplantation of ciliary neurotrophic factor-expressing adult oligodendrocyte precursor cells promotes remyelination and functional recovery after spinal cord injury," *The Journal of Neuroscience*, vol. 30, no. 8, pp. 2989–3001, 2010.

[22] A. R. Harvey, J. W. Ooi, and J. Rodger, "Chapter one - Neurotrophic factors and the regeneration of adult retinal ganglion cell axons," *International Review of Neurobiology*, vol. 106, pp. 1–33, 2012.

[23] J. L. Nielson, I. Sears-Kraxberger, M. K. Strong, J. K. Wong, R. Willenberg, and O. Steward, "Unexpected survival of neurons of origin of the pyramidal tract after spinal cord injury," *The Journal of Neuroscience*, vol. 30, no. 34, pp. 11516–11528, 2010.

[24] S. Hodgetts, P. Simmons, and G. W. Plant, "Human mesenchymal precursor cells (Stro-1⁺) from spinal cord injury patients improve functional recovery and tissue sparing in an acute spinal cord injury rat model," *Cell Transplantation*, vol. 22, no. 3, pp. 393–412, 2013.

[25] S. Hodgetts, P. Simmons, and G. W. Plant, "A comparison of the behavioral and anatomical outcomes in sub-acute and chronic spinal cord injury models following treatment with human mesenchymal precursor cell transplantation and recombinant decorin," *Experimental Neurology*, vol. 248, pp. 343–359, 2013.

[26] E. D. Wirth 3rd, P. J. Reier, R. G. Fessler et al., "Feasibility and safety of neural tissue transplantation in patients with syringomyelia," *Journal of Neurotrauma*, vol. 18, no. 9, pp. 911–929, 2001.

[27] W. Tang, I. Ehrlich, S. B. E. Wolff et al., "Faithful expression of multiple proteins via 2A-peptide self-processing: a versatile and reliable method for manipulating brain circuits," *The Journal of Neuroscience*, vol. 29, no. 27, pp. 8621–8629, 2009.

[28] H. Petrs-Silva and R. Linden, "Advances in recombinant adeno-associated viral vectors for gene delivery," *Current Gene Therapy*, vol. 13, no. 5, pp. 335–345, 2013.

[29] T. H. Hutson, J. Verhaagen, R. J. Yanez-Munoz, and L. D. Moon, "Corticospinal tract transduction: a comparison of seven adeno-associated viral vector serotypes and a non-integrating lentiviral vector," *Gene Therapy*, vol. 19, no. 1, pp. 49–60, 2012.

[30] M. Sendtner, H. Schmalbruch, K. A. Stöckli, P. Carroll, G. W. Kreutzberg, and H. Thoenen, "Ciliary neurotrophic factor prevents degeneration of motor neurons in mouse mutant progressive motor neuronopathy," *Nature*, vol. 358, no. 6386, pp. 502–504, 1992.

[31] A. Harvey, S. Clarkson, and G. Plant, "Corticospinal projections in adult Fischer F344 rats," *Proceedings of the Australian Neuroscience Society*, vol. 16, p. 103, 2005.

[32] F. P. Hamers, G. C. Koopmans, and E. A. Joosten, "CatWalk-assisted gait analysis in the assessment of spinal cord injury," *Journal of Neurotrauma*, vol. 23, no. 3-4, pp. 537–548, 2006.

[33] F. P. Hamers, A. J. Lankhorst, T. J. van Laar, W. B. Veldhuis, and W. H. Gispen, "Automated quantitative gait analysis during overground locomotion in the rat: its application to spinal cord contusion and transection injuries," *Journal of Neurotrauma*, vol. 18, no. 2, pp. 187–201, 2001.

[34] G. D. Muir and A. A. Webb, "Assessment of behavioural recovery following spinal cord injury in rats," *European Journal of Neuroscience*, vol. 12, no. 9, pp. 3079–3086, 2000.

[35] G. W. Plant, P. F. Currier, E. P. Cuervo et al., "Purified adult ensheathing glia fail to myelinate axons under culture conditions that enable Schwann cells to form myelin," *The Journal of Neuroscience*, vol. 22, no. 14, pp. 6083–6091, 2002.

[36] D. M. Basso, M. S. Beattie, and J. C. Bresnahan, "A sensitive and reliable locomotor rating scale for open field testing in rats," *Journal of Neurotrauma*, vol. 12, no. 1, pp. 1–21, 1995.

[37] G. A. Metz and I. Q. Whishaw, "Cortical and subcortical lesions impair skilled walking in the ladder rung walking test: a new task to evaluate fore- and hindlimb stepping, placing, and co-ordination," *Journal of Neuroscience Methods*, vol. 115, no. 2, pp. 169–179, 2002.

[38] M. J. Godinho, L. Teh, M. A. Pollett et al., "Immunohistochemical, ultrastructural and functional analysis of axonal regeneration through peripheral nerve grafts containing Schwann cells expressing BDNF, CNTF or NT3," *PLoS One*, vol. 8, no. 8, article e69987, 2013.

[39] S. G. Leaver, Q. Cui, G. W. Plant et al., "AAV-mediated expression of CNTF promotes long-term survival and regeneration of adult rat retinal ganglion cells," *Gene Therapy*, vol. 13, no. 18, pp. 1328–1341, 2006.

[40] S. T. Mehta, X. Luo, K. K. Park, J. L. Bixby, and V. P. Lemmon, "Hyperactivated Stat3 boosts axon regeneration in the CNS," *Experimental Neurology*, vol. 280, pp. 115–120, 2016.

[41] C. Lang, P. M. Bradley, A. Jacobi, M. Kerschensteiner, and F. M. Bareyre, "STAT3 promotes corticospinal remodelling and functional recovery after spinal cord injury," *EMBO Reports*, vol. 14, no. 10, pp. 931–937, 2013.

[42] D. F. Aschauer, S. Kreuz, and S. Rumpel, "Analysis of transduction efficiency, tropism and axonal transport of AAV serotypes 1, 2, 5, 6, 8 and 9 in the mouse brain," *PLoS One*, vol. 8, no. 9, article e76310, 2013.

[43] A. Watakabe, M. Ohtsuka, M. Kinoshita et al., "Comparative analyses of adeno-associated viral vector serotypes 1, 2, 5, 8 and 9 in marmoset, mouse and macaque cerebral cortex," *Neuroscience Research*, vol. 93, pp. 144–157, 2014.

[44] N. Weishaupt, S. Li, A. Di Pardo, S. Sipione, and K. Fouad, "Synergistic effects of BDNF and rehabilitative training on recovery after cervical spinal cord injury," *Behavioural Brain Research*, vol. 239, pp. 31–42, 2013.

[45] C. A. Danilov and O. Steward, "Conditional genetic deletion of PTEN after a spinal cord injury enhances regenerative growth of CST axons and motor function recovery in mice," *Experimental Neurology*, vol. 266, pp. 147–160, 2015.

[46] E. A. Gallent and O. Steward, "Neuronal *PTEN* deletion in adult cortical neurons triggers progressive growth of cell bodies, dendrites, and axons," *Experimental Neurology*, vol. 303, pp. 12–28, 2018.

[47] E. A. Gutilla, M. M. Buyukozturk, and O. Steward, "Long-term consequences of conditional genetic deletion of PTEN in the sensorimotor cortex of neonatal mice," *Experimental Neurology*, vol. 279, pp. 27–39, 2016.

[48] R. Willenberg, K. Zukor, K. Liu, Z. He, and O. Steward, "Variable laterality of corticospinal tract axons that regenerate after spinal cord injury as a result of PTEN deletion or knock-down," *The Journal of Comparative Neurology*, vol. 524, no. 13, pp. 2654–2676, 2016.

[49] P. Yang, Y. Qin, W. Zhang, Z. Bian, and R. Wang, "Sensorimotor cortex injection of adeno-associated viral vector mediates knockout of PTEN in neurons of the brain and spinal cord of mice," *Journal of Molecular Neuroscience*, vol. 57, no. 4, pp. 470–476, 2015.

[50] Y. Liu, X. Wang, W. Li et al., "A sensitized IGF1 treatment restores corticospinal axon-dependent functions," *Neuron*, vol. 95, no. 4, pp. 817–833.e4, 2017.

[51] J. Rodger, E. S. Drummond, M. Hellstrom, D. Robertson, and A. R. Harvey, "Long-term gene therapy causes transgene-specific changes in the morphology of regenerating retinal ganglion cells," *PLoS One*, vol. 7, no. 2, article e31061, 2012.

[52] C. J. LeVaillant, A. Sharma, J. Muhling et al., "Significant changes in endogenous retinal gene expression assessed 1 year after a single intraocular injection of AAV-CNTF or AAV-BDNF," *Molecular Therapy Methods & Clinical Development*, vol. 3, article 16078, 2016.

[53] S. A. Azizi, D. Stokes, B. J. Augelli, C. DiGirolamo, and D. J. Prockop, "Engraftment and migration of human bone marrow stromal cells implanted in the brains of albino rats—similarities to astrocyte grafts," *Proceedings of the National Academy of Sciences of the United States of America*, vol. 95, no. 7, pp. 3908–3913, 1998.

[54] J. Sanchez-Ramos, S. Song, F. Cardozo-Pelaez et al., "Adult bone marrow stromal cells differentiate into neural cells *in vitro*," *Experimental Neurology*, vol. 164, no. 2, pp. 247–256, 2000.

[55] D. Woodbury, E. J. Schwarz, D. J. Prockop, and I. B. Black, "Adult rat and human bone marrow stromal cells differentiate into neurons," *Journal of Neuroscience Research*, vol. 61, no. 4, pp. 364–370, 2000.

[56] G. C. Kopen, D. J. Prockop, and D. G. Phinney, "Marrow stromal cells migrate throughout forebrain and cerebellum, and they differentiate into astrocytes after injection into neonatal mouse brains," *Proceedings of the National Academy of Sciences of the United States of America*, vol. 96, no. 19, pp. 10711–10716, 1999.

[57] W. Tetzlaff, E. B. Okon, S. Karimi-Abdolrezaee et al., "A systematic review of cellular transplantation therapies for spinal cord injury," *Journal of Neurotrauma*, vol. 28, no. 8, pp. 1611–1682, 2011.

[58] R. S. Oliveri, S. Bello, and F. Biering-Sorensen, "Mesenchymal stem cells improve locomotor recovery in traumatic spinal cord injury: systematic review with meta-analyses of rat models," *Neurobiology of Disease*, vol. 62, pp. 338–353, 2013.

[59] M. Ye, S. Chen, X. Wang et al., "Glial cell line-derived neurotrophic factor in bone marrow stromal cells of rat," *Neuroreport*, vol. 16, no. 6, pp. 581–584, 2005.

[60] R. D. Nandoe, A. Hurtado, A. D. Levi, A. Grotenhuis, and M. Oudega, "Bone marrow stromal cells for repair of the spinal cord: towards clinical application," *Cell Transplantation*, vol. 15, no. 7, pp. 563–577, 2006.

[61] C. M. Kolf, E. Cho, and R. S. Tuan, "Mesenchymal stromal cells. Biology of adult mesenchymal stem cells: regulation of niche, self-renewal and differentiation," *Arthritis Research & Therapy*, vol. 9, no. 1, p. 204, 2007.

[62] S. Hodgetts, G. W. Plant, and A. Harvey, "Chapter 14. Spinal cord injury: experimental animal models and relation to human therapy," in *The Spinal Cord*, H. Watson, G. Paxinos, and G. Kayalioglu, Eds., Elsevier, London, 2009.

[63] A. S. Kramer, A. R. Harvey, G. W. Plant, and S. I. Hodgetts, "Systematic review of induced pluripotent stem cell technology as a potential clinical therapy for spinal cord injury," *Cell Transplantation*, vol. 22, no. 4, pp. 571–617, 2013.

[64] A. Nagai, W. K. Kim, H. J. Lee et al., "Multilineage potential of stable human mesenchymal stem cell line derived from fetal marrow," *PLoS One*, vol. 2, no. 12, article e1272, 2007.

[65] P. Lu, G. Woodruff, Y. Wang et al., "Long-distance axonal growth from human induced pluripotent stem cells after spinal cord injury," *Neuron*, vol. 83, no. 4, pp. 789–796, 2014.

[66] S. Gronthos, A. C. W. Zannettino, S. J. Hay et al., "Molecular and cellular characterisation of highly purified stromal stem cells derived from human bone marrow," *Journal of Cell Science*, vol. 116, no. 9, pp. 1827–1835, 2003.

[67] S. V. White, C. E. Czisch, M. H. Han, C. D. Plant, A. R. Harvey, and G. W. Plant, "Intravenous transplantation of mesenchymal progenitors distribute solely to the lungs and improve outcomes in cervical spinal cord injury," *Stem Cells*, vol. 34, no. 7, pp. 1812–1825, 2016.

4

The Role of Mammalian Glial Cells in Circadian Rhythm Regulation

Donají Chi-Castañeda[1,2] **and Arturo Ortega**[1]

[1]*Laboratorio de Neurotoxicología, Departamento de Toxicología,*
 Centro de Investigación y de Estudios Avanzados del Instituto Politécnico Nacional, Apartado Postal 14-740,
 07000 Ciudad de México, Mexico
[2]*Soluciones para un México Verde S.A. de C.V., 01210 Ciudad de México, Mexico*

Correspondence should be addressed to Arturo Ortega; arortega@cinvestav.mx

Academic Editor: Harry Pantazopoulos

Circadian rhythms are biological oscillations with a period of about 24 hours. These rhythms are maintained by an innate genetically determined time-keeping system called the circadian clock. A large number of the proteins involved in the regulation of this clock are transcription factors controlling rhythmic transcription of *so-called* clock-controlled genes, which participate in a plethora of physiological functions in the organism. In the brain, several areas, besides the suprachiasmatic nucleus, harbor functional clocks characterized by a well-defined time pattern of clock gene expression. This expression rhythm is not restricted to neurons but is also present in glia, suggesting that these cells are involved in circadian rhythmicity. However, only certain glial cells fulfill the criteria to be called glial clocks, namely, to display molecular oscillators based on the canonical clock protein PERIOD, which depends on the suprachiasmatic nucleus for their synchronization. In this contribution, we summarize the current information about activity of the clock genes in glial cells, their potential role as oscillators as well as clinical implications.

1. Introduction

Most light-sensitive organisms have built-in time-measuring devices that are commonly known as circadian clocks. The term *circadian* was introduced by Halberg to describe the biological rhythms that have a period of approximately 24 h and are known as circadian rhythms [1]. Circadian rhythms are present along the phylogenetic scale, in mammals regulate a plethora of functions such as the rest-activity cycle, hormone secretion, and daily variations in metabolism and body temperature [2].

The intracellular circadian clock is based on a transcription-translation feedback system that drive the self-sustaining clock mechanism in the suprachiasmatic nucleus (SCN, the "master clock") and in peripheral tissues ("peripheral clocks") [3, 4]. At the molecular level, the molecular machinery that generates circadian rhythms involves CLOCK- (circadian locomotor output cycles kaput) BMAL1 (brain and

muscle aryl hydrocarbon receptor nuclear translocator-like protein 1) heterodimers that control the periodic expression of *Per* (*periods 1–3*) and *Cry* (*cryptochrome 1,2*) genes. These gene products form the PER-CRY heterodimer that is translocated to the nucleus inhibiting their own transcription. Additionally, an accessory regulatory loop involves the rhythmic regulation of *Bmal1* transcription through the coordinated action of the transcriptional repressor *REV-ERBα* (*Reverse Erb alpha*) and the transcriptional activator *RORα* (*retinoid-related orphan receptor-alpha*) [5–8].

In mammals, the SCN synchronizes multiple peripheral clocks, in numerous tissues and cell types, presumably via the combination of neural and humoral signaling [2, 9]. The general consensus of the cellular identity of the oscillating cells in the brain points to the neurons, although it has been demonstrated that the glial cells are circadian oscillators as well, and their synchronization also depends on the SCN [10–12].

Glial cells make up a large fraction of human nervous system cells, with numbers exceeding those of neurons by a factor of ten, depending on the brain structure studied. Particularly, glial cells occupy about half the volume of the brain and participate in diverse functions, including regulation of synaptic transmission, plasticity, behavior, and synapse development, and these cells are also involved in neurodegeneration [13–17]. Interestingly, it has been described that glial cells also play an important role in the regulation of circadian rhythms [18–23], although little attention has been paid to this function. Accordingly, we summarize here the recent findings about clock genes in glial cells, the plausible role of the glial cells as cellular oscillators, and the possible medical implications of clock genes in this cell type.

2. Clock Genes in Glial Cells

2.1. Astrocytes. This type of glial cell is involved in the buffering of extracellular K^+, regulating neurotransmitter release [24], forming the blood-brain barrier, releasing growth factors, and the regulation of complex brain mechanisms, such as sleep homeostasis [25] and memory [26–28], among other functions.

In 1990, it was suggested that glial cells might express molecular oscillators, which are based on the clock protein PER. Particularly, it was demonstrated that PER was localized both in neurons and glial cells of the fly brain, which showed robust circadian rhythms and abundance [11]. Subsequently, Ewer and coworkers reported that certain weakly rhythmic flies contained detectable PER only in glia, suggesting that glial oscillators play an important role in the pacemaker driving rhythmic behavior [12]. Later, it was confirmed the rhythmic expression of clock genes in rat and mouse astrocytes, indicating that these cells contain a PER-based molecular oscillator that damps in the absence of neuronal signals [29, 30]. These astroglial cultures were capable to display a sustained rhythmicity for 7 days when cocultured with SCN explants, whereas cortical explants did not influence rhythmicity [29], suggesting that the presence of sustained rhythms in glial cells requires a secreted neuronal factor expressed in the SCN. Temperature cycles entrain *Per1* rhythms in astroglial cultures [29] however are unlikely to be a relevant factor, since exposure to SCN explants sustained glial rhythms without any change in temperature.

Several studies have explored the role of the mammalian PER-based oscillator in glial physiology. It has been reported that *Glast* (*glutamate/aspartate transporter*) expression and protein levels within the SCN present a diurnal rhythm in a light/dark (12/12 h) cycle [31]. However, it was not determined whether this rhythm persist or not in nonrhythmic conditions (constant darkness or constant light), in other words in lack of environmental information. Results of Spanagel and collaborators are complementary with the observation concerning to GLAST levels, which do not display an obvious rhythmicity in the *Per2* mutant mice pointing out the presence of a circadian control [31]. Beaulé and colleagues reported that cultured cortical astrocytes from *Clock* mutant animals have reduced *Glast* mRNA and protein levels [32], proposing that the vast majority of glial glutamate (Glu)

uptake activity is a function of the transcription factors *Clock* and *Npas2* (*neuronal PAS domain protein 2*) and of the transcriptional regulator *Per2* [32, 33]. This dependence could be explained by the involvement of CLOCK and NPAS2 in the indirect regulation of *Glast* transcription or in GLAST protein stabilization and/or localization [34]. It should be noted that no evidence has been demonstrated for circadian changes in Glu uptake, suggesting a noncircadian role for clock proteins that might be involved in the regulation of *Glast* gene transcription or *Glast* mRNA translation and/or stability [32, 33].

Concerning Glu, it is known that this neurotransmitter participates in photic entrainment of circadian rhythms. In 2015, it was reported that in cultured Bergmann glial cells, BMAL1 expression is Glu time- and dose-dependent. This phenomena might be a result of stabilization of the protein after it has been phosphorylated by PKA (cyclic AMP-dependent protein kinase) and/or PKC (Ca^{2+}/diacylglycerol-dependent protein kinase), pointing out that Glu is critically involved in glial BMAL1 expression and that glial cells are important in the control of circadian rhythms in the cerebellum [22].

It has been recently demonstrated that not only SCN neurons but also SCN astrocytes possess pacemaking properties [35]. By using long-term live imaging, Brancaccio and colleagues simultaneously codetected circadian oscillations of neuronal and astrocytic intracellular calcium ($[Ca^{2+}]_i$) within the SCN, with $[Ca^{2+}]_i$ levels peaking during the circadian day and night. Thereby, these oscillations of $[Ca^{2+}]_i$ were antiphasic and showed a complementary waveform [35]. In the same study, it was reported widespread circadian oscillations of extracellular Glu ($[Glu]_e$) in the SCN in phase with astrocytic $[Ca^{2+}]_i$. These circadian oscillations of $[Glu]_e$ are generated intrinsically in the SCN and also depend directly on astrocytic metabolism [35]. Using pharmacological inhibition of the glial and neuronal isoforms of the Glu transporters, a continuing circadian oscillation of Glu release by astrocytes is observed. Remarkably, $[Glu]_e$ oscillations are generated by concerted rhythms of release and uptake, and blocking Glu uptake impairs the fine-tuning of the $[Glu]_e$/$[Ca^{2+}]_i$ relationship, reducing the robustness of the rhythms of neuronal $[Ca^{2+}]_i$ across the SCN. Consequently, SCN cellular oscillators progressively desynchronize, until the $[Glu]_e$/$[Ca^{2+}]_i$ alignment is restored. Presynaptic NMDA (N-methyl-D-aspartate) receptors 2C-mediated glutamatergic gliotransmission inhibit neuronal activity during circadian night, and this mechanism is essential to sustain circadian rhythmicity in the dorsal SCN [35]. Accordingly, during the circadian night, SCN astrocytes are metabolically active (high $[Ca^{2+}]_i$) and release high levels (baseline activity) of Glu into the extracellular space, which in turn activates presynaptic NR2C-expressing neurons in the dorsal SCN, thereby increasing GABAergic inhibitory tone across the circuit. In contrast, during the circadian day, $[Glu]_e$ is reduced by diminished glial release and increased EAAT-mediated Glu uptake and consequently, GABAergic tone is reduced, thereby derepressing spontaneous membrane potential, neuronal $[Ca^{2+}]_i$, and facilitating electrical firing [35].

Moreover, it was reported that SCN astrocytes are functional circadian oscillators, which modulate the period of SCN and the rest-activity rhythms [36]. The loss of rhythm in SCN astrocytes by *Bmal1* deletion leads to an extended circadian period of rest-activity rhythms. This *Bmal1* deletion in a small proportion of SCN cells appears to change the period of the SCN and behavior by the loss of rhythmicity in 20% of SCN cells that express AVP (arginine-vasopressin) or 10% of cells that express Aldh1L1 (specific astrocytic marker) or GFAP (glial fibrillary acid protein) [36].

Earlier studies in SCN astrocytes revealed high-amplitude daily rhythms in the expression of GFAP [37] and their coverage of the soma and dendrites of vasointestinal polypeptide- and AVP-expressing SCN neurons, which are related with modifications in synaptic innervation of these neurons [38, 39]. Rhythmic pattern of GFAP was observed in constant darkness in the SCN of hamsters, rats, and mice [37, 40], suggesting that these rhythms are intrinsic and independent of external light cues. Although the role of daily oscillations of GFAP in SCN is unknown, it has been associated with two main aspects of the clock functioning: metabolic exchanges and plasticity [38]. According to this last aspect, it has been demonstrated that mice lacking the *Gfap* show impaired long-term depression in the cerebellum, reduced eye-blink conditioning [41], longer periods of activity, and more arrhythmicity in constant light conditions compared to wild type [40, 42]. These results indicate that GFAP in glial cells plays a role in the regulation of neuronal function.

A daily variation of GFAP in the mouse SCN, as well as the NF-κB (nuclear factor-κB) expression in SCN astrocytes has been documented using tissue slices and primary cell cultures [43]. Particularly, in the latter case, LPS (lipopolysaccharide), IL-1α (interleukin-1 alpha), and TNFα (tumor necrosis factor alpha) promoted the activation of NF-κB, indicating that SCN astrocytes mediate the input signals to the circadian system from the immune system via NF-κB signaling [43].

RORα is expressed in astrocytes but not in microglia. Studies using *staggerer* mice, which have a 122 bp deletion in the *RORα* gene, allowed the identification of several functions of this nuclear receptor, both in the periphery and in the CNS. Interestingly, a massive cerebellar neurodegeneration leading to severe ataxia was also observed in these mice [44].

Furthermore, it has also been reported that *RORα*-deficient mice have abnormal immune responses, associated with increased levels of IL-1β, IL-6, and TNFα [45]. An additional report showed that in primary astrocyte cultures, RORα directly participates in the regulation of the inflammatory reaction via the inhibition of the NF-κB pathway. Thus, in a noninflammatory condition, the nuclear receptor directly increases IL-6 expression, while in an inflammatory condition, RORα reduces cytokine-induced *Il-6* upregulation [46].

Other nuclear receptors involved in the inflammatory response are REV-ERBα and REV-ERBβ; both receptors are expressed in rat C6 cells and in astrocyte cultures derived from rat cortex and spinal cord [47]. Particularly, in rat C6 astroglial cells, it has been reported that TNF significantly increases chemokine *Ccl-2* (*monocyte chemoattractant protein-1*), *Il-6*, *iNOS* (*inducible nitric oxide synthase*), and *Mmp-9* (*matrix metalloprotease-9*) mRNA levels. However, both isoforms of REV-ERB inhibit TNF-induced upregulation of *Ccl-2* and *Mmp-9* mRNA levels. Particularly, REV-ERBα and REV-ERBβ decrease MMP-9 expression via HDAC3 (histone deacetylase 3) [47]. Moreover, it has been shown that REV-ERBα inhibits *Il-6* upregulation in murine skeletal muscle cells and macrophages [48–50], suggesting that the activity of this nuclear receptor is tissue-specific.

Circadian expression of clock genes such as *Per1*, *Per2*, *Cry1*, and *Bmal1* can be observed in mice spinal cord. Surprisingly, circadian expression of *GS* (*glutamine synthetase*, a glial-enriched enzyme) and *COX-1* (*cyclooxygenase-1*) at both mRNA and protein levels was also detected in the same brain area [51]. Moreover, circadian changes in the expression of GS suggest that astrocyte metabolism is subjected to circadian modulation. Whereas, the disruption of astroglial function using fluorocitrate (a glial metabolic inhibitor) led to the suppression of the oscillating expression of not only GS and COX-1 but also the expression of clock genes. These findings suggest that spinal circadian expression of clock genes depends on the activity of astrocytes, since the inhibition of astrocytic function disrupts circadian gene mRNA expression [51].

Gliotransmission is the process by which astrocytes communicate with immediate glia and neurons through the release of transmitters such as ATP and Glu [42, 52, 53]. *In vivo*, a circadian pattern of ATP release appears to derive primarily from astrocytes within the SCN; however, the functional implications of these extracellular ATP rhythms are unknown [54]. Moreover, it has been shown that astrocytes display daily extracellular ATP oscillations that rely on key clock genes (*Clock*, *Per1*, and *Per2*) and inositol triphosphate signaling [55], suggesting that extracellular ATP levels are augmented at specific hours of the day, and probably, a clock-induced increase in energy metabolism and glial activity is present [55].

Mammalian and insect glial cells modulate circadian neuronal circuitry and behavior via glial calcium signaling [19]. Genetic manipulations of glial vesicle trafficking, the membrane ionic gradient, or internal calcium storage all lead to arrhythmic locomotor activity in *Drosophila*, an organism in which astrocytes, but not other glial cell types, are relevant for the circadian modulation of behavior. It should be noted that *Drosophila* and mammalian astrocytes elicit similar functions due to their preserved morphology and molecular signatures. Besides, PER-based glial oscillator is not essential for the free-running behavioral rhythmicity, although the possibility that this oscillator is required for circadian photic sensitivity or the expression of a different rhythm cannot be ruled out [19].

Recently, Xu and colleagues reported the existence of canonical circadian clock genes in mammalian retinal Müller glia. This study not only demonstrated that retinal Müller cells generate molecular circadian rhythms isolated from other retinal cell types but also demonstrated that these retinal cells exhibit unique features of their molecular circadian clock compared to the retina as a complex system. However, it is important to highlight that the authors mention that both mouse and human Müller cells exhibit species-specific differences in the gene dependence of their clocks [56]. Accordingly, it was observed that human Müller cells exhibit *in vitro* circadian rhythms in clock gene expression, although the rhythm in these cells does not seem to depend on *Per1* expression. Whereas, in mouse Müller cells, knockout or knockdown of *Per1* led to arrhythmicity, suggesting that human Müller cells may have a decreased dependence in *Per1* expression to regulate rhythmicity [56]. Additional evidence reported by Tosini and Menaker demonstrates that the mammalian neural retina contains a genetically programmed circadian oscillator [57]. Nevertheless, Xu and coworkers propose to Müller glia as a candidate clock cell population in the mammalian retina [56]. The results obtained in both reports indicate that both neurons and glia play an important role in the generation of circadian rhythms in this autonomous oscillator.

2.2. Microglia. These glial cells are the main innate immune cells of the CNS and play essential functions in the maintenance of neuronal circuitry, regulation of behavior, and functional state of neurotransmission [20, 21].

Knowledge about a molecular clock in this type of glial cells is relatively recent. In 2011, it was demonstrated that the clock genes are constitutively expressed in both cultured murine microglia and the microglial cell line BV-2 cells. In the same study, it was also reported that ATP selectively promotes the expression of mRNA and corresponding protein for *Per1* via P2X7 purinergic receptor subtype in microglial cells [58]. Years later, it was confirmed that cortical microglia contain an intrinsic molecular clock capable of regulating diurnal changes of its morphological aspect [20]. Specifically, it has been demonstrated in mice that microglia controls the sleep-wake cycle-dependent changes in synaptic strength through the extension and retraction of their processes [21]. Hayashi and colleagues showed that CatS (Cathepsin S, a microglia-specific lysosomal cysteine protease in the brain) exhibits a circadian expression in cortical microglia. Such expression of CatS induces diurnal variations in the synaptic strength of the cortical neurons via the proteolytic modification of the perineuronal environment. Conversely, alterations in CatS lead to hyperlocomotor activity, as well as the deletion of the diurnal variations in the synaptic activity and dendritic spine density of the cortical neurons as a consequence of failure to downscale the synaptic strength during sleep [20, 59]. This process is necessary for the acquisition of subsequent novel information after waking [20]; therefore, dysfunction of microglia intrinsic circadian clock could be involved in social behavior abnormalities [59] and neuropsychiatric disorders, including depression and cognitive impairment [60, 61].

In 2015, Fonken and coworkers reported that microglia possesses circadian clock mechanisms and displays rhythmic fluctuations in both basal inflammatory gene expression and inflammatory potential. It is interesting to note that inflammatory potential in microglia is associated with time-of-day differences, this is because of the circadian differences observed in sickness response [23].

Recently, Nakazato and colleagues demonstrated that *Bmal1* modulates *Il-6* upregulation in microglial cells exposed to LPS using siRNA targeting *Bmal1* and *Bmal1*-deficient mice [62]. These results suggest that an intrinsic microglial clock may regulate microglial inflammatory responses under pathological conditions *in vivo*. It was also observed that *Bmal1* bindings to the *Il-6* promoter region only in cells exposed to LPS; for which, they suggest that histone modification occurred at the *Il-6* promoter region with E-box elements [62].

2.3. Oligodendrocytes. These cells are the myelinating glia of the CNS, provide axonal metabolic support [63], and contribute to neuroplasticity [64]. Scarce information regarding clock genes in these cells is available. A previous study suggested that oligodendrocytes' proliferation depends on the time-of-the-day in the hippocampal *hilus*, indicating a close connection between the temporal information and glial cells in this structure [65]. To date, there is no report showing that oligodendrocytes have an internal circadian clock. However, it has been suggested that clock genes might regulate OPC (oligodendrocyte precursor cell) proliferation, since these cells in the hippocampus express cyclin D1 [18], which is regulated by *Per2* gene [66].

3. Clinical Implications

Recent studies indicate that defective clock genes in glial cells participate in diverse brain pathologies, mainly in psychiatric diseases. However, it is important to keep in mind that a single clock gene can have different repercussions on health and that several clock genes may be related to the same pathology (for detailed review, see reference [67]). Particularly, mutations in *Clock*, *Npas2*, and/or *Per2* are all involved in a hyperglutamatergic scenario due to a decrease in GLAST expression and as consequence, a reduction in Glu uptake [31, 32, 68]. In this scenario, astrocytic Glu release has clear pathophysiological implications like stroke, multiple sclerosis, and dementia [69]. Additionally, it has been established that Glu regulates the levels of dopamine and other neurotransmitters and neuropeptides that mediate both positive and negative aspects of drug reinforcement and reward. In this manner, both hyper- and hypoglutamatergic states in specific brain areas are directly involved in different stages of addiction, including development, persistence, and abstinence [68]. Fascinatingly, clock genes participate in the modulation of common mechanisms of drug abuse-related behaviors [31, 70].

Moreover, alterations in *Per1*, *Per3*, and *Bmal1* lead essentially to changes in both short- and long-term memory, chronic oxidative stress in the brain, variations in cocaine sensitization, and association with a number of psychiatric diseases [71–77]. Similarly, *Npas2*, *Gsk3β*, *Dbp*, *Cry1*, and *Clock* are involved in variations in drugs sensitization, as well as in diverse psychiatric diseases, mainly bipolar disorder, schizophrenia, Alzheimer, and unipolar major depressive disorder [32, 78–82].

Nowadays, disturbances in the sleep parameters are common. These disturbances are associated with a spectrum of

TABLE 1: Circadian functions regulated by the glial cells.

CG/CCG/molecule	Circadian functions	References
Astrocytes		
Clock	Regulation of the glutamatergic system (*Glast* mRNA and protein levels)	[32]
	Modulates ATP release	[55]
Npas2	Regulation of the glutamatergic system (*Glast* mRNA and protein levels)	[32]
Per1	Regulation of nociceptive processes	[51]
	Modulates ATP release	[55]
	Regulation of the glutamatergic system (GLAST protein levels)	[31, 32]
Per2	Regulation of nociceptive processes	[51]
	Modulates ATP release	[55]
	Regulates to *cyclin D1*	[66]
Bmal1	Modulates the period of the SCN and behavior	[36]
	Regulation of nociceptive processes	[51]
Cry1	Regulation of nociceptive processes	[51]
Gfap	Participates in metabolic exchanges and plasticity	[38, 40–42]
NF-κB	SCN astrocytes mediate the immune signals to the circadian system via NF-κB signaling	[43]
RORα	Participates in the regulation of the inflammatory response (inhibits NF-κB pathway and regulates IL-6 expression)	[44–46]
REV-ERBα/REV-ERB β	Participates in the regulation of the inflammatory response (both isoforms inhibit TNF-induced upregulation of *Ccl-2* and *Mmp-9*; and *REV-ERBα* inhibits *Il-6* upregulation)	[47–50]
GS	Regulation of the glutamatergic system (glutamate-glutamine metabolic cycle)	[51]
	Regulation of various spinal sensory functions	[51]
COX-1	Regulation of various spinal sensory functions	[51]
IP$_3$	Modulates ATP release (IP$_3$-dependent calcium signaling)	[55]
ATP	Regulation of the energy metabolism and glial activity	[55]
Ca^{2+}	Modulation of circadian behavior	[19]
	Regulates the release of gliotransmitters	[35]
Glu	Regulates BMAL1 expression (Glu time- and dose-dependent)	[22]
	Provides the inhibitory astrocytic-neuronal coupling signal during nighttime in the SCN via NMDAR2C	[35]
Microglia		
ATP	Upregulates the *Per1* mRNA expression via P2X7 purinergic receptor subtype	[58]
CatS	Regulates the synaptic strength, including neuronal transmission and spine density via the proteolytic modification of the perineuronal environment	[20, 21, 59]
Bmal1	Implicated in the inflammatory response (modulates *Il-6* upregulation)	[62]
Oligodendrocytes		
Cyclin D1	Regulation of the OPC proliferation	[18]

ATP: adenosine triphosphate; *Bmal1: brain and muscle ARNT-like protein 1*; Ca^{2+}: calcium; CatS: cathepsin S; CGs: clock genes; CCGs: clock-controlled genes; *Ccl-2: monocyte chemoattractant protein-1*; *Clock: circadian locomotor output cycles kaput*; COX-1: *cyclooxygenase-1*; *Cry1: cryptochrome 1*; *Gfap: glial fibrillary acidic protein*; GLAST: glutamate aspartate transporter; Glu: glutamate; *GS: glutamine synthetase*; *Il-6: interleukin-6*; IP$_3$: inositol triphosphate; *Mmp-9: matrix metalloprotease-9*; NF-κB: nuclear factor-kappaB; NMDAR2C: N-methyl-D-aspartate receptor 2C subunit; *Npas2: neuronal PAS domain protein 2*; P2X7: purinoreceptor; OPCs: oligodendrocyte precursor cells; *Per*: period; *REV-ERB*: reverse Erb; RORα: retinoid-related orphan receptor-alpha; SCN: suprachiasmatic nucleus; TNF: tumor necrosis factor.

neurological and psychiatric disorders. Interestingly, clock genes are also involved in variations related with sleep time, sleep fragmentation, and atypical responses following sleep deprivation [83–85]. However, sleep disruptions also have severe consequences in the immune system, leading to an impaired immune function [86, 87]. In line with these reports, it has been established that immune cells exhibit circadian expression of clock genes, which in turn, participate in the regulation of diverse immunological activities. Particularly, *REV-ERB* is involved in neurodegenerative disorders with an inflammatory component [47]. It has been demonstrated that this clock gene represses macrophage gene expression [88] and targets inflammatory function of macrophages through the direct regulation of *Ccl-2* [50]. On the other hand, *Bmal1* controls rhythmic trafficking of inflammatory monocytes to sites of inflammation [89]. Taking these reports together, it is possible to suggest that circadian disruptions exacerbate inflammatory responses in both periphery [90] and CNS [91].

Additionally, it has been shown that *RORα* is an important molecular player in diverse pathological processes including oxidative stress-induced apoptosis and cerebral hypoxia, both in neurons and astrocytes, due to its neuroprotective properties [44].

Finally, abnormal microglial cells are also associated with neurological disorders [92–94]. Taking into consideration that a risk factor for psychiatric diseases is the dysfunction of the clock system, it is relevant to suggest that the microglial clock might be an interesting target for the development of novel neurological therapeutic agents.

4. Conclusion

The expression of clock genes in glial cells has great importance for the maintenance of a healthy brain (Table 1). Actually, clock genes are relevant for the development of novel strategies for the treatment of a wide range of human diseases such as metabolic and cardiovascular diseases, immune system dysfunction, neuropsychiatric disorders, and even cancer. Specifically, changes in the expression of clock genes in glial cells lead to problems related to an imbalance of the glutamatergic system, resulting in neurological disorders; therefore, understanding the role that glial cells play in brain circadian physiology is extremely relevant.

Acknowledgments

Donají Chi-Castañeda is supported by SNI-CONACYT, and the work in the lab (Arturo Ortega) is supported by CONACYT-México (255087) and "*Soluciones para un México Verde S.A. de C.V.*"

References

[1] F. Halberg, "Physiologic 24-hour periodicity; general and procedural considerations with reference to the adrenal cycle," *Internationale Zeitschrift fur Vitaminforschung Beiheft*, vol. 10, pp. 225–296, 1959.

[2] M. Stratmann and U. Schibler, "Properties, entrainment, and physiological functions of mammalian peripheral oscillators," *Journal of Biological Rhythms*, vol. 21, no. 6, pp. 494–506, 2006.

[3] S. M. Reppert and D. R. Weaver, "Coordination of circadian timing in mammals," *Nature*, vol. 418, no. 6901, pp. 935–941, 2002.

[4] P. L. Lowrey and J. S. Takahashi, "Mammalian circadian biology: elucidating genome-wide levels of temporal organization," *Annual Review of Genomics and Human Genetics*, vol. 5, no. 1, pp. 407–441, 2004.

[5] J. C. Dunlap, "Molecular bases for circadian clocks," *Cell*, vol. 96, no. 2, pp. 271–290, 1999.

[6] S. L. Harmer, S. Panda, and S. A. Kay, "Molecular bases of circadian rhythms," *Annual Review of Cell and Developmental Biology*, vol. 17, no. 1, pp. 215–253, 2001.

[7] S. M. Reppert and D. R. Weaver, "Molecular analysis of mammalian circadian rhythms," *Annual Review of Physiology*, vol. 63, no. 1, pp. 647–676, 2001.

[8] N. Preitner, F. Damiola, Luis-Lopez-Molina et al., "The orphan nuclear receptor REV-ERBα controls circadian transcription within the positive limb of the mammalian circadian oscillator," *Cell*, vol. 110, no. 2, pp. 251–260, 2002.

[9] U. Schibler and P. Sassone-Corsi, "A web of circadian pacemakers," *Cell*, vol. 111, no. 7, pp. 919–922, 2002.

[10] K. K. Siwicki, C. Eastman, G. Petersen, M. Rosbash, and J. C. Hall, "Antibodies to the period gene product of Drosophila reveal diverse tissue distribution and rhythmic changes in the visual system," *Neuron*, vol. 1, no. 2, pp. 141–150, 1988.

[11] D. M. Zerr, J. C. Hall, M. Rosbash, and K. K. Siwicki, "Circadian fluctuations of period protein immunoreactivity in the CNS and the visual system of Drosophila," *The Journal of Neuroscience*, vol. 10, no. 8, pp. 2749–2762, 1990.

[12] J. Ewer, B. Frisch, M. J. Hamblen-Coyle, M. Rosbash, and J. C. Hall, "Expression of the period clock gene within different cell types in the brain of Drosophila adults and mosaic analysis of these cells' influence on circadian behavioral rhythms," *The Journal of Neuroscience*, vol. 12, no. 9, pp. 3321–3349, 1992.

[13] K. R. Jessen and W. D. Richardson, *Glial Cell Development: Basic Principles and Clinical Relevance*, Oxford University Press, 2nd edition, 2001.

[14] K. R. Jessen, "Glial cells," *International Journal of Biochemistry and Cell Biology*, vol. 36, no. 10, pp. 1861–1867, 2004.

[15] T. Stork, R. Bernardos, and M. R. Freeman, "Analysis of glial cell development and function in Drosophila," *Cold Spring Harbor Protocols*, vol. 2012, no. 1, pp. 1–17, 2012.

[16] L. E. Clarke and B. A. Barres, "Emerging roles of astrocytes in neural circuit development," *Nature Reviews Neuroscience*, vol. 14, no. 5, pp. 311–321, 2013.

[17] G. C. Brown and J. J. Neher, "Microglial phagocytosis of live neurons," *Nature Reviews Neuroscience*, vol. 15, no. 4, pp. 209–216, 2014.

[18] Y. Matsumoto, Y. Tsunekawa, T. Nomura et al., "Differential proliferation rhythm of neural progenitor and oligodendrocyte precursor cells in the young adult hippocampus," *PLoS ONE*, vol. 6, no. 11, article e27628, 2011.

[19] F. S. Ng, M. M. Tangredi, and F. R. Jackson, "Glial cells physiologically modulate clock neurons and circadian behavior in a calcium-dependent manner," *Current Biology*, vol. 21, no. 8, pp. 625–634, 2011.

[20] Y. Hayashi, S. Koyanagi, N. Kusunose et al., "The intrinsic microglial molecular clock controls synaptic strength via the circadian expression of cathepsin S," *Scientific Reports*, vol. 3, no. 1, p. 2744, 2013.

[21] Y. Hayashi, S. Koyanagi, N. Kusunose et al., "Diurnal spatial rearrangement of microglial processes through the rhythmic expression of P2Y12 receptors," *Journal of Neurological Disorders*, vol. 01, no. 2, pp. 1–7, 2013.

[22] D. Chi-Castañeda, S. M. Waliszewski, R. C. Zepeda, L. C. R. Hernández-Kelly, M. Caba, and A. Ortega, "Glutamate-dependent BMAL1 regulation in cultured Bergmann glia cells," *Neurochemical Research*, vol. 40, no. 5, pp. 961–970, 2015.

[23] L. K. Fonken, M. G. Frank, M. M. Kitt, R. M. Barrientos, L. R. Watkins, and S. F. Maier, "Microglia inflammatory responses are controlled by an intrinsic circadian clock," *Brain, Behavior, and Immunity*, vol. 45, pp. 171–179, 2015.

[24] N. C. Danbolt, D. N. Furness, and Y. Zhou, "Neuronal vs glial glutamate uptake: resolving the conundrum," *Neurochemistry International*, vol. 98, pp. 29–45, 2016.

[25] M. M. Halassa, C. Florian, T. Fellin et al., "Astrocytic modulation of sleep homeostasis and cognitive consequences of sleep loss," *Neuron*, vol. 61, no. 2, pp. 213–219, 2009.

[26] L. A. Newman, D. L. Korol, and P. E. Gold, "Lactate produced by glycogenolysis in astrocytes regulates memory processing," *PLoS One*, vol. 6, no. 12, article e28427, 2011.

[27] A. Suzuki, S. A. Stern, O. Bozdagi et al., "Astrocyte-neuron lactate transport is required for long-term memory formation," *Cell*, vol. 144, no. 5, pp. 810–823, 2011.

[28] J. Han, P. Kesner, M. Metna-Laurent et al., "Acute cannabinoids impair working memory through astroglial CB1 receptor modulation of hippocampal LTD," *Cell*, vol. 148, no. 5, pp. 1039–1050, 2012.

[29] L. M. Prolo, J. S. Takahashi, and E. D. Herzog, "Circadian rhythm generation and entrainment in astrocytes," *Journal of Neuroscience*, vol. 25, no. 2, pp. 404–408, 2005.

[30] K. Yagita, I. Yamanaka, N. Emoto, K. Kawakami, and S. Shimada, "Real-time monitoring of circadian clock oscillations in primary cultures of mammalian cells using Tol2 transposon-mediated gene transfer strategy," *BMC Biotechnology*, vol. 10, no. 1, p. 3, 2010.

[31] R. Spanagel, G. Pendyala, C. Abarca et al., "The clock gene *Per2* influences the glutamatergic system and modulates alcohol consumption," *Nature Medicine*, vol. 11, no. 1, pp. 35–42, 2005.

[32] C. Beaulé, A. Swanstrom, M. J. Leone, and E. D. Herzog, "Circadian modulation of gene expression, but not glutamate uptake, in mouse and rat cortical astrocytes," *PLoS One*, vol. 4, no. 10, article e7476, 2009.

[33] C. Beaulé, D. Granados-Fuentes, L. Marpegan, and E. D. Herzog, "*In vitro* circadian rhythms: imaging and electrophysiology," *Essays in Biochemistry*, vol. 49, no. 1, pp. 103–117, 2011.

[34] N. C. Danbolt, "Glutamate uptake," *Progress in Neurobiology*, vol. 65, no. 1, pp. 1–105, 2001.

[35] M. Brancaccio, A. P. Patton, J. E. Chesham, E. S. Maywood, and M. H. Hastings, "Astrocytes control circadian timekeeping in the suprachiasmatic nucleus via glutamatergic signaling," *Neuron*, vol. 93, no. 6, pp. 1420–1435.e5, 2017.

[36] C. F. Tso, T. Simon, A. C. Greenlaw, T. Puri, M. Mieda, and E. D. Herzog, "Astrocytes regulate daily rhythms in the suprachiasmatic nucleus and behavior," *Current Biology*, vol. 27, no. 7, pp. 1055–1061, 2017.

[37] M. Lavialle and J. Servière, "Circadian fluctuations in GFAP distribution in the Syrian hamster suprachiasmatic nucleus," *Neuroreport*, vol. 4, no. 11, pp. 1243–1246, 1993.

[38] J. Servière and M. Lavialle, "Chapter 5 astrocytes in the mammalian circadian clock: putative roles," *Progress in Brain Research*, vol. 111, pp. 57–73, 1996.

[39] C. Girardet, D. Becquet, M.-P. Blanchard, A. M. François-Bellan, and O. Bosler, "Neuroglial and synaptic rearrangements associated with photic entrainment of the circadian clock in the suprachiasmatic nucleus," *European Journal of Neuroscience*, vol. 32, no. 12, pp. 2133–2142, 2010.

[40] T. Moriya, Y. Yoshinobu, Y. Kouzu et al., "Involvement of glial fibrillary acidic protein (GFAP) expressed in astroglial cells in circadian rhythm under constant lighting conditions in mice," *Journal of Neuroscience Research*, vol. 60, no. 2, pp. 212–218, 2000.

[41] K. Shibuki, H. Gomi, L. Chen et al., "Deficient cerebellar long-term depression, impaired eyeblink conditioning, and normal motor coordination in GFAP mutant mice," *Neuron*, vol. 16, no. 3, pp. 587–599, 1996.

[42] E. Slat, G. M. Freeman, and E. D. Herzog, "The clock in the brain: neurons, glia, and networks in daily rhythms," *Handbook Experimental Pharmacology*, vol. 217, pp. 105–123, 2013.

[43] M. J. Leone, L. Marpegan, T. A. Bekinschtein, M. A. Costas, and D. A. Golombek, "Suprachiasmatic astrocytes as an interface for immune-circadian signalling," *Journal of Neuroscience Research*, vol. 84, no. 7, pp. 1521–1527, 2006.

[44] S. Jolly, N. Journiac, B. Vernet-der Garabedian, and J. Mariani, "RORalpha, a key to the development and functioning of the brain," *The Cerebellum*, vol. 11, no. 2, pp. 451–452, 2012.

[45] P. Delerive, D. Monté, G. Dubois et al., "The orphan nuclear receptor RORα is a negative regulator of the inflammatory response," *EMBO Reports*, vol. 2, no. 1, pp. 42–48, 2001.

[46] N. Journiac, S. Jolly, C. Jarvis et al., "The nuclear receptor RORα exerts a bi-directional regulation of IL-6 in resting and reactive astrocytes," *Proceedings of the National Academy of Sciences of the United States of America*, vol. 106, no. 50, pp. 21365–21370, 2009.

[47] N. Morioka, M. Tomori, F. F. Zhang, M. Saeki, K. Hisaoka-Nakashima, and Y. Nakata, "Stimulation of nuclear receptor REV-ERBs regulates tumor necrosis factor-induced expression of proinflammatory molecules in C6 astroglial cells," *Biochemical and Biophysical Research Communications*, vol. 469, no. 2, pp. 151–157, 2016.

[48] S. N. Ramakrishnan, P. Lau, L. J. Burke, and G. E. O. Muscat, "Reverb regulates the expression of genes involved in lipid absorption in skeletal muscle cells: evidence for cross-talk between orphan nuclear receptors and myokines," *Journal of Biological Chemistry*, vol. 280, no. 10, pp. 8651–8659, 2005.

[49] S. Sato, T. Sakurai, J. Ogasawara et al., "Direct and indirect suppression of interleukin-6 gene expression in murine macrophages by nuclear orphan receptor REV-ERBα," *The Scientific World Journal*, vol. 2014, pp. 1–10, 2014.

[50] S. Sato, T. Sakurai, J. Ogasawara et al., "A circadian clock gene, Rev-erbα, modulates the inflammatory function of macrophages through the negative regulation of *Ccl2* expression," *The Journal of Immunology*, vol. 192, no. 1, pp. 407–417, 2014.

[51] N. Morioka, T. Sugimoto, M. Tokuhara et al., "Spinal astrocytes contribute to the circadian oscillation of glutamine synthase, cyclooxygenase-1 and clock genes in the lumbar spinal cord of mice," *Neurochemistry International*, vol. 60, no. 8, pp. 817–826, 2012.

[52] P. G. Haydon, "GLIA: listening and talking to the synapse," *Nature Reviews Neuroscience*, vol. 2, no. 3, pp. 185–193, 2001.

[53] V. Parpura and R. Zorec, "Gliotransmission: exocytotic release from astrocytes," *Brain Research Reviews*, vol. 63, no. 1-2, pp. 83–92, 2010.

[54] A. D. Womac, J. F. Burkeen, N. Neuendorff, D. J. Earnest, and M. J. Zoran, "Circadian rhythms of extracellular ATP accumulation in suprachiasmatic nucleus cells and cultured

astrocytes," *European Journal of Neuroscience*, vol. 30, no. 5, pp. 869–876, 2009.

[55] L. Marpegan, A. E. Swanstrom, K. Chung et al., "Circadian regulation of ATP release in astrocytes," *Journal of Neuroscience*, vol. 31, no. 23, pp. 8342–8350, 2011.

[56] L. Xu, G. Ruan, H. Dai, A. C. Liu, J. Penn, and D. G. McMahon, "Mammalian retinal Müller cells have circadian clock function," *Molecular Vision*, vol. 22, pp. 275–283, 2016.

[57] G. Tosini and M. Menaker, "Circadian rhythms in cultured mammalian retina," *Science*, vol. 272, no. 5260, pp. 419–421, 1996.

[58] R. Nakazato, T. Takarada, T. Yamamoto, S. Hotta, E. Hinoi, and Y. Yoneda, "Selective upregulation of Per1 mRNA expression by ATP through activation of P2X7 purinergic receptors expressed in microglial cells," *Journal of Pharmacological Sciences*, vol. 116, no. 4, pp. 350–361, 2011.

[59] F. Takayama, X. Zhang, Y. Hayashi, Z. Wu, and H. Nakanishi, "Dysfunction in diurnal synaptic responses and social behavior abnormalities in cathepsin S-deficient mice," *Biochemical and Biophysical Research Communications*, vol. 490, no. 2, pp. 447–452, 2017.

[60] Y. Bhattacharjee, "Is internal timing key to mental health?," *Science*, vol. 317, no. 5844, pp. 1488–1490, 2007.

[61] Y. Hayashi, Z. Wu, and H. Nakanishi, "A possible link between microglial process dysfunction and neuropsychiatric disorders," *Journal of Neurological Disorders and Stroke*, vol. 2, no. 3, pp. 1–5, 2014.

[62] R. Nakazato, S. Hotta, D. Yamada et al., "The intrinsic microglial clock system regulates interleukin-6 expression," *Glia*, vol. 65, no. 1, pp. 198–208, 2017.

[63] U. Fünfschilling, L. M. Supplie, D. Mahad et al., "Glycolytic oligodendrocytes maintain myelin and long-term axonal integrity," *Nature*, vol. 485, no. 7399, pp. 517–521, 2012.

[64] I. A. McKenzie, D. Ohayon, H. Li et al., "Motor skill learning requires active central myelination," *Science*, vol. 346, no. 6207, pp. 318–322, 2014.

[65] L. J. Kochman, E. T. Weber, C. A. Fornal, and B. L. Jacobs, "Circadian variation in mouse hippocampal cell proliferation," *Neuroscience Letters*, vol. 406, no. 3, pp. 256–259, 2006.

[66] C. C. Lee, "Tumor suppression by the mammalian period genes," *Cancer Causes and Control*, vol. 17, no. 4, pp. 525–530, 2006.

[67] D. Chi-Castañeda and A. Ortega, "Clock genes in glia cells: a rhythmic history," *ASN Neuro*, vol. 8, no. 5, pp. 1–13, 2016.

[68] V. Yuferov, G. Bart, and M. J. Kreek, "Clock reset for alcoholism," *Nature Medicine*, vol. 11, no. 1, pp. 23–24, 2005.

[69] A. M. Domingues, M. Taylor, and R. Fern, "Glia as transmitter sources and sensors in health and disease," *Neurochemistry International*, vol. 57, no. 4, pp. 359–366, 2010.

[70] V. Yuferov, T. Kroslak, K. S. Laforge, Y. Zhou, A. Ho, and M. J. Kreek, "Differential gene expression in the rat caudate putamen after binge cocaine administration: advantage of triplicate microarray analysis," *Synapse*, vol. 48, no. 4, pp. 157–169, 2003.

[71] C. Aston, L. Jiang, and B. P. Sokolov, "Microarray analysis of postmortem temporal cortex from patients with schizophrenia," *Journal of Neuroscience Research*, vol. 77, no. 6, pp. 858–866, 2004.

[72] C. M. Nievergelt, D. F. Kripke, T. B. Barrett et al., "Suggestive evidence for association of the circadian genes *PERIOD3* and *ARNTL* with bipolar disorder," *American Journal of Medical Genetics Part B: Neuropsychiatric Genetics*, vol. 141B, no. 3, pp. 234–241, 2006.

[73] F. Benedetti, S. Dallaspezia, C. Colombo, A. Pirovano, E. Marino, and E. Smeraldi, "A length polymorphism in the circadian clock gene Per3 influences age at onset of bipolar disorder," *Neuroscience Letters*, vol. 445, no. 2, pp. 184–187, 2008.

[74] N. Krishnan, D. Kretzschmar, K. Rakshit, E. Chow, and J. M. Giebultowicz, "The circadian clock gene *period* extends healthspan in aging *Drosophila melanogaster*," *Aging*, vol. 1, no. 11, pp. 937–948, 2009.

[75] J. R. Gerstner, "The aging clock: to 'BMAL'icious toward learning and memory," *Aging*, vol. 2, no. 5, pp. 251–254, 2010.

[76] Z. Gu, B. B. Wang, Y. B. Zhang et al., "Association of *ARNTL* and *PER1* genes with Parkinson's disease: a case-control study of Han Chinese," *Scientific Reports*, vol. 5, no. 1, p. 15891, 2015.

[77] H. Song, M. Moon, H. K. Choe et al., "Aβ-induced degradation of BMAL1 and CBP leads to circadian rhythm disruption in Alzheimer's disease," *Molecular Neurodegeneration*, vol. 10, no. 1, p. 13, 2015.

[78] R. Andretic, S. Chaney, and J. Hirsh, "Requirement of circadian genes for cocaine sensitization in Drosophila," *Science*, vol. 285, no. 5430, pp. 1066–1068, 1999.

[79] A. B. Niculescu 3rd, D. S. Segal, R. Kuczenski, T. Barrett, R. L. Hauger, and J. R. Kelsoe, "Identifying a series of candidate genes for mania and psychosis: a convergent functional genomics approach," *Physiological Genomics*, vol. 4, no. 1, pp. 83–91, 2000.

[80] R. V. Bhat and S. L. Budd, "GSK3β signalling: casting a wide net in Alzheimer's disease," *Neuro-Signals*, vol. 11, no. 5, pp. 251–261, 2002.

[81] V. Soria, E. Martínez-Amorós, G. Escaramís et al., "Differential association of circadian genes with mood disorders: CRY1 and NPAS2 are associated with unipolar major depression and CLOCK and VIP with bipolar disorder," *Neuropsychopharmacology*, vol. 35, no. 6, pp. 1279–1289, 2010.

[82] P. A. Geoffroy, M. Lajnef, F. Bellivier et al., "Genetic association study of circadian genes with seasonal pattern in bipolar disorders," *Scientific Reports*, vol. 5, no. 1, p. 10232, 2015.

[83] E. Naylor, B. M. Bergmann, K. Krauski et al., "The circadian *clock* mutation alters sleep homeostasis in the mouse," *The Journal of Neuroscience*, vol. 20, no. 21, pp. 8138–8143, 2000.

[84] J. P. Wisor, B. F. O'Hara, A. Terao et al., "A role for cryptochromes in sleep regulation," *BMC Neuroscience*, vol. 3, no. 1, p. 20, 2002.

[85] A. Laposky, A. Easton, C. Dugovic, J. Walisser, C. Bradfield, and F. Turek, "Deletion of the mammalian circadian clock gene *BMAL1/Mop3* alters baseline sleep architecture and the response to sleep deprivation," *Sleep*, vol. 28, no. 4, pp. 395–410, 2005.

[86] M. Irwin, J. McClintick, C. Costlow, M. Fortner, J. White, and J. C. Gillin, "Partial night sleep deprivation reduces natural killer and cellular immune responses in humans," *FASEB Journal*, vol. 10, no. 5, pp. 643–653, 1996.

[87] J. Born, T. Lange, K. Hansen, M. Mölle, and H. L. Fehm, "Effects of sleep and circadian rhythm on human circulating immune cells," *The Journal of Immunology*, vol. 158, no. 9, pp. 4454–4464, 1997.

[88] M. T. Y. Lam, H. Cho, H. P. Lesch et al., "Rev-Erbs repress macrophage gene expression by inhibiting enhancer-directed transcription," *Nature*, vol. 498, no. 7455, pp. 511–515, 2013.

[89] K. D. Nguyen, S. J. Fentress, Y. Qiu, K. Yun, J. S. Cox, and A. Chawla, "Circadian gene *Bmal1* regulates diurnal oscillations of Ly6C^{hi} inflammatory monocytes," *Science*, vol. 341, no. 6153, pp. 1483–1488, 2013.

[90] O. Castanon-Cervantes, M. Wu, J. C. Ehlen et al., "Dysregulation of inflammatory responses by chronic circadian disruption," *Journal of Immunology*, vol. 185, no. 10, pp. 5796–5805, 2010.

[91] L. K. Fonken, Z. M. Weil, and R. J. Nelson, "Mice exposed to dim light at night exaggerate inflammatory responses to lipopolysaccharide," *Brain, Behavior, and Immunity*, vol. 34, pp. 159–163, 2013.

[92] K. Saijo and C. K. Glass, "Microglial cell origin and phenotypes in health and disease," *Nature Reviews Immunology*, vol. 11, no. 11, pp. 775–787, 2011.

[93] J.-P. Louboutin and D. S. Strayer, "Relationship between the chemokine receptor CCR5 and microglia in neurological disorders: consequences of targeting CCR5 on neuroinflammation, neuronal death and regeneration in a model of epilepsy," *CNS and Neurological Disorders Drug Targets*, vol. 12, no. 6, pp. 815–829, 2013.

[94] Y. Nakagawa and K. Chiba, "Diversity and plasticity of microglial cells in psychiatric and neurological disorders," *Pharmacology and Therapeutics*, vol. 154, pp. 21–35, 2015.

5

Cardiac Arrest Induces Ischemic Long-Term Potentiation of Hippocampal CA1 Neurons That Occludes Physiological Long-Term Potentiation

James E. Orfila,[1] **Nicole McKinnon,**[2] **Myriam Moreno,**[1] **Guiying Deng,**[3] **Nicholas Chalmers,**[1] **Robert M. Dietz,**[2] **Paco S. Herson,**[1,3] **and Nidia Quillinan**[1]

[1]*Neuronal Injury Program, Department of Anesthesiology, University of Colorado, Anschutz Medical Campus, Aurora, CO 80045, USA*

[2]*Department of Pediatrics, University of Colorado, Anschutz Medical Campus, Aurora, CO 80045, USA*

[3]*Department of Pharmacology, University of Colorado, Anschutz Medical Campus, Aurora, CO 80045, USA*

Correspondence should be addressed to Nidia Quillinan; nidia.quillinan@ucdenver.edu

Academic Editor: Paola Bonsi

Ischemic long-term potentiation (iLTP) is a form of synaptic plasticity that occurs in acute brain slices following oxygen-glucose deprivation. *In vitro*, iLTP can occlude physiological LTP (pLTP) through saturation of plasticity mechanisms. We used our murine cardiac arrest and cardiopulmonary resuscitation (CA/CPR) model to produce global brain ischemia and assess whether iLTP is induced *in vivo*, contributing to the functionally relevant impairment of pLTP. Adult male mice were subjected to CA/CPR, and slice electrophysiology was performed in the hippocampal CA1 region 7 or 30 days later. We observed increased miniature excitatory postsynaptic current amplitudes, suggesting a potentiation of postsynaptic AMPA receptor function after CA/CPR. We also observed increased phosphorylated GluR1 in the postsynaptic density of hippocampi after CA/CPR. These data support the *in vivo* induction of ischemia-induced plasticity. Application of a low-frequency stimulus (LFS) to CA1 inputs reduced excitatory postsynaptic potentials in slices from mice subjected to CA/CPR, while having no effects in sham controls. These results are consistent with a reversal, or depotentiation, of iLTP. Further, depotentiation with LFS partially restored induction of pLTP with theta burst stimulation. These data provide evidence for iLTP following *in vivo* ischemia, which occludes pLTP and likely contributes to network disruptions that underlie memory impairments.

1. Introduction

Ischemic long-term potentiation (iLTP) is an increase in excitatory synaptic strength that occurs immediately following oxygen and glucose deprivation (OGD) in acute brain slices [1–6]. Elevations in extracellular glutamate during OGD cause prolonged activation of postsynaptic α-amino-3-hydroxy-5-methyl-4-isoxazolepropionic acid (AMPA) and N-methyl-D-aspartic acid (NMDA) receptors, resulting in an influx of sodium and calcium. Rises in intracellular calcium stimulate calcium/calmodulin-dependent protein kinase (CAMKII) signaling, which potentiates postsynaptic excitatory function via increased AMPA receptor phosphorylation and expression at the synapse. There is some indirect evidence to support that iLTP occurs following *in vivo* ischemia. Previously, we demonstrated increased activation of CAMKII within hours of global ischemia induced by cardiac arrest [7]. There is also evidence to support acute activation of CAMKII and increased NMDA receptor expression in the hippocampus within hours of *in vivo* focal ischemia [8]. However, it is unknown whether acute activation of CAMKII seen following *in vivo* ischemia causes synaptic potentiation in the hippocampus or whether ischemic LTP is maintained for days beyond the ischemic event.

Shared mechanisms between ischemic and physiologic LTP suggest that it is likely these plasticity processes would occlude one another, as has been described in studies where acute hippocampal brain slices were subjected to *in vitro* ischemia [3, 4]. Physiological hippocampal long-term potentiation (pLTP) is an experience- or frequency-dependent increase in synaptic strength and is a cellular substrate for learning and memory. Similar to iLTP, pLTP occurs through an NMDA and CAMKII-dependent increase in synaptic AMPA receptor function [9–12]. Memory deficits in cardiac arrest survivors are attributed to ischemic injury to the hippocampus that causes loss of pyramidal CA1 neurons [13, 14]. In addition to neuronal cell death, global ischemia causes persistent deficits in pLTP in surviving neurons of the CA1 [7, 15–19]. Therefore, pLTP deficits caused by brain ischemia likely contribute to memory deficits, and therapies that restore pLTP have the potential to improve cognitive function after CA/CPR. Acute neuroprotective interventions that reduce CA1 injury can also prevent pLTP deficits; however, there is no strategy that targets LTP deficits at delayed time points and that is independent of preventing neuronal cell death [7, 15, 19, 20]. The goal of this study was to determine whether *in vivo* global ischemia from cardiac arrest causes ischemic LTP that prevents physiological LTP.

2. Methods

2.1. Experimental Animals and Cardiac Arrest Model. The Institutional Animal Care and Use Committee (IACUC) at the University of Colorado approved all experimental protocols in accordance with the National Institutes of Health and guidelines for the care and use of animals in research. Analysis was performed with investigators blinded to experimental groups. Adult (8–12-week-old) male C57Bl6 (Charles River, Wilmington, MA) mice were subjected to CA/CPR as previously described during the ON light cycle [21–23]. A total of 54 animals were included in this study.

Briefly, anesthesia was induced with 3% isoflurane and maintained with 1.5–2% isoflurane in oxygen-enriched air using a nose cone. Temperature probes were inserted in the left ear and rectum to monitor tympanic (head) and body temperature simultaneously. A PE-10 catheter was inserted into the right internal jugular vein for drug administration. Needle electrodes were placed subcutaneously on the chest for continuous electrocardiogram (EKG) monitoring. Animals were endotracheally intubated and connected to a mouse ventilator (MiniVent Ventilator, Harvard Apparatus). Cardiac arrest was induced with injection of 50 μl KCl (0.5 M) via the jugular catheter and confirmed by asystole on EKG. During cardiac arrest, the endotracheal tube was disconnected, anesthesia stopped, and body temperature was allowed to spontaneously decrease to a minimum of 35.5°C, and head temperature was maintained at 37.5°C. Resuscitation began eight minutes after induction of cardiac arrest by slow injection of 0.5–1.0 ml epinephrine solution (16 μg epinephrine/ml 0.9% saline), chest compressions, and ventilation with 100% oxygen at a respiratory rate of 200 breaths/min. Chest compressions were stopped as soon as spontaneous circulation was restored. Resuscitation was abandoned if spontaneous circulation was not restored within 2.5 minutes. Mice were extubated after they recovered an adequate respiratory rate and effort. Sham controls

underwent the same procedures as mice undergoing cardiac arrest including anesthesia, intubation, placement of the jugular catheter, EKG leads, and temperature management. Sham controls did not receive KCl or epinephrine injections or chest compressions. The animals were placed in a single-housed static recovery cage on a heated water blanket (35°C) for the first 24 hours of recovery and at ambient room temperature for long-term recovery (up to 30 days). Mice received soft food and subcutaneous saline for 3 days after surgery and had free access to water and regular chow.

2.2. Acute Slice Preparation. Following CA/CPR or sham surgery, mice were anesthetized with isoflurane (3.5%) and transcardially perfused with ice-cold artificial cerebral spinal fluid (ACSF) containing (in mmol/l) 126 NaCl, 2.5 KCl, 2.5 CaCl$_2$, 1.2 MgCl$_2$, 1.2 NaH$_2$PO$_4$, 21.4 NaHCO$_3$, and 11 D-glucose, bubbled with 95% O$_2$/5% CO$_2$ to maintain pH of 7.4. Mice were decapitated and brains were rapidly removed. Horizontal hippocampal sections (300 μM) were cut in ice-cold ACSF using a VT1200S Vibratome (Leica, Buffalo Grove, IL, USA) and then maintained at room temperature for at least 30 minutes prior to recording.

2.3. Miniature Excitatory Postsynaptic Currents (mEPSCs). Whole-cell recordings were performed at room temperature (22°C) in a submersion chamber and were continuously perfused with ACSF containing picrotoxin (PTX, 100 μM) and tetrodotoxin (TTX, 250 nM). Recordings were obtained using borosilicate glass pipettes that were fabricated using a Flaming/Brown heat puller (Sutter Instruments, Novato, CA, USA) to a resistance of 2–4 MΩ. Internal recording solution contained (in mmol/l) 120 K-gluconate, 9 KCl, 10 KOH, 4 NaCl, 10 HEPES, 0.05 EGTA, 1 MgCl$_2$, 4 Na$_2$ATP, and 0.4 Na$_2$GTP. Series resistance was <20 MΩ and did not change more than 20% during the experiment. Whole-cell voltage-clamp recordings were performed at a holding potential of −70 mV. Gap-free continuous recordings were acquired in 3-minute sweeps. Miniature events were identified using Clampfit software with template event detection, and mEPSC amplitude and frequency were quantified for each cell. To generate cumulative probability histograms events from all sham or CA/CPR, mice were pooled.

2.4. Extracellular Field Recording. For extracellular recordings, slices were transferred to an interface recording chamber that was continuously perfused with ACSF (1.5 ml/min) and warmed to 32°C. Extracellular field excitatory postsynaptic potentials (fEPSPs) recorded in the stratum radiatum were evoked with a bipolar stimulus electrode positioned in the stratum molecularae/luminaris to evoke glutamate release from Schaffer collaterals (0.05 Hz). Input-output curves were generated by increasing stimulus intensity in 10 μA increments and recording fEPSP slopes. Stimulus intensity was adjusted to produce a fEPSP with a slope that was 50% of the maximum. A stable baseline fEPSP was recorded for 20 minutes before theta burst stimulation (TBS; 10 trains of 4–100 Hz pulses) was applied to Schaffer collaterals. fEPSPs were recorded for 60 minutes following TBS, and percent change from baseline was calculated for the last 10 minutes of the recording. Low-frequency stimulation (LFS) was delivered for 10 minutes (900 pulses at 0.5 Hz), and percent change from baseline was analyzed 20 minutes after LFS. Data were compressed to 1-minute averages, and the extent of LTP or depotentiation was measured as percentage of the baseline fEPSP slope during the last 10 minutes of the recording.

2.5. Western Blot Analysis. Following CA/CPR or sham surgery, mice were deeply anesthetized with isoflurane (3.5%), heads were decapitated and brains were rapidly removed. Hippocampi were isolated and rapidly frozen with 2-methylbutane on dry ice. Individual hippocampi were homogenized in sucrose buffer containing protease and phosphatase inhibitors using a PTFE tissue grinder in a glass tube. Homogenates were centrifuged at 1000 ×g for 10 minutes to remove cellular debris and nuclei. Supernatant was removed and spun at 10,000 ×g for 15 minutes. This supernatant was collected and spun at 100,000 ×g for 60 minutes, yielding a supernatant that contains the cytosolic cellular fraction (S3). The pellet (P2) was resuspended in triton buffer and then centrifuged at 32,000 ×g for 20 minutes, yielding a pellet (P4) that contains the postsynaptic density (PSD) fraction. This pellet was resuspended in N-PER buffer (Thermo Fisher, Waltham, MA) containing protease and phosphatase inhibitors. The PSD protein concentration was quantified using a BCA kit, and samples were diluted in 4x denaturing sample buffer to a final concentration of 1 μg/μl. Protein (20 μg) was loaded onto a polyacrylamide gel for protein electrophoresis and transferred to a PVDF membrane. Membranes were blocked in Tris-buffered saline with Tween (TBS-T) containing 5% BSA or milk. Primary antibody incubations were performed overnight at 4°C and detected using horseradish peroxidase-conjugated secondary antibodies. Bands were visualized using a maximum sensitivity-enhanced chemiluminescence substrate with the ChemiDoc Gel Imaging System (Bio-Rad, Hercules, CA). Multiple antibodies were probed on each membrane by stripping with Restore Plus stripping buffer after chemiluminescent detection. Integrated volume of bands was normalized to beta-actin integrated volume for that sample. Normalized protein expression is presented relative to sham controls.

2.6. Statistics. For electrophysiology experiments, n indicates the number of recordings with no more than two recordings for a given experiment from a single animal. Data are presented as mean ± SEM. Statistical comparisons were made between two groups using Student's t-test and multiple groups using one-way analysis of variance (ANOVA) followed by Dunnett's post hoc comparison of groups relative to control. Statistical comparisons were performed using GraphPad Prism 7.0. Differences with a p value of <0.05 were considered significant.

3. Results

3.1. Increased AMPA Receptor Function following In Vivo Ischemia. The expression of LTP occurs through an increase in AMPA receptor function resulting from phosphorylation and increased synaptic expression. To directly measure postsynaptic AMPA receptor function, we performed whole-cell recording of miniature EPSCs (mEPSCs) in CA1 neurons 7 days after CA/CPR. Delayed neuronal cell death occurs at 2-3 days postinjury; therefore, by 7 days postinjury, cell death processes are complete and electrophysiology can be performed in surviving neurons that exhibit LTP deficits [7, 19, 22, 24]. Miniature excitatory events were isolated using tetrodotoxin (TTX, 250 nM) and picrotoxin (PTX, 100 μM) (Figure 1(a)). Mean mEPSC amplitude, kinetics, and frequency were analyzed using Clampfit template event detection. Cumulative frequency distributions of mEPSC amplitudes were generated by pooling events from recordings in sham ($n = 2,729$ events) and CA/CPR ($n = 3,213$ events). The cumulative frequency curve was right-shifted in mice after CA/CPR compared to sham controls, with larger maximum amplitudes (110.7 pA versus 56.2 pA) (Figure 1(b)). The shift to larger events was also detected as an increase in the mean mEPSC amplitude from $16.43 ± 0.94$ ($n = 12$) to $20.74 ± 1.1$ ($n = 15$; $p = 0.008$) (Figure 1(c)). Rise and decay kinetics of mEPSCs were not different between shams and controls (Table 1). There were also no changes in the biophysical properties of neurons that would account for the larger amplitude mEPSCs observed after CA/CPR (Table 1). Event frequency was similar in sham ($1.4 ± 0.4$, $n = 12$) and cardiac arrest mice ($1.4 ± 0.3$, $n = 15$; $p = 0.95$) (Figure 1(d)), indicating no change in synapse number. These data suggest there is increased postsynaptic AMPA receptor function at CA1 synapses following CA/CPR.

Synaptic potentiation results from NMDA receptor-dependent activation of CAMKII and the subsequent increase in AMPA receptor phosphorylation and expression at postsynaptic sites. Previously, we reported an acute increase in CAMKII activity (T286 phosphorylation) in the hippocampus 3-hour post-CA/CPR, suggesting an ischemia-induced increase in CAMKII activation [7]. To determine whether there are changes in glutamate receptor phosphorylation and expression at delayed time points after cardiac arrest, we isolated the hippocampus from shams and 7 days after CA/CPR, and protein fractions enriched for postsynaptic densities were subjected to Western blot analysis (Figure 2(a)). We observed an increase in levels of phosphorylated AMPA receptors (GluR1 pS831) from $1.01 ± 0.03$ ($n = 7$) in shams to $1.23 ± 0.1$ ($n = 6$) at 7 days postinjury ($p = 0.047$), consistent with an increase in receptor function (Figure 2(b)). GluR1 AMPA receptor expression (sham: $1 ± 0.16$, $n = 7$; CA/CPR: $1.28 ± 0.22$, $n = 7$) and GluR2/3 expression (sham: $1 ± 0.2$, $n = 5$; CA/CPR: $1.25 ± 0.16$, $n = 4$) were not different after cardiac arrest ($p = 0.312$ and $p = 0.36$, resp.) (Figures 2(c) and 2(d)). Ischemic LTP caused by *in vitro* ischemia can increase NMDA expression [8]. We observed a small increase in NMDA receptor (GluN1) from $1 ± 0.14$ ($n = 5$) to $1.38 ± 0.21$ ($n = 4$) expression that was not significant ($p = 0.1675$) (Figure 2(e)). Finally, we saw no change in PSD-95 levels after cardiac arrest (sham: $1 ± 0.1$, $n = 7$; CA/CPR: $1.05 ± 0.21$, $n = 7$; $p = 0.823$), suggesting no changes in the overall synapse density (Figure 2(f)). These data are consistent with our mEPSC data

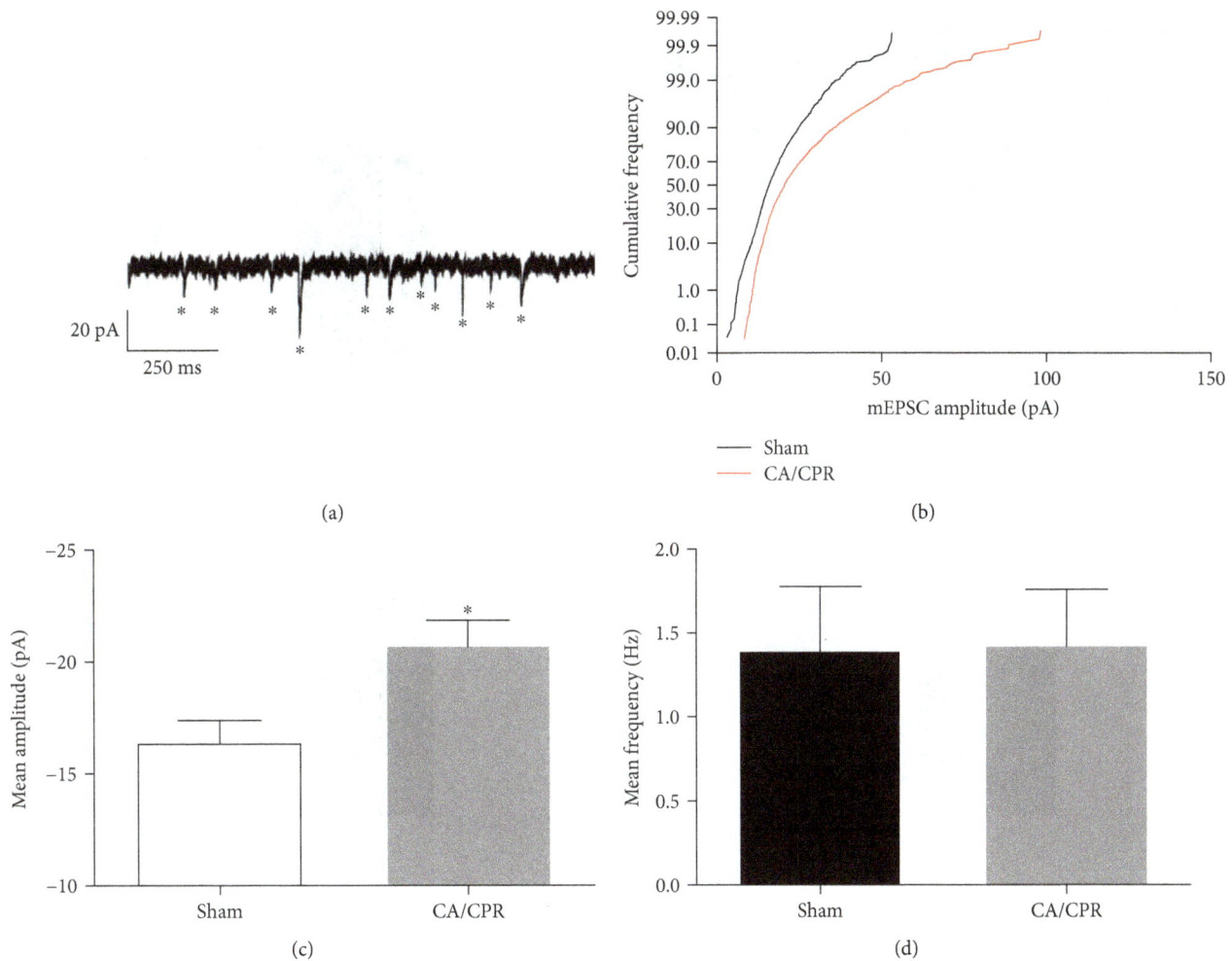

(a)

(b)

(c)

(d)

FIGURE 1: Lasting potentiation of miniature excitatory postsynaptic currents (mEPSCs) induced by cardiac arrest. (a) A representative trace from a sham control of whole-cell voltage clamp recording of mEPSC events recorded from CA1 neurons in acute brain slices. Events were detected with Clampfit software and are indicated with an asterisk. (b) CA/CPR produced a rightward shift in the cumulative frequency distribution of mEPSC amplitudes relative to shams. Events from sham (black, $n = 2729$ events) or CA/CPR (red, $n = 3213$ events) mice were pooled to generate histograms. (c) CA/CPR produced an increase in mean mEPSC amplitudes compared to sham. Mean mEPSC amplitude was calculated for each recording (sham: $n = 12$; CA/CPR: $n = 15$), and means for groups were compared using Student's unpaired t-test ($*$ indicates $p < 0.05$). (d) CA/CPR did not alter synaptic density in CA1 neurons. No change in mean mEPSC frequency was observed between sham and CA/CPR mice. Mean mEPSC frequency was calculated for each recording (sham: $n = 12$; CA/CPR: $n = 15$), and means for groups were compared using Student's unpaired t-test.

TABLE 1

	Sham	7 days	30 days	p value
R_m (MW)	281.0 ± 30.85 ($n = 10$)	230.6 ± 38.65 ($n = 16$)		0.367
C_m (pF)	5.738 ± 1.360 ($n = 10$)	9.224 ± 1.845 ($n = 16$)		0.1893
PPR (pulse 1/pulse 2)	1.32 ± 0.1 ($n = 5$)	1.30 ± 0.08 ($n = 8$)	1.33 ± 0.07 ($n = 4$)	0.889
I/O (slope)	3.65 ± 0.59 ($n = 6$)	4.57 ± 0.33 ($n = 6$)	3.85 ± 0.78 ($n = 6$)	0.548
EPSC rise time (ms)	2.68 ± 0.27 ($n = 12$)	2.37 ± 0.17 ($n = 15$)		0.3271
EPSC decay time (ms)	11.60 ± 1.08 ($n = 12$)	12.55 ± 0.99 ($n = 15$)		0.5273

showing increased amplitude and no change in frequency of mEPSC events.

3.2. Depotentiation Restores the Ability to Induce Physiological LTP in Postischemic Neurons. Depotentiation,

which is the reversal of LTP, is induced with low-frequency stimulation of synapses that were previously given high-frequency stimulation to induce LTP [25–28]. We hypothesized that ischemic LTP following CA/CPR would be reversed with a depotentiation stimulus.

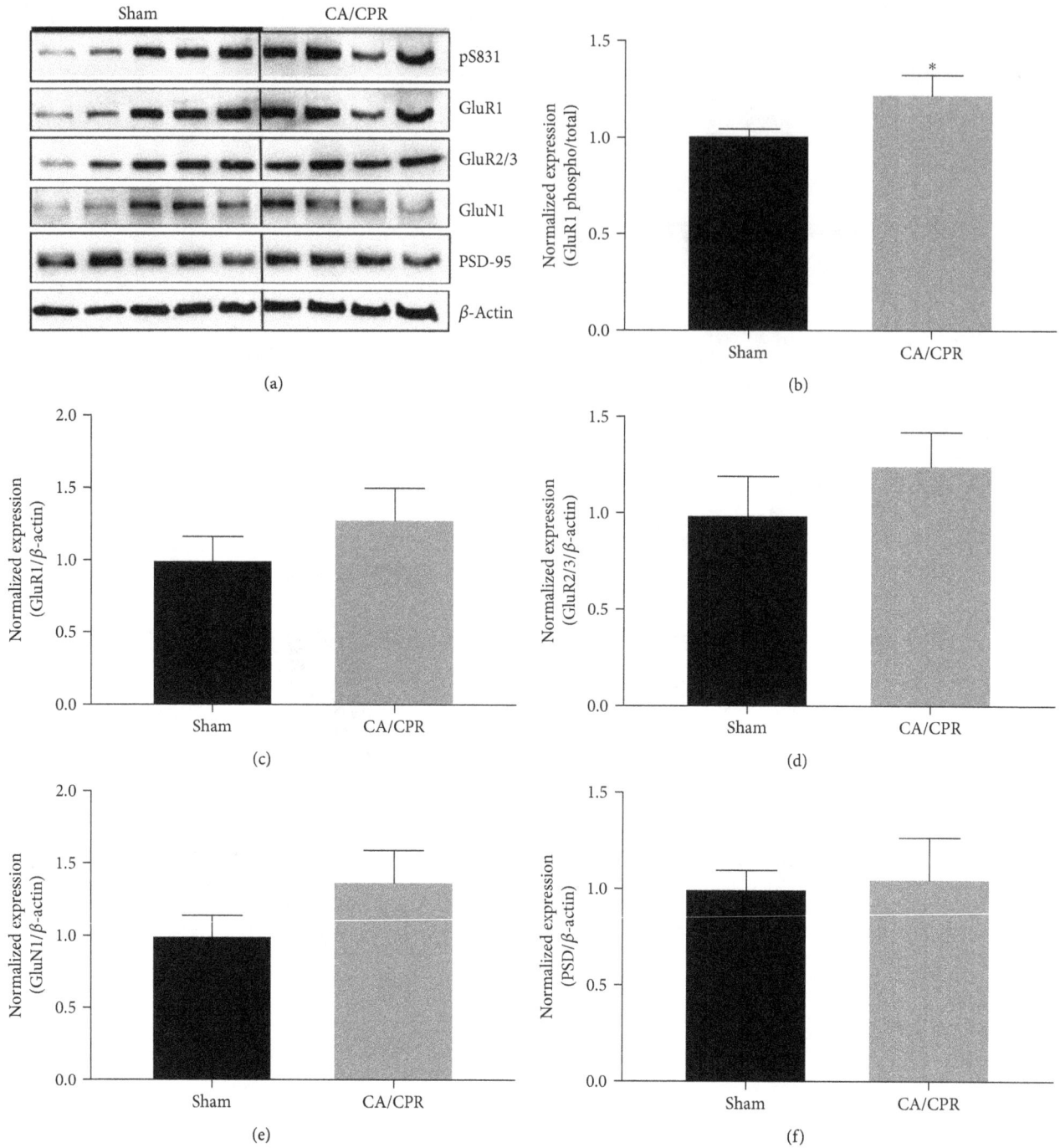

(a)

(b)

(c)

(d)

(e)

(f)

FIGURE 2: Increased AMPA receptor phosphorylation after CA/CPR. (a) Representative blots of protein expression from synaptic fractions of sham and CA/CPR hippocampus. Blots were cropped to show bands at molecular weight for indicated proteins. (b) Normalized phosphorylated S831: total GluR1 expression was calculated for each sample by dividing optical density of phosphoS831 by total GluR1 density within the same blot. (c) Normalized GluR1 expression was calculated for each sample by dividing optical density of total GluR1 by β-actin density within the same blot. (d) Normalized GluR2/3 expression was calculated for each sample by dividing optical density of total GluR2/3 by β-actin density within the same blot. (e) Normalized GluN1 expression was calculated for each sample by dividing optical density of total GluN1 by β-actin density within the same blot. (f) Normalized PSD-95 expression was calculated for each sample by dividing optical density of PSD-95 by β-actin density within the same blot. Values were normalized to sham controls. Shams ($n = 7$) and CA/CPR ($n = 6$) groups were compared using Student's t-test. $*$ indicates $p < 0.05$.

Previous studies use stimulation frequencies ranging between 0.5 and 2 Hz to depotentiate pLTP without inducing long-term depression (LTD). We found that 900 pulses, delivered at 0.5 Hz, reversed LTP that was induced by a previous theta burst stimulation (TBS) from $182.5 \pm 7.7\%$ to $132.7 \pm 15.4\%$ of baseline amplitude ($n = 5$). Importantly, this LFS protocol did not induce LTD in naive controls, having no effect on fEPSP slope from baseline following LFS ($n = 6$; $p = 0.13$) (Figure 3(a)), thus fitting the definition of a depotentiation protocol.

We next tested whether a depotentiation LFS protocol was capable of reducing synaptic strength in mice subjected to CA/CPR, thus providing further evidence of sustained iLTP. In sham controls, fEPSP slopes were $110 \pm 4.2\%$ ($n = 6$) of baseline after LFS, an increase that was not statistically significant ($p = 0.06$) (Figure 3(b)). Acute slices prepared 7 days after CA/CPR showed a decrease in fEPSP slope to $83 \pm 10.6\%$ ($n = 7$) of baseline after LFS, a change that was not statistically different from baseline ($p = 0.2$) but was significantly different than the change observed in controls ($p = 0.007$). At 30 days after CA/CPR, the change in fEPSP slope to $75.73 \pm 7.0\%$ ($n = 5$) of baseline after LFS was significantly different from baseline ($p = 0.015$) and from the change observed in controls ($p = 0.002$). This provides additional evidence for CA1 synapses being in a potentiated state following *in vivo* ischemia.

The induction of ischemic LTP by CA/CPR may occlude physiological LTP. To test this, we delivered LFS to induce depotentiation and followed this with TBS in slices from mice at 7 days postinjury. After acquiring a stable 10-minute baseline, we delivered LFS, resulting in a decrease of fEPSP slope to $87.7 \pm 0.4\%$ ($n = 5$) of baseline (Figure 3(c), dotted line). After 20 minutes, we delivered TBS, which increased fEPSP slope to $115.1 \pm 6.1\%$ of original baseline, a potentiation of 28% ($p = 0.015$) (Figure 3(c), shaded blue). These data suggest that LTP mechanisms are saturated, and that reversal of ischemic LTP with LFS partially restores the capacity to induce physiological LTP.

4. Discussion

We have provided several pieces of evidence for the presence of sustained ischemic LTP subsequent to *in vivo* global ischemia caused by cardiac arrest: (1) increased postsynaptic glutamate receptor function, (2) increased postsynaptic glutamate receptor phosphorylation, and (3) the ability to depotentiate CA1 synapses after cardiac arrest. Further, we have shown that ischemic LTP occludes physiological LTP, providing a possible target for interventional strategies to improve memory function after cardiac arrest.

To our knowledge, this is the first study to demonstrate that *in vivo* ischemia causes synaptic alterations that are consistent with ischemic LTP. Until now, all electrophysiological evidence for this phenomenon comes from *in vitro* studies using oxygen and glucose deprivation in slices. Therefore, by showing that this phenomenon occurs in vivo, we suggest that this is a mechanism through which memory impairment occurs. Ischemic LTP is similar to physiological LTP in its NMDA receptor dependence, activation of intracellular signaling, and an increase in postsynaptic AMPA receptor function [3, 5]. The stimulus for inducing ischemic LTP is the massive increase in extracellular glutamate that occurs within minutes of the onset of ischemia [29–33]. Importantly, it is this massive increase in extracellular glutamate that stimulates excitotoxic cell death. By enhancing postsynaptic responses to extracellular glutamate, ischemic LTP likely amplifies excitotoxicity mechanisms [34, 35], but it is unclear

from *in vitro* studies what contribution this phenomenon has to CA1 injury after CA/CPR. Similarly, it is difficult to disentangle ischemic LTP and excitotoxicity *in vivo*, as they have similar induction mechanisms. Previous work from our laboratory and others has shown that pharmacological or genetic interventions reduce NMDA receptor activation or CAMKII activation, not only reducing neuronal cell death but also preserving physiological LTP [7, 19]. It is possible that neuroprotective strategies prevent LTP impairments, in part, by blocking ischemic LTP.

Our strongest evidence for ischemic LTP comes from electrophysiological recordings that demonstrate increased miniature EPSC amplitude. The advantage of this method is that we can specifically assess postsynaptic receptor function in CA1 region of the hippocampus. In our recording conditions, increased mEPSC amplitudes likely represent increased AMPA rather than NMDA receptor function. Other groups have reported that iLTP observed at acute time points is a result of increased expression and function of NMDA receptors [1, 3, 8]. However, we have previously demonstrated no change in NMDA receptor function or expression at 7 days after CA/CPR, consistent with our results here [19, 20]. These differences may be due to the use of *in vivo* versus *in vitro* models, or that our studies were performed days, rather than hours after the ischemic insult. Analysis of glutamate receptor expression performed here was from the synaptic fraction of the entire hippocampus, not just the CA1 region. Therefore, increases in CA1 receptor expression may be underrepresented within this pool. Regardless, our Western blot data provided evidence for increased phosphorylation of the GluR1 AMPA receptor subunit, which is consistent with our electrophysiological data. There have been mixed results as to whether iLTP has a presynaptic mechanism [3, 6]. We failed to detect differences in paired-pulse ratio, suggesting a postsynaptic mechanism for iLTP induced by CA/CPR. Others have reported that impaired hippocampal LTP following global ischemia is associated with reduced spine densities [36–38]. However, we did not detect a reduction in mEPSC frequency and PSD-95 expression, which are indirect measures of the number of synapses. Therefore, our data is consistent with ischemia-induced changes in plasticity without changes in the number of functional synapses. However, further experiments are needed to rule out an ischemia effect on spine density that may contribute to impaired synaptic plasticity.

Physiological LTP and ischemic LTP have shared mechanisms and, therefore, have the ability to occlude one another. Indeed, tetanic stimulation delivered just prior to OGD prevents ischemic LTP and vice versa [4–6]. Remarkably, we saw that depotentiation prior to theta burst stimulation allowed for the induction of physiological LTP. Therefore, these results support in vitro findings that ischemic LTP saturates plasticity mechanisms to occlude physiological LTP. The stimulus frequency used to depotentiate had no effect on naive control slices, giving us confidence that we induced the depotentiation of synapses, rather than inducing long-term depression, which has different signaling mechanisms. While there was some physiological LTP following depotentiation, LFS did not restore completely back

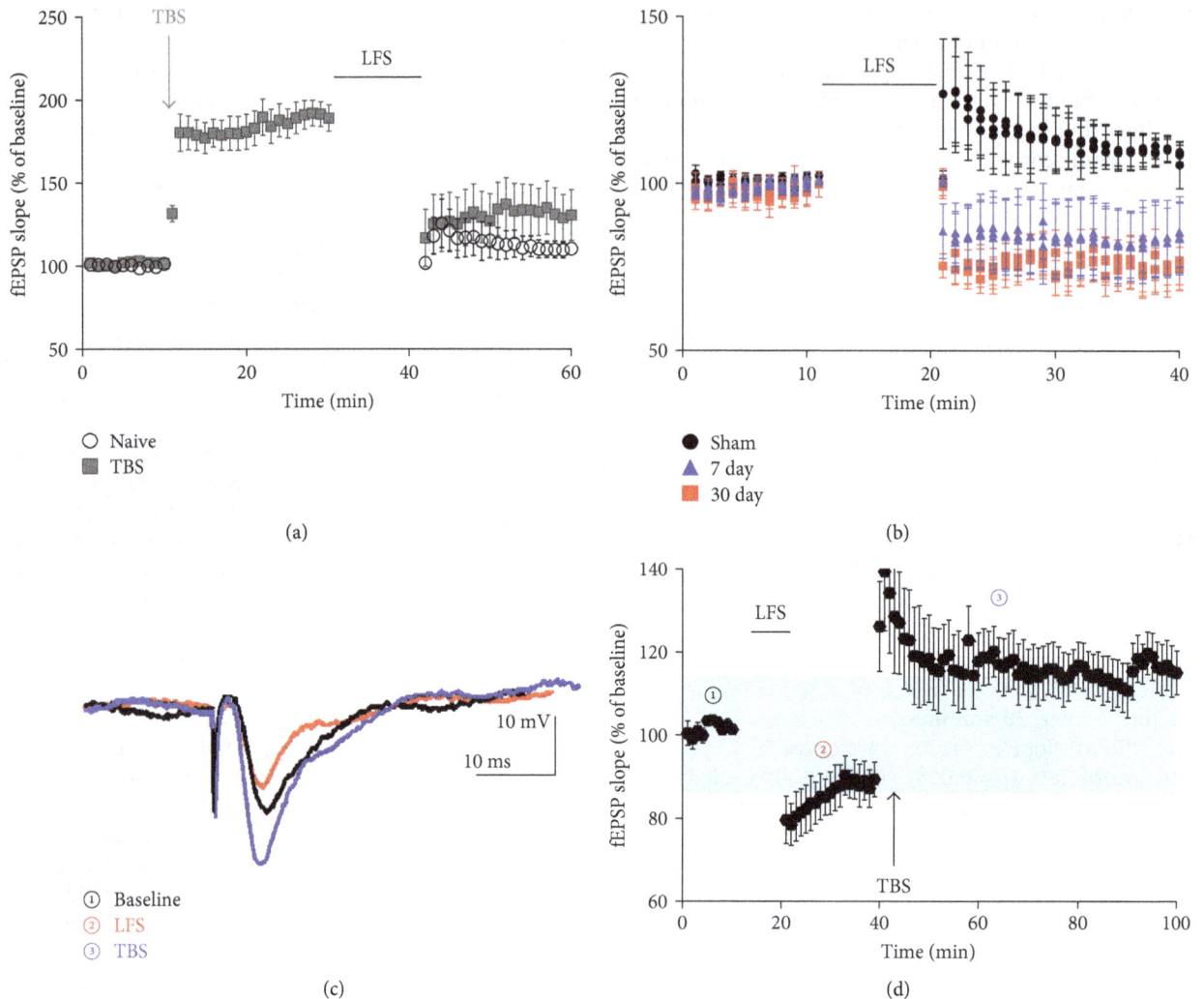

FIGURE 3: Depotentiation with low-frequency stimulation (LFS) reversed ischemic LTP and partially restored physiological LTP. (a) LFS depotentiates physiological LTP. 20 minutes after theta burst stimulation (TBS), LFS was delivered for 10 minutes (900 pulses at 0.5 Hz), resulting in a significant reduction in fEPSP slope (grey squares). LFS delivered to naive slices that did not receive TBS did not alter fEPSP slope (black circles). (b) LFS was delivered to slices from sham control (black circles) or 7 (blue triangles) or 30 days (red squares) after CA/CPR. LFS reduces fEPSC only in mice that were subjected to CA/CPR, indicating a reversal of iLTP. (c) Representative trace in recordings where we obtained a baseline (black trace) delivered LFS which reduced fEPSP amplitude (red trace) and subsequent TBS, which induced LTP (blue trace). (d) Summary of recordings in which we first delivered LFS then delivered TBS. Numbers on graph correlate with traces in panel (c). Magnitude of pLTP is shaded in blue.

to naive control levels. Therefore, it is likely that there are additional mechanisms that contribute to the LTP impairments in the hippocampus after cerebral ischemia. Regardless, these data suggest that induction of depotentiation to restore physiological plasticity may be a relevant therapy for improving memory function after ischemic brain injury. Future studies should address whether *in vivo* low-frequency electrical stimulation of the hippocampus, with implanted electrodes or through transmagnetic stimulation, can produce depotentiation and reduce memory deficits *in vivo*.

In vitro studies have been limited in their ability to record ischemic LTP for only the first hours after ischemia. Here, we are able to show that ischemic LTP is maintained for weeks after injury onset. At 7 and 30 days of postinjury, cell death

mechanisms have subsided and recordings are from the surviving hippocampal network. Our ability to depotentiate ischemic LTP and then induce physiological LTP at these delayed time points demonstrates that LTP impairments can be targeted to improve synaptic function, independent of acute neuroprotection. This is an important advance, as acute neuroprotective strategies have failed to improve cognitive outcomes in clinical trials. Cognitive impairments are present in patients that receive therapeutic hypothermia, the only strategy that has given positive results in cardiac arrest victims [39–41]. Therefore, strategies that can provide additional benefit to therapeutic hypothermia have promised to improve neurological function and quality of life for patients. Interestingly, rodent studies have shown that exposure of animals to novel environments can depotentiate previously acquired experience-dependent LTP, indicating the potential for novel rehabilitation strategies to reverse iLTP [28]. Future studies should determine whether such a behavioral paradigm could depotentiate ischemic LTP in the intact animal and improve future memory behavior.

In summary, we have demonstrated that *in vivo* global ischemia produces ischemic LTP which is the result of increased postsynaptic AMPA receptor function. Is iLTP beneficial or detrimental to hippocampal function? Our data demonstrating no change in input-output relations or synaptic density suggest that the hippocampal network is able to compensate for the loss of CA1 neurons after CA/CPR. Ischemic LTP may contribute to this normalization and therefore may have some benefit to the hippocampal network. However, the maintenance of iLTP for weeks after the ischemic insult is detrimental to physiological plasticity and likely worsens memory impairments. Thus, it appears that iLTP may serve as a beneficial compensatory mechanism following brain ischemia that if sustained during the chronic phase is detrimental to long-term recovery. Importantly, we show that this pathological form of plasticity is reversible and thus may be a therapeutic target for cognitive deficits after brain ischemia.

Acknowledgments

This work was supported by AHA BGIA25670032 (Nidia Quillinan) and R01 NS046072 (Nidia Quillinan) and NINDS R01 NS080851 (Paco S. Herson) and R01 NS092645 (Paco S. Herson).

References

[1] V. Crepel, C. Hammond, P. Chinestra, D. Diabira, and Y. Ben-Ari, "A selective LTP of NMDA receptor-mediated currents induced by anoxia in CA1 hippocampal neurons," *Journal of Neurophysiology*, vol. 70, no. 5, pp. 2045–2055, 1993.

[2] V. Crepel, C. Hammond, K. Krnjevic, P. Chinestra, and Y. Ben-Ari, "Anoxia-induced LTP of isolated NMDA receptor-mediated synaptic responses," *Journal of Neurophysiology*, vol. 69, no. 5, pp. 1774–1778, 1993.

[3] K. S. Hsu and C. C. Huang, "Characterization of the anoxia-induced long-term synaptic potentiation in area CA1 of the rat hippocampus," *British Journal of Pharmacology*, vol. 122, no. 4, pp. 671–681, 1997.

[4] M. Lyubkin, D. M. Durand, and M. A. Haxhiu, "Interaction between tetanus long-term potentiation and hypoxia-induced potentiation in the rat hippocampus," *Journal of Neurophysiology*, vol. 78, no. 5, pp. 2475–2482, 1997.

[5] N. Maggio, E. Shavit Stein, and M. Segal, "Ischemic LTP: NMDA-dependency and dorso/ventral distribution within the hippocampus," *Hippocampus*, vol. 25, no. 11, pp. 1465–1471, 2015.

[6] P. Quintana, S. Alberi, D. Hakkoum, and D. Muller, "Glutamate receptor changes associated with transient anoxia/ hypoglycaemia in hippocampal slice cultures," *European Journal of Neuroscience*, vol. 23, no. 4, pp. 975–983, 2006.

[7] G. Deng, J. E. Orfila, R. M. Dietz et al., "Autonomous CaMKII activity as a drug target for histological and functional nuroprotection after resuscitation from cardiac arrest," *Cell Reports*, vol. 18, no. 5, pp. 1109–1117, 2017.

[8] N. Wang, L. Chen, N. Cheng, J. Zhang, T. Tian, and W. Lu, "Active calcium/calmodulin-dependent protein kinase II (CaMKII) regulates NMDA receptor mediated post-ischemic long-term potentiation (i-LTP) by promoting the interaction between CaMKII and NMDA receptors in ischemia," *Neural Plasticity*, vol. 2014, Article ID 827161, 10 pages, 2014.

[9] I. Buard, S. J. Coultrap, R. K. Freund et al., "CaMKII "autonomy" is required for initiating but not for maintaining neuronal long-term information storage," *The Journal of Neuroscience*, vol. 30, no. 24, pp. 8214–8220, 2010.

[10] V. Derkach, A. Barria, and T. R. Soderling, "Ca^{2+}/calmodulin-kinase II enhances channel conductance of α-amino-3-hydroxy-5-methyl-4-isoxazolepropionate type glutamate receptors," *Proceedings of the National Academy of Sciences of the United States of America*, vol. 96, no. 6, pp. 3269–3274, 1999.

[11] C. E. Herron, R. A. J. Lester, E. J. Coan, and G. L. Collingridge, "Frequency-dependent involvement of NMDA receptors in the hippocampus: a novel synaptic mechanism," *Nature*, vol. 322, no. 6076, pp. 265–268, 1986.

[12] R. C. Malenka and R. A. Nicoll, "Long-term potentiation–a decade of progress?," *Science*, vol. 285, no. 5435, pp. 1870–1874, 1999.

[13] M. Horn and W. Schlote, "Delayed neuronal death and delayed neuronal recovery in the human brain following global ischemia," *Acta Neuropathologica*, vol. 85, no. 1, pp. 79–87, 1992.

[14] T. Ng, D. I. Graham, J. H. Adams, and I. Ford, "Changes in the hippocampus and the cerebellum resulting from hypoxic insults: frequency and distribution," *Acta Neuropathologica*, vol. 78, no. 4, pp. 438–443, 1989.

[15] X. Dai, L. Chen, and M. Sokabe, "Neurosteroid estradiol rescues ischemia-induced deficit in the long-term potentiation of rat hippocampal CA1 neurons," *Neuropharmacology*, vol. 52, no. 4, pp. 1124–1138, 2007.

[16] F. Gillardon, I. Kiprianova, J. Sandkuhler, K. A. Hossmann, and M. Spranger, "Inhibition of caspases prevents cell death of hippocampal CA1 neurons, but not impairment of hippocampal long-term potentiation following global ischemia," *Neuroscience*, vol. 93, no. 4, pp. 1219–1222, 1999.

[17] I. Kiprianova, J. Sandkühler, S. Schwab, S. Hoyer, and M. Spranger, "Brain-derived neurotrophic factor improves long-term potentiation and cognitive functions after transient forebrain ischemia in the rat," *Experimental Neurology*, vol. 159, no. 2, pp. 511–519, 1999.

[18] K. Mori, M. Yoshioka, N. Suda et al., "An incomplete cerebral ischemia produced a delayed dysfunction in the rat hippocampal system," *Brain Research*, vol. 795, no. 1-2, pp. 221–226, 1998.

[19] J. E. Orfila, K. Shimizu, A. K. Garske et al., "Increasing small conductance Ca^{2+}–activated potassium channel activity reverses ischemia-induced impairment of long-term potentiation," *European Journal of Neuroscience*, vol. 40, no. 8, pp. 3179–3188, 2014.

[20] R. M. Dietz, G. Deng, J. E. Orfila, X. Hui, R. J. Traystman, and P. S. Herson, "Therapeutic hypothermia protects against ischemia-induced impairment of synaptic plasticity following juvenile cardiac arrest in sex-dependent manner," *Neuroscience*, vol. 325, pp. 132–141, 2016.

[21] M. P. Hutchens, R. J. Traystman, T. Fujiyoshi, S. Nakayama, and P. S. Herson, "Normothermic cardiac arrest and cardiopulmonary resuscitation: a mouse model of ischemia-reperfusion injury," *Journal of Visualized Experiments*, vol. 54, no. 54, article e3116, 2011.

[22] J. Kofler, K. Hattori, M. Sawada et al., "Histopathological and behavioral characterization of a novel model of cardiac arrest and cardiopulmonary resuscitation in mice," *Journal of Neuroscience Methods*, vol. 136, no. 1, pp. 33–44, 2004.

[23] N. Quillinan, G. Deng, K. Shimizu et al., "Long-term depression in Purkinje neurons is persistently impaired following cardiac arrest and cardiopulmonary resuscitation in mice," *Journal of Cerebral Blood Flow & Metabolism*, vol. 37, no. 8, pp. 3053–3064, 2016.

[24] G. Deng, J. C. Yonchek, N. Quillinan et al., "A novel mouse model of pediatric cardiac arrest and cardiopulmonary resuscitation reveals age-dependent neuronal sensitivities to ischemic injury," *Journal of Neuroscience Methods*, vol. 222, pp. 34–41, 2014.

[25] Z. I. Bashir and G. L. Collingridge, "An investigation of depotentiation of long-term potentiation in the CA1 region of the hippocampus," *Experimental Brain Research*, vol. 100, no. 3, pp. 437–443, 1994.

[26] X. Guli, T. Tokay, T. Kirschstein, and R. Kohling, "Status epilepticus enhances depotentiation after fully established LTP in an NMDAR-dependent but GluN2B-independent manner," *Neural Plasticity*, vol. 2016, Article ID 6592038, 10 pages, 2016.

[27] C. C. Huang, Y. C. Liang, and K. S. Hsu, "Characterization of the mechanism underlying the reversal of long term potentiation by low frequency stimulation at hippocampal CA1 synapses," *Journal of Biological Chemistry*, vol. 276, no. 51, pp. 48108–48117, 2001.

[28] Y. Qi, N. W. Hu, and M. J. Rowan, "Switching off LTP: mGlu and NMDA receptor–dependent novelty exploration–induced depotentiation in the rat hippocampus," *Cerebral Cortex*, vol. 23, no. 4, pp. 932–939, 2013.

[29] A. J. Baker, M. H. Zornow, M. R. Grafe et al., "Hypothermia prevents ischemia-induced increases in hippocampal glycine concentrations in rabbits," *Stroke*, vol. 22, no. 5, pp. 666–673, 1991.

[30] D. Jabaudon, M. Scanziani, B. H. Gahwiler, and U. Gerber, "Acute decrease in net glutamate uptake during energy deprivation," *Proceedings of the National Academy of Sciences of the United States of America*, vol. 97, no. 10, pp. 5610–5615, 2000.

[31] D. J. Rossi, T. Oshima, and D. Attwell, "Glutamate release in severe brain ischaemia is mainly by reversed uptake," *Nature*, vol. 403, no. 6767, pp. 316–321, 2000.

[32] N. Shimada, R. Graf, G. Rosner, A. Wakayama, C. P. George, and W. D. Heiss, "Ischemic flow threshold for extracellular glutamate increase in cat cortex," *Journal of Cerebral Blood Flow & Metabolism*, vol. 9, no. 5, pp. 603–606, 1989.

[33] K. Takata, Y. Takeda, T. Sato, H. Nakatsuka, M. Yokoyama, and K. Morita, "Effects of hypothermia for a short period on histologic outcome and extracellular glutamate concentration during and after cardiac arrest in rats," *Critical Care Medicine*, vol. 33, no. 6, pp. 1340–1345, 2005.

[34] P. Calabresi, D. Centonze, A. Pisani, L. M. Cupini, and G. Bernardi, "Synaptic plasticity in the ischaemic brain," *The Lancet Neurology*, vol. 2, no. 10, pp. 622–629, 2003.

[35] M. Di Filippo, A. Tozzi, C. Costa et al., "Plasticity and repair in the post-ischemic brain," *Neuropharmacology*, vol. 55, no. 3, pp. 353–362, 2008.

[36] K. Kocsis, L. Knapp, L. Gellert et al., "Acetyl-L-carnitine normalizes the impaired long-term potentiation and spine density in a rat model of global ischemia," *Neuroscience*, vol. 269, pp. 265–272, 2014.

[37] D. Nagy, K. Kocsis, J. Fuzik et al., "Kainate postconditioning restores LTP in ischemic hippocampal CA1: onset-dependent second pathophysiological stress," *Neuropharmacology*, vol. 61, no. 5-6, pp. 1026–1032, 2011.

[38] G. N. Neigh, E. R. Glasper, J. Kofler et al., "Cardiac arrest with cardiopulmonary resuscitation reduces dendritic spine density in CA1 pyramidal cells and selectively alters acquisition of spatial memory," *European Journal of Neuroscience*, vol. 20, no. 7, pp. 1865–1872, 2004.

[39] Hypothermia after Cardiac Arrest Study Group, "Mild therapeutic hypothermia to improve the neurologic outcome after cardiac arrest," *The New England Journal of Medicine*, vol. 346, no. 8, pp. 549–556, 2002.

[40] G. Lilja, N. Nielsen, H. Friberg et al., "Cognitive function in survivors of out-of-hospital cardiac arrest after target temperature management at 33°C versus 36°C," *Circulation*, vol. 131, no. 15, pp. 1340–1349, 2015.

[41] M. Tiainen, E. Poutiainen, T. Kovala, O. Takkunen, O. Happola, and R. O. Roine, "Cognitive and neurophysiological outcome of cardiac arrest survivors treated with therapeutic hypothermia," *Stroke*, vol. 38, no. 8, pp. 2303–2308, 2007.

6

Impact of Global Mean Normalization on Regional Glucose Metabolism in the Human Brain

Kristian N. Mortensen,[1,2] Albert Gjedde,[2,3] Garth J. Thompson,[1] Peter Herman,[1] Maxime J. Parent,[1] Douglas L. Rothman,[1,4] Ron Kupers,[2] Maurice Ptito,[2,3,5,6] Johan Stender,[2,7] Steven Laureys,[7] Valentin Riedl,[8] Michael T. Alkire,[9] and Fahmeed Hyder[1,4]

[1]*Department of Radiology & Biomedical Imaging and Magnetic Resonance Research Center, Yale University, New Haven, CT, USA*
[2]*Department of Neuroscience, University of Copenhagen, Copenhagen, Denmark*
[3]*Departments of Nuclear Medicine and Clinical Research, Odense University Hospital, University of Southern Denmark, Odense, Denmark*
[4]*Department of Biomedical Engineering, Yale University, New Haven, CT, USA*
[5]*Chaire de Recherche Harland Sanders, School of Optometry, University of Montreal, Montreal, Canada*
[6]*Neuropsychiatry Laboratory, Psychiatric Centre, Rigshospitalet, Copenhagen, Denmark*
[7]*GIGA-Consciousness, Coma Science Group, Université de Liège, Liège, Belgium*
[8]*Departments of Neuroradiology, Nuclear Medicine and Neuroimaging Center, Technische Universität München, München, Germany*
[9]*Department of Anesthesiology, University of California, Irvine, CA, USA*

Correspondence should be addressed to Fahmeed Hyder; fahmeed.hyder@yale.edu

Academic Editor: J. Michael Wyss

Because the human brain consumes a disproportionate fraction of the resting body's energy, positron emission tomography (PET) measurements of absolute glucose metabolism (CMR_{glc}) can serve as disease biomarkers. Global mean normalization (GMN) of PET data reveals disease-based differences from healthy individuals as fractional changes across regions relative to a global mean. To assess the impact of GMN applied to metabolic data, we compared CMR_{glc} with and without GMN in healthy awake volunteers with eyes closed (i.e., control) against specific physiological/clinical states, including healthy/awake with eyes open, healthy/awake but congenitally blind, healthy/sedated with anesthetics, and patients with disorders of consciousness. Without GMN, global CMR_{glc} alterations compared to control were detected in all conditions except in congenitally blind where regional CMR_{glc} variations were detected in the visual cortex. However, GMN introduced regional and bidirectional CMR_{glc} changes at smaller fractions of the quantitative delocalized changes. While global information was lost with GMN, the quantitative approach (i.e., a validated method for quantitative baseline metabolic activity without GMN) not only preserved global CMR_{glc} alterations induced by opening eyes, sedation, and varying consciousness but also detected regional CMR_{glc} variations in the congenitally blind. These results caution the use of GMN upon PET-measured CMR_{glc} data in health and disease.

1. Introduction

Noninvasive neuroimaging with positron emission tomography (PET) and functional magnetic resonance imaging (fMRI) provide the foundations of human brain mapping, as practiced in the past four decades for PET and three decades for fMRI [1–4]. Early PET studies concentrated on quantitative imaging of resting-state blood flow and metabolism [2, 5], whereas later PET and then fMRI studies used tools with some form of global mean normalization

(GMN), most notably statistical parametric mapping (SPM), or the Scaled Subprofile Model of principal component analysis (SSM-PCA), to obtain regional differences among control and metabolically/functionally perturbed states. When these methods are applied to PET metabolic radiotracers, such as [18F]fluorodeoxyglucose (FDG), the application of these analysis tools often proceeded with the assumption that global brain metabolic activity, defined as the mean metabolic rate of gray matter or the entire brain, is a valid basis for normalization of regional values, in part because it is held to facilitate group comparisons in the presence of physiological and/or experimental intraindividual and interindividual differences [6, 7]. GMN yields parametric images of fractional or percentage differences from a variably defined global mean. While it is not a formal requirement for either SPM or SSM-PCA, GMN has become an almost routine and a necessary preparatory step in analyses of neuroimaging data. For example, in the SSM-PCA method, the global effects are removed by log transformation and centering, but this procedure has a similar effect to GMN in that it removes any scalar multiplicative parameters at the individual level. Many PET studies exemplify the use of GMN to reveal differences of cerebral metabolic rate of glucose (CMR_{glc}) across states of health and different diseases. However, to validate the metabolic differences, it is necessary to adequately account for the substantial variability of resting metabolic rates of human brain among individuals and brain states [8].

The covariance pattern extraction can be independent of the normalization process on PET data. For example, SSM-PCA analysis does not proceed as a form of GMN of the data. Steps like log transformation and centering can, on certain conditions, be used to remove scalar factors from the underlying disease patterns, which may be caused by variable spatial covariance. Thus, it is important to differentiate univariate assessment of CMR_{glc} from voxel weights of disease pattern derived as principal components of multivariate spatial covariance. Effects of absolute quantification on SSM derivation of disease-specific network profiles were reported by Strother et al. [9] and more recently by Borghammer et al. [10–14], who concluded that GMN can yield spurious interpretations of perturbed measures of brain activity. Commonly used PCA analysis methods focus on regional differences at the group level, beyond differences in global brain function. However, we contest that analysis methods which assume that global differences do not exist may cause global effects to contaminate "local" results, and thus, global effects should be separately evaluated to avoid this concern.

Several decades after the advent of PET, fMRI became the common method of choice to detect functional differences among brain regions and/or, differences between control and patient groups, and for mapping of functional connectivity in resting brain [15]. The fMRI approach reveals resting-state correlations of the somewhat poorly defined regional blood oxygenation level-dependent (BOLD) signal among brain regions. Thus "functional connectivity networks" are derived by searching for significant correlations from the spontaneous fluctuations of the BOLD signal. However, the BOLD signal itself is a nontrivial function of oxygen extracted from the circulation and, therefore, reflects changes in rates of both cerebral blood flow (CBF) and oxidative metabolism (CMR_{O2}) [16]. Most analysis methods of resting-state fMRI remove, among other variables, the global BOLD signal to reveal the networks [17]. Results are then inferred within these so-called resting-state networks from the remaining fluctuations, where the amplitude of the spontaneous BOLD signal is significantly reduced upon regression [17, 18]. In contrast, FDG-PET reveals resting-state network activity by calculation of differences among the regional CMR_{glc} of a group of subjects or across different metabolic states, with subsequent application of network analysis to the regions that differ among groups and/or conditions [19]. Most resting-state fMRI and PET studies thus use some form of GMN prior to comparison of the data for network determination. However, our focus here is only the effects of GMN upon PET imaging.

The validity of the GMN procedure for creating metabolic maps originally remained uncontested on the assumption that most glucose and oxygen consumed in the resting-state served "nonfunctional" mechanisms which are uncorrelated with cognitive activity [20]. However, results from both early and more recent studies challenge this assumption [18, 21]. The resting brain is the most energy-demanding organ in the human body [22], the energy turnover due to Na^+,K^+-ATPase function that sustains membrane repolarization and ion gradient restoration for continuous neuronal activity [23–25]. It is well accepted that energy demands of neuronal activity in the resting awake human brain by far exceed the magnitude of the additional energy turnover associated with evoked or spontaneous changes of functional activity [26]. Yet, the fraction of the total metabolic rate altered by spontaneous or evoked events remains uncertain, and the extent to which GMN obscures differences of the energy demand across functional states thus still remains uncertain. In this context, CBF and CMR_{O2} values measured in healthy aging and in Parkinson's disease show that conventional GMN obscures evidence of metabolic changes in the brain [27, 28]. Borghammer et al. showed that GMN of quantitative PET-measured CBF measurements can yield false positive findings of perfusion changes [10], but the methods are nonetheless being generalized to metabolic PET scans [29]. Borghammer et al. also demonstrated that foci of elevated CBF attributed to small brain regions actually can arise as a consequence of normalization applied only to gray matter [11]. In an examination of simulated reduction of cortical metabolism, Borghammer et al. further noted that GMN generally only recovered a few percent of the original signal and conversely led to artifactual findings of relative increases [12]. Thus, there are two issues that potentially affect the use of PET images as biomarkers of disease; the raising of regional differences to significance and the removal of global differences among individuals and groups that results from GMN.

Prompted by this evidence, we sought to test the hypothesis that GMN may not only artificially raise minor regional variations to significance but also may significantly obscure global metabolic effects when PET images of the resting brain in specific disorders are compared. We used FDG-PET to measure CMR_{glc} at different sites, where the control states (of resting healthy awake volunteers with eyes closed) were compared to subjects in states established by conditions ranging from normal sensory input to sedation by anesthesia to different clinical states. While some experiments involved blood sampling of the FDG tracer's supply to the brain, necessary to obtain absolute values of CMR_{glc} ($aCMR_{glc}$), others did not. To compare FDG-PET images from different sites, we developed a new method allowing quantitative measures of CMR_{glc} ($qCMR_{glc}$) by a calibration procedure that is based on comparison of $qCMR_{glc}$ data with $aCMR_{glc}$ data for a control state (i.e., healthy awake with eyes closed). We then validated the method, which is aimed for quantitative baseline metabolic activity without GMN, by first comparing $qCMR_{glc}$ values found in control experiments from different sites and then comparing $qCMR_{glc}$ to $aCMR_{glc}$ for experiments with blood sampling. We tested conditions that included awake and eyes open states (presence of sensory input), pharmacological intervention (anesthesia), disorders of consciousness, and congenital blindness (clinical states), in comparison to resting healthy awake subjects with eyes closed (control). Comparison of t-maps of CMR_{glc} without GMN reveal heuristically important and pathognomonic evidence of perturbations of brain metabolism across states or among groups. However, GMN induced artificial relative increases in states that are generally accepted as only inducing metabolic decreases.

2. Materials and Methods

2.1. Subjects. Participants underwent tomography at four sites, and imaging at each site included a control group. FDG-PET measures were collected in a total of nine different resting states (Table 1) and compiled as anonymized data, most of which previously had been published prior to the present analysis. A group of healthy awake subjects imaged with eyes closed (HAEC) was recorded at each site. Each site's HAEC served as control for the other groups recorded at that site. There were 8 other groups: healthy awake subjects with eyes open (HAEO) [30]; healthy subjects sedated with 1% desflurane (Des1%), 0.25% sevoflurane (Sev0.25%) [31], or 0.5% sevoflurane (Sev0.5%); awake congenitally blind (CB) subjects [32]; and patients with disorders of consciousness, including unresponsive wakefulness syndrome (UWS), minimally conscious state (MCS), and emergence from MCS (EMCS) [33]. The diagnostic criteria for the selected disorders of consciousness have been described earlier [34]. All healthy participants were right-handed.

Among the five groups of healthy volunteers, two without sedation (HAEC and HAEO) underwent tomography in Munich, Germany, and those with sedation (Sev0.25%, Sev0.5%, and Des1%) in Irvine, CA, USA. Among the four groups with some form of disability, the CB underwent tomography in Copenhagen, Denmark. All three groups with disorders of consciousness had tomography in Liège, Belgium. All tomograms were acquired upon obtaining written informed consent from participants or from caregivers (in the case of disorders of consciousness), in accordance with the Helsinki Protocol, and all studies were approved by the appropriate ethical review board per institution; the Ethics

Committee of the University Hospital of Liège (Belgium), the Research Ethics Committee of the University of Copenhagen and Frederiksberg (Denmark); the Institutional Review Board at the University of California, Irvine (USA); and the ethics review board of the Klinikum Rechts der Isar, Technische Universität München (Germany).

2.2. Tomography. All subjects underwent FDG-PET and MRI scanning. Details of FDG-PET and MRI acquisition are described in the original studies [30–34]. Briefly, tomographies in USA and Denmark were performed on Siemens ECAT high-resolution research tomographs (HRRT), in Germany on a Siemens Biograph mMR PET/MRI, and in Belgium on a Philips GEMINI TF PET/CT. Blood sampling in USA subjects allowed calculation of absolute values of CMR_{glc} ($aCMR_{glc}$) [31].

2.2.1. Tomography (Site Number 1). The two healthy groups without any sedation, consisting of 11 HAEO subjects (aged 52 ± 10 years, 7 males) and 11 different HAEC subject (aged 57 ± 10 years, 8 males; i.e., $HAEC_{GER}$), all used an MRI/PET tomograph (Siemens Biograph mMR) at the Neuroimaging Center of Technical University of Munich, Germany (Table 1). Subjects held their eyes closed or open depending on their assigned group; details of the scans have been published elsewhere [30]. Structural MRI data were acquired (magnetization-prepared 180-degree radiofrequency pulses and rapid gradient-echo (MP-RAGE), repetition time (TR) 2.3 s, echo time (TE) 2.98 ms, 160 slices with 0.5 mm gap, 256×256 mm field of view (FOV), 256×256 matrix size, and 5 minutes and 3 seconds). About 30 minutes after the bolus FDG injection, a 10-minute emission recording was acquired (saturated list mode, 128 slices with 0.5 mm gap, 192×192 mm matrix, and $3.7 \times 2.3 \times 2.7$ mm voxel).

2.2.2. Tomography (Site Number 2). The three sedated groups (age range 18–22 years), consisting of 8 Sev0.25% subjects, 8 Sev0.5% subjects (same cases as Sev0.25%), and 7 Des1% subjects, were all scanned using the Siemens ECAT high-resolution research tomograph (HRRT) at the Department of Anesthesiology of the University of California, Irvine, California, USA, and also underwent MRI (Table 1). Details of the tomographies of the Sev0.25% group, same as the other groups, have been published elsewhere [31]. Two intravenous catheters were inserted, one for arterialized venous blood sampling and the other for FDG infusion (203.5 MBq) enabling measurement of absolute CMR_{glc}. A brief attenuation scan was obtained using a Cs-137 source, and a ten-minute emission recording was obtained (207 slices at 1.2 mm gap) beginning 32 min after FDG application; participants were still for the tracer uptake interval, except when asked to perform a hand gesture as a test of alertness/sedation. The tomograph had an effective resolution of 3.3 mm full width at half maximum (FWHM). Participants had tomographies on different occasions for the selected doses of anesthetic gases, delivered with standard calibrated vaporizers in 100% oxygen via a standard semicircle breathing circuit using a Dräger AV anesthesia machine. A Datex Ohmeda Capnomac Ultima (Helsinki, Finland) was

TABLE 1: Details of different groups imaged at the various sites (Germany, USA, Denmark, and Belgium; see text for details).

PET imaging site	Experimental group	Control group
Site number 1, Germany (Technical University of Munich)	HAEO ($n = 11$)	HAEC$_{GER}$ ($n = 11$)
Site number 2, USA (University of California, Irvine)	* Sev0.25% ($n = 8$) * Sev0.5% ($n = 8$) * Des1% ($n = 7$)	* HAEC$_{sev}$ ($n = 8$) * HAEC$_{des}$ ($n = 7$)
Site number 3, Denmark (Rigshospitalet, Copenhagen University Hospital)	CB ($n = 7$)	HAEC$_{DEN}$ ($n = 7$)
Site number 4, Belgium (University Hospital of Liege)	UWS ($n = 65$) MCS ($n = 65$) EMCS ($n = 17$)	HAEC$_{BEL}$ ($n = 28$)

* indicates that both absolute CMR$_{glc}$ (aCMR$_{glc}$) and quantified CMR$_{glc}$ (qCMR$_{glc}$) were obtained from the USA site, enabling comparison between them (see Figures 1(b) and 1(c)). aCMR$_{glc}$: absolute CMR$_{glc}$ with blood sampling of the tracer FDG supply to the brain; qCMR$_{glc}$: calibration of quantified comparing qCMR$_{glc}$ with aCMR$_{glc}$ for HAEC only eqs. (1 and 2); HAEC: healthy people awake with eyes closed (control condition); HAEO: healthy people awake with eyes open; Des1%: healthy people sedated with 1% desflurane; Sev0.25%: healthy people sedated with 0.25% sevoflurane; Sev0.50%: healthy people sedated with 0.5% sevoflurane; CB: awake people with congenital blindness; UWS: patients who were unresponsive wakefulness syndrome; MCS: patients who were in a minimally conscious state; EMCS: patients who emerged from MCS.

used to monitor expired CO_2 and anesthetic gas levels. This HAEC group consisted of the participants who received 0% sevoflurane (HAEC$_{sev}$; $n = 8$; Table 1) and 0% desflurane (HAEC$_{des}$; $n = 7$; Table 1).

2.2.3. Tomography (Site Number 3). PET data were acquired in a group of 7 CB participants (three males aged 41 ± 8 years) and 7 HEAC (aged 25 ± 5 years, four males; HAEC$_{DEN}$) using a Siemens ECAT HRRT at Rigshospitalet in Copenhagen, Denmark (Table 1). Participants' MRIs were acquired using a 3 T Siemens Trio MRI scanner at the Danish Research Centre for Magnetic Resonance, Hvidovre Hospital, Hvidovre, Denmark. Details of the scans have been published elsewhere [32]. One among the seven CB participants had limited vision at birth that progressed to complete blindness at the age of seven; all others were completely blind from birth. Structural MRI data were acquired (MP-RAGE, TR 1.5 s, TE 3.93 ms, inversion recovery time (TI) 0.8 s, 256 slices with no gap, 192×256 mm FOV, and 6 minutes 36 seconds). PET data were acquired forty minutes after bolus injection of approximately 210 MBq FDG (single frame, OSEM3D mode, 207 slices with no gap, $1.2 \times 1.2 \times 1.2$ mm voxels, and 40 minutes). During the tracer uptake period, control participants were blindfolded and all participants rested in a dimly lit room without falling asleep.

2.2.4. Tomography (Site Number 4). The groups with disorders of consciousness consisted of (i) 49 UWS patients (aged 46 ± 16, 31 males; mean time since injury 1.7 ± 3.2 years), (ii) 65 MCS patients (aged 40 ± 16, 41 males; mean time since injury 3.3 ± 4.3 years), and (iii) 17 EMCS patients (aged 35 ± 15, 15 males; mean time since injury 3.0 ± 3.7 years). The control group (HAEC$_{BEL}$) consisted of 28 participants (aged 44 ± 16, 16 males). All participants were scanned using the Philips GEMINI TF PET/CT device at the University Hospital of Liege, Liege, Belgium (Table 1), according to procedures described in detail elsewhere [33–35]. About 30 min after intravenous FDG injection, a single 12-minute emission frame was recorded (90 slices with no gap, 256×256 matrix, and $2 \times 2 \times 2$ mm voxels). The control subjects were kept awake in a dimly lit room during the FDG uptake, and all patients were kept awake during FDG uptake.

2.3. Registration. All PET images were registered to the Montreal Neurological Institute (MNI) space ($3 \times 3 \times 3$ mm) using a combination of linear and nonlinear registration tools on publicly available platforms (i.e., advanced normalization tools (ANTs) from http://stnava.github.io/ANTs, or Bio-Image Suite from http://bioimagesuite.yale.edu). PET images from Germany, USA, and Denmark were first registered to their corresponding MRI image using a rigid body transformation and then carried to the MNI template by computed affine and nonlinear transformations, with interpolation to a $3 \times 3 \times 3$ mm^3 voxel size. Belgian PET images were directly registered to a common PET template created from the HAEC$_{DEN}$ group, using a combination of linear and nonlinear registrations applying very restrictive and highly regularized registration parameters.

2.4. Calibrating Quantified Measures of CMR$_{glc}$ (qCMR$_{glc}$). As shown in Table 1, only the USA site had blood sampling data to enable FDG-PET counts to be converted into "absolute CMR$_{glc}$" units of μmol/g/min (aCMR$_{glc}$). To compare metabolic measurements recorded from different sites (where blood sampling data were unavailable), we developed a new method for calibrating quantified measures of CMR$_{glc}$ (qCMR$_{glc}$) that targets quantitative baseline metabolic activity without GMN. This method is based on the comparison of qCMR$_{glc}$ data with aCMR$_{glc}$ data also for the HAEC condition from Hyder et al. study (aCMR$_{glc}$-HYD), with a mean male age of 26.1 ± 3.8 years [36]. For consistency of the data from the USA site with data from other sites, we also calculated qCMR$_{glc}$ for these five USA datasets, which in turn provided the validation for our procedure (see below).

Our goal was to preserve between-state global differences in metabolism, which are believed to be removed by GMN. Previous work has demonstrated that for identical conditions (i.e., HAEC), region-to-region aCMR$_{glc}$ variation is proportional to region-to-region PET radiation counts [37]. We opted to apply per-site fitting procedure by using the same linear model for all individuals at a given site. Assuming HAEC groups are comparable across sites [19], then this procedure would have the potential to compare metabolic differences between states recorded at different sites.

The "quantified CMR_{glc}" metric, referred to as $qCMR_{glc}$ to focus on quantitative baseline metabolic activity without GMN, was obtained in two steps. First, a linear intensity transformation of the original tissue radioactivity values was computed on a per-site basis, such that the distribution of voxels in the mean across the gray and white matter of the cerebrum (excluding the cerebellum) from each site was matched in intensity to the distribution of voxels from the published $aCMR_{glc}$-HYD database [36]. The similarity between the distributions was calculated as the Jensen-Shannon Divergence [38] (JSD), where the per-site linear intensity transformation was calculated as the minimization of the following expression:

$$JSD\left[dist\left(<aCMR_{glc}-HYD>\right)-dist\left(a_{site}\cdot<FDG_{HAEC}>+b_{site}\right)\right],$$
$$(1)$$

where dist ($<aCMR_{glc}-HYD>$) and dist ($<FDG_{HAEC}>$), respectively, refer to the distribution of voxels in the mean across the gray and white matter of the cerebrum (excluding the cerebellum) of the published $aCMR_{glc}$-HYD database [36] and the original tissue-radioactivity values for each HAEC group (FDG_{HAEC}) from any site (Table 1), and a_{site} and b_{site} are, respectively, the resultant slope and intercept from the fit, unique for the specific site. Prior to minimization of eq. (1), $<FDG_{HAEC}>$ was spatially smoothed to match the point-spread function of $<aCMR_{glc}$-HYD$>$ as computed by the 3dFWHMx program from the AFNI software package. Then, the $qCMR_{glc}$ maps for each subject were computed by applying the a_{site} and b_{site} from eq. (1) as follows:

$$qCMR_{glc}=a_{site}\cdot FDG+b_{site},\qquad(2)$$

where FDG refers to tissue-radioactivity concentrations from any individual voxel for any single subject in any group and only for the specific site for which a_{site} and b_{site} were calculated. The calculated $qCMR_{glc}$ was used throughout this study as fitted between each site's HAEC group and all other groups from that site. The $qCMR_{glc}$ calculation was carried out using the distributions of only intracranial voxels.

Two tests were run to validate $qCMR_{glc}$. First, if comparable $qCMR_{glc}$ values exist in HAEC groups from different sites, this would indicate that between-site comparisons are possible. To test this, the mean $qCMR_{glc}$ within 41 gray matter regions (Table S1) drawn in the MNI reference space was calculated for the five control groups ($HAEC_{DEN}$, $HAEC_{GER}$, $HAEC_{sev}$, $HAEC_{des}$, and $HAEC_{BEL}$) and $aCMR_{glc}$-HYD from Hyder et al. [36] that also represented the HAEC condition. Pearson correlation and Euclidean distance were calculated between the group means of $aCMR_{glc}$-HYD and $qCMR_{glc}$ in their respective 41 gray matter regions repeated for each pair of groups. Then, p values for statistical significance were calculated with permutation testing across the 41 gray matter regions with 1000 repetitions and rerunning the correlation and distance

calculations then taking the percentile of the actual correlation/distance based on the randomly permuted correlations/distances as a null distribution (one-sided test, Pearson correlation higher than the null hypothesis and Euclidean distance lower than the null hypothesis).

Second, as a further test of the ability to compare $qCMR_{glc}$ between groups, we used $aCMR_{glc}$ data that was available from the USA site. The Des1% and $HAEC_{des}$ groups had the same subjects, as did the Sev0.25%, Sev0.5%, and $HAEC_{sev}$ groups. The same data were also used to calculate $qCMR_{glc}$ (see above). Means of $aCMR_{glc}$ and $qCMR_{glc}$ were calculated within each gray matter region across all subjects. Treating the respective HAEC group as the x-axis and the respective anesthetized group as the y-axis, a linear fit was calculated. The slopes from the linear fits from $aCMR_{glc}$ were compared to those from $qCMR_{glc}$ to establish the validity of our calibration method.

2.5. Image Analysis. Mean $qCMR_{glc}$ maps were computed as the voxel-by-voxel average across each group of subjects and for the combined group of control subjects from all tomography sites. Statistical t-maps were computed using an unpaired voxel-wise two-sample two-tailed Student's t-test, assuming equal variance for $qCMR_{glc}$ images following smoothing with an 8 mm Gaussian kernel. Statistical t-maps were also generated with the same parameters following GMN images, with individual scaling to the whole-brain mean of $qCMR_{glc}$. Statistics were computed both for $qCMR_{glc}$ and GMN images using the gray matter regions (Table S1) for difference of each state from the HAEC condition.

3. Results

3.1. Validating Quantified Measures of CMR_{glc} ($qCMR_{glc}$). We compared the mean quantified estimates of CMR_{glc} ($qCMR_{glc}$) across 41 gray matter regions for the five HAEC groups listed in Table 1 to absolute CMR_{glc} ($aCMR_{glc}$) of the HAEC group from Hyder et al. [36] ($aCMR_{glc}$-HYD), as shown in Figure 1(a). The Pearson correlation and Euclidean distance between each pair of groups are listed in Table 2. All correlations were highly significant, and Euclidean distances were less than half of the mean in even one dimension, despite there being 41 dimensions. Although $HAEC_{sev}$ and $HAEC_{des}$ correlated the highest because the subjects in these groups overlapped, different groups of subjects (e.g., $HAEC_{des}$ and $HAEC_{DEN}$ or $HAEC_{sev}$ and $HAEC_{DEN}$) had similarly high correlation. We attribute the high correlation among control subjects to the tight age group. The p values resulting from comparing actual correlations and distances to an artificially generated null distribution were zero (for Pearson correlation, the value is higher than for 1000 random permutations; for Euclidean distance, the value is lower than for 1000 random permutations). The values indicate that all HAEC groups, whether associated with $aCMR_{glc}$ or $qCMR_{glc}$, were highly similar in terms of both spatial extent (correlation) and actual value (distance), confirming that it is valid to compare the HAEC groups from different sites.

Figure 1(b) shows the linear fit between the states of anesthesia and respective control states using the $aCMR_{glc}$

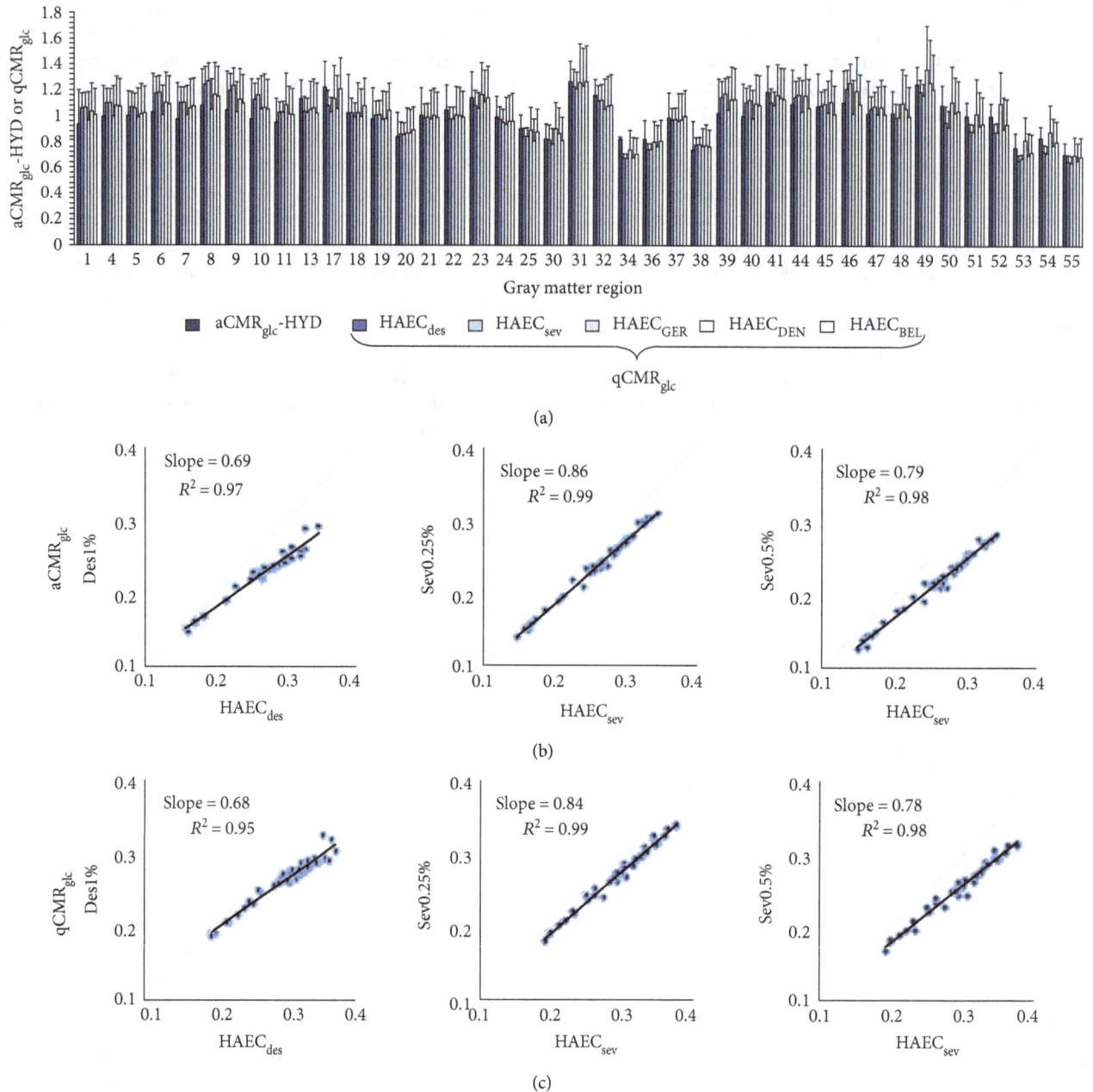

FIGURE 1: Validation of quantified CMR_{glc} ($qCMR_{glc}$). (a) Comparison of absolute CMR_{glc} from Hyder et al. [36] ($aCMR_{glc}$-HYD) with $qCMR_{glc}$ from five sites for the HAEC condition (Table 1). Bars represent the mean across all subjects in each group for gray matter regions (Table S1), where error bars are one standard deviation. All $qCMR_{glc}$ and $aCMR_{glc}$-HYD values were very similar both relatively between regions and in terms of mean value, suggesting across-site comparisons are possible with our procedure for quantified CMR_{glc}. The Pearson correlation and the Euclidean distance (Table 2) suggest high similarity and low difference of CMR_{glc} for the HAEC group across all sites. (b) Scatter plots, from left to right, for $aCMR_{glc}$ between Des1%, Sev0.25%, or Sev0.5% groups and equivalent HAEC groups (Table 1). Each point is one gray matter region (Table S1). Slope and R^2 from a linear fit are shown, and units are μmol/g/min, where a slope of less than 1 corresponds to a lower CMR_{glc} in the anesthetized group compared to the control. (c) Same as in (b), except using $qCMR_{glc}$ from each group. The slopes are almost identical in (b) and (c), indicating that the calculation of $qCMR_{glc}$ does not alter the relationship between groups for $aCMR_{glc}$.

estimates from site number 2, while Figure 1(c) shows the same fit for $qCMR_{glc}$ estimates where a slope of less than 1 in both Figures 1(b) and 1(c) corresponds to a lower $qCMR_{glc}$ in the anesthetized group compared to the control group. All linear fits had $R^2 \geq 0.95$. The slopes of the linear

fits were nearly identical for $aCMR_{glc}$ and $qCMR_{glc}$ (Des1%: 0.69 versus 0.68; Sev0.25%: 0.86 versus 0.84; and Sev0.5%: 0.79 versus 0.78). We also noted small but consistent shifts of intercepts between the healthy awake and sedated, which were reproducible for $aCMR_{glc}$ and $qCMR_{glc}$ (Des1%: 0.045

TABLE 2: Results of quantified CMR_{glc} ($qCMR_{glc}$) from Figure 1(a), where HAEC groups from different sites are compared to absolute CMR_{glc} from Hyder et al. [36] ($aCMR_{glc}$-HYD). The upper triangular half is Pearson correlation (italicized), whereas the lower triangular half is Euclidean distance (non-italicized). In the table $p = 0$ for all entries. The Pearson correlations were highly significant, and all the Euclidean distances were less than even one despite a total of 41 dimensions' means. The high similarity between $qCMR_{glc}$ in the HAEC groups measured at different sites indicates that comparisons between sites are possible using our procedure for quantified CMR_{glc}.

		$aCMR_{glc}$-HYD	$HAEC_{des}$	$HAEC_{sev}$	$qCMR_{glc}$ $HAEC_{GER}$	$HAEC_{DEN}$	$HAEC_{BEL}$
	$aCMR_{glc}$-HYD		*0.82*	*0.771*	*0.908*	*0.878*	*0.912*
	$HAEC_{des}$	0.233		*0.993*	*0.763*	*0.973*	*0.942*
	$HAEC_{sev}$	0.246	0.0401		*0.712*	*0.956*	*0.905*
$qCMR_{glc}$	$HAEC_{GER}$	0.213	0.202	0.228		*0.851*	*0.876*
	$HAEC_{DEN}$	0.243	0.0851	0.11	0.154		*0.946*
	$HAEC_{BEL}$	0.177	0.108	0.137	0.135	0.111	

versus 0.062; Sev0.25%: 0.013 versus 0.024; and Sev0.5%: 0.011 versus 0.0.024). The largely consistent slope estimates for $aCMR_{glc}$ and $qCMR_{glc}$ in Figures 1(b) and 1(c) demonstrate that group-to-group differences present in $aCMR_{glc}$ estimates were preserved after calculating $qCMR_{glc}$.

3.2. $qCMR_{glc}$ across Different States.
Compared to the eyes closed condition of the HAEC control group members ($0.31 \pm 0.06 \,\mu mol/g/min$), the eyes open HAEO group members had higher global estimates of $qCMR_{glc}$ ($0.34 \pm 0.06 \,\mu mol/g/min$) and the CB members had similar global gray matter estimates of $qCMR_{glc}$ ($0.31 \pm 0.05 \,\mu mol/g/min$), as shown in Figure 2(a). The HAEO group members had 8–12% higher global $qCMR_{glc}$ estimates ($0.34 \pm 0.06 \,\mu mol/g/min$) compared to the members of the HAEC control group in both gray and white matter regions (Figures S1A and S2A, resp.). The $qCMR_{glc}$ differences between HAEC and HAEO match reports of simple radiation counts [37]. In contrast, members of the CB group revealed only insignificant differences of global $qCMR_{glc}$ estimates across gray and white matter regions, compared with members of the HAEC groups (Figures S1B and S2B, resp.). Table 3 shows the relationship of $qCMR_{glc}$ when comparing different states to the control condition as assessed by linear regression analysis with intercept at zero (intercept = 0) and a floating intercept (intercept $\neq$ 0). Compared to HAEC, decreasing slopes were observed from HAEO to CB to Sev0.25% to Sev0.5% to Des1% to EMCS to MCS to UWS in both gray and white matter, and this pattern did not change with the regression method. There were minimal differences in the slopes (less than 16%) between the two regression methods except for UWS, which also had the largest intercept (0.07 in gray matter and 0.05 in white matter). The intercepts in all other cases were much smaller in comparison, suggesting that intercept at zero is a sufficient approximation for most of the states examined (Figures S1 and S2).

Compared to HAEC controls, the groups of individuals under sedation (Sev0.25%, Sev0.5%, and Des1%) had lower global $qCMR_{glc}$ estimates (0.29 ± 0.06, 0.27 ± 0.05, and $0.27 \pm 0.05 \,\mu mol/g/min$ in gray matter, respectively; Figure 2(b)). Compared to the HAEC control group members, members of the three sedation groups had 8–15% lower $qCMR_{glc}$

estimates in gray matter (Figure S1C) and 8–12% lower estimates in white matter (Figure S2C).

Compared to the HAEC group of control subjects, patients with disorders of consciousness (UWS, MCS, and EMCS) all had significantly lower $qCMR_{glc}$ estimates (0.20 ± 0.04, 0.19 ± 0.04, and $0.14 \pm 0.02 \,\mu mol/g/min$ in gray matter, resp.; Figure 2(c)). Compared to the HAEC control group, the clinical states had 36–54% lower estimates of $qCMR_{glc}$ in gray matter (Figure S1D) and 29–43% lower estimates in white matter (Figure S2D).

3.3. Statistical t-Maps for $qCMR_{glc}$ and GMN Data across States.
Relative to the HAEC control group, the statistical t-maps for the disorders of consciousness groups (UWS, MCS, and EMCS), sedated groups (Des1%, Sev0.25%, and Sev0.5%), healthy participants with eyes open group (HAEO), and the group of congenitally blind subjects (CB), respectively, are shown in Figures 3–6, respectively.

The UWS, MCS, and EMCS group members all had global declines, judging from the $qCMR_{glc}$t-maps (Figure 3(a)), consistent with the greatest decrease in subcortical regions. In contrast, judged from the GMN t-maps, the UWS, MCS, and EMCS group members had subcortical hypometabolism, whereas other regions had relative hypermetabolism (Figure 3(b)). Compared to the MCS and EMCS group members, the UWS group had areas of relative hypermetabolism in subcortical gray matter (Figure 3(b)).

The Sev0.25%, Sev0.5%, and Des1% groups all showed global metabolic decrease in the $qCMR_{glc}$t-maps (Figure 4(a)), with the Des1% group having less of a decline in white matter than the Sev0.25% and Sev0.5% groups. In contrast, using GMN t-maps, the Sev0.25%, Sev0.5%, and Des1% groups all had a regional pattern of both hypometabolism and hypermetabolism (Figure 4(b)). The Des1% group had relative hypermetabolism of deep brain regions, whereas the Sev0.25% and Sev0.5% groups had common patterns of bidirectional change that were most pronounced and of greatest spatial extent in the Sev0.5% group.

The HAEO group had diffuse global increases, estimated from the $qCMR_{glc}$t-maps with the greatest increase in the occipital cortex (Figure 5(a)), while GMN t-maps in contrast showed relative white matter hypermetabolism and gray

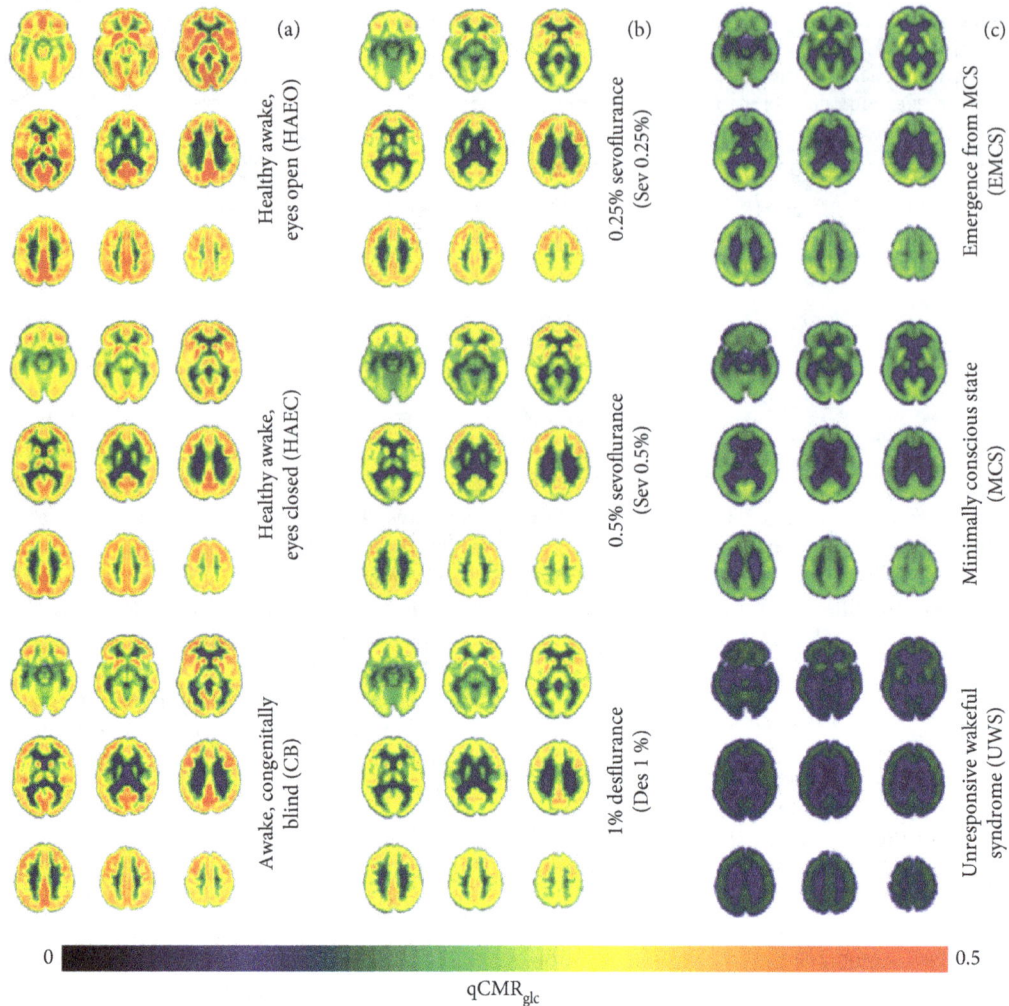

FIGURE 2: Quantified CMR_{glc} ($qCMR_{glc}$) maps of the human brain across nine different states (Table 1), which are (a) healthy awake sighted people with eyes closed (HAEC) or with eyes open (HAEO), as well as healthy awake people who are congenitally blind (CB), (b) healthy people under sedation with gaseous anesthetics (i.e., 0.25% sevoflurane (Sev0.25%), 0.5% sevoflurane (Sev0.5%), and 1% desflurane (Des1%)), and (c) patients with disorders of consciousness (i.e., unresponsive wakefulness syndrome (UWS), minimally conscious state (MCS), and emergence from minimally conscious state (EMCS)). Global increases in $qCMR_{glc}$ were observed proceeding from bottom to top in each column, which is in general agreement with prior PET studies [19, 45–50, 53]. The units are in μmol/g/min. With HAEC as the control condition, all other groups (except the CB group) showed significant global differences in gray matter (Figure S1) and white matter (Figure S2). These and all other images are in the coordinates of the MNI template: left column (from top to bottom) with z values of −15 mm, −12 mm, and −39 mm; middle column (from top to bottom) with z values of −6 mm, −21 mm, and −48 mm; and right column (from top to bottom) with z values of −3 mm, −30 mm, and −57 mm.

matter hypometabolism, except in the visual cortex, which had hypermetabolism (Figure 5(b)).

Only the CB group members had brain regions of both metabolic increases and decreases (albeit of smaller magnitudes) in the $qCMR_{glc}t$-maps, with the increases mainly in the visual cortex and the decreases beyond the visual cortex (Figure 6(a)). This pattern was repeated when the GMN t-maps revealed large domains of hypometabolic and hypermetabolic cortices, with vision areas showing the strongest relative hypermetabolism (Figure 6(b)). While in the $qCMR_{glc}t$-maps the hypometabolic (green in Figure 6(a)) and hypermetabolic (red in Figure 6(a)) regions revealed homogenous activities, in the GMN t-maps the hypometabolic (blue and green in Figure 6(b)) and hypermetabolic

(red and yellow in Figure 6(b)) regions showed heterogeneous activities.

The hot and cold colors in Figures 3–6 enabled visualization of the effect upon thresholding. However, we could not apply the same statistical threshold across all conditions because of large variation of groups' sizes (Table 1). Thus, we used thresholding as a means to reveal positive and negative clusters with GMN versus $qCMR_{glc}$ images, when compared to the control condition of eyes closed (Table 4). With disorders of consciousness (Figure S3), for the $qCMR_{glc}$ images there were only large-sized negative clusters (>98% of voxels), whereas in GMN images there were many smaller-sized negative (6–7% of voxels) and positive (0.1–14% of voxels) clusters. With anesthesia sedation (Figure S4), for the

TABLE 3: Relationship of quantified CMR$_{glc}$ (qCMR$_{glc}$) in gray and white matter of the human brain, comparing different states to the control condition, as assessed by linear regression analysis with (intercept = 0) and without (intercept ≠ 0) an intercept at the origin. See Table 1 for abbreviations of conditions. See Figures S1 and S2 for details on intercept = 0.

HAEC versus	Intercept ≠ 0			Intercept = 0	
	Slope	Intercept	R^2	Slope	R^2
Gray matter					
HAEO	1.12	0.00	0.93	1.12	0.93
CB	0.87	0.03	0.87	0.97	0.89
Sev0.25%	0.87	0.02	0.98	0.92	0.98
Sev0.5%	0.79	0.02	0.98	0.85	0.97
Des1%	0.73	0.04	0.95	0.86	0.94
EMCS	0.54	0.03	0.8	0.64	0.83
MCS	0.49	0.04	0.73	0.6	0.78
UWS	0.26	0.07	0.65	0.46	0.73
White matter					
HAEO	1.10	0.00	0.95	1.08	0.95
CB	0.90	0.02	0.92	0.98	0.93
Sev0.25%	0.88	0.01	0.99	0.99	0.92
Sev0.5%	0.81	0.01	0.98	0.88	0.98
Des1%	0.77	0.03	0.97	0.91	0.96
EMCS	0.61	0.02	0.81	0.71	0.84
MCS	0.59	0.02	0.73	0.69	0.77
UWS	0.35	0.05	0.64	0.57	0.73

qCMR$_{glc}$ images there were only large-sized negative clusters (71–96% of voxels), whereas in GMN images there were many smaller-sized negative (0.2–13% of voxels) and positive (0.3–11% of voxels) clusters. With eyes open in awake/healthy (Figure S5), for the qCMR$_{glc}$ images there was only one large-sized positive cluster (60% of voxels), whereas in GMN images there were many smaller-sized negative (2–20% of voxels) and positive (0.1–9% of voxels) clusters. With congenitally blind (Figure S6), for the qCMR$_{glc}$ images there was only one small-sized positive cluster and two small-sized negative clusters (each 1% of voxels), whereas in GMN images there was one large-sized negative cluster (45% of voxels) and three smaller-sized positive clusters (0.2–27% of voxels) clusters. In brief, the thresholded t-maps showed that the number of positive/ negative clusters in the GMN images were much greater (Table 4). Thus, all groups, except CB, had globally unidirectional metabolic offsets in qCMR$_{glc}$ t-maps, whereas regionally bidirectional differences were seen for all groups in GMN t-maps. In addition, the hypometabolism and hypermetabolic regions identified by GMN t-maps depict metabolic changes that are substantially smaller in magnitude (i.e., 3–6 times) than the global differences captured by the qCMR$_{glc}$$t$-maps (Figure S7).

4. Discussion

Absolute quantification of brain glucose metabolism with FDG-PET requires continuous arterial blood sampling throughout the imaging procedure [1, 39]. As arterial blood sampling in clinical settings is difficult or logistically impossible, alternative approaches are commonly used to determine relative differences among groups or conditions. The complementary approaches for quantitative PET generally involve a form of interindividual normalization, based on the ratio of dose injected and body weight as a proportional index of arterial input [40] or on the average uptake in whole brain, gray matter, or a preselected reference region inside [10] or outside [33] the brain. Moreover, there are considerations of arterialized venous sampling [41, 42] and image-derived input functions [43, 44]. The validity of any normalization approach relies on specific assumptions that usually are not readily testable, such as the linearity of the relationship between body weight and distribution volume, the expected range of metabolic changes (i.e., regional versus global), or the validity of a chosen reference region for the population being examined.

Here, we used a new validated method for deriving quantitative baseline metabolic activity from FDG-PET without individual normalization [37], but where the quantified measure of CMR$_{glc}$ (qCMR$_{glc}$) for the HAEC condition was compared to the absolute CMR$_{glc}$ (aCMR$_{glc}$) from Hyder et al. (aCMR$_{glc}$-HYD), also for the HAEC condition [36]. The process consisted of two steps. First, an intensity transformation was computed on a per-site basis for all HAEC datasets, using the Jensen-Shannon divergence method [38], to match the distribution of voxel intensities to the aCMR$_{glc}$-HYD database [36]. This enabled the original tissue-radioactivity values for each HAEC group to be converted to aCMR$_{glc}$ units on a per-site basis. This procedure also created a per-site intensity transformation that maps the original PET radioactivity counts to qCMR$_{glc}$, which can be used to

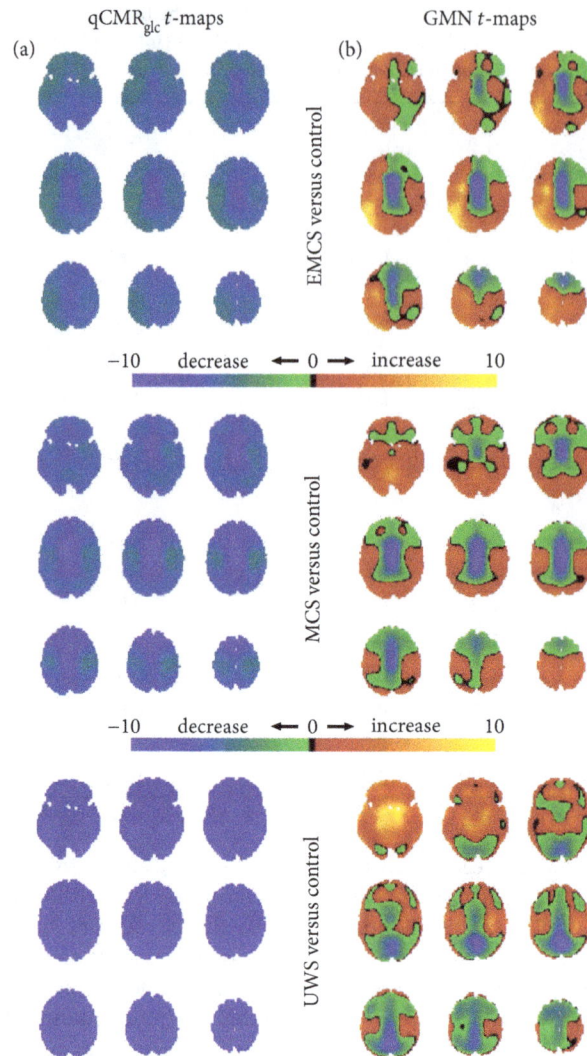

FIGURE 3: Spatial distributions of metabolic variations in patients with disorders of consciousness (i.e., UWS, MCS, and EMCS in Figure 2(c)) versus the control group (i.e., HAEC in Figure 2(a)), shown with respect to unthresholded Student's t-maps using (a) qCMR$_{glc}$ images and (b) GMN images. (a) For the UWS, MCS, and EMCS groups, the unthresholded t-maps with qCMR$_{glc}$ indicated globally unidirectional metabolic decreases in patients with disorders of consciousness. (b) But the unthresholded t-maps with GMN demonstrated the presence of regionally bidirectional metabolic changes in disorders of consciousness. Based on validation of qCMR$_{glc}$ to aCMR$_{glc}$-HYD (Figures 1 and 2; Table 2), without GMN the global decreases corresponded to about 0.15 μmol/g/min (UWS < MCS ≈ EMCS) and with GMN the global changes were diminished to put overemphasis on the regional differences. See Figure S3 for thresholded maps (Table 4).

convert radioactivity values for other conditions (i.e., conditions without lesions) scanned at that site using the same scanning parameters into aCMR$_{glc}$ units. Finally, we validated this procedure by comparing qCMR$_{glc}$ to aCMR$_{glc}$, on a voxel-by-voxel basis using Pearson correlation and Euclidean distance for all gray matter regions between the two datasets.

Our goal was to compare glucose metabolism measured by PET from a large number of conditions, including specific levels of sedation depth induced by anesthesia, several levels of disorder of consciousness, awake/healthy with eyes open, and congenital blindness. Each cohort included a control group of healthy, awake individuals resting with eyes closed, which were all comparable across sites. The validated qCMR$_{glc}$ group data led to new insights into the effects of

GMN on the detection and interpretation of global versus regional metabolic estimates.

The qCMR$_{glc}$ maps for all states (except the congenitally blind) revealed significant global differences relative to the eyes closed control group, which ranged in magnitude from ~10% increase for the awake, eyes open group to ~60% decrease in the unresponsive wakefulness syndrome. These global changes of qCMR$_{glc}$ are in good agreement with previous findings of changes with eyes open versus eyes closed states [45, 46], congenitally blind versus healthy sighted subjects [47, 48], effects of halogenated anesthetics [49–52], and findings in disorders of consciousness [35, 53]. Specifically, various anesthetics and disorders of consciousness have largely reported globally depressed metabolism compared to the healthy condition (see references within [19, 33]).

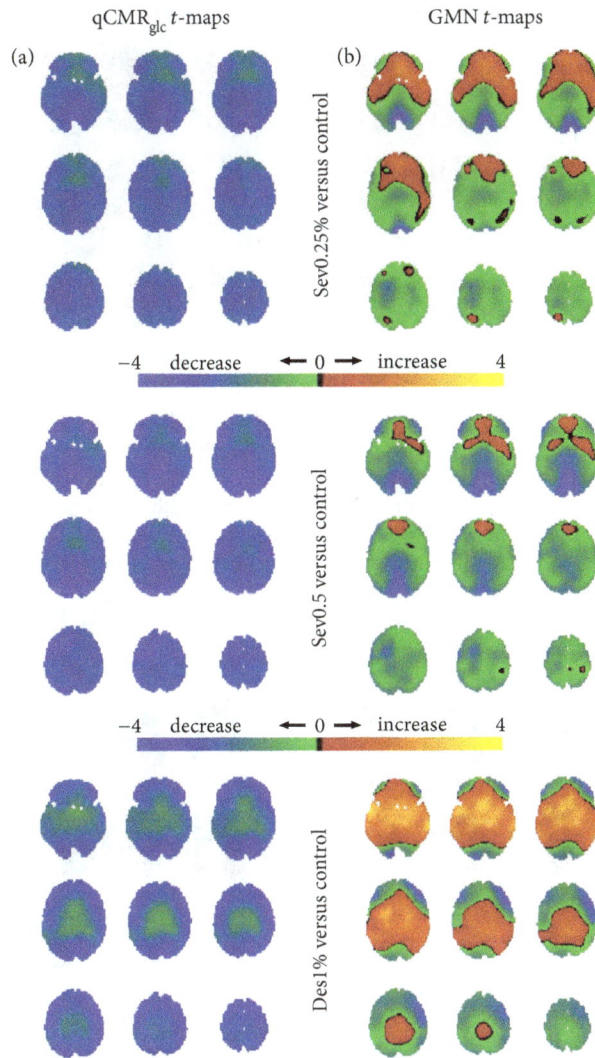

FIGURE 4: Spatial distributions of metabolic variations with sedation (i.e., Des1%, Sev0.25%, and Sev0.5% in Figure 2(b)) versus the control group (i.e., HAEC in Figure 2(a)), shown with respect to unthresholded Student's t-maps using (a) qCMR$_{glc}$ images and (b) GMN images. (a) For Des1%, Sev0.25%, and Sev0.5% groups, the unthresholded t-maps with qCMR$_{glc}$ indicated globally unidirectional metabolic decreases with sedation. (b) However, the unthresholded t-maps with GMN depicted regions with metabolic increases and decreases upon sedation. Based on validation of qCMR$_{glc}$ to aCMR$_{glc}$-HYD (Figures 1 and 2; Table 2), without GMN the global decreases corresponded to about $0.05\,\mu$mol/g/min (Des1% $\approx$ Sev0.5% < Sev1%) and with GMN the deemphasis on global changes put the focus on the regional differences. See Figure S4 for thresholded maps (Table 4).

After GMN, these large global changes were absent from the GMN t-maps due to regression to the mean value. Consequently, the GMN t-maps showed patterns of regional increase and decrease in metabolism among different states, suggesting that significant global information is not captured with the GMN procedure. Although increases/decreases were observed in congenitally blind with/without GMN, both the hypometabolic and hypermetabolic regions showed heterogeneous activities upon GMN. These results suggest that global normalization puts an overemphasis on regional differences.

4.1. GMN Eliminates Global Metabolic Changes across States.
In all conditions other than congenitally blind, we found globally unidirectional changes of qCMR$_{glc}$ estimates compared to the control group, with metabolic differences among states distributed within a large range (i.e., 0.14 to $0.34\,\mu$mol/g/min). In sharp contrast, GMN yielded regional increases and decreases compared to the eyes closed control group, with relative metabolic rate differences among states distributed within a narrow range (i.e., $\pm0.05\,\mu$mol/g/min). These results suggest that the global component of FDG-PET images contains state-dependent metabolic information that is lost upon GMN. Moreover, the present work shows that the hypometabolism and hypermetabolic regions revealed by GMN depict metabolic changes that are substantially smaller in magnitude than the inherent global metabolic differences. Although the regional pattern of deviations from the global mean of normalized FDG conveys important information about metabolic networks, exclusion

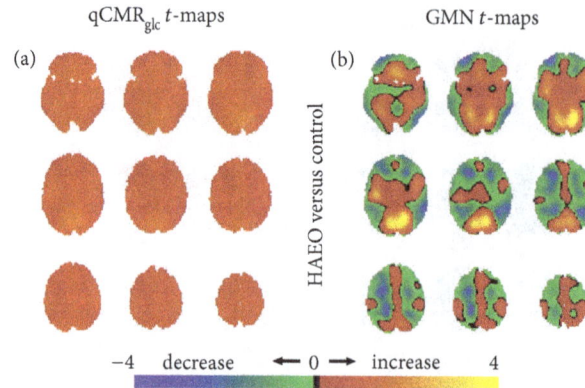

FIGURE 5: Spatial distributions of metabolic variations with healthy participants with eyes open (i.e., HAEO in Figure 2(a)) versus the eyes closed control group (i.e., HAEC in Figure 2(a)), shown with respect to unthresholded Student's t-maps using (a) qCMR$_{glc}$ images and (b) GMN images. (a) For the HAEO group, the unthresholded t-maps with qCMR$_{glc}$ indicated the presence of globally unidirectional metabolic increases with eyes open. (b) Conversely, the unthresholded t-maps with GMN revealed regions of increased and decreased metabolism with eyes open. Based on validation of qCMR$_{glc}$ to aCMR$_{glc}$-HYD (Figures 1 and 2; Table 2), without GMN the global increases corresponded to about 0.05 μmol/g/min while with GMN, the global changes were minute. See Figure S5 for thresholded maps (Table 4).

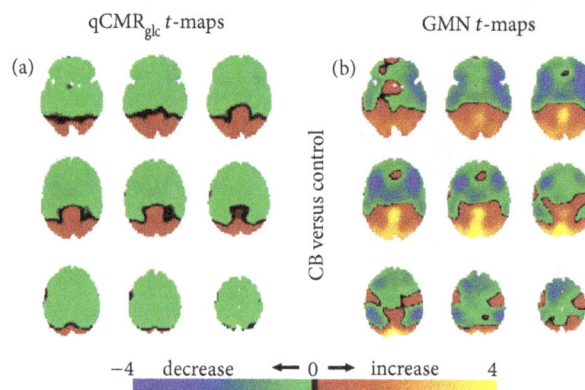

FIGURE 6: Spatial distributions of metabolic variations in the congenitally blind (i.e., CB in Figure 2(a)) versus the eyes closed control group (i.e., HAEC in Figure 2(a)), shown with respect to unthresholded Student's t-maps using (a) qCMR$_{glc}$ images and (b) GMN images. (a) For the CB group, the unthresholded t-maps with qCMR$_{glc}$ images indicated both regions with increased and decreased metabolism in association with blindness. Unidirectional metabolic decreases were observed in CB in most regions other than visual areas. (b) Similarly, the unthresholded t-maps with GMN indicated regionally bidirectional metabolic changes with blindness and unidirectional metabolic increases were observed in regions associated with vision. Based on validation of qCMR$_{glc}$ to aCMR$_{glc}$-HYD (Figures 1 and 2; Table 2), with and without GMN the global changes were essentially negligible. There were increases/decreases in visual/nonvisual areas, either with or without GMN. See Figure S6 for thresholded maps (Table 4).

of the global mean can yield different interpretations such as the regionally increased metabolic activity to disease states, a concern previously raised in the context of neurodegenerative diseases [12, 54].

However, when absolute differences are of small magnitude and regionalized, as in the present comparison of congenitally blind to the sighted control group, images with and without GMN showed very similar patterns of hypometabolism and hypermetabolic areas. In this particular case, the GMN procedure exposed the differences only after removal of interindividual global variations, without any penalty for misrepresentation of the magnitude of the differences. Overall, these comparisons, especially with that of the congenitally blind group versus the other groups, strongly suggest that there are new insights to be gained by inclusion

of both absolute and GMN analysis for PET-FDG data of neuropsychiatric and neurodegenerative diseases.

4.2. Study Limitations and Future Directions. The main limitation of the current study is the acquisition of PET-FDG images from multiple sites that were calibrated to produce qCMR$_{glc}$ comparisons across the different groups, thereby limiting the statistical significance of state-dependent variations. The high similarity between qCMR$_{glc}$ in the resting awake eyes closed (control) state across five different sites, which were nearly identical to aCMR$_{glc}$ region-to-region variations, suggests that qCMR$_{glc}$ maps from the different sites indeed were comparable. While the qCMR$_{glc}$ measure proved stable on a per-group basis, this report did not investigate its validity on a per-subject basis, specifically for conditions with

TABLE 4: Thesholding t-maps in Figures 3–6 revealed unidirectional and bidirectional changes, which is illustrated in terms of the number of positive (P) and negative (N) clusters, where they, respectively, correspond to areas of higher and lower intensities compared to control. See Table 1 for abbreviations of conditions. The positive clusters in the thresholded GMN (P_{GMN}) versus qCMR$_{glc}$ (P_{qCMR}) t-maps were 8 times greater, whereas negative clusters in the thresholded GMN (N_{GMN}) versus qCMR$_{glc}$ (N_{qCMR}) t-maps were 2 times greater. Similarity between thresholded GMN and qCMR$_{glc}$ t-maps was assessed by several metrics: (i) the total number of clusters given by the sum of P and N clusters, for qCMR$_{glc}$ ($T_{qCMR} = P_{qCMR} + N_{qCMR}$) and GMN ($T_{GMN} = P_{GMN} + N_{GMN}$) thresholded t-maps; (ii) the difference between the P clusters (D_P) for GMN and qCMR$_{glc}$ thresholded t-maps ($D_P = P_{GMN} - P_{qCMR}$); (iii) the difference between the N clusters (D_N) for GMN and qCMR$_{glc}$ thresholded t-maps ($D_N = N_{GMN} - N_{qCMR}$). Analysis shows that T_{GMN} was about 4 times greater than T_{qCMR}, whereas both D_P and D_N were greater than 0, signifying that GMN thresholded t-maps consistently revealed more bidirectional changes. For thresholded t-maps, see Figure S3 for EMCS, MCS, and UWS versus control (HAEC); Figure S4 for Sev0.25, Sev0.5, and Des1 versus control (HAEC); Figure S5 for HAEO versus control (HAEC); and Figure S6 for CB versus control (HAEC).

Condition versus control	Threshold (t-value)	Number of clusters				Similarity between GMN and qCMR$_{glc}$			
		P_{qCMR}	N_{qCMR}	P_{GMN}	N_{GMN}	T_{qCMR}	T_{GMN}	D_P	D_N
EMCS	4	0	1	2	1	1	3	2	0
MCS	4	0	1	5	1	1	6	5	0
UWS	4	0	1	2	1	1	3	2	0
Sev0.25%	2	0	1	1	2	1	3	1	1
Sev0.5%	2	0	1	0	4	1	4	0	3
Des1%	2	0	1	2	3	1	5	2	2
HAEO	1	1	0	3	2	1	5	2	2
CB	0.5	1	2	3	1	3	4	2	−1
Mean ± standard deviation		0.3 ± 0.5	1.0 ± 0.5	2.3 ± 1.5	1.9 ± 1.1	1.3 ± 0.7	4.1 ± 1.1	2.0 ± 1.4	0.9 ± 1.4

brain lesions. Future FDG-PET studies quantified with arterial sample inputs can improve aCMR$_{glc}$ estimates to reduce the intersubject variation among groups. Notwithstanding this conclusion, the present qCMR$_{glc}$ estimates had excellent correlations among all five control groups in this study. In the brain regions least vulnerable to effects of partial volume effects (i.e., regions defined by wide swathes of cortex with net spillover to and from adjacent tissues due to the inherent spatial smoothness of PET data is low), gray matter qCMR$_{glc}$ exceeded the estimates in white matter by 2–3-fold for the control state, in good agreement with prior studies [19, 55, 56]. However, different magnetic resonance spectroscopy (MRS) methods (e.g., ^{17}O MRS, ^{31}P MRS, ^{13}C MRS) and calibrated fMRI can be used to obtain absolute maps of CMR$_{glc}$ or CMR$_{O2}$ across these tissues for further validation [57].

Another concern of this study is the small sample sizes in three out of four sites and which limited the types of image analysis techniques we could employ. Variations in the Pearson correlation and the Euclidean distance for comparing across the control groups could be due to the multicenter data being heterogeneous (e.g., data acquired with different PET cameras). This and other weaknesses of the study limit the validity of the qCMR$_{glc}$ method for imaging others brain disorders (e.g., Alzheimer's disease and Parkinson's disease) at this stage, and thus, this procedure could be considered if aCMR$_{glc}$ comparisons are made for groups imaging across different brain states and/or PET scanners.

As noted above, qCMR$_{glc}$ for gray and white matter is sensitive to partial volume effects because the thickness of the cerebral cortex is close to the spatial resolution delivered by current PET instruments [58]. Higher spatial resolution, such as that from the Siemens HRRT used to acquire FDG-

derived images in the USA and Denmark sites, as well as improved MRI-based detection of cortical thickness, will provide better partial volume correction [59], propagating to increased accuracy of global versus regional metabolic differences measured across disease states. Using an HRRT scanner with sufficient resolution to measure the PET signal from the human globus pallidus, Borghammer et al. [14] employed reference cluster normalization to report that only the globus pallidus showed significant hypermetabolism in Parkinson's disease. A review of 2-deoxy-glucose studies of rodent and nonhuman primate models of Parkinson's disease showed that the globus pallidus most consistently reported true hypermetabolism [60]. Subsequent studies have dealt with the issue of normalization as raised by Borghammer et al. [14]. Dhawan et al. [61] reported that the spatial covariance pattern was not induced by reductions in global activity, opposing Borghammer et al. [14], whereas Dukart et al. [62] examined usefulness of different normalization procedures, and their findings do not contradict Borghammer et al. [14]. Since the sample sizes in some of our groups were small, we could not compare the results from different types of normalization methods (e.g., reference cluster and data-driven) and instead chose to compare effects on PET data with and without GMN.

Based on our results, and previous work, we thus caution that comparing any disease with the healthy condition should not begin with the assumption that global changes do not exist or, if they do exist, that they are not relevant to alterations in brain function (and behavior). We observed global changes across the entire brain without GMN in nearly all the states examined herein, but with GMN, these global changes were diminished showing bidirectional changes in all conditions examined. In one condition, the global changes appeared quite similar with and without GMN, but there was no assumption made about global or regional changes despite both analysis methods revealing nearly the same regional changes. Existing statistical analysis methods can undermine the relevance of global changes. For example, the Gaussian random field theory is optimized to detect small spatial regions of activity differences, defining "signal" as a limited spatial region whereas "noise" is defined as the background in large swathes of tissue. Also, if the global mean is used as a nuisance variable in techniques such as analysis of covariance, global changes will, by definition, be obscured. While our current work is focused on univariate analysis, if one includes the global signal as a "covariate of no interest," it does not matter whether the analysis is univariate or multivariate, the procedure still effectively removes global effects. For example, if the total signal (and underlying neuronal activity) from all brain regions were reduced by a factor of 2, both univariate and multivariate analysis would conclude no difference across regions, unless an absolute measure of the global component was included. The basic idea that the global signal should not be discarded applies to both univariate and multivariate analysis. Thus, to adequately measure signal versus noise in global as well as regional brain metabolism with the highest level of confidence, higher-sensitivity imaging methods are needed in combination with different statistical analysis methods, which are beyond the scope of the current work and are issues for future studies.

5. Conclusions

At present, analysis of PET data generally ignores the global baseline signal. However, both the baseline neuronal activity and the requisite energy demands supporting the activity of the cerebral cortex of awake humans are substantial [25, 26, 63]. Removing the global PET signal prior to comparison with the resting awake eyes closed (control) state exposed regionally bidirectional metabolic effects, along with some regional changes observed upon normalization. Improper use of global signal normalization may thus lead to the incorrect assignment of elevated metabolism to regions and, by inference, the presence of elevated neuronal activity despite an impaired state of consciousness. Conversely, the approach used here (i.e., without GMN) not only preserved the global alteration caused by sedation and consciousness disorders but also detected localized abnormalities in the context of the congenitally blind. In light of the current findings, we recommend that the baseline metabolic activity be included in the analysis of PET neuroimaging data, and only then is it possible to discern global and regional metabolic differences between healthy and diseased states.

Abbreviations

BOLD: Blood oxygen level-dependent
CBF: Cerebral blood flow
CMR_{glc}:   Cerebral metabolic rate of glucose metabolism
CMR_{O2}:   Cerebral metabolic rate of oxygen metabolism
GMN: Global mean normalization
MNI: Montreal Neurological Institute
PET: Positron emission tomography.

Disclosure

Garth J. Thompson's current address is iHuman Institute, ShanghaiTech University, Shanghai 201210, China

Authors' Contributions

Ron Kupers, Maurice Ptito, Steven Laureys, Valentin Riedl, Michael T. Alkire, Albert Gjedde, and Fahmeed Hyder conceived of, designed, and performed the research. Kristian N. Mortensen, Garth J. Thompson, Peter Herman, and Fahmeed Hyder analyzed the data. Kristian N. Mortensen, Garth J. Thompson, Peter Herman, Maxime J. Parent, Douglas L. Rothman, Johan Stender, Albert Gjedde, Ron Kupers, Maurice Ptito, Steven Laureys, Valentin Riedl, Michael T. Alkire, and Fahmeed Hyder wrote the paper.

Acknowledgments

This study was supported by National Institutes of Health grants (R01 MH-067528, R01 NS-100106, and P30 NS-052519) and the Lundbeckfonden fellowship (to Ron Kupers).

Supplementary Materials

Figure S1: voxel-to-voxel correlations of qCMRglc in gray matter of the human brain. Figure S2: voxel-to-voxel correlations of qCMRglc in white matter of the human brain. Figure S3: thresholded t-maps of metabolic variations in disorders of consciousness. Figure S4: thresholded t-maps of metabolic variations in anesthetic sedation. Figure S5: thresholded t-maps of metabolic variations with eyes open. Figure S6: thresholded t-maps of metabolic variations in congenital blindness. Figure S7: magnitude of metabolic variations with and without GMN. Table S1: description of human gray matter regions. (*Supplementary Materials*)

References

[1] A. Gjedde, K. Wienhard, W. D. Heiss et al., "Comparative regional analysis of 2-fluorodeoxyglucose and methylglucose uptake in brain of four stroke patients. With special reference to the regional estimation of the lumped constant," *Journal of Cerebral Blood Flow & Metabolism*, vol. 5, no. 2, pp. 163–178, 1985.

[2] A. Gjedde, "Functional brain imaging celebrates 30th anniversary," *Acta Neurologica Scandinavica*, vol. 117, no. 4, pp. 219–223, 2008.

[3] K. J. Friston, "Modalities, modes, and models in functional neuroimaging," *Science*, vol. 326, no. 5951, pp. 399–403, 2009.

[4] D. Eidelberg, "Metabolic brain networks in neurodegenerative disorders: a functional imaging approach," *Trends in Neurosciences*, vol. 32, no. 10, pp. 548–557, 2009.

[5] M. E. Raichle, "A brief history of human brain mapping," *Trends in Neurosciences*, vol. 32, no. 2, pp. 118–126, 2009.

[6] D. Eidelberg, J. R. Moeller, V. Dhawan et al., "The metabolic topography of parkinsonism," *Journal of Cerebral Blood Flow & Metabolism*, vol. 14, no. 5, pp. 783–801, 1994.

[7] K. J. Friston, A. P. Holmes, K. J. Worsley, J. P. Poline, C. D. Frith, and R. S. J. Frackowiak, "Statistical parametric maps in functional imaging: a general linear approach," *Human Brain Mapping*, vol. 2, no. 4, pp. 189–210, 1994.

[8] F. Hyder and D. L. Rothman, "Neuronal correlate of BOLD signal fluctuations at rest: err on the side of the baseline," *Proceedings of the National Academy of Sciences of the United States of America*, vol. 107, no. 24, pp. 10773–10774, 2010.

[9] S. C. Strother, J. S. Liow, J. R. Moeller, J. J. Sidtis, V. J. Dhawan, and D. A. Rottenberg, "Absolute quantitation in neurological PET: do we need it?," *Journal of Cerebral Blood Flow & Metabolism*, vol. 11, no. 1, pp. A3–16, 1991.

[10] P. Borghammer, K. Y. Jonsdottir, P. Cumming et al., "Normalization in PET group comparison studies–the importance of a valid reference region," *NeuroImage*, vol. 40, no. 2, pp. 529–540, 2008.

[11] P. Borghammer, J. Aanerud, and A. Gjedde, "Data-driven intensity normalization of PET group comparison studies is superior to global mean normalization," *NeuroImage*, vol. 46, no. 4, pp. 981–988, 2009.

[12] P. Borghammer, P. Cumming, J. Aanerud, S. Förster, and A. Gjedde, "Subcortical elevation of metabolism in Parkinson's disease–a critical reappraisal in the context of global mean normalization," *NeuroImage*, vol. 47, no. 4, pp. 1514–1521, 2009.

[13] P. Borghammer, M. Chakravarty, K. Y. Jonsdottir et al., "Cortical hypometabolism and hypoperfusion in Parkinson's disease is extensive: probably even at early disease stages," *Brain Structure and Function*, vol. 214, no. 4, pp. 303–317, 2010.

[14] P. Borghammer, P. Cumming, K. Østergaard et al., "Cerebral oxygen metabolism in patients with early Parkinson's disease," *Journal of the Neurological Sciences*, vol. 313, no. 1-2, pp. 123–128, 2012.

[15] B. B. Biswal, "Resting state fMRI: a personal history," *NeuroImage*, vol. 62, no. 2, pp. 938–944, 2012.

[16] R. D. Hoge, "Calibrated fMRI," *NeuroImage*, vol. 62, no. 2, pp. 930–937, 2012.

[17] R. Vos de Wael, F. Hyder, and G. J. Thompson, "Effects of tissue-specific functional magnetic resonance imaging signal regression on resting-state functional connectivity," *Brain Connectivity*, vol. 7, no. 8, pp. 482–490, 2017.

[18] F. Hyder and D. L. Rothman, "Quantitative fMRI and oxidative neuroenergetics," *NeuroImage*, vol. 62, no. 2, pp. 985–994, 2012.

[19] F. Hyder, R. K. Fulbright, R. G. Shulman, and D. L. Rothman, "Glutamatergic function in the resting awake human brain is supported by uniformly high oxidative energy," *Journal of Cerebral Blood Flow & Metabolism*, vol. 33, no. 3, pp. 339–347, 2013.

[20] O. D. Creutzfeldt, "Neurophysiological correlates of different functional states of the brain, in Brain Work," in *The Coupling of Function, Metabolism and Blood Flow in the Brain*, A. B. S. VIII, D. H. Ingvar, and N. A. Lassen, Eds., pp. 21–46, Blackwell Munksgaard Publishing, Copenhagen, Denmark, 1975.

[21] K. Hoedt-Rasmussen, E. Sveinsdottir, and N. A. Lassen, "Regional cerebral blood flow in man determined by intra-arterial injection of radioactive inert gas," *Circulation Research*, vol. 18, no. 3, pp. 237–247, 1966.

[22] L. C. Aiello and P. Wheeler, "The expensive-tissue hypothesis - the brain and the digestive-system in human and primate evolution," *Current Anthropology*, vol. 36, no. 2, pp. 199–221, 1995.

[23] A. Gjedde, P. Johannsen, G. E. Cold, and L. Østergaard, "Cerebral metabolic response to low blood flow: possible role of cytochrome oxidase inhibition," *Journal of Cerebral Blood Flow & Metabolism*, vol. 25, no. 9, pp. 1183–1196, 2005.

[24] F. Hyder, D. L. Rothman, and M. R. Bennett, "Cortical energy demands of signaling and nonsignaling components in brain are conserved across mammalian species and activity levels," *Proceedings of the National Academy of Sciences of the United States of America*, vol. 110, no. 9, pp. 3549–3554, 2013.

[25] Y. Yu, P. Herman, D. L. Rothman, D. Agarwal, and F. Hyder, "Evaluating the gray and white matter energy budgets of human brain function," *Journal of Cerebral Blood Flow & Metabolism*, 2017.

[26] R. G. Shulman, F. Hyder, and D. L. Rothman, "Insights from neuroenergetics into the interpretation of functional neuroimaging: an alternative empirical model for studying the brain's support of behavior," *Journal of Cerebral Blood Flow & Metabolism*, vol. 34, no. 11, pp. 1721–1735, 2014.

[27] J. Aanerud, P. Borghammer, M. M. Chakravarty et al., "Brain energy metabolism and blood flow differences in healthy aging," *Journal of Cerebral Blood Flow & Metabolism*, vol. 32, no. 7, pp. 1177–1187, 2012.

[28] J. Aanerud, P. Borghammer, A. Rodell, K. Y. Jónsdottir, and A. Gjedde, "Sex differences of human cortical blood flow and energy metabolism," *Journal of Cerebral Blood Flow & Metabolism*, vol. 37, no. 7, pp. 2433–2440, 2017.

[29] P. G. Spetsieris and D. Eidelberg, "Scaled subprofile modeling of resting state imaging data in Parkinson's disease: methodological issues," *NeuroImage*, vol. 54, no. 4, pp. 2899–2914, 2011.

[30] V. Riedl, K. Bienkowska, C. Strobel et al., "Local activity determines functional connectivity in the resting human brain: a simultaneous FDG-PET/fMRI study," *The Journal of Neuroscience*, vol. 34, no. 18, pp. 6260–6266, 2014.

[31] M. T. Alkire, R. Gruver, J. Miller, J. R. McReynolds, E. L. Hahn, and L. Cahill, "Neuroimaging analysis of an anesthetic gas that blocks human emotional memory," *Proceedings of the National Academy of Sciences of the United States of America*, vol. 105, no. 5, pp. 1722–1727, 2008.

[32] R. Kupers, P. Pietrini, E. Ricciardi, and M. Ptito, "The nature of consciousness in the visually deprived brain," *Frontiers in Psychology*, vol. 2, p. 19, 2011.

[33] J. Stender, K. N. Mortensen, A. Thibaut et al., "The minimal energetic requirement of sustained awareness after brain injury," *Current Biology*, vol. 26, no. 11, pp. 1494–1499, 2016.

[34] J. Stender, O. Gosseries, M. A. Bruno et al., "Diagnostic precision of PET imaging and functional MRI in disorders of consciousness: a clinical validation study," *The Lancet*, vol. 384, no. 9942, pp. 514–522, 2014.

[35] J. Stender, R. Kupers, A. Rodell et al., "Quantitative rates of brain glucose metabolism distinguish minimally conscious from vegetative state patients," *Journal of Cerebral Blood Flow & Metabolism*, vol. 35, no. 1, pp. 58–65, 2015.

[36] F. Hyder, P. Herman, C. J. Bailey et al., "Uniform distributions of glucose oxidation and oxygen extraction in gray matter of

normal human brain: no evidence of regional differences of aerobic glycolysis," *Journal of Cerebral Blood Flow & Metabolism*, vol. 36, no. 5, pp. 903–916, 2016.

[37] G. J. Thompson, V. Riedl, T. Grimmer, A. Drzezga, P. Herman, and F. Hyder, "The whole-brain "global" signal from resting state fMRI as a potential biomarker of quantitative state changes in glucose metabolism," *Brain Connectivity*, vol. 6, no. 6, pp. 435–447, 2016.

[38] J. Lin, "Divergence measures based on the Shannon entropy," *IEEE Transactions on Information Theory*, vol. 37, no. 1, pp. 145–151, 1991.

[39] C. S. Patlak, R. G. Blasberg, and J. D. Fenstermacher, "Graphical evaluation of blood-to-brain transfer constants from multiple-time uptake data," *Journal of Cerebral Blood Flow & Metabolism*, vol. 3, no. 1, pp. 1–7, 1983.

[40] S.-C. Huang, "Anatomy of SUV. Standardized uptake value," *Nuclear Medicine and Biology*, vol. 27, no. 7, pp. 643–646, 2000.

[41] A. P. van der Weerdt, L. J. Klein, C. A. Visser, F. C. Visser, and A. A. Lammertsma, "Use of arterialised venous instead of arterial blood for measurement of myocardial glucose metabolism during euglycaemic-hyperinsulinaemic clamping," *European Journal of Nuclear Medicine and Molecular Imaging*, vol. 29, no. 5, pp. 663–669, 2002.

[42] L. M. Wahl, M. C. Asselin, and C. Nahmias, "Regions of interest in the venous sinuses as input functions for quantitative PET," *Journal of Nuclear Medicine*, vol. 40, no. 10, pp. 1666–1675, 1999.

[43] G. Xiong, C. Paul, A. Todica, M. Hacker, P. Bartenstein, and G. Böning, "Noninvasive image derived heart input function for CMRglc measurements in small animal slow infusion FDG PET studies," *Physics in Medicine & Biology*, vol. 57, no. 23, pp. 8041–8059, 2012.

[44] F. O'Sullivan, J. Kirrane, M. Muzi et al., "Kinetic quantitation of cerebral PET-FDG studies without concurrent blood sampling: statistical recovery of the arterial input function," *IEEE Transactions on Medical Imaging*, vol. 29, no. 3, pp. 610–624, 2010.

[45] M. E. Phelps, J. C. Mazziotta, D. E. Kuhl et al., "Tomographic mapping of human cerebral metabolism visual stimulation and deprivation," *Neurology*, vol. 31, no. 5, pp. 517–529, 1981.

[46] C. Veraart, A. G. de Volder, M. C. Wanet-Defalque, A. Bol, C. Michel, and A. M. Goffinet, "Glucose utilization in human visual cortex is abnormally elevated in blindness of early onset but decreased in blindness of late onset," *Brain Research*, vol. 510, no. 1, pp. 115–121, 1990.

[47] M. C. Wanet-Defalque, C. Veraart, A. de Volder et al., "High metabolic activity in the visual cortex of early blind human subjects," *Brain Research*, vol. 446, no. 2, pp. 369–373, 1988.

[48] A. G. De Voldera, A. Bol, J. Blin et al., "Brain energy metabolism in early blind subjects: neural activity in the visual cortex," *Brain Research*, vol. 750, no. 1-2, pp. 235–244, 1997.

[49] M. T. Alkire, R. J. Haier, N. K. Shah, and C. T. Anderson, "Positron emission tomography study of regional cerebral metabolism in humans during isoflurane anesthesia," *Anesthesiology*, vol. 86, no. 3, pp. 549–557, 1997.

[50] M. T. Alkire, C. J. D. Pomfrett, R. J. Haier et al., "Functional brain imaging during anesthesia in humans: effects of halothane on global and regional cerebral glucose metabolism," *Anesthesiology*, vol. 90, no. 3, pp. 701–709, 1999.

[51] L. Schlunzen, M. S. Vafaee, G. E. Cold, M. Rasmussen, J. F. Nielsen, and A. Gjedde, "Effects of subanaesthetic and anaesthetic doses of sevoflurane on regional cerebral blood flow in healthy volunteers. A positron emission tomographic study," *Acta Anaesthesiologica Scandinavica*, vol. 48, no. 10, pp. 1268–1276, 2004.

[52] L. Schlünzen, N. Juul, K. V. Hansen, A. Gjedde, and G. E. Cold, "Regional cerebral glucose metabolism during sevoflurane anaesthesia in healthy subjects studied with positron emission tomography," *Acta Anaesthesiologica Scandinavica*, vol. 54, no. 5, pp. 603–609, 2010.

[53] S. Laureys, A. M. Owen, and N. D. Schiff, "Brain function in coma, vegetative state, and related disorders," *The Lancet Neurology*, vol. 3, no. 9, pp. 537–546, 2004.

[54] I. Yakushev, A. Hammers, A. Fellgiebel et al., "SPM-based count normalization provides excellent discrimination of mild Alzheimer's disease and amnestic mild cognitive impairment from healthy aging," *NeuroImage*, vol. 44, no. 1, pp. 43–50, 2009.

[55] B. Horwitz, R. Duara, and S. I. Rapoport, "Intercorrelations of glucose metabolic rates between brain regions: application to healthy males in a state of reduced sensory input," *Journal of Cerebral Blood Flow & Metabolism*, vol. 4, no. 4, pp. 484–499, 1984.

[56] J. M. Rumsey, R. Duara, C. Grady et al., "Brain metabolism in autism. Resting cerebral glucose utilization rates as measured with positron emission tomography," *Archives of General Psychiatry*, vol. 42, no. 5, pp. 448–455, 1985.

[57] F. Hyder and D. L. Rothman, "Advances in imaging brain metabolism," *Annual Review of Biomedical Engineering*, vol. 19, no. 1, pp. 485–515, 2017.

[58] C. la Fougère, S. Grant, A. Kostikov et al., "Where *in-vivo* imaging meets cytoarchitectonics: the relationship between cortical thickness and neuronal density measured with high-resolution [18F]flumazenil-PET," *NeuroImage*, vol. 56, no. 3, pp. 951–960, 2011.

[59] M. C. Huisman, L. W. van Golen, N. J. Hoetjes et al., "Cerebral blood flow and glucose metabolism in healthy volunteers measured using a high-resolution PET scanner," *EJNMMI Research*, vol. 2, no. 1, p. 63, 2012.

[60] P. Borghammer, "Perfusion and metabolism imaging studies in Parkinson's disease," *Danish Medical Journal*, vol. 59, no. 6, article B4466, 2012.

[61] V. Dhawan, C. C. Tang, Y. Ma, P. Spetsieris, and D. Eidelberg, "Abnormal network topographies and changes in global activity: absence of a causal relationship," *NeuroImage*, vol. 63, no. 4, pp. 1827–1832, 2012.

[62] J. Dukart, R. Perneczky, S. Förster et al., "Reference cluster normalization improves detection of frontotemporal lobar degeneration by means of FDG-PET," *PLoS One*, vol. 8, no. 2, article e55415, 2013.

[63] A. Gjedde and S. Marrett, "In search of baseline: absolute and relative measures of blood flow and oxidative metabolism in visual cortex stimulated at three levels of complexity," *Journal of Experimental & Clinical Neurosciences*, vol. 3, no. 1, 2016.

7

Botulinum Neurotoxin Application to the Severed Femoral Nerve Modulates Spinal Synaptic Responses to Axotomy and Enhances Motor Recovery in Rats

Marcel Irintchev, Orlando Guntinas-Lichius⊙, and Andrey Irintchev⊙

Department of Otorhinolaryngology, Jena University Hospital, Am Klinikum 1, 07747 Jena, Germany

Correspondence should be addressed to Andrey Irintchev; andrey.irintchev@med.uni-jena.de

Academic Editor: Laura Baroncelli

Botulinum neurotoxin A (BoNT) and brain-derived neurotrophic factor (BDNF) are known for their ability to influence synaptic inputs to neurons. Here, we tested if these drugs can modulate the deafferentation of motoneurons following nerve section/suture and, as a consequence, modify the outcome of peripheral nerve regeneration. We applied drug solutions to the proximal stump of the freshly cut femoral nerve of adult rats to achieve drug uptake and transport to the neuronal perikarya. The most marked effect of this application was a significant reduction of the axotomy-induced loss of perisomatic cholinergic terminals by BoNT at one week and two months post injury. The attenuation of the synaptic deficit was associated with enhanced motor recovery of the rats 2–20 weeks after injury. Although BDNF also reduced cholinergic terminal loss at 1 week, it had no effect on this parameter at two months and no effect on functional recovery. These findings strengthen the idea that persistent partial deafferentation of axotomized motoneurons may have a significant negative impact on functional outcome after nerve injury. Intraneural application of drugs may be a promising way to modify deafferentation and, thus, elucidate relationships between synaptic plasticity and restoration of function.

1. Introduction

Injury to peripheral nerves in adult mammals causes deafferentation of the axotomized motoneurons, a phenomenon known as "synaptic stripping" [1]. Synaptic terminals are removed from cell bodies and dendrites of motoneurons by activated microglial and astroglial cells [1–6]. The overall posttraumatic loss is reversed to a large extent if muscles become reinnervated [3, 6, 7], but restoration of some synaptic inputs is incomplete [8–11]. Such deficits, for example, in cholinergic and glutamatergic innervation, may contribute to functional deficits after muscle reinnervation as they are well correlated with functional performance after long-term reinnervation [9, 12].

Here, we pursued to influence synaptic responses after peripheral nerve injury and, thus, eventually alter the outcome by using botulinum neurotoxin A (BoNT) or brain-derived neurotrophic factor (BDNF). When applied intramuscularly, BoNT blocks synaptic transmission at the neuromuscular junction and, in addition, is transported retrogradely to the motoneuron cell body and possibly also transcytosed to afferent synaptic terminals [13–16]. BoNT causes progressive synaptic stripping detectable at 4 days after intramuscular injection and abolishes excitatory and inhibitory synaptic transmission on motoneurons at 1-2 weeks after application [17]. Rather than intramuscularly, we applied BoNT to the proximal nerve stump immediately after nerve transection similar to the application of retrograde tracers assuming that this type of application will enhance synaptic stripping similar to intramuscular BoNT application. In other animals, we applied BDNF to the proximal stump of the freshly cut nerve hoping to achieve an effect opposite to that of BoNT, that is, attenuation of synaptic loss. When administered to cut proximal axons immediately after transection, BNDF reduces synaptic stripping and enhances recovery of tonic firing of regenerating motoneurons [18].

Synaptotrophic effects of exogenous BDNF have also been reported after ventral root avulsion [19]. Finally, a single session of brief electrical stimulation (20 Hz, 1 hour) of the proximal stump of the freshly transected femoral nerve in rats leads to enhanced nerve regeneration over weeks and this effect is apparently associated with an upregulation of BDNF and its cognitive receptor TrkB in the motoneuron cell body [20, 21]. It is possible, though not proven, that this enhanced BDNF signaling leads to, among other mechanisms, better regeneration via synaptotrophic effects. We measured the effects of BoNT or BDNF application using stereological estimates of chemically defined nerve terminal densities in motor nuclei, a motor recovery test, and retrograde labeling of motoneurons. For this first experiment using intraneural drug application, we selected the femoral nerve model in rats for a practical reason: the anatomy in this model allows work with a longer proximal trunk after nerve transection as compared with, for example, the facial nerve and, thus, easier application of BoNT or BDNF solutions to the severed nerve using plastic mini cups. The well-established femoral nerve model is a valuable alternative to other spinal nerve models like the sciatic one offering the possibility to analyze precision of target reinnervation, reliable functional assessments, and a straightforward search of anatomical deficits and structure-function correlations [22]. Helpful for this study was also previous data on long-term functional recovery, precision of motor reinnervation, and correlations between these measures after section/suture of the femoral nerve in adult rats [23].

2. Materials and Methods

2.1. Animals and Experimental Design. Ten-week-old female Wistar Unilever rats ($N = 65$) from Charles River Laboratories (Sulzfeld, Germany) were used. To monitor short-term numerical changes in synaptic terminal populations, retrograde neuronal tracer (Fluoro-Gold, FG) was injected unilaterally into the quadriceps muscles of 20 animals (experiment I). Four days later, the femoral nerve on the injected side was cut and solutions containing bovine serum albumin (BSA), BoNT, or BDNF were applied to the proximal nerve stump (5 rats per group, see details on application below). Synaptic populations in the quadriceps motor nucleus, defined by the retrograde labeling, were studied one week after nerve transection. The rest five rats served as an "intact" control, that is, they were similarly treated and analyzed with the exception of nerve injury. To analyze long-term synaptic alterations, the rats in experiment II were subjected to nerve lesion and application of BSA ($N = 6$), BoNT type A ($N = 7$), or BDNF ($N = 7$). Intramuscular (i.m.) injections of FG were performed two months after injury followed by, one week later, video recordings for single-frame motion analysis (SFMA) and tissue sampling for synaptic terminal analyses. Analysis of long-term functional effects was done in experiment III. After nerve injury and application of BSA ($N = 7$), BoNT ($N = 10$), or BDNF ($N = 8$), the animals were repeatedly video recorded over a 20-week observation period and then subjected to retrograde

labeling of motoneurons regenerated beyond the injury site to analyze "preferential motor reinnervation" [24]. The animals were housed under standard conditions and received food and water ad libitum. Visual examinations for complications like BoNT-induced muscle paralysis, abnormal grooming, or self-mutilations were performed regularly (once daily in the first week, once or twice weekly at later time periods). Such complications were not observed. Experiments were performed according to the animal protection laws of Germany and the European Community. Experiments were blinded.

2.2. Surgery and Drug Application. Rats were anesthetized with fentanyl (Fentanyl Janssen, Janssen, Neuss, Germany, 0.005 mg/kg i.m.), midazolam (Dormicum-R, Roche, Basel, Switzerland, 2 mg/kg i.m.), and medetomidine (Domitor-R, Orion Pharma, Espoo, Finland, 0.15 mg/kg i.m.). The trunk of the right nerve was exposed under an operation microscope and cut at approximately 7 mm proximal to the bifurcation of the saphenous and quadriceps muscle branches (Figure 1(a)). The proximal nerve stump was inserted for 30 min into a cup containing 0.1% BSA (Sigma, Taufkirchen, Germany) in saline, 100 U/ml BoNT (Xeomin, Merz Pharma, Frankfurt, Germany), or 20 μg/ml human recombinant BDNF (Biomol, Hamburg, Germany) in 0.1% BSA saline (Figure 1(b)). As a rough orientation for the drug concentrations served previous in vivo studies on synaptic effects using BoNT [13, 17] and BDNF [18]. The cups were cut from standard yellow pipette tips after their distal ends were heat-sealed using a lighter (Figure 1(b), capacity ~10 μl). After drug treatment, the nerve trunks and their surroundings were thoroughly rinsed with saline and the nerve ends were aligned using two epineural 10–0 sutures (Ethicon, Norderstedt, Germany). Finally, the skin was closed with 4–0 sutures (Ethicon) and the rats received subcutaneously an antidote cocktail consisting of atipamezole (Antisedan, Orion Pharma, 0.75 mg/kg), flumazenil (Anexate, Roche, 0.2 mg/kg), and naloxone (Naloxon, CuraMed Pharma, Karlsruhe, Germany, 0.12 mg/kg).

2.3. Single-Frame Motion Analysis (SFMA). SFMA was performed as described previously [23]. Briefly, the rats (experiments II and III) were video recorded prior to nerve injury from behind and from the left and right side during walking along a wooden plate (1500 mm long, 120 mm wide, and 20 mm thick) using a video camera (100 frames per second, Pike F-032, Allied Vision Technologies, Stadtroda, Germany). The video recordings were repeated 8 weeks (experiment II) or at 1, 2, 4, 8, 12, 16, and 20 weeks (experiment III) after injury. At least three walking trials were recorded per rear, left and right side view of each animal per time point. Analyses were performed using noncommercial software packages: VirtualDub 1.6.19 (http://www.virtualdub.org) and Image Tool 3.0 (University of Texas Health Science Center at San Antonio, TX, USA, http://compdent.uthscsa.edu/imagetool.asp). Two parameters were measured: the foot-base angle (FBA) and the step length ratio (SLR). The FBA is measured at toe-off position on the side ipsilateral to injury as an angle between the line dividing the sole surface

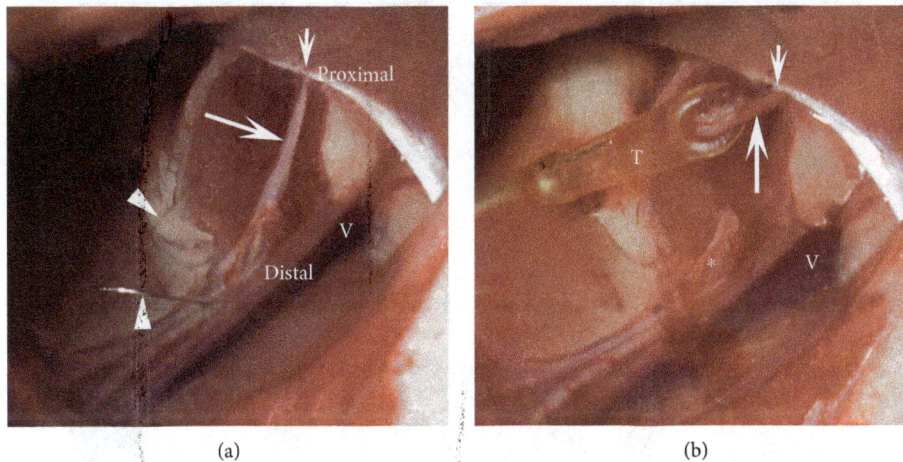

FIGURE 1: Drug application to the severed nerve. (a) The right femoral nerve trunk (arrow) prior to nerve injury. Proximally, the nerve is fixed by an epineural suture (short arrow) to the nearby muscle aponeurosis to prevent withdrawal of the proximal stump after nerve cut. Seen are also the 10–0 thread (upper arrowhead) used to fix the nerve and its needle (lower arrowhead), as well as the femoral vein (V). (b) The femoral nerve is transected, and the proximal stump is inserted in a self-made cup (T, see Materials and Methods) filled with drug solution. The distal nerve stump is marked by an asterisk.

into two halves and the horizontal line (minimum of 3 measurements per animal and time point). The SLR is calculated as ratio of the lengths of two successive steps (minimum of 6 SLR values per animal and time point). Using the FBA and SLR values, two additional parameters were calculated: (1) the product FBA × SLR and (2) the FBA × SLR recovery index [23].

2.4. Retrograde Labeling of Motoneurons.

To label the quadriceps motor nucleus (experiments I and II), 125 μl of 1% Fluoro-Gold (Fluorochrome, Denver, CO, USA) in saline was injected into the right quadriceps muscle without anesthesia of the rats (Figure 2(a)). For analysis of "preferential motor reinnervation" [23], 20 weeks after injury, the rats in experiment III were anesthetized as described above. The quadriceps and the saphenous branches were cut approximately 5 mm distal to the bifurcation. Fluoro-Ruby (tetramethylrhodamine dextran, MW 10,500, Molecular Probes/Life Technologies, Darmstadt, Germany) and Fluoro-Emerald (fluorescein dextran, MW 10,000, Molecular Probes) crystals were applied for 30 min to the proximal stumps of the quadriceps and the saphenous branch, respectively. Labeling was considered successful if no leakage of dye beyond the parafilm sheaths underlying the nerve ends was noticed after the 30 min application period. Six days later, the rats were anaesthetized and perfused with 4% formaldehyde in 0.1 M sodium cacodylate buffer, pH 7.3. The lumbar spinal cords were removed, postfixed overnight, and cut transversely (serial sections of 40 μm thickness) on a cryostat (CM1850, Leica Microsystems, Wetzlar, Germany). The sections were collected on SuperFrost Plus glass slides (Carl Roth, Karlsruhe, Germany) and coverslipped using Fluoromount G (Southern Biotechnology Associates/Biozol, Eching, Germany). Counting was based on stereological principles and done on an Axiophot 2 fluorescence microscope [25].

2.5. Immunofluorescence.

Tissue processing and staining were performed as previously described [26]. Under anesthesia (see above), the rats were perfused with 4% formaldehyde in 0.1 M cacodylate buffer, pH 7.3, for 15 min at room temperature (RT). The lumbar spinal cords were then postfixed in the same fixative overnight at 4°C and cryoprotected by infiltration with 15% sucrose in cacodylate buffer for 2 days at 4°C. The samples were frozen in precooled 2-methyl-butane (isopentane, −80°C) for 2 min and stored in liquid nitrogen until sectioned. Transverse sections of 25 μm thickness were obtained using a cryostat (CM1850, Leica Microsystems, Wetzlar, Germany) such that 6 spaced serial sections 250 μm apart were present on each slide. Immunofluorescence staining was performed after antigen retrieval (30 min at 80°C in 10 mM sodium citrate solution, pH 9.0). Nonspecific binding was blocked for 1 hour at RT with phosphate-buffered saline (PBS, pH 7.3) containing 0.2% Triton X-100 (Sigma), 0.02% sodium azide (Sigma), and 5% normal serum (Jackson ImmunoResearch Europe, Suffolk, UK) from the species in which the secondary antibody was raised (Table 1). The primary antibodies were diluted in PBS containing 0.5% lambda-carrageenan (Sigma) and 0.2% sodium azide and applied to the sections for 3 days at 4°C (Table 1). Cy3-conjugated secondary antibodies, diluted in PBS containing 0.5% lambda-carrageenan and 0.2% sodium azide, were applied for 2 hours at RT (Table 1). Cell nuclei were stained for 10 min at RT with bis-benzimide solution (Hoechst 33258 dye, 5 μg ml^{-1} in PBS, Sigma). For each antigen, all sections were stained in the same primary and secondary antibody solutions stabilized by the nongelling vegetable gelatin lambda-carrageenan and kept in screw-capped staining plastic jars (capacity 35 ml, 10 slides, Carl Roth). This method enables repeated long-term usage and high reproducibility of the immunohistochemical staining [26–28]. Staining controls included omitting the first antibody or replacing it by normal serum or IgG. These controls

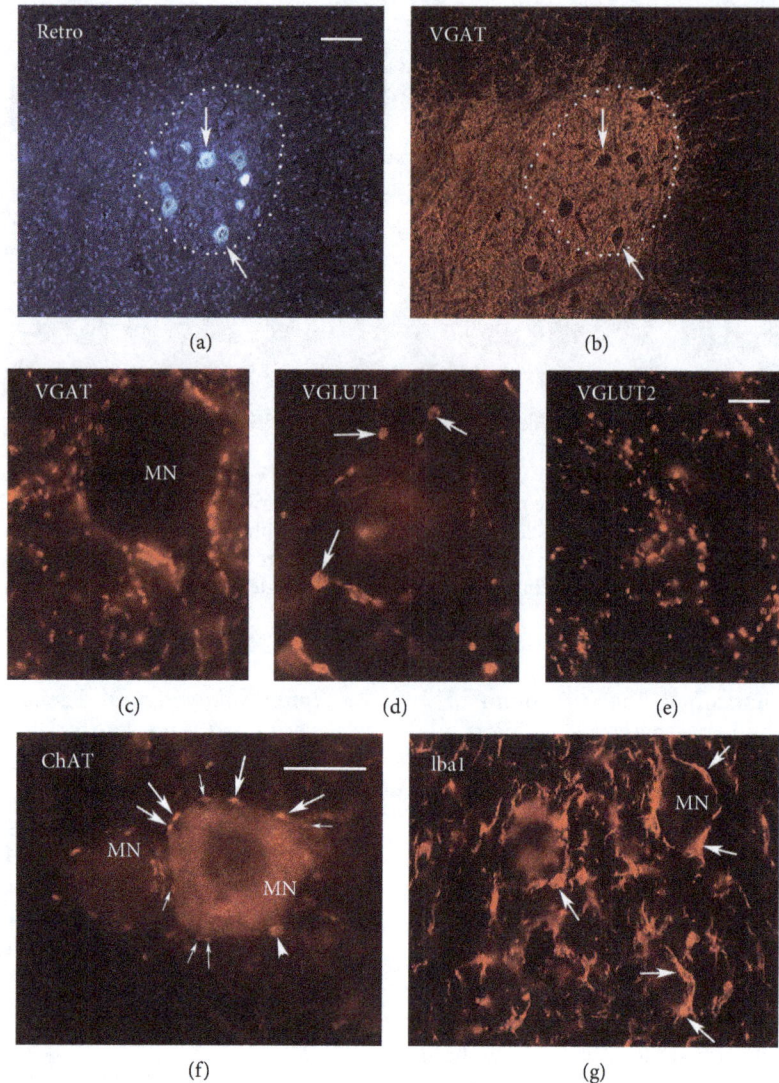

FIGURE 2: Images of synaptic terminals and Iba1$^+$ cells in the quadriceps motor nucleus. (a-b) A section containing back-labeled cell bodies of femoral motoneurons (a, arrows) is additionally stained for nuclei (a) and VGAT (b). The boundary of the quadriceps motor nucleus is indicated by a dotted line. Scale bar = 100 μm for (a-b). (c–e) VGAT$^+$ and VGLUT 2$^+$ axonal terminals (c, e) and VGLUT1$^+$ varicosities (arrows, d). Scale bar = 10 μm for (c–e). (f) ChAT staining of two motoneuron cell bodies (MN) surrounded by cholinergic terminals (arrows). Counted were terminals around the MN soma with a visible nucleus (pale area in the center of the MN on the right hand side) which were in focus (thick arrows). Terminals out of focus or only partially seen in the focus plane (thin arrows) were not counted. No quantification was undertaken for the second MN profile (on the left hand side) since it had no visible nucleus. The arrowhead points to a ChAT$^+$ cross-sectional profile of a dendrite close to the MN cell body. Such "perisomatic" dendritic profiles could be traced for long distances throughout the section thickness in contrast to the limited extent of the perisomatic terminals in the z-axis. (g) Iba1$^+$ cells (arrows) some of which surround a motoneuron cell body (MN). Scale bar indicates 25 μm and 50 μm for panels (f) and (g), respectively. (a–g) Shown are representative images from tissue sections after different treatments to illustrate the quality of each staining which was similar in all experimental groups and time points.

were negative. Examples of immunohistochemical stainings are shown in Figures 2(b)–2(g).

2.6. Quantitative Immunohistochemical Analyses. Quantitative analyses were performed using the Stereo Investigator 8.1 software (MicroBrightField Europe, Magdeburg, Germany) and a fluorescence microscope (Axioskop 2 mot plus, Zeiss, Oberkochen, Germany) equipped with a motorized stage (Zeiss) and a CX 9000 digital camera (MicroBrightField) as described [9, 12]. Cell and synaptic terminal densities were estimated using the optical disector in every 10th spaced serial section (250 μm apart) in which back-labeled femoral motoneurons were visible (Figure 2(a)). The boundaries of the quadriceps motor nucleus were outlined (Plan Neofluar 5x objective, Zeiss, Figure 2(a)), and cell or synaptic terminal densities (N_v) were estimated using randomly placed disectors. For VGAT$^+$ (Figures 2(b) and 2(c)), VGLUT1$^+$ (Figure 2(d)), and VGLUT2$^+$ terminals (Figure 2(e)), the disectors had a 100 μm^2 base and a 5 μm height with an interdisector spacing of 100 μm. Individually

TABLE 1: Antibodies used for immunohistochemistry.

Antigen	Species and type, dilution	Supplier, code	Structures labeled by primary antibodies	References
Choline acetyltransferase	Goat polyclonal, 1:500	Chemicon/Millipore, Schwalbach, Germany, AB144P	Cholinergic cells, axons and axon terminals, large perisomatic terminals on motoneurons	Hellström et al. [44], Nagy et al. [45], Wilson et al. [46]
Iba1 (ionized calcium binding adaptor molecule 1)	Rabbit polyclonal, 1:1500	Wako Chemicals, Neuss, Germany, 019-19741	Microglial cells	Imai et al. [64], Ito et al. [65]
VGAT (vesicular GABA transporter)	Mouse monoclonal, 1:500	Synaptic Systems, Gottingen, Germany, 131 011	Inhibitory (GABAergic and glycinergic) axon terminals	Chaudhry et al. [66], McIntire et al. [67], Wojcik et al. [68]
VGLUT1 (vesicular glutamate transporter 1)	Rabbit polyclonal, 1:1000	Synaptic Systems, 135 303	Excitatory (glutamatergic) axon terminals of primary (Ia) afferents	Alvarez et al. [69], Oliveira et al. [70], Rotterman et al. [10]
VGLUT2 (vesicular glutamate transporter 2)	Rabbit polyclonal, 1:1000	Synaptic Systems, 135 403	Excitatory (glutamatergic) axon terminals of spinal cord interneurons	Alvarez et al. [69], Oliveira et al. [70]
SNAP-25 BoTox-A cleaved	Mouse monoclonal (4F3-2C1), 1:200	MyBioSource, San Diego, CA, USA, MBS350064	Synaptic terminals containing SNAP-25 (synaptosomal-associated protein 25) cleaved by botulinum toxin A	Manufacturer's data sheet, Rheaume et al. [32]
Goat IgG	Cy3-conjugated donkey polyclonal, 1:200	Jackson ImmunoResearch Europe, Suffolk, UK, 705-165-003		
Mouse IgG	Cy3-conjugated goat polyclonal, 1:200	Jackson ImmunoResearch, 115-165-003		
Rabbit IgG	Cy3-conjugated goat polyclonal, 1:200	Jackson ImmunoResearch, 111-165-003		

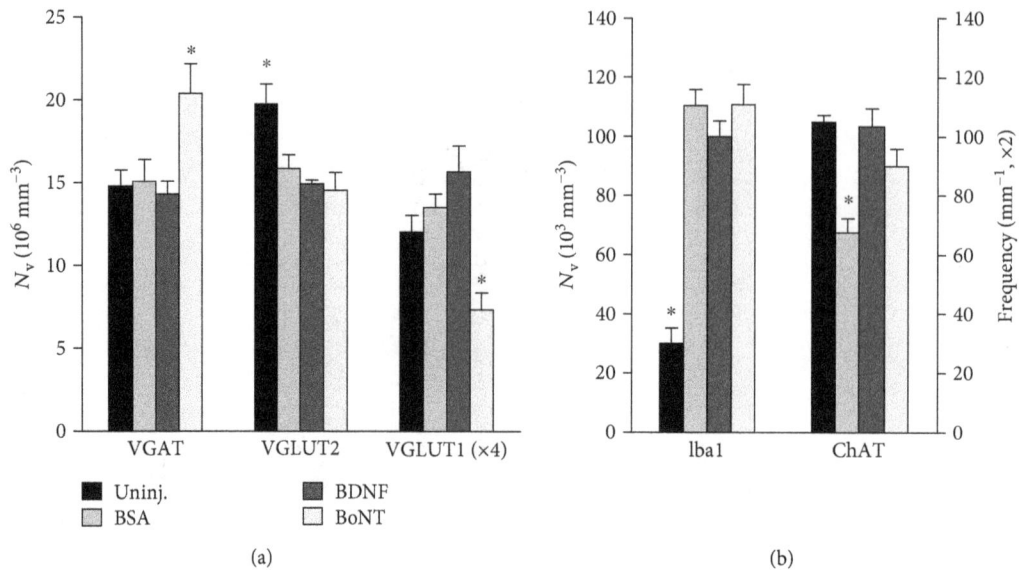

FIGURE 3: Analysis of synaptic terminals and microglia in the quadriceps motor nucleus 1 week after femoral nerve injury and drug application. Included are also values from control rats without nerve injury and drug treatment ("Uninj."). Shown are numerical densities (number per unit volume) of VGAT$^+$, VGLUT1$^+$, and VGLUT2$^+$ terminals and Iba1$^+$ microglial cells, as well as frequency (number per unit length) of ChAT$^+$ perisomatic terminals (mean values + SEM). Asterisks indicate mean values significantly different from all other groups (one-way ANOVA, $F_{3,16} = 4.87$–44.8, $p = 0.014$ – <0.001) with Holm-Sidak post hoc tests ($p = 0.042$ – <0.001). $N = 5$ per group.

discernible immunopositive puncta were counted using a Plan Neofluar 100x oil objective (Zeiss). For Iba1$^+$ cells (Figure 2(g)), the size of the disectors was $3600\,\mu m^2$ base and $10\,\mu m$ height and the spacing between disectors was $100\,\mu m$.

Analyses of cholinergic perisomatic terminals were performed on ChAT-immunostained sections using the Stereo Investigator (Figure 2(f), [9]). All motoneuron profiles with discernible nucleus in a quadriceps motor column transect were analyzed. Each motoneuron, visualized at 100x magnification, was focused at the level of its largest cell body cross-sectional area, and its cell body perimeter and number of perisomatic terminals were determined (Figure 2(f)). Frequency of perisomatic ChAT$^+$ terminals was calculated as number of perisomatic terminals per unit perimeter length. Mean values of individual animals were used to calculate group mean values.

2.7. Statistical Analyses. Data were analyzed using one-way analysis of variance (ANOVA) or two-way ANOVA for repeated measures followed by Holm-Sidak multiple comparison tests (SigmaPlot 12, SPSS, Chicago, IL, USA). Regression analyses were performed using SigmaPlot. The threshold value for acceptance of differences was 5%.

3. Results and Discussion

3.1. Short-Term Effects on Synaptic Terminal Numbers. We initially tested whether intraneural drug applications alter short-term synaptic responses to nerve injury in the spinal motor nucleus (experiment I). We estimated the effects of nerve injury and application of BSA as compared to rats

without nerve lesions ("BSA" versus "Uninj." in Figure 3) using antibodies against synaptic terminal markers (Table 1). Numbers of microglial cells were also analyzed since these cells are activated after injury and are involved in synaptic remodeling [29–31]. The observed effects included reduced density of excitatory VGLUT2$^+$ terminals (−20%, Figure 3(a)), increased density of Iba1$^+$ microglia (+267%, Figure 3(b)), and decrease in modulatory perisomatic ChAT$^+$ terminals (−36%, Figure 3(b)). Inhibitory VGAT$^+$ and excitatory VGLUT1$^+$ Ia boutons were not significantly affected (+2% and +13%, resp., Figures 3(a) and 3(b)). Assuming that BSA has no measurable influence on these variables, the differences found between the two groups represent axotomy-related responses. In line with this notion is the finding of similar changes in the rat facial nucleus 1 week after axotomy [9]. Compared with BSA, BDNF had only one effect: attenuation of injury-induced ChAT$^+$ terminal loss (Figure 3(b)). A similar protective effect on ChAT$^+$ terminals had also BoNT (Figure 3(b)). In addition, BoNT application resulted, again as compared with BSA, in increased density of VGAT$^+$ terminals (+35%) and reduced density of VGLUT1$^+$ boutons (−46%), while VGLUT2$^+$ terminals and Iba1$^+$ cells were not significantly affected (−9% and 0%, resp., Figure 3(a)).

To test if the BoNT effects could be related to its retrograde transport into the spinal cord, we performed immunohistochemistry for BoNT-cleaved SNAP-25 (SNAP-25$_{197}$) which labels sites of BoNT proteolytic activity [32]. One week after nerve injury and BoNT application, immunofluorescence labeling was present around back-labeled somata and in the neuropil of the femoral motor nucleus (Figure 4). This pattern of labeling is similar to that previously observed by

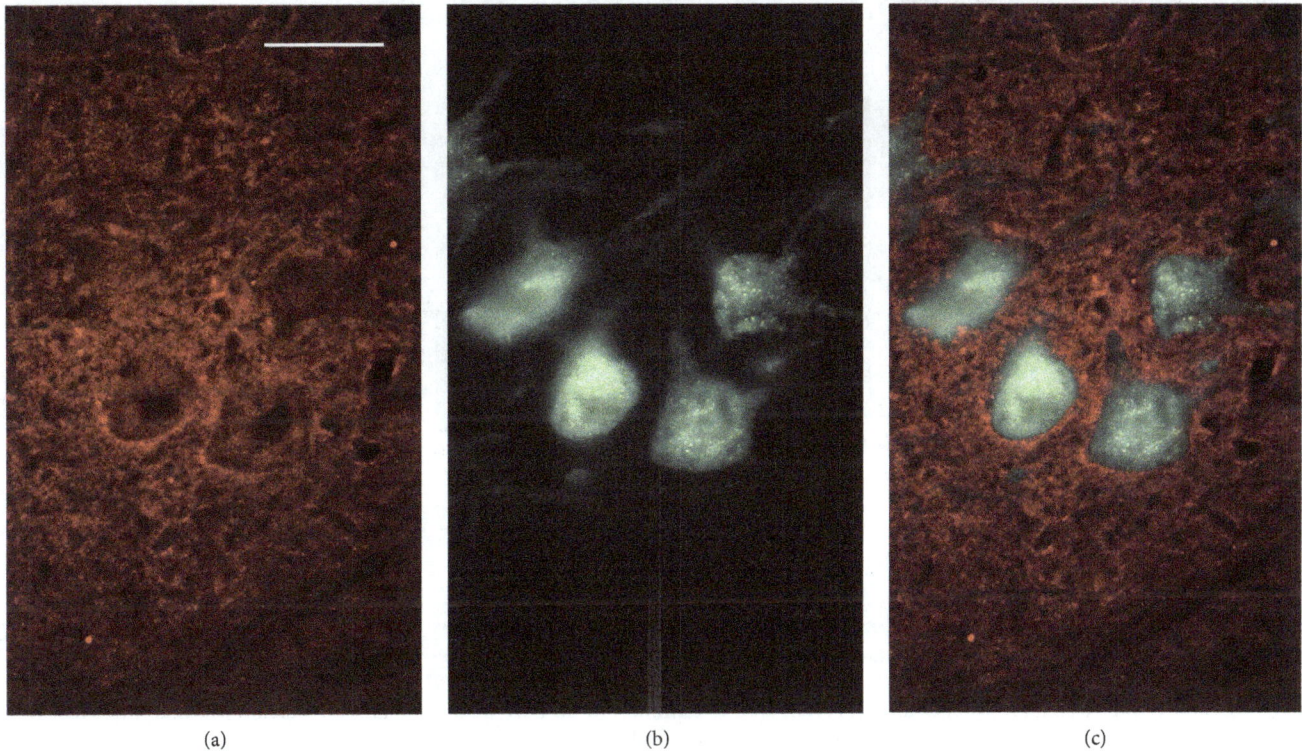

| (a) | (b) | (c) |

FIGURE 4: Cleaved SNAP-25 staining of a spinal cord section one week after injury and BoNT application. Immunostaining (a) is seen around the somata of back-labeled motoneurons and in the neuropil among them (b, c). Scale bar = 50 μm.

other groups [13, 14] and suggests that BoNT action has been transported into the spinal cord and could possibly be active in afferent terminals.

Overall, these findings show that the drug applications altered some synaptic responses to axotomy. Our working hypothesis was (see Introduction) that BDNF would have synaptotrophic effects and, indeed, injury-related loss of ChAT$^+$ perisomatic boutons was prevented. At the same time, however, other major inputs, excitatory VGLUT2$^+$ and inhibitory VGAT$^+$ terminals, were not affected as initially hypothesized. It is possible that the intracellular concentration of active exogenous BDNF achieved in our experiment has not been optimal to produce pronounced, long-term effects. BDNF appears to have a dose-dependent influence on nerve regeneration, that is, facilitation at low doses and inhibition at higher ones [33]. Therefore, we do not assume that BDNF is inefficient in our model unless this proves true in a future dose-dependence study.

In contrast to BDNF, we expected that BoNT would enhance loss of terminals after axotomy with a more pronounced effect on excitatory (VGLUT1$^+$ and VGLUT2$^+$) than on inhibitory (VGAT$^+$) terminals [34, 35]. This appeared true for VGLUT1$^+$ terminals, but the effects on VGAT$^+$ and ChAT$^+$ terminals were, on the opposite, synaptotrophic (Figure 3). This heterogeneity of effects suggests also other mechanisms of action in addition to inhibition of synaptic vesicle exocytosis by cleaving SNAP-25 [35]. It is possible, for example, that the increase in inhibitory VGAT$^+$ terminals results from inhibition of some of these heterogeneous in origin terminals [36] and subsequent sprouting of

unaffected inhibitory axons. Partial inhibition and reactive sprouting could also affect the cholinergic input to motoneurons. Alternatively or in addition, it is possible that BoNT has neurotrophic effects achieved via colocalization and signaling through the p75 receptor [15, 37]. This notion is not necessarily in disagreement with the limited effects of BDNF described above since different receptors (p75 versus TrkB) and neurotrophins may be involved.

3.2. Long-Term Synaptic Effects and Recovery of Function. We further investigated whether drug-related synaptic alterations persist after a longer reinnervation period, two months after injury (experiment II). We found, again compared with a BSA control group, that the BDNF effect on ChAT$^+$ terminals at 1-week post injury has disappeared while a previously nonexisting deficit in VGLUT1$^+$ terminals was now present (Figures 5(a) and 5(b)). BoNT-related differences in VGAT$^+$ and VGLUT1$^+$ terminal numbers had also disappeared at two months after injury, but the ChAT$^+$ terminal frequency was still higher similar to 1 week after lesion (Figures 5(a) and 5(b)). Immunohistochemistry for cleaved SNAP-25 in the spinal cord at two months after injury showed labeling similar to the one observed at 1 week (data not shown). This observation suggests that BoNT enzymatic activity is present for a long period of time after application.

Functional analysis performed in the same animal groups revealed significantly lower foot-base angle (FBA) and step length ratio (SLR) in the BoNT group as compared to BSA- and BDNF-treated rats (Figure 6(a)). This finding indicates better functional recovery as both parameters increase after

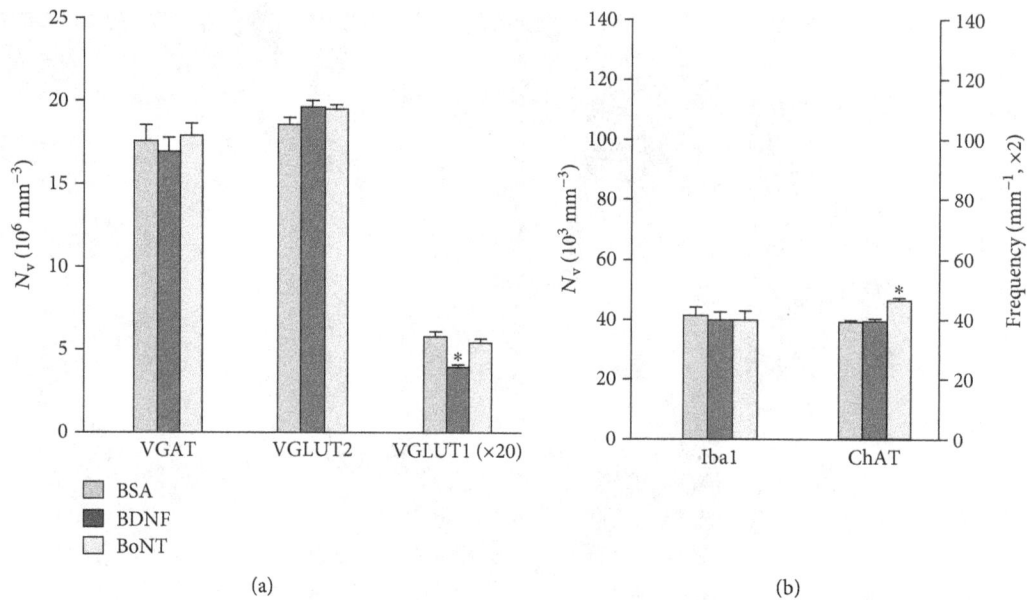

(a)

(b)

FIGURE 5: Analysis of synaptic terminals and microglia in the quadriceps motor nucleus two months after femoral nerve injury and drug application. Asterisks indicate mean values significantly different from all other groups (one-way ANOVA, $F_{2,16} = 11.4$ and 30.4, $p < 0.002$ and 0.001 for VGLUT1 and ChAT, resp.) with Holm-Sidak post hoc tests ($p = 0.005 - <0.001$). $N = 5 - 7$ per group. Note that numbers of Iba1$^+$ cells and ChAT$^+$ terminals (b) and numbers of VGLUT1$^+$ terminals (a) in BSA-treated animals are much lower than these at 1 week after injury (Figures 3(a) and 3(b)). This is consistent with previous findings [9, 10].

injury and decrease as reinnervation and recovery proceed (see Figures 7(a) and 7(b)). Regression analysis did not indicate any significant statistical relationship between individual structural parameters (Figure 5) and functional measures (Figure 6(a)) with the exception of ChAT$^+$ terminal densities (Figures 6(b)–6(d)). Higher frequencies of cholinergic perisomatic terminals appeared to be associated with lower ("better") functional values. The coefficients of determination (r^2, values shown in Figures 6(b)–6(d)) indicate that some 70% of the variability in functional parameters may be explained, in statistical terms, by variability in numbers of ChAT$^+$ terminals. Previous work using facial nerve or spinal cord injury models has also shown strong statistical relationships between degree of functional recovery, on one side, and degree of preservation/recovery of ChAT$^+$ terminal frequency on facial [9, 12] or spinal motoneurons [38–40], on the other side. These large cholinergic terminals form C-type synapses on motoneuronal perikarya and proximal dendrites and utilize M2 muscarinic receptors for acetylcholine in the postsynaptic membrane [41–46]. Although not that numerous, these synapses strongly influence motoneuron function by regulating action potential after hyperpolarization in a way that, under normal conditions, ensures sufficient motoneuron output to drive motor behavior [47, 48]. We can, therefore, assume that partial loss of perisomatic cholinergic terminals, associated with a reduced expression of postsynaptic receptors [49, 50], may significantly impair motor behaviors such as walking, whisking, and blinking [51].

3.3. Long-Term Functional Effects.
Finally, we were interested whether functional effects of drug application could appear

later or earlier than the analyzed postinjury time point (two months), a time period when reinnervation and recovery are well advanced but not completed. We performed experiment III in which rats were treated similarly to experiment II but monitored functionally between the first and the 20th week after injury. Time course and degree of recovery were very similar between BSA- and BDNF-treated animals (Figures 7(a)–7(d)) and in agreement with previous observations after transection and suture of the femoral nerve in adult rats [23]. In contrast, recovery after BoNT application was accelerated between the 2nd and 12th week (Figures 7(a)–7(d)) and advantages of this treatment were even present at the final time point studied, 20 weeks (Figure 7(a)).

After the 20-week observation period, the animals in experiment III were subjected to retrograde labeling to assess precision of reinnervation (Figures 8(a)–8(c)), a factor that can influence the functional outcome after femoral nerve injury and regeneration in rats [23]. The numbers of motoneurons projecting into the appropriate quadriceps nerve only, into the inappropriate saphenous nerve, or into both nerves ("Muscle," "Skin," and "Both" in Figure 8(d), resp.) were similar in the three groups of rats. This finding suggests that the functional improvements seen in the BoNT group are not related to an enhanced preferential reinnervation of the muscle. This notion is supported by the lack of significant covariations between numbers of back-labeled motoneurons and functional parameters.

3.4. Possible Mechanisms of Drug Effects.
We applied BoNT only once using the time frame between axonal membrane damage and sealing to load the proximal axon and cell body

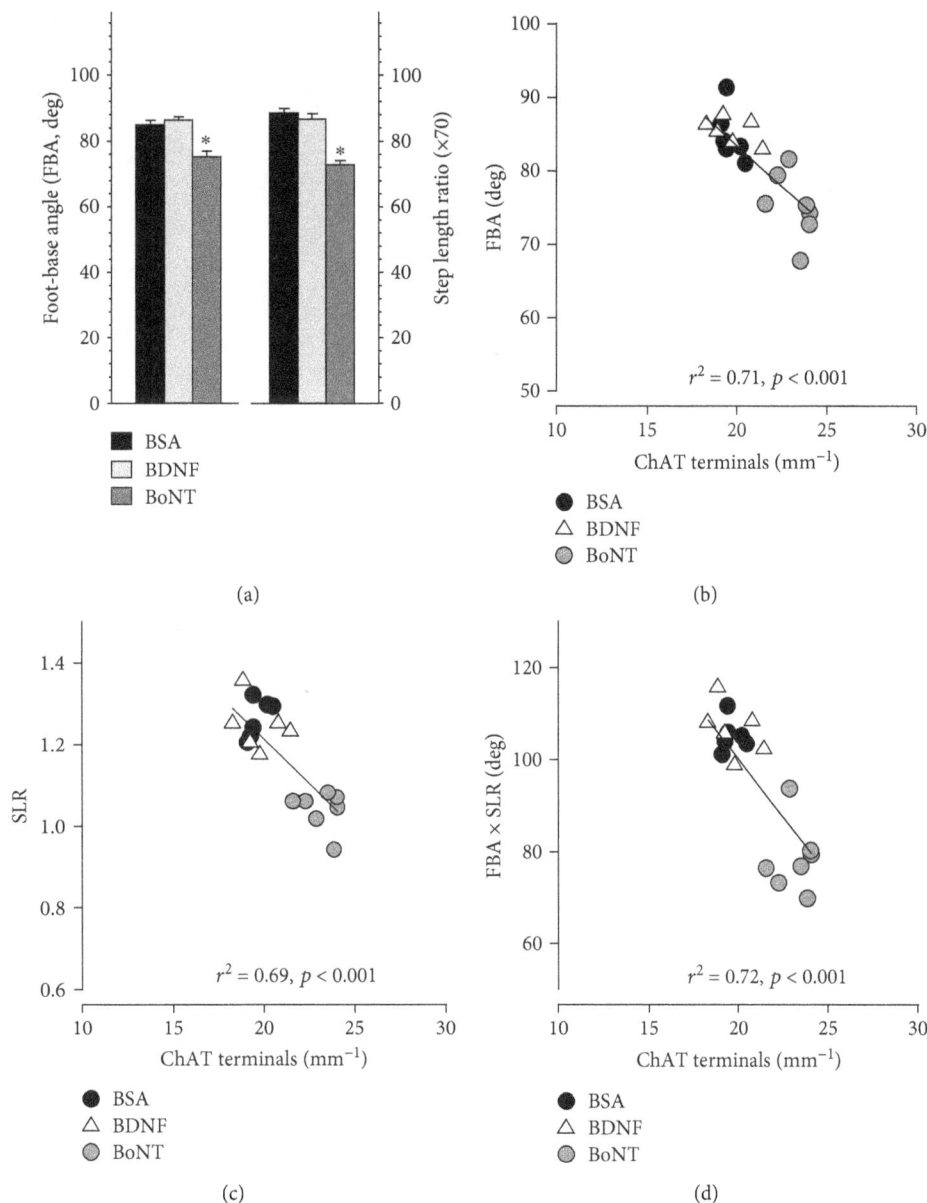

FIGURE 6: Motor recovery and correlations between functional parameters and ChAT terminal frequency two months after femoral nerve lesion and drug application. (a) Shown are mean values + SEM of foot-base angle (FBA) on the operated side and step length ratio (SLR). $N = 6$, 7, and 7 for BSA, BDNF, and BoNT, respectively. For both parameters, one-way ANOVA showed effects of treatment ($F_{2,17} = 18.4$ and 38.0 for FBA and SLR, respectively, $p < 0.001$ for both parameters). The BoNT group mean values were significantly different from the values of the BSA and BDNF groups (asterisks, $p < 0.001$, Holm-Sidak test). (b–d) Individual values of functional parameters plotted against numbers of ChAT terminals. Shown are regression lines, coefficients of determination (r^2), and probability values (p).

with toxin similar to retrograde tracers (Figures 8(a)–8(c)). Our expectation was that this uptake will be sufficient to "prime" the initial responses of motoneurons to injury, in particular their deafferentation, and, thus, eventually achieve long-term effects on regeneration without need of repeated drug delivery to the injury site. As estimated by gait analysis, our experiment was successful as functional regeneration was enhanced already at two weeks after injury and recovery remained accelerated for months thereafter. Enhancement of axonal regrowth in the crushed sciatic nerve of mice by a single low-dose intraneural application of BoNT has been

just reported, but the underlying mechanisms for these effects have remained unclear [37]. Here, we propose that the improvement of regeneration in our model is a consequence of attenuated loss of cholinergic modulatory input to femoral motoneurons (Table 2). In addition, it is possible that BoNT has an additional neuroprotective effect. At one week after injury, we found, compared with control rats, an increase in VGAT$^+$ inhibitory afferents in the quadriceps motor nucleus, reduced numbers of excitatory VGLUT1$^+$ Ia afferents, and no change in excitatory VGLUT2$^+$ terminals (Figure 3, Table 2). We can speculate that this constellation

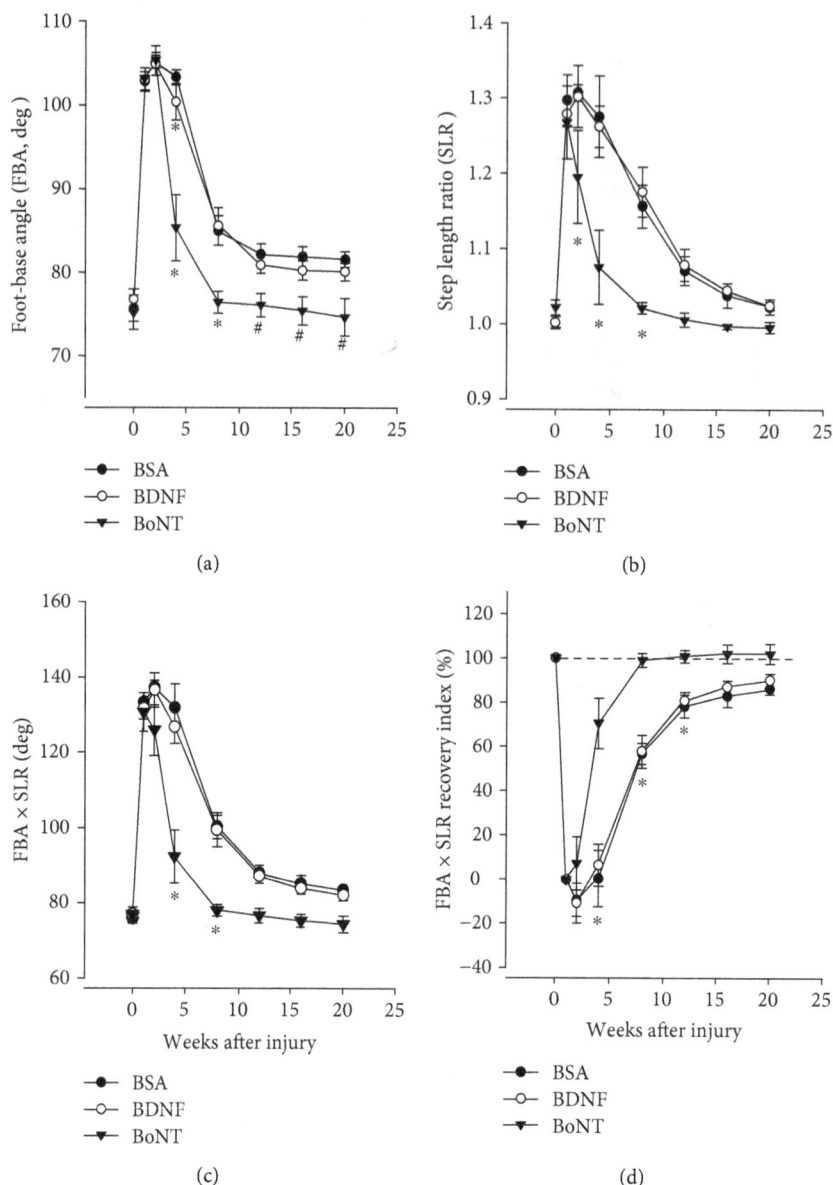

FIGURE 7: Time course and degree of motor recovery after femoral nerve lesion and drug application. Shown are mean values ± SEM of foot-base angle on the operated side (FBA, a), step length ratio (SLR, b), product FBA × SLR (c), and recovery index for the product FBA × SLR (d) prior to injury (0 week) and 1–20 weeks p.o. The dashed horizontal line in (d) is drawn at 100%, a value indicating full degree of recovery. $N = 7$, 8, and 9 for BSA, BDNF, and BoNT, respectively. For all parameters shown, two-way ANOVA for repeated measures showed effects of time ($F_{7,147} = 52.4$–209, $p < 0.001$) and treatment ($F_{2,21} = 9.51$–15.6, $p = 0.003$ – <0.001). Indicated by symbols are group mean values significantly different from * the corresponding postoperative values of the BSA and BDNF groups and # the corresponding value of the BSA group ($p < 0.05$, Holm-Sidak post hoc procedure).

attenuates the increased excitability of the axotomized motoneurons and, thus, allows better recovery of the motoneuron and its better regeneration [18, 52]. It is also thinkable that BoNT-related modulations of reflexes and/or pain-related transmission may have also positive functional consequences [53–56]. A major unresolved issue in this study is why BoNT had synaptotrophic effects on some types of synapses. The unexpected observation, which is unrelated to the main goal and achievement of this work, has to be explained by future experiments.

Similar to BoNT, BDNF is retrogradely transported from the periphery to the cell body of motoneurons and then transcytosed to afferent presynaptic terminals [57]. Exogenous BDNF has already shown synaptotrophic properties in injury models [18, 19, 58], and exogenous BDNF can improve axonal regeneration [59, 60]. We indeed found a BDNF effect at one week after injury—prevention of injury-induced ChAT+ terminal loss (Figure 3, Table 2), but no functional effects were seen (Figures 6(a) and 7). This may be related to lack of a prolonged protective effect on ChAT+

(a)   (b)

(c)   (d)

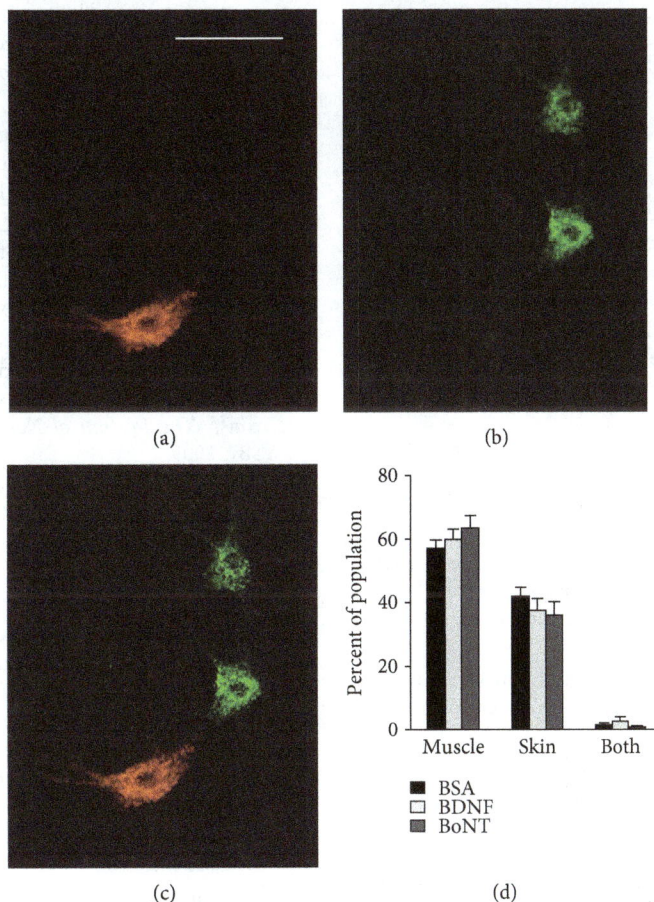

Figure 8: Retrograde labeling of motoneurons 20 weeks after lesion. (a–c) Representative images of motoneurons back-labeled through the muscle (quadriceps) and the skin (saphenous) branch of the femoral nerve ("Muscle" and "Skin") using Fluoro-Ruby and Fluoro-Emerald (red and green fluorescence), (a) and (b), respectively, overlay in (c). Scale bar = 100 μm. (d) Quantitative analysis of retrogradely labeled cells including double-labeled motoneurons ("Both"). Shown are mean values + SEM. One-way ANOVA showed no effect of treatment on any of the motoneuron categories ($F_{2,18} = 0.95$–1.14, $p = 0.342$–0.533). $N = 7$ animals per group.

Table 2: Summary of effects of drug application on VGLUT1$^+$, VGLUT2$^+$, ChAT$^+$, and VGAT$^+$ synaptic terminals and Iba1$^+$ cells one week and two months after injury. Arrows indicate increase ($\uparrow$), decrease ($\downarrow$), or no difference (=) compared to BSA treatment.

	BoNT versus BSA		BDNF versus BSA	
	1 week	2 months	1 week	2 months
VGLUT1	$\downarrow$	=	=	$\downarrow$
VGLUT2	=	=	=	=
ChAT	$\uparrow$	$\uparrow$	$\uparrow$	=
VGAT	$\uparrow$	=	=	=
Iba1	=	=	=	=

terminals as observed two months after BoNT application (Figure 5, Table 2).

4. Conclusions

The results of this study provide further support to the notion that insufficient recovery of synaptic inputs to motoneurons, in particular, perisomatic cholinergic terminals, may be an essential factor limiting recovery after peripheral nerve injury and regeneration. In addition, it appears encouraging that single intraoperative application of drugs to the severed nerve can be a useful way to modify neuronal responses to axotomy and, thus, modulate regeneration and eventually improve functional outcome of nerve injury. The list of candidates for such applications may be long, ranging from other neurotrophins or combinations of neurotrophins (e.g., BDNF and neurotrophin-3 [18], NGF [61]) or growth factors (e.g., vascular endothelial growth factor (VEGF) [62]) to small bioactive molecules [63].

Acknowledgments

The authors are grateful to Frau Heike Thieme for excellent technical assistance.

References

[1] K. Blinzinger and G. Kreutzberg, "Displacement of synaptic terminals from regenerating motoneurons by microglial cells," *Zeitschrift für Zellforschung und Mikroskopische Anatomie*, vol. 85, no. 2, pp. 145–157, 1968.

[2] R. C. Borke, R. S. Bridwell, and M. E. Nau, "The progression of deafferentation as a retrograde reaction to hypoglossal nerve injury," *Journal of Neurocytology*, vol. 24, no. 10, pp. 763–774, 1995.

[3] D. H. Chen, "Qualitative and quantitative study of synaptic displacement in chromatolyzed spinal motoneurons of the cat," *The Journal of Comparative Neurology*, vol. 177, no. 4, pp. 635–663, 1978.

[4] J. M. Kerns and E. J. Hinsman, "Neuroglial response to sciatic neurectomy. I. Light microscopy and autoradiography," *Journal of Comparative Neurology*, vol. 151, no. 3, pp. 237–253, 1973.

[5] G. W. Kreutzberg, "Dynamic changes in motoneurons during regeneration," *Restorative Neurology and Neuroscience*, vol. 5, no. 1, pp. 59-60, 1993.

[6] B. E. H. Sumner and F. I. Sutherland, "Quantitative electron microscopy on the injured hypoglossal nucleus in the rat," *Journal of Neurocytology*, vol. 2, no. 3, pp. 315–328, 1973.

[7] B. E. H. Sumner, "A quantitative analysis of boutons with different types of synapse in normal and injured hypoglossal nuclei," *Experimental Neurology*, vol. 49, no. 2, pp. 406–417, 1975.

[8] T. Brännström and J. O. Kellerth, "Recovery of synapses in axotomized adult cat spinal motoneurons after reinnervation into muscle," *Experimental Brain Research*, vol. 125, no. 1, pp. 19–27, 1999.

[9] A. Raslan, P. Ernst, M. Werle et al., "Reduced cholinergic and glutamatergic synaptic input to regenerated motoneurons after facial nerve repair in rats: potential implications for recovery of motor function," *Brain Structure & Function*, vol. 219, no. 3, pp. 891–909, 2014.

[10] T. M. Rotterman, P. Nardelli, T. C. Cope, and F. J. Alvarez, "Normal distribution of VGLUT1 synapses on spinal motoneuron dendrites and their reorganization after nerve injury," *The Journal of Neuroscience*, vol. 34, no. 10, pp. 3475–3492, 2014.

[11] A. J. Schultz, T. M. Rotterman, A. Dwarakanath, and F. J. Alvarez, "VGLUT1 synapses and P-boutons on regenerating motoneurons after nerve crush," *The Journal of Comparative Neurology*, vol. 525, no. 13, pp. 2876–2889, 2017.

[12] G. Hundeshagen, K. Szameit, H. Thieme et al., "Deficient functional recovery after facial nerve crush in rats is associated with restricted rearrangements of synaptic terminals in the facial nucleus," *Neuroscience*, vol. 248, pp. 307–318, 2013.

[13] F. Antonucci, C. Rossi, L. Gianfranceschi, O. Rossetto, and M. Caleo, "Long-distance retrograde effects of botulinum neurotoxin A," *The Journal of Neuroscience*, vol. 28, no. 14, pp. 3689–3696, 2008.

[14] I. Matak, P. Riederer, and Z. Lackovic, "Botulinum toxin's axonal transport from periphery to the spinal cord," *Neurochemistry International*, vol. 61, no. 2, pp. 236–239, 2012.

[15] L. Restani, F. Giribaldi, M. Manich et al., "Botulinum neurotoxins A and E undergo retrograde axonal transport in primary motor neurons," *PLoS Pathogens*, vol. 8, no. 12, article e1003087, 2012.

[16] L. Restani, E. Novelli, D. Bottari et al., "Botulinum neurotoxin A impairs neurotransmission following retrograde transsynaptic transport," *Traffic*, vol. 13, no. 8, pp. 1083–1089, 2012.

[17] A. M. Pastor, B. Moreno-Lopez, R. R. De La Cruz, and J. M. Delgado-Garcia, "Effects of botulinum neurotoxin type A on abducens motoneurons in the cat: ultrastructural and synaptic alterations," *Neuroscience*, vol. 81, no. 2, pp. 457–478, 1997.

[18] M. A. Davis-López de Carrizosa, C. J. Morado-Diaz, J. J. Tena et al., "Complementary actions of BDNF and neurotrophin-3 on the firing patterns and synaptic composition of motoneurons," *The Journal of Neuroscience*, vol. 29, no. 2, pp. 575–587, 2009.

[19] L. N. Novikov, L. N. Novikova, P. Holmberg, and J.-O. Kellerth, "Exogenous brain-derived neurotrophic factor regulates the synaptic composition of axonally lesioned and normal adult rat motoneurons," *Neuroscience*, vol. 100, no. 1, pp. 171–181, 2000.

[20] A. Al-Majed, T. Brushart, and T. Gordon, "Electrical stimulation accelerates and increases expression of BDNF and trkB mRNA in regenerating rat femoral motoneurons," *The European Journal of Neuroscience*, vol. 12, no. 12, pp. 4381–4390, 2000.

[21] A. A. al-Majed, C. M. Neumann, T. M. Brushart, and T. Gordon, "Brief electrical stimulation promotes the speed and accuracy of motor axonal regeneration," *The Journal of Neuroscience*, vol. 20, no. 7, pp. 2602–2608, 2000.

[22] A. Irintchev, "Potentials and limitations of peripheral nerve injury models in rodents with particular reference to the femoral nerve," *Annals of Anatomy*, vol. 193, no. 4, pp. 276–285, 2011.

[23] M. Kruspe, H. Thieme, O. Guntinas-Lichius, and A. Irintchev, "Motoneuron regeneration accuracy and recovery of gait after femoral nerve injuries in rats," *Neuroscience*, vol. 280, pp. 73–87, 2014.

[24] T. Brushart, "Preferential reinnervation of motor nerves by regenerating motor axons," *The Journal of Neuroscience*, vol. 8, no. 3, pp. 1026–1031, 1988.

[25] O. Simova, A. Irintchev, A. Mehanna et al., "Carbohydrate mimics promote functional recovery after peripheral nerve repair," *Annals of Neurology*, vol. 60, no. 4, pp. 430–437, 2006.

[26] A. Irintchev, A. Rollenhagen, E. Troncoso, J. Z. Kiss, and M. Schachner, "Structural and functional aberrations in the cerebral cortex of tenascin-C deficient mice," *Cerebral Cortex*, vol. 15, no. 7, pp. 950–962, 2005.

[27] A. Irintchev, M. Zeschnigk, A. Starzinski-Powitz, and A. Wernig, "Expression pattern of M-cadherin in normal, denervated, and regenerating mouse muscles," *Developmental Dynamics*, vol. 199, no. 4, pp. 326–337, 1994.

[28] M. V. Sofroniew and U. Schrell, "Long-term storage and regular repeated use of diluted antisera in glass staining jars for increased sensitivity, reproducibility, and convenience of single- and two-color light microscopic immunocytochemistry," *The Journal of Histochemistry and Cytochemistry*, vol. 30, no. 6, pp. 504–511, 1982.

[29] S. Cullheim and S. Thams, "The microglial networks of the brain and their role in neuronal network plasticity after lesion," *Brain Research Reviews*, vol. 55, no. 1, pp. 89–96, 2007.

[30] D. Gomez-Nicola and V. H. Perry, "Microglial dynamics and role in the healthy and diseased brain: a paradigm of functional plasticity," *The Neuroscientist*, vol. 21, no. 2, pp. 169–184, 2015.

[31] G. W. Kreutzberg, "Microglia: a sensor for pathological events in the CNS," *Trends in Neurosciences*, vol. 19, no. 8, pp. 312–318, 1996.

[32] C. Rheaume, B. B. Cai, J. Wang et al., "A highly specific monoclonal antibody for botulinum neurotoxin type A-cleaved SNAP25," *Toxins*, vol. 7, no. 7, pp. 2354–2370, 2015.

[33] M. Richner, M. Ulrichsen, S. L. Elmegaard, R. Dieu, L. T. Pallesen, and C. B. Vaegter, "Peripheral nerve injury modulates neurotrophin signaling in the peripheral and central nervous system," *Molecular Neurobiology*, vol. 50, no. 3, pp. 945–970, 2014.

[34] C. Verderio, C. Grumelli, L. Raiteri et al., "Traffic of botulinum toxins A and E in excitatory and inhibitory neurons," *Traffic*, vol. 8, no. 2, pp. 142–153, 2007.

[35] C. Verderio, D. Pozzi, E. Pravettoni et al., "SNAP-25 modulation of calcium dynamics underlies differences in GABAergic and glutamatergic responsiveness to depolarization," *Neuron*, vol. 41, no. 4, pp. 599–610, 2004.

[36] P. H. Beske, S. M. Scheeler, M. Adler, and P. M. McNutt, "Accelerated intoxication of GABAergic synapses by botulinum neurotoxin A disinhibits stem cell-derived neuron networks prior to network silencing," *Frontiers in Cellular Neuroscience*, vol. 9, p. 159, 2015.

[37] S. Cobianchi, J. Jaramillo, S. Luvisetto, F. Pavone, and X. Navarro, "Botulinum neurotoxin A promotes functional recovery after peripheral nerve injury by increasing regeneration of myelinated fibers," *Neuroscience*, vol. 359, pp. 82–91, 2017.

[38] I. Apostolova, A. Irintchev, and M. Schachner, "Tenascin-R restricts posttraumatic remodeling of motoneuron innervation and functional recovery after spinal cord injury in adult mice," *The Journal of Neuroscience*, vol. 26, no. 30, pp. 7849–7859, 2006.

[39] I. Jakovcevski, J. F. Wu, N. Karl et al., "Glial scar expression of CHL1, the close homolog of the adhesion molecule L1, limits recovery after spinal cord injury," *The Journal of Neuroscience*, vol. 27, no. 27, pp. 7222–7233, 2007.

[40] H. J. Lee, I. Jakovcevski, N. Radonjic, L. Hoelters, M. Schachner, and A. Irintchev, "Better functional outcome of compression spinal cord injury in mice is associated with enhanced H-reflex responses," *Experimental Neurology*, vol. 216, no. 2, pp. 365–374, 2009.

[41] Z. Csaba, E. Krejci, and V. Bernard, "Postsynaptic muscarinic m2 receptors at cholinergic and glutamatergic synapses of mouse brainstem motoneurons," *The Journal of Comparative Neurology*, vol. 521, no. 9, pp. 2008–2024, 2013.

[42] M. S. Davidoff and A. P. Irintchev, "Acetylcholinesterase activity and type C synapses in the hypoglossal, facial and spinal-cord motor nuclei of rats. An electron-microscope study," *Histochemistry*, vol. 84, no. 4-6, pp. 515–524, 1986.

[43] J. Hellström, U. Arvidsson, R. Elde, S. Cullheim, and B. Meister, "Differential expression of nerve terminal protein isoforms in VAChT-containing varicosities of the spinal cord ventral horn," *The Journal of Comparative Neurology*, vol. 411, no. 4, pp. 578–590, 1999.

[44] J. Hellström, A. L. R. Oliveira, B. Meister, and S. Cullheim, "Large cholinergic nerve terminals on subsets of motoneurons and their relation to muscarinic receptor type 2," *The Journal of Comparative Neurology*, vol. 460, no. 4, pp. 476–486, 2003.

[45] J. I. Nagy, T. Yamamoto, and L. M. Jordan, "Evidence for the cholinergic nature of C-terminals associated with subsurface cisterns in alpha-motoneurons of rat," *Synapse*, vol. 15, no. 1, pp. 17–32, 1993.

[46] J. M. Wilson, J. Rempel, and R. M. Brownstone, "Postnatal development of cholinergic synapses on mouse spinal motoneurons," *The Journal of Comparative Neurology*, vol. 474, no. 1, pp. 13–23, 2004.

[47] G. B. Miles, R. Hartley, A. J. Todd, and R. M. Brownstone, "Spinal cholinergic interneurons regulate the excitability of motoneurons during locomotion," *Proceedings of the National Academy of Sciences of the United States of America*, vol. 104, no. 7, pp. 2448–2453, 2007.

[48] L. Zagoraiou, T. Akay, J. F. Martin, R. M. Brownstone, T. M. Jessell, and G. B. Miles, "A cluster of cholinergic premotor interneurons modulates mouse locomotor activity," *Neuron*, vol. 64, no. 5, pp. 645–662, 2009.

[49] D. B. Hoover, R. H. Baisden, and J. V. Lewis, "Axotomy-induced loss of m2 muscarinic receptor mRNA in the rat facial motor nucleus precedes a decrease in concentration of muscarinic receptors," *The Histochemical Journal*, vol. 28, no. 11, pp. 771–778, 1996.

[50] D. B. Hoover and J. C. Hancock, "Effect of facial nerve transection on acetylcholinesterase, choline acetyltransferase and [^{3}H] quinuclidinyl benzilate binding in rat facial nuclei," *Neuroscience*, vol. 15, no. 2, pp. 481–487, 1985.

[51] E. C. Witts, L. Zagoraiou, and G. B. Miles, "Anatomy and function of cholinergic C bouton inputs to motor neurons," *Journal of Anatomy*, vol. 224, no. 1, pp. 52–60, 2014.

[52] D. Gonzalez-Forero and B. Moreno-Lopez, "Retrograde response in axotomized motoneurons: nitric oxide as a key player in triggering reversion toward a dedifferentiated phenotype," *Neuroscience*, vol. 283, pp. 138–165, 2014.

[53] M. Kerzoncuf, L. Bensoussan, A. Delarque, J. Durand, J. M. Viton, and C. Rossi-Durand, "Plastic changes in spinal synaptic transmission following botulinum toxin A in patients with post-stroke spasticity," *Journal of Rehabilitation Medicine*, vol. 47, no. 10, pp. 910–916, 2015.

[54] R. Kumar, H. P. Dhaliwal, R. V. Kukreja, and B. R. Singh, "The botulinum toxin as a therapeutic agent: molecular structure and mechanism of action in motor and sensory systems," *Seminars in Neurology*, vol. 36, no. 01, pp. 010–019, 2016.

[55] R. Mazzocchio and M. Caleo, "More than at the neuromuscular synapse: actions of botulinum neurotoxin A in the central nervous system," *The Neuroscientist*, vol. 21, no. 1, pp. 44–61, 2015.

[56] G. Sandrini, R. De Icco, C. Tassorelli, N. Smania, and S. Tamburin, "Botulinum neurotoxin type A for the treatment of pain: not just in migraine and trigeminal neuralgia," *The Journal of Headache and Pain*, vol. 18, no. 1, p. 38, 2017.

[57] H. B. Rind, R. Butowt, and C. S. von Bartheld, "Synaptic targeting of retrogradely transported trophic factors in motoneurons: comparison of glial cell line-derived neurotrophic factor, brain-derived neurotrophic factor, and cardiotrophin-1 with tetanus toxin," *The Journal of Neuroscience*, vol. 25, no. 3, pp. 539–549, 2005.

[58] J. Krakowiak, C. Liu, C. Papudesu, P. J. Ward, J. C. Wilhelm, and A. W. English, "Neuronal BDNF signaling is necessary

for the effects of treadmill exercise on synaptic stripping of axotomized motoneurons," *Neural Plasticity*, vol. 2015, Article ID 392591, 11 pages, 2015.

[59] M. Gao, P. Lu, D. Lynam et al., "BDNF gene delivery within and beyond templated agarose multi-channel guidance scaffolds enhances peripheral nerve regeneration," *Journal of Neural Engineering*, vol. 13, no. 6, article 066011, 2016.

[60] D. Santos, F. Gonzalez-Perez, X. Navarro, and J. Del Valle, "Dose-dependent differential effect of neurotrophic factors on in vitro and in vivo regeneration of motor and sensory neurons," *Neural Plasticity*, vol. 2016, Article ID 4969523, 13 pages, 2016.

[61] M. A. Davis-Lopez de Carrizosa, C. J. Morado-Diaz, S. Morcuende, R. R. de la Cruz, and A. M. Pastor, "Nerve growth factor regulates the firing patterns and synaptic composition of motoneurons," *The Journal of Neuroscience*, vol. 30, no. 24, pp. 8308–8319, 2010.

[62] P. M. Calvo, R. R. de la Cruz, and A. M. Pastor, "Synaptic loss and firing alterations in axotomized motoneurons are restored by vascular endothelial growth factor (VEGF) and VEGF-B," *Experimental Neurology*, vol. 304, pp. 67–81, 2018.

[63] K. W.-H. Lo, T. Jiang, K. A. Gagnon, C. Nelson, and C. T. Laurencin, "Small-molecule based musculoskeletal regenerative engineering," *Trends in Biotechnology*, vol. 32, no. 2, pp. 74–81, 2014.

[64] Y. Imai, I. Ibata, D. Ito, K. Ohsawa, and S. Kohsaka, "A novel gene iba1 in the major histocompatibility complex class III region encoding an EF hand protein expressed in a monocytic lineage," *Biochemical and Biophysical Research Communications*, vol. 224, no. 3, pp. 855–862, 1996.

[65] D. Ito, Y. Imai, K. Ohsawa, K. Nakajima, Y. Fukuuchi, and S. Kohsaka, "Microglia-specific localisation of a novel calcium binding protein, Iba1," *Molecular Brain Research*, vol. 57, no. 1, pp. 1–9, 1998.

[66] F. A. Chaudhry, R. J. Reimer, E. E. Bellocchio et al., "The vesicular GABA transporter, VGAT, localizes to synaptic vesicles in sets of glycinergic as well as GABAergic neurons," *The Journal of Neuroscience*, vol. 18, no. 23, pp. 9733–9750, 1998.

[67] S. L. McIntire, R. J. Reimer, K. Schuske, R. H. Edwards, and E. M. Jorgensen, "Identification and characterization of the vesicular GABA transporter," *Nature*, vol. 389, no. 6653, pp. 870–876, 1997.

[68] S. M. Wojcik, S. Katsurabayashi, I. Guillemin et al., "A shared vesicular carrier allows synaptic corelease of GABA and glycine," *Neuron*, vol. 50, no. 4, pp. 575–587, 2006.

[69] F. J. Alvarez, R. M. Villalba, R. Zerda, and S. P. Schneider, "Vesicular glutamate transporters in the spinal cord, with special reference to sensory primary afferent synapses," *The Journal of Comparative Neurology*, vol. 472, no. 3, pp. 257–280, 2004.

[70] A. L. R. Oliveira, F. Hydling, E. Olsson et al., "Cellular localization of three vesicular glutamate transporter mRNAs and proteins in rat spinal cord and dorsal root ganglia," *Synapse*, vol. 50, no. 2, pp. 117–129, 2003.

8

The Neural and Behavioral Correlates of Anomia Recovery following Personalized Observation, Execution, and Mental Imagery Therapy: A Proof of Concept

Edith Durand (ID), Pierre Berroir, and Ana Inés Ansaldo

Centre de Recherche de l'Institut Universitaire de Gériatrie de Montréal (CRIUGM), École d'Orthophonie, Faculté de Médecine, Université de Montréal, Montreal, QC, Canada

Correspondence should be addressed to Edith Durand; edith.durand@umontreal.ca

Academic Editor: Ambra Bisio

The impact of sensorimotor strategies on aphasia recovery has rarely been explored. This paper reports on the efficacy of personalized observation, execution, and mental imagery (POEM) therapy, a new approach designed to integrate sensorimotor and language-based strategies to treat verb anomia, a frequent aphasia sign. Two participants with verb anomia were followed up in a pre-/posttherapy fMRI study. POEM was administered in a massed stimulation schedule, with personalized stimuli, resulting in significant improvement in both participants, with both trained and untrained items. Given that the latter finding is rarely reported in the literature, the evidence suggests that POEM favors the implementation of a word retrieval strategy that can be integrated and generalized. Changes in fMRI patterns following POEM reflect a reduction in the number of recruited areas supporting naming and the recruitment of brain areas that belong to the language and mirror neuron systems. The data provide evidence on the efficacy of POEM for verb anomia, while pointing to the added value of combined language and sensorimotor strategies for recovery from verb anomia, contributing to the consolidation of a word retrieval strategy that can be better generalized to untrained words. Future studies with a larger sample of participants are required to further explore this avenue.

1. Introduction

Aphasia is an acquired language impairment following brain damage, such as stroke, whose consequences can be devastating [1]. Anomia is the most frequent and pervasive symptom for people with aphasia, regardless of the aphasia type. Anomia is described as difficulty in retrieving words in structured tasks, such as picture naming, sentence completion, or spontaneous speech. Anomia can affect different types of words, including nouns and verbs. Research has long focused on noun retrieval, while therapies targeting verb anomia remain rare [2]. This is somewhat surprising, considering the central role of verbs in sentence and speech production [3].

In recovery from aphasia, the attempt to compensate for anomia may be related to the concept of neuroplasticity. Neuroplasticity refers to a number of brain mechanisms involved in learning and relearning and is reflected in changes in brain activation patterns highlighted by functional magnetic resonance imaging (fMRI). Two main forms of neuroplasticity have been studied in the context of aphasia recovery: functional reactivation, which occurs when previously damaged and inactive areas recover their function after a latency period, and functional reorganization, which reflects compensation for the permanent damage of specific brain areas by the recruitment of other areas not previously involved in the given function [4]. Different types of neuroplasticity may be involved in recovery from anomia; adaptive neuroplasticity results in functional recovery, whereas maladaptive neuroplasticity results in persistence of errors [4, 5]. There is a long-standing debate in the anomia recovery literature regarding functional reorganization: Is better recovery supported by perilesional left hemisphere (LH) language processing areas or right hemisphere (RH) homologues of those areas? However, the extent to which an RH shift reflects adaptive or maladaptive neuroplasticity remains controversial (Anglade et al., 2014). Moreover, the impact that different therapy procedures may have on the recruitment of canonical or noncanonical language processing circuits remains to be explored.

With regard to verb anomia, therapy approaches have been designed with reference to models of word processing that view the phonological and semantic processing of words as key elements for word retrieval (see [2], for a review). Thus, phonological approaches use sound cues and rhymes to elicit words, whereas semantic approaches use semantic cues and reinforce the semantic features of a given word to facilitate word naming. The efficacy of both approaches has been proven, in particular with treated items [2]. Conversely, poor generalization of treatment effects to untrained verbs has been consistently reported [6–12]. Furthermore, none of these studies have explored the neural substrates sustaining recovery from verb anomia. Regarding the lack of generalization of therapy effects to untrained verbs, it should be noted that none of the publications cited took into consideration the dynamic component of verb processing. The meaning of an action verb includes a dynamic semantic feature that an object does not require. This assumption—grounded in embodied cognition theory—implies that word meaning depends on modal experiences. Thus, semantic processing of a given word—noun or verb—will depend upon the sensory and motor modalities by which objects and actions corresponding to those words are learned and how this learning impacts the functional brain networks supporting word processing ([13, 14]; Pulvermüller et al., 1996). In other words, the learning modality and features of a given word will determine the conceptual and brain-related substrates supporting word retrieval; with verbs, particularly action verbs, these should include sensorimotor features and brain processing areas [15].

An interesting example of how word encoding influences the efficacy of a given strategy for word retrieval comes from the work by Marangolo et al. showing that action observation on its own can represent a useful tool for verb retrieval [16, 17]. Action observation therapy (AOT) principles were first developed for stroke patients who suffered from a motor deficit affecting the upper limbs. Several studies have consistently shown that AOT is an effective way to enhance motor function [18–21]. Ertelt et al. [18] first showed that patients in the chronic stage after stroke experienced significantly improved motor function following a four-week video therapy program compared with a control therapy; additionally, neural activations associated with the AOT showed a significant rise in activity in areas sustaining the action observation/action execution matching system [18]. This system includes the mirror neuron system, which will be discussed below.

In the language rehabilitation domain, Marangolo et al. [17] administered AOT to stroke patients who suffered from aphasia in order to improve verb retrieval. They compared action observation with action observation and execution and found that the mere observation of the performed action was sufficient to activate the corresponding sensorimotor representation in the semantic system, which served as input at the lexical level facilitating verb retrieval. However, their results were not replicated by another recent work [22] and the effect was restricted to trained items. Moreover, the neural substrate underlying recovery with AOT has not yet been investigated.

Several studies have examined the efficacy of other sensorimotor strategies to facilitate verb retrieval. For example, Raymer et al. (2006) examined the effect of gesture execution in aphasia treatment, using pantomimes paired with verbal training for noun and verb retrieval in a group of aphasic patients. Their results showed improved naming of trained nouns and verbs but no generalization of treatment effects to untrained words. Similarly, Rose and Sussmilch [23] obtained significant results following therapy combining verb naming and gesture production; again, the results were restricted to trained items. In sum, observation of action and gesture execution, both associated with verb naming, yielded positive results with trained verbs but not with untrained ones. None of those studies included fMRI segregation analysis of areas sustaining recovery, and thus the behavioral changes observed cannot be linked to any specific neural substrate. Thus, while functional neuroimaging data on verb processing have mostly been related to healthy populations, very little is known about therapy-induced neuroplasticity in the recovery from verb anomia.

In healthy adults, action verb naming has been shown to be supported by left frontal cortical areas, including the left prefrontal cortex (Shapiro et al., 2001), the left superior parietal lobule, the left superior temporal gyrus (Shapiro et al., 2006), the left superior frontal gyrus (Shapiro et al., 2005), and the primary motor cortex in the posterior portion of the precentral gyrus (Porro et al., 1996, [13], and Pulvermüller et al., 2005). As discussed by Durand and Ansaldo [15], these areas have also been associated with the so-called mirror neuron system (MNS), which is thought to support AOT in motor neurorehabilitation after stroke. Mirror neurons are a particular class of visuomotor neurons, originally discovered in area F5 of the monkey premotor cortex, that discharge both when a monkey does a particular action and when it observes another monkey or a human doing a similar action [24]. The MNS is a mechanism that unifies perception and action, transforming sensory representations of the behavior of others into motor representations of the same behavior in the observer's brain [25]. From this perspective, some authors have suggested that language evolved from a gestural system, first as pantomime and gradually as conventional gestures, eventually developing into a symbolic code [24, 26, 27]. This sensorimotor system is considered to be the structure underlying vocabulary and grammar development [26, 28]. In this view, mirror neurons are considered to be embodied cognitive agents, as they coordinate multimodal information resulting from an individual's interaction with the environment. According to such theories, the MNS may play a central role in the development of language in humans [24, 26, 27] and in semantic processing, especially action semantic processing.

Apart from the MNS, several links can be made between vision and action. The cortical visual system is known to be segregated into two anatomically and functionally distinct pathways: a ventral occipitotemporal pathway that subserves object perception and a dorsal occipitoparietal pathway that subserves object localization and visually guided action [29–31]. Goodale and Goodale and Milner [30, 32] proposed a model in which the perceptual detection of possible actions in the environment involves the dorsal stream, stretching from the primary visual cortex to the posterior parietal lobe and reaching the premotor areas and a distributed network of areas in the caudal frontal cortex. More than just a visual detection system, the dorsal stream allows action selection with continuous matching between the visual and motor areas [33]. A recent study has shown that, along the dorsal pathway, the anterior intraparietal area and the ventral premotor cortex extract sensorimotor information from perceptual stimuli, making it possible to detect action possibilities from the information detected through the retinotopic map [33].

Recent research shows that sensorimotor processes play a crucial role in language processing. Thus, both behavioral studies [34] and neurofunctional studies [35–44] suggest that the understanding of action words recruits motor areas. Along the same lines, Tremblay and Small [44] showed that functional specialization of specific premotor areas is involved in both action observation and execution. Moreover, Tomasino and Rumiati (2013) showed that the involvement of sensorimotor areas depends on the strategy used to perform the task. Specifically, if the task requires a person to imagine actions, sensorimotor areas will be involved. Visual mental imagery allows one to obtain an internal representation that functions as a weak form of perception [45]. Mental imagery is known to be an efficient therapy tool for rehabilitation of motor impairments. In language rehabilitation, mental imagery is a relatively new tool, though some studies on aphasia recovery report the activation of visual mental imagery processing areas, such as the inferior occipital gyrus [46].

Taking into account the promising but limited results obtained with anomia therapy approaches based on action observation, gesture, or mental imagery used separately, we designed a new therapy approach combining three sensorimotor strategies previously used to treat verb anomia, namely, action observation, gesture execution, and mental imagery, and combined the three of them in a massed practice format. Thus, personalized observation, execution, and mental imagery therapy (POEM therapy) was designed based on principles of experience-dependent neuroplasticity, namely, stimulus specificity and salience, and a time/frequency ratio corresponding to massed stimulation (for a review of this issue, see [5]). Several studies have shown the benefits of massed practice, defined as practice of a given number of trials in a short time [47–49].

In sum, POEM therapy was developed based on evidence, while incorporating principles of experience-dependent neuroplasticity and targeted, repetitive, and intensive practice of action naming, with the purpose of contributing to strategy development and integration [5]. Moreover, to identify the neural substrates associated with the outcomes of POEM therapy, we used fMRI to assess functional brain activity before and after intervention with POEM therapy and thus assess treatment-induced neuroplasticity.

The purpose of this study is to examine the effects of POEM therapy on the recovery from verb anomia in the context of chronic aphasia and to identify the neural changes associated with behavioral improvement. Two participants with chronic nonfluent aphasia were examined before and after POEM therapy, and behavioral and event-related fMRI measures were taken. Participants received three sessions of POEM therapy per week over five weeks, in line with a massed therapy approach [47, 48, 50]. Activation maps obtained in the context of oral verb naming were obtained before and after POEM therapy. It was expected that

(1) POEM therapy would result in significant recovery of verb naming;

(2) a series of motor and premotor areas would sustain the observed recovery.

2. Material and Methods

2.1. Participants. Aphasia severity and typology were determined by an experienced speech-language pathologist (SLP: ED). Inclusion criteria were (1) a single LH stroke, (2) a diagnosis of moderate-to-severe aphasia according to the Montreal-Toulouse Battery (Nespoulous et al., 1986), (3) the presence of anomia according to a standardized naming task [51], (4) having French as their mother tongue, and (5) being right-handed prior to the stroke (Edinburgh Inventory; Oldfield, 1971). Exclusion criteria were (1) the presence of a neurological or psychiatric diagnosis other than stroke, (2) incompatibility with fMRI testing, or (3) diagnosis of mild cognitive impairment or dementia prior to stroke [52]. Participants gave written informed consent according to the Declaration of Helsinki. This study was approved by the Ethics Committee of the Regroupement de Neuroimagerie Québec. Table 1 contains sociodemographic information on the two participants, and Figure 1 shows their structural magnetic resonance imaging (MRI) results.

2.1.1. Participant 1. P1 is a 65-year-old right-handed woman, who was 7 years postonset from a left temporal stroke, which resulted in nonfluent aphasia and right hemiparesis. She benefited from individual language therapy for a short time just after the stroke; since then, she has participated in activities organized by the association for persons with aphasia. At the beginning of the study, she was not receiving any language therapy. Aphasia testing conducted at that point showed moderate transcortical motor aphasia with moderate apraxia of speech.

2.1.2. Participant 2. P2 is a 72-year-old right-handed woman, who was 34 years postonset from a left temporal stroke, which resulted in nonfluent aphasia and right upper limb hemiplegia. She had received individual language therapy intermittently over the previous 20 years, particularly during the first years after the stroke. She often participates in activities organized by the association for persons with aphasia. At the beginning of the study, she was not receiving any language therapy. Aphasia testing conducted at that point showed severe transcortical motor aphasia with mild apraxia of speech.

2.2. Experimental Procedure. The experimental protocol is similar to previous studies conducted in our lab (Marcotte and Ansaldo, 2010, 2012, and 2013). A baseline language assessment was conducted prior to therapy, followed by an initial fMRI session (T1), which identified the neural substrate of spontaneous correct naming. Afterward, patients received therapy from a trained SLP (ED). A second fMRI session (T2) was performed after five weeks of therapy. This session allowed us to identify the brain areas that subserved therapy-induced neuroplasticity. During both fMRI sessions, patients performed an overt naming task. (See Table 2 for the MRI results.)

2.2.1. Language Assessment. Before therapy, the participants were examined with subtests from Montreal-Toulouse 86 Beta version (Nespoulous et al., 1986) to assess global comprehension, repetition, and fluency; the kissing and dancing test (KDT) for verb comprehension [53]; the dénomination de verbes lexicaux (DVL38) for verb naming [51]; the test de dénomination de Québec (TDQ) for noun naming [54]; and three subtests of the Apraxia Battery for Adults—Second Edition [55]—to measure the presence and severity of verbal, limb, and oral apraxia. These tests allow a complete description of the aphasia profile.

2.2.2. Baseline and Items for fMRI Session and Therapy. Stimuli used for the baseline, the fMRI naming task, and the therapy sessions were 5-second action videos (Durand et al., in prep.). Before therapy, the participant underwent three baseline naming assessments using 134 action videos. Baselines were separated by at least four days; the participant had to show stable oral naming performance. In order to provide more individualized therapy, a set of stimuli was created for the participants on the basis of individual performance on the baseline as follows: correctly named (spontaneous, $n = 20$) and incorrectly named ($n = 60$). Of the incorrectly named items, only 20 were trained and the remaining 40 items allowed us to measure the generalization of therapy effects to untrained items. All sets of items (spontaneous, trained, and untrained) were matched for word frequency, number of phonemes, and syllabic complexity. Statistical analysis of the lists showed nonsignificant differences regarding these variables.

Before the first fMRI session, each participant took part in a practice session in a mock scanner. They could therefore become accustomed to the scanner noise and environment.

For the pretherapy fMRI sessions, a set of items was developed including correctly named (spontaneous, $n = 20$) and incorrectly named ($n = 60$) items and scrambled videos that were optimized to fit the same parameters (motion, colors) as the videos for the control conditions ($n = 40$). For the posttherapy fMRI session, the same set was presented, but this time, the incorrectly named items ($n = 60$) were divided into trained items ($n = 20$) and untrained items ($n = 40$) to measure generalization.

TABLE 1: Sociodemographic, clinical, and cognitive data for the 2 participants.

Patient ID	P1	P2
Sociodemographic data		
Age (years)	65	72
Gender	F	F
Education (years)	18	11
Clinical data		
Handedness	R	R
Etiology	Ischemia	Ischemia
Months postonset	84	408
Aphasia type	Transcortical motor	Transcortical motor
Lesion volume (cm^3)	38	132
Level of verb anomia	68%	55%
Cognitive data (CASP)		
Language (max. 6)	5	6
Visuoconstructive functions (max. 6)	6	5
Executive functions (max. 6)	6	6
Memory (max. 6)	6	6
Praxis (max. 6)	6	5
Orientation (max. 6)	4	6
Total CASP (max. 36)	33	34

CASP: Cognitive Assessment scale for Stroke Patients (Benaim et al., 2015).

During the fMRI scanning, participants were instructed to name the randomly presented videos and to say "baba" in response to scrambled videos. After therapy, the same set of items was presented. Oral responses were audio-recorded with Audacity software.

2.2.3. fMRI Sessions. Participants lay in a supine position on the MRI scanner bed with their head stabilized by foam. Stimuli were pseudorandomly displayed in an optimized order projected by means of E-Prime software (Psychology Software Tools) from a computer onto a screen at the head of the bore and were visible in a mirror attached to the head coil. Each video and picture was presented for 5000 ms, with an interstimulus interval (ISI) ranging from 1104 to 10,830 ms. As shown in Figure 2, participants were instructed to name each action and object, as clearly and accurately as possible, and to say "baba" each time they saw a distorted picture, while avoiding head movements. An MRI-compatible microphone was placed close to the participant's mouth, and Audacity software (http://www.audacityteam.org) was used to record oral responses.

2.2.4. Functional Neuroimaging Parameters. Images were acquired using a 3T MRI Siemens Trio scanner, which was updated (Prisma Fit) during our data collection, with a standard 32-channel head coil. The image sequence was a $T2^*$-weighted pulse sequence (TR = 2200 ms; TE = 30 ms; matrix = 64×64 voxels; FOV = 210 mm; flip angle = 90°; slice thickness = 3 mm; and acquisition = 36 slides in the axial

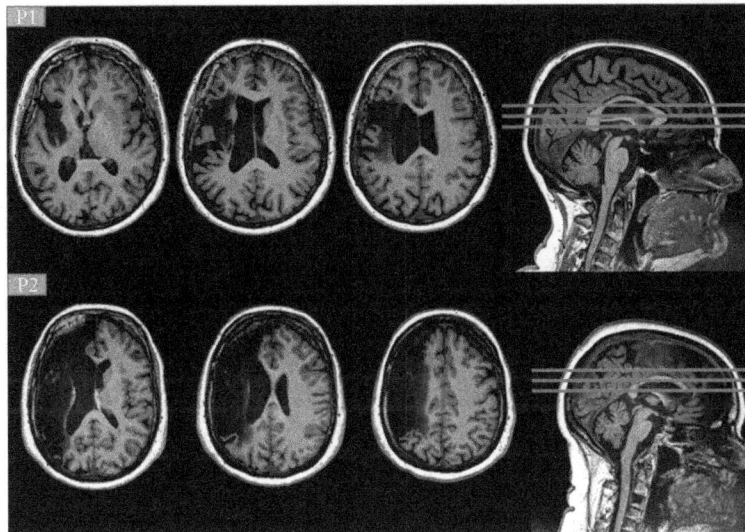

FIGURE 1: Lesion location on anatomical MRI for P1 (top three slices) and for P2 (bottom three slices).

TABLE 2: Language assessment and verb naming scores during the pre- and posttherapy MRI sessions for both participants.

Patient ID	P1		P2	
	Pre	Post	Pre	Post
Language assessment				
Comprehension (max. 47)	46	45	32	N/A
Repetition (max. 33)	30	30	N/A	N/A
Fluency	11	5	15	16
TDQ (max. 60)	40	47	52	57
KDT (max. 52)	51	49	48	N/A
DVL38 (max. 114)	77	81	63	65
Verb naming scores during fMRI session	Pre	Post	Pre	Post
Score for trained items (/20)	9	16	10	19
Score for untrained items (/40)	24	30	15	13

Pre: pre-POEM therapy; Post: post-POEM therapy.

plane with a distance factor of 25% in order to scan the whole brain, including the cerebellum). A high-resolution structural image was obtained before the two functional runs using a 3D T1-weighted imaging sequence using an MP-RAGE (TFE) sequence (TR = 2300 ms; TE = 2.98 ms; 192 slices; matrix = 256 × 256 mm; voxel size = 1 × 1 × 1 mm; and FOV = 256 mm).

2.2.5. Language Therapy with POEM. A trained SLP (ED) provided the POEM therapy, which lasted for one hour and was provided three times per week, over five weeks. During each session, participants were trained to name 20 actions presented in 5-second videos. If the participant could not name the action within 5 to 10 s, she was asked to make the gesture associated with this action, helped by the SLP. If she could not name the action, the participant was asked to imagine the action in a personal context. For instance, with the action *to water*, the following sequence can be produced after the action observation: the SLP says "Show me what the person is doing with your hands," and the participant can imitate someone who is watering. If the action is still not named, the SLP says "Imagine this action in your garden." After these prompts, the word was given to the participant, who was asked to repeat it once.

2.3. Behavioral and fMRI Data Analysis. Responses to the fMRI naming task were recorded and coded offline by an experienced SLP (ED), in order to build the design matrices. Preprocessing and statistical analyses were performed using SPM12 software (Wellcome Trust Centre for Neuroimaging, Institute of Neurology, University College London), running on MATLAB_R2016b (MathWorks Inc., MA, USA). fMRI images were preprocessed with the usual spatial realignment and slice timing. Motion was assessed to ensure that the naming task did not involve head motion exceeding 3 mm. Because precise, valid normalization is critical to understanding the neural substrates of treatment-induced recovery, we used the "Clinical toolbox" extension [56]. This toolbox allows optimal segmentation and registration of brains with distorted anatomy due to lesions. Lesion masks (PB) hand-traced on T1-weighted images were used to minimize the impact of the lesion on the normalization estimates, by substituting healthy tissue for homologous regions of the intact hemisphere [57]. This yields transformation matrices for normalization into the standard stereotaxic space (MNI space) with $3 \times 3 \times 3$ mm^3 voxel size. A spatially smoothed 8 mm Gaussian filter was chosen for the smoothing step. Preprocessed data were analyzed using the general linear model implemented in SPM12. Statistical parametric maps were obtained for each subject and each measurement period (first and second fMRI sessions), by applying linear contrasts to the parameter estimates for the conditions of interest (successful naming with trained/untrained items). Neuroimaging data analyses were performed only on correct responses. Individual maps were calculated for each condition for the whole brain with cluster size superior to 10 voxels and $p < 0.001$ uncorrected.

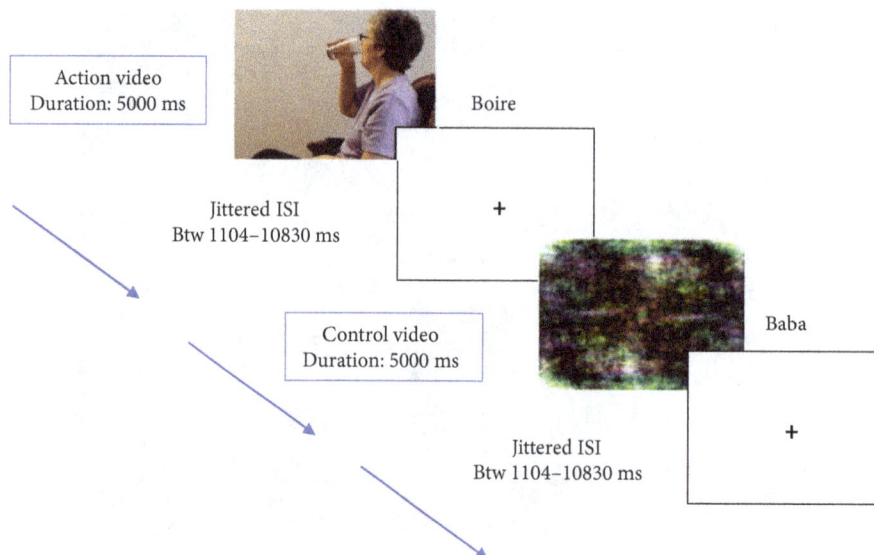

FIGURE 2: Naming task during fMRI acquisition.

Furthermore, a Lehéricy index (LI) was calculated for each participant to estimate the relative contribution of the LH and RH to verb naming in each condition, pre- and posttherapy. We applied Lehéricy's algorithm, defined as follows: $(L - R)/(L + R)$, where L represents the number of activated voxels in the LH and R represents the number of activated voxels in the RH. LIs were calculated using voxels in clusters ($k \geq 10$) that exceeded the threshold ($p < 0.001$ uncorrected). LIs can range from -1.0 to $+1.0$. By convention, values between -0.2 and $+0.2$ represent bilateral language distribution, values between -0.2 and -1.0 represent RH dominance, and values between $+0.2$ and $+1.0$ represent LH dominance. Values between ± 0.5 and ± 1.0 are considered to reflect strong hemisphere dominance [58].

3. Results

3.1. Participant 1. By the end of the therapy period, P1 was able to name all of the 20 trained items. However, her performance in the scanner was less accurate than that at the last therapy session, as she named 16 trained items in the posttherapy fMRI session, which occurred one day after the end of therapy. In addition, P1 named 30 of the 40 untrained items that she was unable to name before therapy. Moreover, P1 showed improved verb naming on the DVL38 and noun naming on the TDQ.

As for her fMRI results, spontaneous correct naming before therapy significantly activated the left primary motor cortex, left angular gyrus, and right fusiform gyrus, with predominant LH activation according to the LI. (See Table 3 for fMRI results and Table 4 for LIs.)

Regarding trained items after the therapy, the activation map revealed significant activation in the left cerebellum, left and right middle temporal gyri, and right fusiform gyrus. Moreover, the LI indicated an increase in predominant LH activation (0.17).

Finally, with untrained items, the posttherapy activation map showed significant activation of regions similar to those activated for the trained items, namely, the left middle temporal gyrus and right fusiform gyrus, with the addition of the right inferior frontal gyrus. The LI in this case showed a shift to predominant RH recruitment.

3.2. Participant 2. Following therapy, P2 was able to name all of the 20 trained items and correctly named 19 trained items in the posttherapy fMRI session. P2 also named 13 of the 40 untrained items she had been unable to name before therapy. Again, her performance outside the scanner was better for untrained items. Finally, like P1, P2 showed improved verb naming ability on the DVL38 and noun naming ability on the TDQ.

The activation map for correct naming before therapy showed the recruitment of a large set of areas, including bilateral activation of the angular gyrus, superior parietal lobule, premotor cortex, left middle and inferior occipital gyri, and right cerebellum. The LI (0.6) corresponded to a predominant LH activation. (See Table 3 for fMRI results and Table 4 for LIs.)

With trained items, posttherapy activation maps were much smaller, as fewer areas were recruited, namely, the right premotor cortex and left cerebellum, and the LI showed predominant RH activation (-0.58). Unfortunately, it was not possible to obtain an activation map for untrained items, due to the lack of a suprathreshold cluster number.

4. Discussion

This study examined the behavioral and neural correlates of personalized observation, execution, and mental imagery (POEM) therapy, a new approach combining sensorimotor and language-based strategies to treat verb anomia, which was delivered in a massed stimulation format. Two participants with nonfluent chronic aphasia were examined

TABLE 3: Significantly activated areas associated with the production of correct verbs for the two participants.

Pretherapy

Patient ID	Condition	Left hemisphere SPM results							Right hemisphere SPM results						
		Region	BA	X	Y	Z	T-score	Cluster size	Region	BA	X	Y	Z	T-score	Cluster size
P1	Spontaneously named > baba	Primary motor	4	−39	−25	65	4.82	20	Fusiform	37	60	−46	5	4.79	28
		Angular gyrus	39	−60	−49	35	3.74	13							
	Incorrectly named > baba	Angular gyrus	39	−60	−43	26	3.49	10	Fusiform	37	60	−46	5	4.2	15
			39	−60	−52	32	3.37								
P2	Spontaneously named > baba	Angular gyrus	39	−27	−67	32	5.2	1117	Superior parietal lobule	7	33	−55	53	4.35	117
		Superior parietal lobule	7	−27	−67	44	5.08		Angular gyrus	39	30	−67	26	3.64	
		Superior parietal lobule	7	−21	−61	35	4.84		Angular gyrus	39	33	−64	35	3.47	
		Inferior occipital gyrus	19	−33	−73	−4	4.76	167	Cerebellum		−18	−76	−19	3.95	115
		Middle occipital gyrus	18	−24	−97	−1	4.23				−24	−70	−25	3.91	
		Premotor cortex	6	−15	14	47	4.22	100			−33	−70	−28	3.67	
			6	−12	8	62	4.09		Cerebellum	6	12	−39	−49	3.97	69
			6	−21	11	56	3.92		Premotor cortex	6	54	−4	35	5.03	56
		Fusiform	37	−51	−40	−10	4.09	46	Prefrontal cortex-SMA	8	42	5	35	3.74	11
		Fusiform		−48	−52	−19	3.19								
		Middle occipital gyrus	18	−3	−70	2	3.75	33							
		Striate cortex	17	−18	−79	14	3.78	17							
	Incorrectly named > baba	Superior parietal lobule	7	−21	−61	35	5.59	1273	Cerebellum		18	−25	−34	5.58	471
		Primary motor	4	−3	−28	74	4.96		Cerebellum		9	−37	−49	4.75	
		Middle occipital gyrus	18	−27	−85	5	4.34		Angular gyrus	39	36	−58	44	3.91	76
		Premotor cortex	6	−3	8	65	4.58	230	Superior parietal lobule	7	30	−61	35	3.6	
			6	−15	14	47	4.13		Primary motor	4	57	−1	32	4.37	39
									Middle frontal gyrus	9	54	26	20	3.91	22
									Inferior frontal gyrus	45	54	29	11	3.69	
									Anterior middle frontal gyrus	46	48	35	17	3.25	

Posttherapy

Patient ID	Condition	Left hemisphere SPM results							Right hemisphere SPM results						
		Region	BA	X	Y	Z	T-score	Cluster size	Region	BA	X	Y	Z	T-score	Cluster size
P1	Spontaneously named > baba								Middle temporal gyrus	21	60	−43	2	4.2	19
	Trained > baba	Cerebellum		−24	−88	−28	4.6	31	Fusiform	37	60	−49	5	4.42	32
		Middle temporal gyrus	21	−60	−22	−4	4.02	14	Middle temporal gyrus	21	48	−40	5	3.46	
		Middle temporal gyrus	21	−54	−31	−1	3.52								
	Untrained > baba	Middle temporal gyrus	21	−60	−25	−4	4.68	21	Fusiform	37	60	−46	5	5.04	82
		Middle temporal gyrus	21	−54	−31	−1	3.81		Inferior frontal gyrus	44	39	11	17	4.32	54
P2	Spontaneously named > baba	Premotor cortex	6	−15	−19	50	4.5	59	Premotor cortex	6	51	−4	35	5.56	114
		Middle occipital gyrus	18	−24	−94	2	3.49	20	Cerebellum		15	−73	−31	3.56	12
		Middle occipital gyrus	18	−12	−85	−10	3.47	14							
		Cerebellum		−33	−73	−28		16							
				−27	−64	−25									
	Trained > baba	Cerebellum		15	−73	−31	3.75	10	Premotor cortex	6	51	−4	35	4.25	38
	Untrained > baba	No suprathreshold cluster							No suprathreshold cluster						

BA: Brodmann area; baba: condition control.

TABLE 4: Lateralization indexes related to successful verb naming in the different conditions pre- and posttherapy for P1 and P2.

Lehéricy index	P1	P2
Spontaneous pretherapy	0.08	0.6
Spontaneous posttherapy	−1	−0.07
Incorrect pretherapy	−0.2	0.42
Incorrect—trained posttherapy	0.17	−0.58
Incorrect—untrained posttherapy	−0.73	N/A

with a verb naming task during event-related fMRI scanning, before and after therapy. Both participants benefited from POEM, with improvements observed with both trained and untrained items. Concurrently with the behavioral improvement, changes in the neural substrates sustaining verb naming were observed in both participants, with distinctive activation patterns observed posttherapy, including areas related to the nature of POEM therapy.

As hypothesized, the outcomes revealed the positive effects of POEM therapy on verb naming for both participants. The results are in line with previous studies showing that sensorimotor strategies are efficient therapy tools for recovery from verb anomia secondary to aphasia [16, 17, 22, 23]. However, none of those studies found positive therapy effects on untrained items. Two possible interpretations of these results were considered: on the one hand, they could be due to the origins of verb anomia; on the other hand, they could be due to the types of strategies used. In their study using semantic plus gesture treatments for verb anomia, Rose and Sussmilch [23] reported significant improvement for two participants with lexical-phonological-based anomia, but there is no improvement for the participant with semantic-based anomia. Similarly, Marangolo et al. [17] obtained positive results with AOT on verb retrieval for participants with lexical-phonological-based verb anomia, but there is no improvement for those who presented semantic-based verb anomia. The authors of those studies suggested that the severity of the semantic impairment underlying the anomia was responsible for the lack of improvement after the therapy. In our study, the semantic processing assessment showed that each participant had a preserved semantic system before the therapy. Because sensorimotor strategies are related to the semantic component of action, the improvement in verb retrieval would have been facilitated by preserved semantic abilities.

Furthermore, improvement was also observed on the untrained list after POEM therapy. Although this result was limited for P2 in the context of fMRI, the improvement was noted behaviorally and the same result has been found consistently with a group of 10 participants who have received POEM therapy (Durand et al., in prep). However, a generalization to untrained items was not found in several earlier studies using sensorimotor strategies. The sensorimotor strategies applied by Marangolo et al. [17], Raymer et al. (2007), and Rose and Sussmilch [23] used only one type of sensorimotor cue—gesture or observation in association with verb naming—whereas with POEM therapy, several sensorimotor cues were provided—observation of the action,

gesture, and mental imagery—which may have facilitated word retrieval. According to cognitive models of word naming, this combination of semantic inputs could increase activation at the semantic level and facilitate the flow to the lexical and articulation levels and verb naming [59, 60]. Moreover, in line with the embodied theory, the various sensorimotor cues in POEM therapy tap into the specific encoding features of verbs [14, 26, 36, 42, 44], thus enhancing the therapy's specificity, another factor that has been shown to contribute to therapy efficacy [2].

The personalized approach potentially contributes to POEM's efficacy and generalization effects. Thus, verbs targeted with POEM were selected according to each participant's naming performance before therapy. Personalization of therapy items is considered to increase motivation, and thus attention focus, and has been shown to contribute to therapy efficacy [61].

Finally, as shown by previous works [47–49], massed stimulation with the POEM protocol may also explain the differences observed between our study and the other studies considered. The structured and massed practice on a limited number of items may have contributed to the implementation of a naming strategy that could be generalized to untreated items.

The improvement observed for our two participants occurred concomitantly with changes in neural recruitment. As hypothesized, the recovery following POEM therapy involves the recruitment of an alternative circuit, including the activation of motor and premotor areas. Although the behavioral improvement looks the same for both participants, two different patterns appeared after the POEM therapy.

In the case of P1, the pretherapy fMRI session showed bilateral distribution according to the LI. More specifically, considering the activation maps for spontaneously named items to be trained or untrained, the recruitment includes the left primary motor area, left angular gyrus, and right fusiform gyrus. The left primary motor area and left angular gyrus are canonical areas, part of the dorsal stream pathway of language [62], that reveal the perilesional recruitment associated with aphasia recovery. These two areas are also known to be involved in verb naming [13, 63]. The angular gyrus, which is an associative area between somatosensory information and visual information, participates in the processing of sequence actions, which may be related to the processing of the action videos (Crozier et al., 1999). The recruitment of the right fusiform gyrus can also be related to the processing of visual stimuli. The fusiform gyrus is involved in lexical-semantic association, that is, associating words with visual stimuli [64]. To summarize, for P1, the pretherapy fMRI session revealed the recruitment of canonical areas for verb naming, including perilesional areas, in line with a functional reactivation.

After the POEM therapy, the activation map for trained items reveals that distribution is still bilateral (LI = 0.17), including the right fusiform gyrus and the bilateral middle temporal gyri and left cerebellum. The bilateral middle temporal gyri participate in semantic processing, word generation, and observation of motion [65]. Classically, the cerebellum is known to regulate motor movement and be involved in motor speech planning. But recent fMRI studies have revealed the contribution of the cerebellum to other kinds of language processing [66, 67], namely, verb generation [68]. To sum up, post-POEM therapy, the activation pattern is consistent with the sensorimotor nature of POEM therapy and therefore is likely to have been therapy-induced.

More interestingly, in P1, the activation patterns for trained and untrained items posttherapy included common areas, with the activation of the left middle temporal gyrus, right fusiform gyrus, and right inferior frontal gyrus. The similarity of neural recruitment for trained and untrained items after POEM therapy suggests that the same kind of processing was used to name the verbs. Furthermore, these similar activations occur concomitantly with the generalization observed in behavioral results. The behavioral and neural results are evidence of the potential application of the same strategies to retrieve verbs.

In the case of P2, the pretherapy fMRI session showed dominant LH activation according to the LI. Considering the large lesion on the left hemisphere, it is not surprising that the activation for spontaneously named items included posterior visual processing areas such as the striate cortex and middle and inferior occipital gyri. But canonical areas for verb naming were also recruited, namely, the angular gyrus and premotor cortex bilaterally. These areas are known to be part of the action naming network in the LH [13, 14, 44]. The bilateral activations on the activation map pretherapy revealed adaptive neuroplasticity with a functional reorganization, which included the homologous areas for verb naming.

After P2's POEM therapy, there was a dramatic decrease in the number of areas recruited for verb naming. The posttherapy activation is supported exclusively by the right premotor area and the left cerebellum. As discussed above, these two areas are involved in action observation and verb naming [44, 66, 67]. This significant reduction in the number of brain areas supporting correct naming suggests that POEM therapy could lead to a more economical use of brain resources. Moreover, considering the LI (−0.58), there was a shift to the RH. This shift is related to adaptive neuroplasticity and is not surprising considering P2's large lesion. This result is in line with the suggested complementary role of the RH in the context of large lesions proposed by Anglade et al. (2013) who argued that, when there is a large lesion with near-complete destruction of the primary language processing areas, significant RH activation is involved.

Our preliminary results showed that neural changes appeared together with behavioral improvements in verb naming after POEM therapy was applied. Although neurorehabilitation studies in the physical domain had provided convincing evidence that action observation and motor imagery might enhance the efficacy of motor training and/or motor recovery by stimulating the activity of the sensorimotor system [69–72], no studies had explored this combination in the case of language rehabilitation. However, the link between action observation, motor imagery, and the sensorimotor system through the MNS system may apply to language too. As discussed by Durand and Ansaldo [15], the MNS is considered to have provided a natural platform for the development of language in humans. Several studies in the field of embodied cognition have provided evidence that the sensorimotor system can be considered an embodied cognitive agent, as it coordinates multimodal information resulting from an individual's interaction with the environment and constitutes a physiological substrate for empirical data linking language and motor processing [24, 26, 27].

Several fMRI studies have shown links between language and motor processing areas within the MNS. Specifically, language comprehension and production tasks engage somatotopic activations, that is, the recruitment of specific motor areas, depending on the body part involved in the action associated with the language target [35, 43]. These findings suggest that the MNS plays an important role in the reintegration of sensorimotor representations during the conceptual processing of actions evoked by linguistic stimuli. Thus, the cooccurrence of these activations weaves connections between motor and language processing areas. These connections represent an interesting framework devoted to the enhancement of skill recovery in language rehabilitation. They were exploited through the application of POEM therapy, leading to preliminary results with two participants.

This work concerns two case studies, and thus, it represents a proof of concept for further investigation of the effects of POEM. Thus, larger experimental samples are required to test for the external validity of these findings. This being said, the two single-case studies reported here concern two different cases, in terms of lesion size, location, and volume, thus providing evidence for the efficacy of POEM in more than one type of aphasia patients. Hence, while group study strength lies on statistical power, single-case studies are informative in terms of the variables that can influence recovery. In particular, group studies average activations, while single-case studies show different patterns of neurofunctional changes, in particular perilesional activations, which are known to better correlate with functional recovery [73]. The present study shows how similar behavioral improvement across the two participants is observed in the context of different lesion volumes and neurofunctional patterns.

Another potential caveat of the present study concerns sociodemographic differences between the two participants, in particular, time poststroke, lesion volume, and education level. Specifically, P2 was 408 months poststroke, while P1 was 84 months poststroke. Time elapsed after stroke has been shown to play an important role in treatment-related changes, but this concerns particularly the acute or subacute phase of recovery, as opposed to the chronic state, which is generally considered to go beyond 6–12 months after stroke [74, 75]. Consequently, we do not think that differences in neurofunctional patterns observed in P1 and P2 can be accounted for by time elapsed after stroke but reflect the influence of lesion size and volume, while these two factors do not seem to modulate POEM therapy efficacy, as documented by equivalent improvement across the two participants.

In all, the results of this study provide evidence for the efficacy of POEM and its neural correlates, in two cases of chronic verb anomia, resulting from lesions varying in size, location, and volume, and in participants with different educational backgrounds. Future studies will examine the effects of POEM on larger samples (Durand et al., in prep.) and gather both the anatomical and functional correlates of language and motor networks sustaining its efficacy. It will possibly increase our understanding of the mechanisms underlying the recovery from verb anomia, so that more efficient and synergistic rehabilitative interventions based on the links between motricity and language can be designed.

Disclosure

The results of this study will be presented as a scientific poster at the Tenth Annual Meeting of the Society for the Neurobiology of Language (Québec, Canada, August 16–18, 2018).

Acknowledgments

The authors wish to thank the participants for their contribution to this study. This research was supported by the Heart and Stroke Foundation of Canada research grant to Ana Inés Ansaldo and a Fonds de Recherche du Québec-Santé doctoral grant to Edith Durand.

References

[1] J. M. C. Lam and W. P. Wodchis, "The relationship of 60 disease diagnoses and 15 conditions to preference-based health-related quality of life in Ontario hospital-based long-term care residents," *Medical Care*, vol. 48, no. 4, pp. 380–387, 2010.

[2] J. Webster and A. Whitworth, "Treating verbs in aphasia: exploring the impact of therapy at the single word and sentence levels," *International Journal of Language and Communication Disorders*, vol. 47, no. 6, pp. 619–636, 2012.

[3] P. Conroy, K. Sage, and M. A. Lambon Ralph, "Towards theory-driven therapies for aphasic verb impairments: a review of current theory and practice," *Aphasiology*, vol. 20, no. 12, pp. 1159–1185, 2006.

[4] J. Grafman, "Conceptualizing functional neuroplasticity," *Journal of Communication Disorders*, vol. 33, no. 4, pp. 345–356, 2000.

[5] J. A. Kleim and T. A. Jones, "Principles of experience-dependent neural plasticity: implications for rehabilitation after brain damage," *Journal of Speech, Language and Hearing Research*, vol. 51, pp. S225–S239, 2008.

[6] R. S. Berndt, C. C. Mitchum, A. N. Haendiges, and J. Sandson, "Verb retrieval in aphasia. 1. Characterizing single word impairments," *Brain and Language*, vol. 56, no. 1, pp. 68–106, 1997.

[7] P. Conroy, K. Sage, and M. A. Lambon Ralph, "The effects of decreasing and increasing cue therapy on improving naming speed and accuracy for verbs and nouns in aphasia," *Aphasiology*, vol. 23, no. 6, pp. 707–730, 2009.

[8] P. Conroy, K. Sage, and M. L. Ralph, "Improved vocabulary production after naming therapy in aphasia: can gains in picture naming generalise to connected speech?," *International Journal of Language and Communication Disorders*, vol. 44, no. 6, pp. 1036–1062, 2009.

[9] J. Marshall, T. Pring, and S. Chiat, "Verb retrieval and sentence production in aphasia," *Brain and Language*, vol. 63, no. 2, pp. 159–183, 1998.

[10] A. M. Raymer, M. Ciampitti, B. Holliway et al., "Semantic-phonologic treatment for noun and verb retrieval impairments in aphasia," *Neuropsychological Rehabilitation*, vol. 17, no. 2, pp. 244–270, 2007.

[11] A. M. Raymer and L. Rothi, "Clinical diagnosis and treatment of naming disorders," in *The Handbook of Adult Language Disorders: Integrating Cognitive Neuropsychology, Neurology and Rehabilitation*, A. E. Hillis, Ed., pp. 163–182, Psychology Press, New York and East Sussex, 2002.

[12] J. L. Wambaugh and M. Ferguson, "Application of semantic feature analysis to retrieval of action names in aphasia," *Journal of Rehabilitation Research and Development*, vol. 44, no. 3, pp. 381–394, 2007.

[13] F. Pulvermüller, "Brain mechanisms linking language and action," *Nature Reviews Neuroscience*, vol. 6, no. 7, pp. 576–582, 2005.

[14] F. Pulvermüller, "Meaning and the brain: the neurosemantics of referential, interactive, and combinatorial knowledge," *Journal of Neurolinguistics*, vol. 25, no. 5, pp. 423–459, 2012.

[15] E. Durand and A. I. Ansaldo, "Recovery from anomia following semantic feature analysis: therapy-induced neuroplasticity relies upon a circuit involving motor and language processing areas," *The Mental Lexicon*, vol. 8, no. 2, pp. 195–215, 2013.

[16] S. Bonifazi, F. Tomaiuolo, G. Altoè, M. Ceravolo, L. Provinciali, and P. Marangolo, "Action observation as a useful approach for enhancing recovery of verb production: new evidence from aphasia," *European Journal of Physical and Rehabilitation Medicine*, vol. 49, 2013.

[17] P. Marangolo, S. Bonifazi, F. Tomaiuolo et al., "Improving language without words: first evidence from aphasia," *Neuropsychologia*, vol. 48, no. 13, pp. 3824–3833, 2010.

[18] D. Ertelt, S. Small, A. Solodkin et al., "Action observation has a positive impact on rehabilitation of motor deficits after stroke," *NeuroImage*, vol. 36, pp. T164–T173, 2007.

[19] M. Franceschini, M. Agosti, A. Cantagallo, P. Sale, M. Mancuso, and G. Buccino, "Mirror neurons: action observation treatment as a tool in stroke rehabilitation," *European Journal of Physical and Rehabilitation Medicine*, vol. 46, no. 4, pp. 517–523, 2010.

[20] M. Franceschini, M. G. Ceravolo, M. Agosti et al., "Clinical relevance of action observation in upper-limb stroke rehabilitation: a possible role in recovery of functional dexterity. A randomized clinical trial," *Neurorehabilitation and Neural Repair*, vol. 26, no. 5, pp. 456–462, 2012.

[21] M.-H. Zhu, J. Wang, X. D. Gu et al., "Effect of action observation therapy on daily activities and motor recovery in stroke patients," *International Journal of Nursing Sciences*, vol. 2, no. 3, pp. 279–282, 2015.

[22] S. Routhier, N. Bier, and J. Macoir, "The contrast between cueing and/or observation in therapy for verb retrieval in

post-stroke aphasia," *Journal of Communication Disorders*, vol. 54, pp. 43–55, 2015.

[23] M. Rose and G. Sussmilch, "The effects of semantic and gesture treatments on verb retrieval and verb use in aphasia," *Aphasiology*, vol. 22, no. 7-8, pp. 691–706, 2008.

[24] G. Rizzolatti and L. Craighero, "The mirror-neuron system," *Annual Review of Neuroscience*, vol. 27, no. 1, pp. 169–192, 2004.

[25] G. Rizzolatti and C. Sinigaglia, "The functional role of the parieto-frontal mirror circuit: interpretations and misinterpretations," *Nature Reviews Neuroscience*, vol. 11, no. 4, pp. 264–274, 2010.

[26] M. C. Corballis, "Mirror neurons and the evolution of language," *Brain and Language*, vol. 112, no. 1, pp. 25–35, 2010.

[27] M. Gentilucci and G. C. Campione, "From action to speech," in *Language and Action in Cognitive Neuroscience*, Y. Coello and A. Bartolo, Eds., pp. 59–79, Psychology press Taylor & Francis Group, London and New York, 2012.

[28] V. Gallese and G. Lakoff, "The brain's concepts: the role of the sensory-motor system in conceptual knowledge," *Cognitive Neuropsychology*, vol. 22, no. 3-4, pp. 455–479, 2005.

[29] E. Freud, D. C. Plaut, and M. Behrmann, "'What' is happening in the dorsal visual pathway," *Trends in Cognitive Sciences*, vol. 20, no. 10, pp. 773–784, 2016.

[30] M. A. Goodale, "Transforming vision into action," *Vision Research*, vol. 51, no. 13, pp. 1567–1587, 2011.

[31] R. D. McIntosh and T. Schenk, "Two visual streams for perception and action: current trends," *Neuropsychologia*, vol. 47, no. 6, pp. 1391–1396, 2009.

[32] M. A. Goodale and A. D. Milner, "Separate visual pathways for perception and action," *Trends in Neurosciences*, vol. 15, no. 1, pp. 20–25, 1992.

[33] S. Zipoli Caiani and G. Ferretti, "Semantic and pragmatic integration in vision for action," *Consciousness and Cognition*, vol. 48, pp. 40–54, 2017.

[34] P. Aravena, Y. Delevoye-Turrell, V. Deprez et al., "Grip force reveals the context sensitivity of language-induced motor activity during "action words" processing: evidence from sentential negation," *PLoS One*, vol. 7, no. 12, article e50287, 2012.

[35] L. Aziz-Zadeh, S. M. Wilson, G. Rizzolatti, and M. Iacoboni, "Congruent embodied representations for visually presented actions and linguistic phrases describing actions," *Current Biology*, vol. 16, no. 18, pp. 1818–1823, 2006.

[36] M. Bedny, A. Caramazza, A. Pascual-Leone, and R. Saxe, "Typical neural representations of action verbs develop without vision," *Cerebral Cortex*, vol. 22, no. 2, pp. 286–293, 2012.

[37] J. R. Binder, R. H. Desai, W. W. Graves, and L. L. Conant, "Where is the semantic system? A critical review and meta-analysis of 120 functional neuroimaging studies," *Cerebral Cortex*, vol. 19, no. 12, pp. 2767–2796, 2009.

[38] V. Boulenger, O. Hauk, and F. Pulvermüller, "Grasping ideas with the motor system: semantic somatotopy in idiom comprehension," *Cerebral Cortex*, vol. 19, no. 8, pp. 1905–1914, 2009.

[39] G. Buccino, F. Lui, N. Canessa et al., "Neural circuits involved in the recognition of actions performed by nonconspecifics: an fMRI study," *Journal of Cognitive Neuroscience*, vol. 16, no. 1, pp. 114–126, 2004.

[40] S. Caspers, K. Zilles, A. R. Laird, and S. B. Eickhoff, "ALE meta-analysis of action observation and imitation in the human brain," *NeuroImage*, vol. 50, no. 3, pp. 1148–1167, 2010.

[41] L. Fernandino, L. L. Conant, J. R. Binder et al., "Parkinson's disease disrupts both automatic and controlled processing of action verbs," *Brain and Language*, vol. 127, no. 1, pp. 65–74, 2013.

[42] D. Jirak, M. M. Menz, G. Buccino, A. M. Borghi, and F. Binkofski, "Grasping language – a short story on embodiment," *Consciousness and Cognition*, vol. 19, no. 3, pp. 711–720, 2010.

[43] M. Tettamanti, G. Buccino, M. C. Saccuman et al., "Listening to action-related sentences activates fronto-parietal motor circuits," *Journal of Cognitive Neuroscience*, vol. 17, no. 2, pp. 273–281, 2005.

[44] P. Tremblay and S. L. Small, "From language comprehension to action understanding and back again," *Cerebral Cortex*, vol. 21, no. 5, pp. 1166–1177, 2011.

[45] J. Pearson, T. Naselaris, E. A. Holmes, and S. M. Kosslyn, "Mental imagery: functional mechanisms and clinical applications," *Trends in Cognitive Sciences*, vol. 19, no. 10, pp. 590–602, 2015.

[46] E. Gleichgerrcht, J. Fridriksson, C. Rorden, T. Nesland, R. Desai, and L. Bonilha, "Separate neural systems support representations for actions and objects during narrative speech in post-stroke aphasia," *NeuroImage: Clinical*, vol. 10, pp. 140–145, 2016.

[47] E. Maas, D. A. Robin, S. N. Austermann Hula et al., "Principles of motor learning in treatment of motor speech disorders," *American Journal of Speech-Language Pathology*, vol. 17, no. 3, pp. 277–298, 2008.

[48] E. L. Middleton, M. F. Schwartz, K. A. Rawson, H. Traut, and J. Verkuilen, "Towards a theory of learning for naming rehabilitation: retrieval practice and spacing effects," *Journal of Speech, Language, and Hearing Research*, vol. 59, no. 5, pp. 1111–1122, 2016.

[49] F. Pulvermüller and M. L. Berthier, "Aphasia therapy on a neuroscience basis," *Aphasiology*, vol. 22, no. 6, pp. 563–599, 2008.

[50] F. Pulvermüller and L. Fadiga, "Chapter 26 - brain language mechanisms built on action and perception," in *Neurobiology of Language*, G. Hickok and S. L. Small, Eds., Academic Press, San Diego, 2016.

[51] C. Hammelrath, *DVL 38: test de dénomination des verbes lexicaux en images*, Ortho éd, 1999.

[52] J. L. Barnay, G. Wauquiez, H. Y. Bonnin-Koang et al., "Feasibility of the Cognitive Assessment scale for Stroke Patients (CASP) vs. MMSE and MoCA in aphasic left hemispheric stroke patients," *Annals of Physical and Rehabilitation Medicine*, vol. 57, no. 6-7, pp. 422–435, 2014.

[53] T. H. Bak and J. R. Hodges, *Kissing and Dancing Test Sydney (Australia) Neuroscience Research Australia*, Neuroscience Research Australia NeuRA, 2003.

[54] J. Macoir, C. Beaudoin, J. Bluteau, O. Potvin, and M. A. Wilson, "TDQ-60-a color picture-naming test for adults and elderly people: validation and normalization data," *Aging, Neuropsychology, and Cognition*, vol. 24, pp. 1–14, 2017.

[55] B. L. Dabul, *Apraxia Battery for Adults*, Pro-ed, 2nd edition, 2000.

[56] C. Rorden, L. Bonilha, J. Fridriksson, B. Bender, and H.-O. Karnath, "Age-specific CT and MRI templates for

spatial normalization," *NeuroImage*, vol. 61, no. 4, pp. 957–965, 2012.

[57] P. Nachev, E. Coulthard, H. R. Jäger, C. Kennard, and M. Husain, "Enantiomorphic normalization of focally lesioned brains," *NeuroImage*, vol. 39, no. 3, pp. 1215–1226, 2008.

[58] M. Catani, D. K. Jones, and D. H. Ffytche, "Perisylvian language networks of the human brain," *Annals of Neurology*, vol. 57, no. 1, pp. 8–16, 2005.

[59] M. Goldrick and B. Rapp, "A restricted interaction account (RIA) of spoken word production: the best of both worlds," *Aphasiology*, vol. 16, no. 1-2, pp. 20–55, 2002.

[60] W. J. M. Levelt, "Spoken word production: a theory of lexical access," *Proceedings of the National Academy of Sciences*, vol. 98, no. 23, pp. 13464–13471, 2001.

[61] K. Marcotte, D. Adrover-Roig, B. Damien et al., "Therapy-induced neuroplasticity in chronic aphasia," *Neuropsychologia*, vol. 50, no. 8, pp. 1776–1786, 2012.

[62] G. Hickok and D. Poeppel, "Dorsal and ventral streams: a framework for understanding aspects of the functional anatomy of language," *Cognition*, vol. 92, no. 1-2, pp. 67–99, 2004.

[63] K. Herholz, A. Thiel, K. Wienhard et al., "Individual functional anatomy of verb generation," *NeuroImage*, vol. 3, no. 3, pp. 185–194, 1996.

[64] S. Abrahams, L. H. Goldstein, A. Simmons et al., "Functional magnetic resonance imaging of verbal fluency and confrontation naming using compressed image acquisition to permit overt responses," *Human Brain Mapping*, vol. 20, no. 1, pp. 29–40, 2003.

[65] G. Rizzolatti, L. Fadiga, M. Matelli et al., "Localization of grasp representations in humans by PET: 1. Observation versus execution," *Experimental Brain Research*, vol. 111, no. 2, pp. 246–252, 1996.

[66] H. J. De Smet, P. Paquier, J. Verhoeven, and P. Mariën, "The cerebellum: its role in language and related cognitive and affective functions," *Brain and Language*, vol. 127, no. 3, pp. 334–342, 2013.

[67] P. Mariën, H. Ackermann, M. Adamaszek et al., "Consensus paper: language and the cerebellum: an ongoing enigma," *The Cerebellum*, vol. 13, no. 3, pp. 386–410, 2014.

[68] M. Frings, A. Dimitrova, C. F. Schorn et al., "Cerebellar involvement in verb generation: an fMRI study," *Neuroscience Letters*, vol. 409, no. 1, pp. 19–23, 2006.

[69] M. Bassolino, M. Campanella, M. Bove, T. Pozzo, and L. Fadiga, "Training the motor cortex by observing the actions of others during immobilization," *Cerebral Cortex*, vol. 24, no. 12, pp. 3268–3276, 2014.

[70] M. Bassolino, G. Sandini, and T. Pozzo, "Activating the motor system through action observation: is this an efficient approach in adults and children?," *Developmental Medicine and Child Neurology*, vol. 57, pp. 42–45, 2015.

[71] A. Bisio, L. Avanzino, N. Gueugneau, T. Pozzo, P. Ruggeri, and M. Bove, "Observing and perceiving: a combined approach to induce plasticity in human motor cortex," *Clinical Neurophysiology*, vol. 126, no. 6, pp. 1212–1220, 2015.

[72] R. Gentili, C. Papaxanthis, and T. Pozzo, "Improvement and generalization of arm motor performance through motor imagery practice," *Neuroscience*, vol. 137, no. 3, pp. 761–772, 2006.

[73] M. Meinzer, P. M. Beeson, S. Cappa et al., "Neuroimaging in aphasia treatment research: consensus and practical guidelines for data analysis," *NeuroImage*, vol. 73, pp. 215–224, 2013.

[74] M. Meinzer and C. Breitenstein, "Functional imaging studies of treatment-induced recovery in chronic aphasia," *Aphasiology*, vol. 22, no. 12, pp. 1251–1268, 2008.

[75] D. Saur, R. Lange, A. Baumgaertner et al., "Dynamics of language reorganization after stroke," *Brain*, vol. 129, no. 6, pp. 1371–1384, 2006.

Electroacupuncture Improves Baroreflex and γ-Aminobutyric Acid Type B Receptor-Mediated Responses in the Nucleus Tractus Solitarii of Hypertensive Rats

Qi Zhang ⓘ,[1] Ying-Ying Tan,[1] Xiao-hua Liu,[1] Fan-Rong Yao,[2] and Dong-Yuan Cao ⓘ[3]

[1]*Shaanxi Key Laboratory of Chinese Medicine Encephalopathy, Shaanxi University of Chinese Medicine, Xianyang, Shaanxi 712046, China*

[2]*Department of Pharmacology & Toxicology, Brody School of Medicine, East Carolina University, Greenville, NC 27834, USA*

[3]*Key Laboratory of Shaanxi Province for Craniofacial Precision Medicine Research, Research Center of Stomatology, Xi'an Jiaotong University College of Stomatology, Xi'an, Shaanxi 710004, China*

Correspondence should be addressed to Qi Zhang; zhangqi@sntcm.edu.cn

Academic Editor: J. Michael Wyss

Electroacupuncture (EA) has been reported to benefit hypertension, but the underlying mechanisms are still unclear. We hypothesized that EA attenuates hypertension, in part, through modulation of γ-aminobutyric acid (GABA) receptor function in the nucleus tractus solitarii (NTS). In the present study, the long-term effect of EA on GABA receptor function and expression was examined in the NTS of two-kidney, one-clip (2K1C) renovascular hypertensive rats. EA (0.1–0.4 mA, 2 and 15 Hz) was applied at Zusanli (ST36) acupoints overlying the deep fibular nerve for 30 min once a day for two weeks. The results showed that long-term EA treatment improved blood pressure (BP) and markedly restored the baroreflex response in 2K1C hypertensive rats. The increased pressor and depressor responses to microinjection of $GABA_B$ receptor agonist and antagonist into the NTS in the hypertensive rats were blunted by the EA treatment. Moreover, EA treatment attenuated the increased $GABA_B$ receptor expression in the NTS of hypertensive rats. In contrast, EA had no significant effect on the $GABA_A$ receptor function and expression in the NTS of 2K1C hypertensive rats. These findings suggest that the beneficial effects of EA on renovascular hypertension may be through modulation of functional $GABA_B$ receptors in the NTS.

1. Introduction

Acupuncture has been used for centuries in treatment of various disorders, including cardiovascular disease (for review, see [1, 2]). Electroacupuncture (EA) is a more effective way of administering acupuncture, which applies a pulsating electrical current to acupuncture needles for acupoint stimulation. Clinical and experimental studies indicate that low-frequency EA at Zusanli (ST36) acupoint may have therapeutic and modulatory effects on some types of hypertension [1, 3–5]. It has been demonstrated that the nervous system, neurotransmitters, and endogenous substances are

involved in EA treatment [6–8]. However, the underlying mechanisms for beneficial antihypertensive responses of EA are unclear.

It is well known that elevated sympathetic outflow and impaired baroreflex function contribute to the development of hypertension [9]. The evidence suggests that EA could lower sympathetic activity and significantly inhibit the sympathoexcitatory reflex responses in rats [10–12]. It has also been reported that sensory stimulation of the hindlimb somatic afferent modifies neuronal activity of the nucleus tractus solitarii (NTS) [13]. The NTS is the main integration center for regulating autonomic reflex and sympathetic outflow [14]. Thus, neuronal activity in the NTS is one of the important targets of EA for modulating sympathoexcitatory reflex function.

Within the NTS, GABAergic inhibition plays an important role in baroreflex signal processing. There is considerable evidence suggesting increased GABAergic inhibition in the NTS contributes to the development of hypertension [14–16]. Moreover, the NTS contains a high density of both $GABA_B$ and $GABA_A$ receptors [17]. $GABA_B$ receptors are metabotropic G protein-coupled receptors that mediate presynaptic and postsynaptic inhibitions by reductions in calcium conductance or increases in potassium conductance. Our previous studies and others showed that hypertensive rats exhibit enhanced $GABA_B$ receptor function and regulation within the NTS [18–21]. Thus, manipulations resulting in changes in $GABA_B$ receptor function in the NTS may have a greater effect on blood pressure (BP) regulation in hypertension. However, whether alterations in $GABA_B$ function contribute to the antihypertensive effect of EA is unknown.

In the present study, we tested the hypothesis that EA reduced BP and improved baroreflex response in renovascular hypertensive rats, as well as the beneficial antihypertensive effect of EA was associated with modulation of functional $GABA_B$ receptors within the NTS of hypertensive rats.

2. Methods

2.1. Animals. Adult male Sprague-Dawley rats, weighing 200–210 g, were used in this study. All animals were provided by the Laboratory Animal Center of Xi'an Jiaotong University and housed under controlled conditions with a 12 : 12-h light-dark cycle. Food and water were available to the animals ad libitum. All protocols were approved by the Institutional Animal Care and Use Committee of Shaanxi University of Chinese Medicine.

2.2. Blood Pressure Measurement. Conscious BP recording was carried out with a radiotelemetry system, as described previously [21]. Ten days before making a two-kidney, one-clip (2K1C) model or sham operation, the rats were anesthetized with isoflurane (3%), which was delivered through a nose cone. A telemetry BP probe (model TA11PA-C40, Data Sciences International, St. Paul, MN, USA) was positioned intra-abdominally and secured to the ventral abdominal muscle with the catheter inserted into the lower abdominal aorta. The telemetry signals received by the device were processed and digitized as radiofrequency data, which were recorded and stored in a computer using the Dataquest IV system (Data Sciences International, St. Paul, MN, USA), and the mean values of BP and heart rate (HR) were calculated in a conscious state. Continuous recordings were started 4 days after the probe implantation.

For the microinjection studies, acute BP recording was performed using PE50 catheters under isoflurane (3%) anesthesia. PE50 catheters filled with heparinized saline (100 IU/mL) were placed in the right femoral artery and connected to a BP transducer and a bridge amplifier (AD Instrument,

Bella Vista, Australia). The BP and HR data were collected and analyzed with PowerLab software (AD Instrument, Bella Vista, Australia).

2.3. Experimental Group. Male rats were randomly divided into four groups after one week of adaptation: the sham group, 2K1C hypertensive group, 2K1C plus EA treatment group (2K1C + EA), and 2K1C plus sham EA treatment group (2K1C + SEA). The 2K1C hypertensive model was established as previously described [22]. Briefly, after basal BP recording for a 3-day control period using radiotelemetry, the rats were anesthetized with pentobarbital (i.p., 40 mg/kg). The left kidney was accessed through a left lateral incision and partly obstructed with a silver clip with an internal diameter of 0.20 mm. Sham-operated rats were performed the same surgical procedures without clip placement.

2.4. EA Application. Fourteen days after 2K1C or sham surgery, the EA application was performed as previously described [5, 11]. Rats were adapted and handled gently for 30 min each day, for 3 days before the beginning of the experiment. BP was recorded using radiotelemetry each day before EA treatment. Stainless steel needles (0.16 mm diameter) were inserted bilaterally in the ST36 acupoint, which was located in the anterolateral portion of the hindlimb, in the middle of the cranial tibial muscle, 5 mm below the capitulum fibulae, 7 mm deep from the skin surface, and is innervated by the deep fibular nerve [23]. As the sham EA control group, a nonacupuncture point located at the junction between the tail and buttock was applied stimulation by the needle just inserting into the epidermis of the skin. The electrical stimulation was performed using Hans-200A electrostimulator (Beijing Sheng Da Medical Instrument Center, Beijing, China) at alternate frequencies (2 Hz and 15 Hz), with 0.5 ms in duration and certain intensity (≤4 mA) which elicited slight muscle contraction or movement of the paw. Either EA or SEA stimulation was applied for 30 min once a day for 2 weeks. In the sham control group and 2K1C group, rats were stayed for a 30-minute period with needle insertion but without electrical stimulation of ST36 acupoints. All procedures were performed by the same researcher.

2.5. Baroreflex Responses. At the end of the EA treatment, rats were anesthetized with inhalation of isoflurane (3%). PE50 catheters filled with heparinized saline (100 IU/mL) were placed in the right femoral artery for BP monitoring, and the ipsilateral femoral vein was inserted with the PE10 venous cannula for intravenous administration. Following the baseline BP and HR recordings, baroreflex sensitivity was evaluated by administration of phenylephrine ($5 \mu g \, kg^{-1}$, i.v.) and sodium nitroprusside ($30 \mu g \, kg^{-1}$, i.v.) by intravenous bolus injections to induce either an increase or decrease in BP, respectively, and subsequent bradycardic or tachycardic responses. A 10 min interval between injections was necessary for blood pressure to return to baseline. The one second mean HR values in response to 10 mmHg incremental changes in MAP (from 5 mmHg to 35 mmHg) were analyzed. The values were plotted; the differences between groups were calculated as described previously [24].

Spontaneous baroreflex sensitivity was assessed by the sequence method using the radiotelemetry data as previously described [25–27]. Analysis was performed with HemoLab Software Ver. 20.5. Baroreflex sequence was identified as the correlation coefficient (r) between systolic blood pressure and pulse interval values greater than or equal to 0.8. Baroreflex sensitivity was calculated from the slope of the linear regression lines between systolic blood pressure and the pulse interval of each baroreflex sequence, and the up sequence gain (in ms/mmHg), down sequence gain (in ms/mmHg), and overall baroreflex gain (in ms/mmHg) were determined.

2.6. Measurement of Urinary Norepinephrine Excretion. Urinary norepinephrine (NE) content was measured at 12 days after EA treatment. Urinary samples were collected after rats were placed in metabolism cages for 24 h, and NE enzyme immunoassay kit (Labor Diagnostika Nord KG, Nordhorn, Germany) was used to detect NE content in 24 h urinary excretion, as described previously. The sensitivity of this kit is 1.5 pg/sample.

2.7. Microinjection Experiments. At the end of the 14-day EA treatment, the BP and HR data were collected and analyzed with PowerLab software (AD Instrument, Bella Vista, Australia). GABA$_B$ receptor agonist or antagonist was microinjected bilaterally into the NTS according to the procedures described previously [21]. In brief, the anesthetized animal was placed in a stereotaxic frame. After surgical exposure of the dorsal medulla oblongata, a multiple-barrel glass injection pipette (tip size 20–40 μm) was positioned in the NTS. The coordinates for the NTS were determined from the Paxinos and Watson rat atlas, which is 0.5 mm rostral to the caudal tip of the area postrema, 0.5 mm lateral to the midline, and 0.5 mm below the dorsal surface. Proper placement was confirmed by checking for an L-glutamate-induced (300 pmol, in 50 nL) depressor response, which induced a characteristically abrupt decrease in BP (ΔBP > 35 mmHg) and HR (ΔHR > 30 beats/min) if the needle tip was located precisely in the NTS. After a responsive site was identified by L-glutamate, the probe remained in this site throughout the remainder of the experiment. The volume of microinjection was determined by the displacement of fluid meniscus in the micropipette barrel under a microscope. The GABA$_B$ receptor antagonist (CGP-35348, 100 pmol in 50 nL, Sigma-Aldrich), GABA$_B$ receptor agonist (baclofen, 50 pmol in 50 nL, Sigma-Aldrich), GABA$_A$ receptor antagonist (bicuculline, 10 pmol in 50 nL, Sigma-Aldrich), or GABA$_A$ receptor agonist (muscimol, 100 pmol in 50 nL, Sigma-Aldrich) was dissolved in saline and microinjected bilaterally into the NTS. Each dose for microinjection study was determined by preliminary experiments and our previous studies [18, 21]. The duration of each injection was 15 s. For bilateral microinjections of a given drug, the time interval between the two microinjections was <1 min. Rat body temperature was maintained in the range of 36.5–37.5°C with a heating pad. After the protocol, injection sites were marked with methylene blue dye (50 nL) and verified histologically.

2.8. Real-Time RT-PCR. The animals were killed with an excessive dose of sodium pentobarbital, and the NTS tissues were obtained using the micropunch technique as described previously [21]. In brief, using a rodent brain slicer (Rui-WoDe Inc., RWD68709), 1 mm thick sections were obtained from the NTS caudal to calamus. The coordinates for the NTS were approximately −13.6 to −14.6 from the bregma, 0.5 mm lateral to the midline, and 0.5 mm below the dorsal surface of the brain stem. The NTS samples were identified and collected bilaterally from the section under a microscope by a punch made of 20-gauge stainless steel tubing. Real-time PCR was used to detect changes in the GABA$_B$ and GABA$_A$ receptor mRNA as detailed by us previously [18]. The total RNA was isolated from NTS tissue lysates using an RNeasy kit (Qiagen, Valencia, CA, USA) according to the manufacturer's instructions. TaqMan PCR probes for rat GABA$_B$ (Rn00578911_m1), GABA$_A$ (Rn01464079_m1), and 18 S rRNA (Rn03928990_g1) were obtained from Thermo Fisher Scientific (Carlsbad, CA, USA). Amplification was performed in an Applied Biosystems PRISM 7000 sequence detection system. A comparative cycle of threshold (CT) fluorescence method was applied with 18 S rRNA as the internal control. The final data of real-time PCR were presented as the ratio of the mRNA of interest to 18 S rRNA.

2.9. Western Blotting. The procedures were as described previously [21]. NTS samples were homogenized in an ice-cold lysing buffer containing 20 mM Tris·HCl (pH 6.8), 150 mM NaCl, 10% glycerol, 1% NP-40, and 8 μL/mL inhibitor cocktail (125 mM PMSF, 2.5 mg/mL aprotinin, 2.5 mg/mL leupeptin, 2.5 mg/mL antipain, and 2.5 mg/mL chymostatin). The homogenate was centrifuged, and the supernatant was collected. The protein concentration was measured using a protein assay kit (Bio-Rad Laboratories, Hercules, CA, USA). The samples were boiled for 5 minutes, followed by loading on the SDS-PAGE gel (10 μg of protein, 20 μL per well) for electrophoresis using a Bio-Rad minigel apparatus at 100 V for 60 minutes. The fractionized protein on the gel was electrophoretically transferred onto the nitrocellulose membranes at 350 mA for 90 minutes. After blocking for 1 hour with 5% milk in Tris-buffered saline at room temperature, the membrane was probed with primary antibody (GABA$_B$ rabbit polyclonal antibody, #AB5850, Chemicon, 1:1000; or GABA$_A$ receptor rabbit polyclonal antibody, #AB5954, Chemicon, 1:500) and secondary antibody (goat anti-rabbit IgG horseradish peroxidase, Bio-Rad, 1:3000). Then the membrane was treated with enhanced chemiluminescence substrate (ECL Western blotting detection kit, Amersham Pharmacia Biotechnology, Piscataway, NJ, USA) for 5 minutes at room temperature. The specificity of GBR and GAR was tested by preincubation of the antibodies with the blocking peptides for 2 h at room temperature. The subsequent incubation steps were carried out as usual. The bands in the film were visualized and analyzed using Quantity One Software (Bio-Rad).

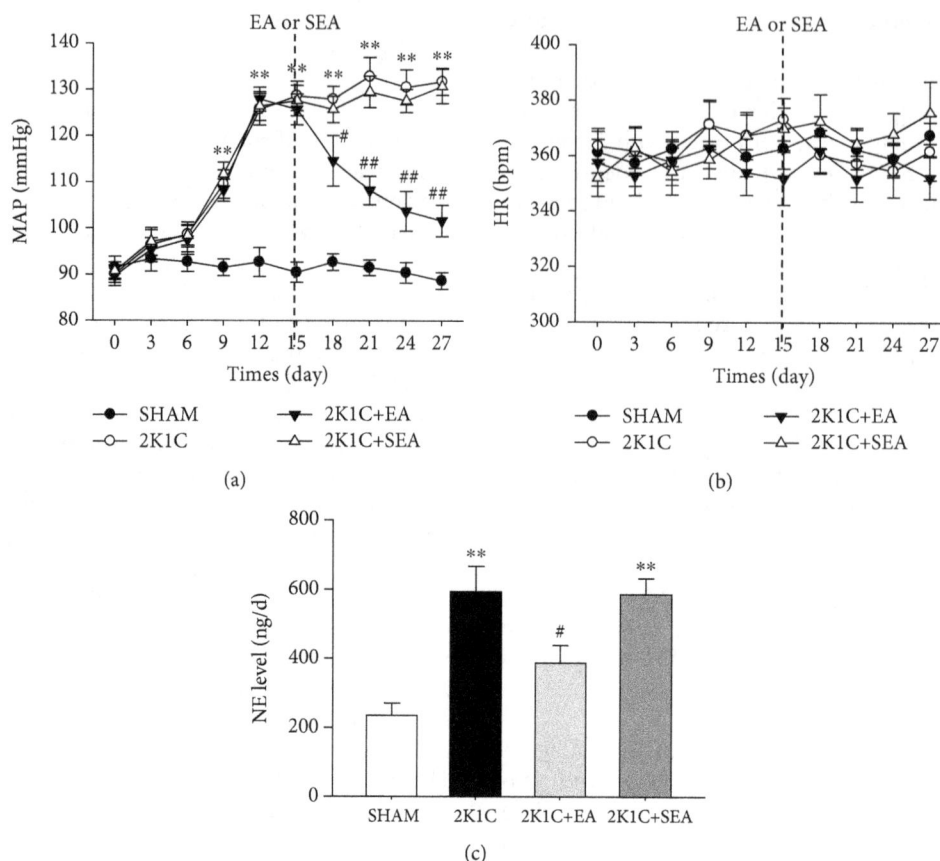

(a)

(b)

(c)

FIGURE 1: Long-term EA treatment attenuates hypertension in 2K1C hypertensive rats. (a) Time course of mean arterial pressure (MAP) in each group over 27 days. (b) Time course of heart rate (HR) in each group over 27 days. MAP and HR were measured by radiotelemetry. (c) The change in the urinary norepinephrine excretion at day 27 after the 2K1C hypertensive model was established. Data are presented as mean $\pm$ SE; $n = 7 - 9$ rats; $^{*}P < 0.05$, $^{**}P < 0.01$ vs. the sham group; $^{\#}P < 0.05$, $^{\#\#}P < 0.01$ vs. 2K1C group.

2.10. Statistical Analyses. All data are expressed as means $\pm$ SE. Comparisons between experimental groups were performed with ANOVA followed by a Newman-Keuls test. Differences were considered significant at $P < 0.05$.

3. Results

3.1. Effect of EA Treatment on the Development of 2K1C Hypertension and Baroreflex Response. Mean arterial BP (MAP) and HR were measured via radiotelemetry. The baseline MAP and HR values were similar between the sham, 2K1C, 2K1C + EA, and 2K1C + SEA groups. As shown in Figure 1(a), the MAP was increased in the 2K1C group compared with that in the sham group. After 14 days of EA treatment, the 2K1C + EA group showed reduced MAP compared with the 2K1C group. However, the 2K1C + SEA group maintained high MAP compared with the sham group. In addition, no significant alterations in HR were observed in all groups (Figure 1(b)).

To determine whether chronic EA treatment altered sympathetic activities, urinary NE excretion was evaluated. As shown in Figure 1(c), urinary NE excretion markedly increased in the 2K1C group at day 27 after the 2K1C hypertensive model was established, and EA

treatment significantly lowered the NE excretion in the 2K1C + EA group.

The 2K1C group presented a reduction in baroreflex gain after administration of phenylephrine and sodium nitroprusside compared with the sham group, and the 2K1C + EA group exhibited the restored baroreflex sensitivity compared with the 2K1C group. However, the 2K1C + SEA group maintained the depressed baroreflex sensitivity compared with the sham group (Figures 2(a) and 2(b)). The assessment of baroreflex gain by means of the sequence method (total gain, up sequence gain, and down sequence gain) also revealed an improvement in baroreflex function in the 2K1C + EA group compared to the 2K1C group (Figures 2(c)–2(e)).

3.2. Effect of EA Treatment on GABA$_B$ Receptor-Mediated Responses in NTS. To investigate the effect of EA treatment on GABA$_B$ receptor function in the NTS, GABA$_B$ receptor antagonist CGP-35348 or GABA$_B$ receptor agonist baclofen was microinjected into the NTS of rats. As shown in Figure 3, the microinjection sites in the NTS were identified. Bilateral microinjection of CGP-35348 (100 pmol, 50 nL) into the NTS decreased MAP and HR in varying degrees in different groups (Figure 4(a)). The response to CGP-35348 microinjected into the NTS was greater in the 2K1C group

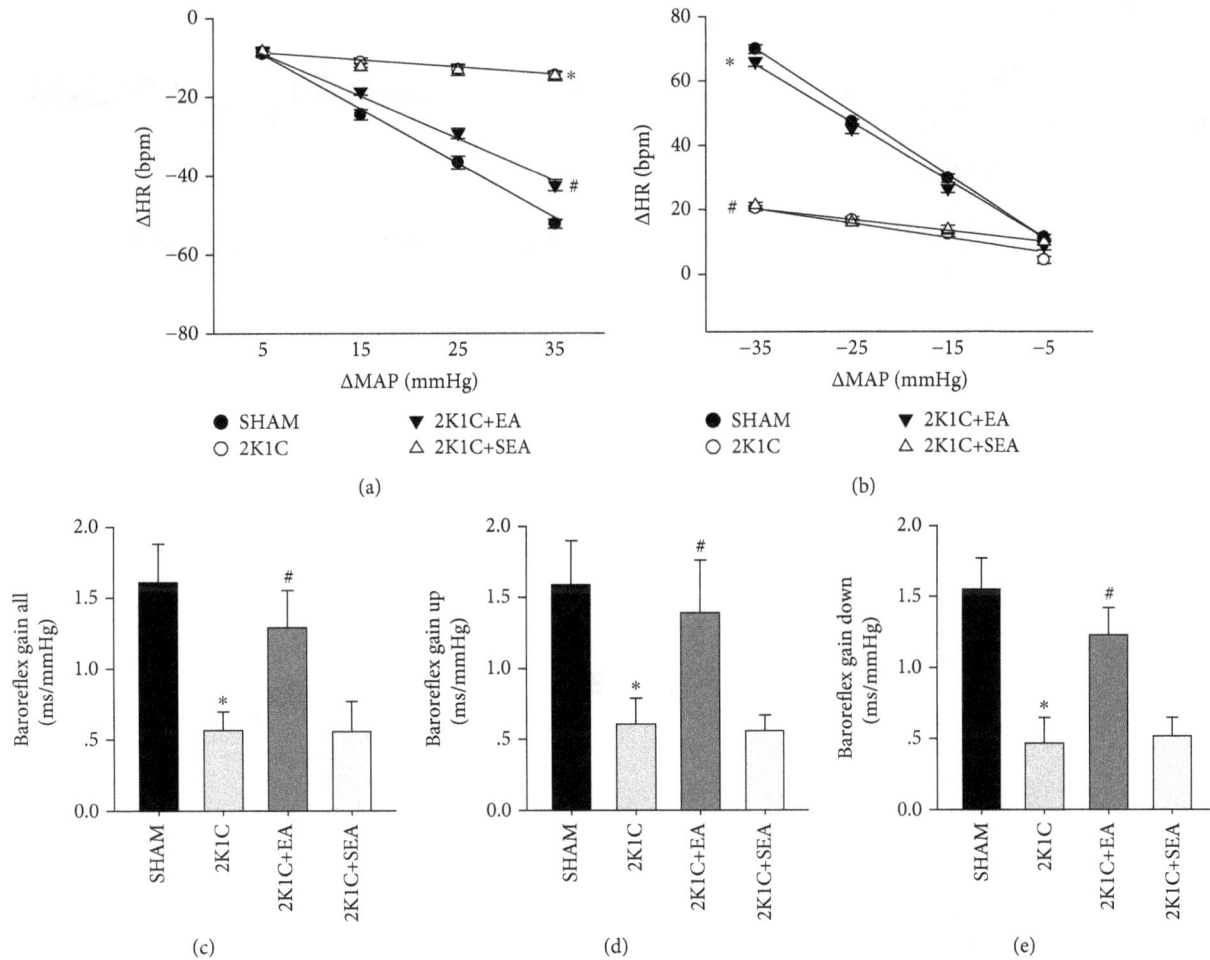

FIGURE 2: Long-term EA treatment restores the baroreflex response in 2K1C hypertensive rats. (a) Grouped heart rate (HR) baroreflex response to each 10 mmHg change in mean arterial pressure (MAP) elicited by phenylephrine. (b) Grouped heart rate (HR) baroreflex response to each 10 mmHg change in mean arterial pressure (MAP) evoked by sodium nitroprusside. (c–e) Spontaneous baroreflex analysis with overall baroreflex gain (combination of up and down sequences), up sequence gain, and down sequence gain (in ms/mmHg). Data are presented as mean ± SE; $n = 7 - 9$ rats; $^*P < 0.05$ vs. the sham group; $^\#P < 0.05$ vs. the 2K1C group.

when compared with that in the sham group. Treatment with EA for 14 days normalized the response to CGP-35348 in 2K1C hypertensive rats (Figure 4(b)). No differences in MAP change were found between the 2K1C + SEA group and the 2K1C group. Changes in HR after microinjection of CGP-35348 into the NTS followed the same pattern as MAP (Figure 4(c)).

As shown in Figures 5(a) and 5(b), microinjection of baclofen into the NTS induced an elevation in BP in varying degrees in different groups. The amplitudes of MAP change induced by baclofen in the 2K1C group were significantly greater than those in the sham group. In contrast, treatment with EA for 14 days significantly reduced the MAP change in the 2K1C + SEA group when compared with the 2K1C group. Changes in HR after microinjection of baclofen into NTS followed the same pattern as MAP (Figure 5(c)).

3.3. Effect of EA Treatment on GABA_A Receptor-Mediated Responses in NTS.

3.3. Effect of EA Treatment on $GABA_A$ Receptor-Mediated Responses in NTS. To investigate the effect of EA treatment on $GABA_A$ receptor function in the NTS, the bicuculline or muscimol was microinjected into the NTS of rats.

Microinjection of bicuculline (10 pmol in 50 nL) into the NTS decreased MAP and HR in all investigated groups. As shown in Figures 6(a) and 6(b), there were no significant differences in peak MAP and HR changes after bicuculline microinjection among the sham, 2K1C, 2K1C + EA, and 2K1C + SEA groups. In addition, microinjection of muscimol (100 pmol in 50 nL) into the NTS significantly increased MAP and HR in rats of all four groups. As shown in Figures 6(c) and 6(d), similar to bicuculline response, the peak MAP and HR changes after muscimol microinjection exhibited no significant differences among the sham, 2K1C, 2K1C + EA, and 2K1C + SEA groups.

3.4. Effect of EA Treatment on $GABA_B$ and $GABA_A$ Receptor Expressions in NTS. $GABA_B$ and $GABA_A$ receptor mRNA levels in the NTS were detected with real-time RT-PCR. The results shown in Figure 7(a) demonstrate that $GABA_B$ receptor mRNA levels in the NTS increased in the 2K1C group, and EA attenuated this change. There were no differences in the levels of $GABA_A$ receptor mRNA among groups. In addition, $GABA_B$ and $GABA_A$ receptor protein levels were

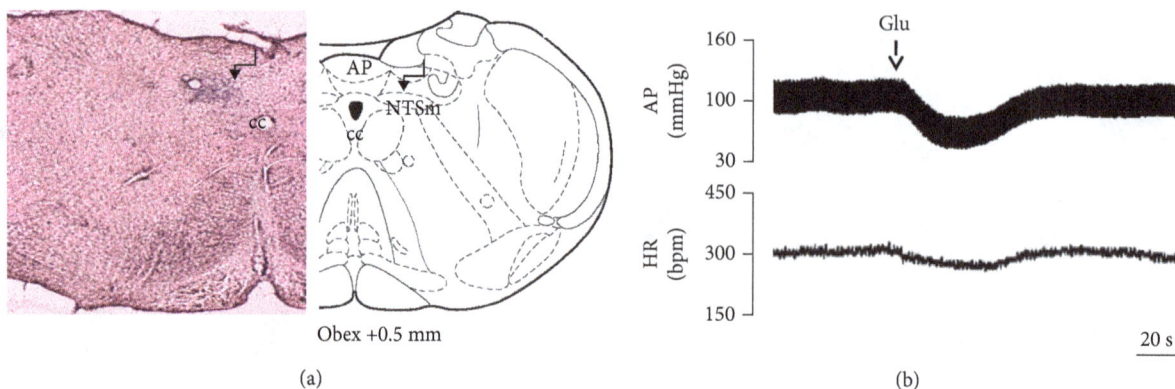

(a)   (b)

FIGURE 3: Identification of the microinjection sites in the nucleus tractus solitarii (NTS). (a) A representative photomicrograph showing the NTS microinjection site and the location of this microinjection site based on the rat brain atlas. The arrow indicates the injection site. (b) Functional identification of the NTS with microinjections of glutamate (Glu; 300 pmol in 50 nL) in one rat. Unilateral glutamate produced decreases in arterial pressure (AP) and HR.

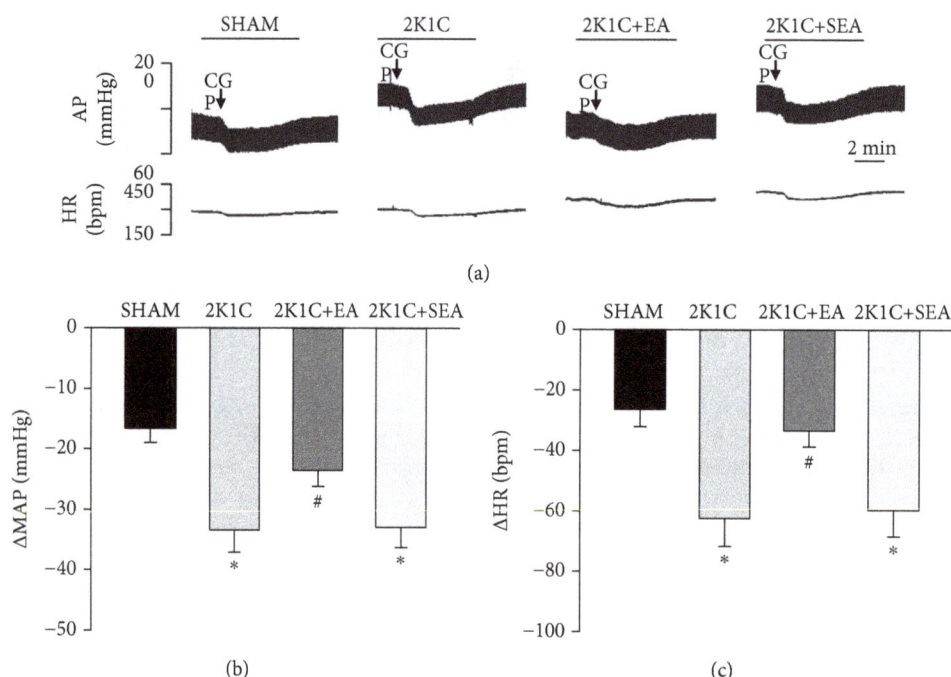

(a)

(b)   (c)

FIGURE 4: Effect of the GABA$_B$ receptor antagonist, CGP-35348, microinjected into the NTS on MAP and HR in the sham, 2K1C, 2K1C + EA, and 2K1C + SEA groups. (a) Representative original tracings showing AP and HR changes evoked by microinjection of CGP-35348 (100 pmol in 50 nL) into the NTS in the sham, 2K1C, 2K1C + EA, and 2K1C + SEA groups. The horizontal bar represents recording duration of 2 min. Arrows indicates the injection of CGP-35348 (CGP). The peak alteration (Δ) of MAP (b) and peak alteration (Δ) of HR (c) after microinjection of CGP-35348 (100 pmol in 50 nL) into the NTS of the sham, 2K1C, 2K1C + EA, and 2K1C + SEA groups. Values are means $\pm$ SE ($n = 7 - 8$ in each group). *$P < 0.05$ vs. sham group; #$P < 0.05$ vs. 2K1C group.

determined by Western blot analysis in the micropunched NTS in rats. Data in Figure 7(c) demonstrate that the 2K1C group presented a twofold increase in GABA$_B$ expression levels compared with the sham group, and EA treatment significantly reduced GABA$_B$ expression in the 2K1C + EA group when compared to the 2K1C group. In contrast, the expression of GABA$_A$ receptor was comparable between the sham, 2K1C, 2K1C + EA, and 2K1C + SEA groups (Figures 7(b) and 7(d)).

4. Discussion

The main findings of our present study demonstrated that (1) long-term EA treatment at ST36 lowers the increased blood pressure and improves the depressed baroreflex response in 2K1C hypertensive rats, (2) the enhanced responses to a GABA$_B$ receptor antagonist or an agonist microinjected into the NTS of hypertensive rats were significantly reversed by long-term EA treatment at ST36, and (3) EA treatment

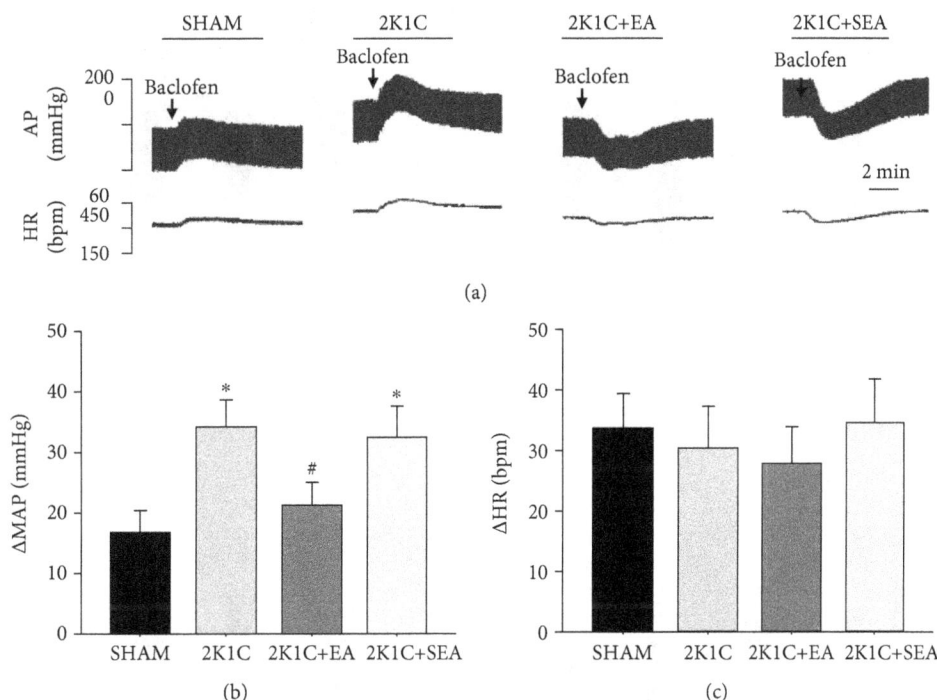

FIGURE 5: Effect of the GABA$_B$ receptor agonist baclofen on MAP and HR in the sham, 2K1C, 2K1C + EA, and 2K1C + SEA groups. (a) Representative original tracings showing AP and HR changes evoked by microinjection of baclofen (50 pmol in 50 nL) into the NTS in the sham, 2K1C, 2K1C + EA, and 2K1C + SEA groups. The peak alteration (Δ) of MAP (b) and peak alteration (Δ) of HR (c) after microinjection of baclofen (50 pmol in 50 nL) into the NTS. Values are means ± SE ($n = 7 - 8$ in each group). *$P < 0.05$ vs. sham group; #$P < 0.05$ vs. 2K1C group.

reduced the increased GABA$_B$ receptor expression in the NTS of the hypertensive rat. These results suggest that the BP-lowering action of EA treatment is related to the modulation of functional GABA$_B$ receptor expression and inhibitory GABAergic neurotransmission in the NTS.

Both clinical and animal studies indicate that acupuncture at certain acupoints is capable of reducing arterial BP and ameliorating end-organ damage in hypertension and has been recommended as an effective nonpharmacological treatment [1, 2]. It has been demonstrated that EA at the ST36 acupoint is most effective in treating cardiovascular diseases. For example, stimulation of the ST36 acupoint overlying the deep peroneal nerves inhibits sympathoexcitatory reflex responses induced by gastric distension and gall bladder stimulation [12, 28, 29]. Therefore, the ST36 point was chosen in the present study to investigate the long-term effect of EA on 2K1C hypertensive rats, and we demonstrated that two-week acupuncture significantly decreased high BP in 2K1C rats.

The baroreflex is one of the most powerful and rapidly acting mechanisms for controlling arterial BP. It has been suggested that arterial baroreflex is involved in the long-term control of BP [30]. Several studies have shown that the sensitivity of the baroreflex is diminished in several forms of hypertension [22, 31, 32]. In addition, patients with baroreflex failure suffer from a volatile hypertension with sympathetic nerve activity increased for years [33]. The results from the present study supported the insights

that 2K1C hypertensive rats exhibit the reduced baroreflex sensitivity and that treatment with EA at the ST36 point could restore this sensitivity. Similar results have been reported for aortic-denervated rabbits and heart failure rats [10, 34, 35], supporting the notion that EA-induced changes in baroreceptor activity may be involved in blunted sympathoexcitation responses.

The NTS is the primary termination site for a variety of cardiovascular afferents. Incremental evidence indicates that the NTS is involved in mediating the central interaction between baroreceptor and somatosensory receptor inputs [13, 14, 36, 37]. This information is integrated and via projections to the rostral and caudal ventrolateral medulla or to the ambiguous nucleus, and then the reflex control of autonomic nerve activity occurs. It has been demonstrated that sensory stimulation of the hindlimb somatic afferent modifies neuronal activities in the NTS [13], and resection of the deep peroneal nerve eliminates the therapeutic effect of EA on the ST36 acupoint [29, 35, 38]. However, the precise route by which sensory signals elicited from acupuncture transits the NTS to activate outgoing regulation signals needs further investigation. GABA appears to be the primary inhibitory neurotransmitter in the NTS, and enhancement of GABAergic neurotransmission in the NTS tends to increase sympathetic outflow and has been implicated in various forms of experimental hypertension [15, 16]. In the present study, we confirmed that 2K1C rats had enhanced responses of GABA$_B$ receptors in the

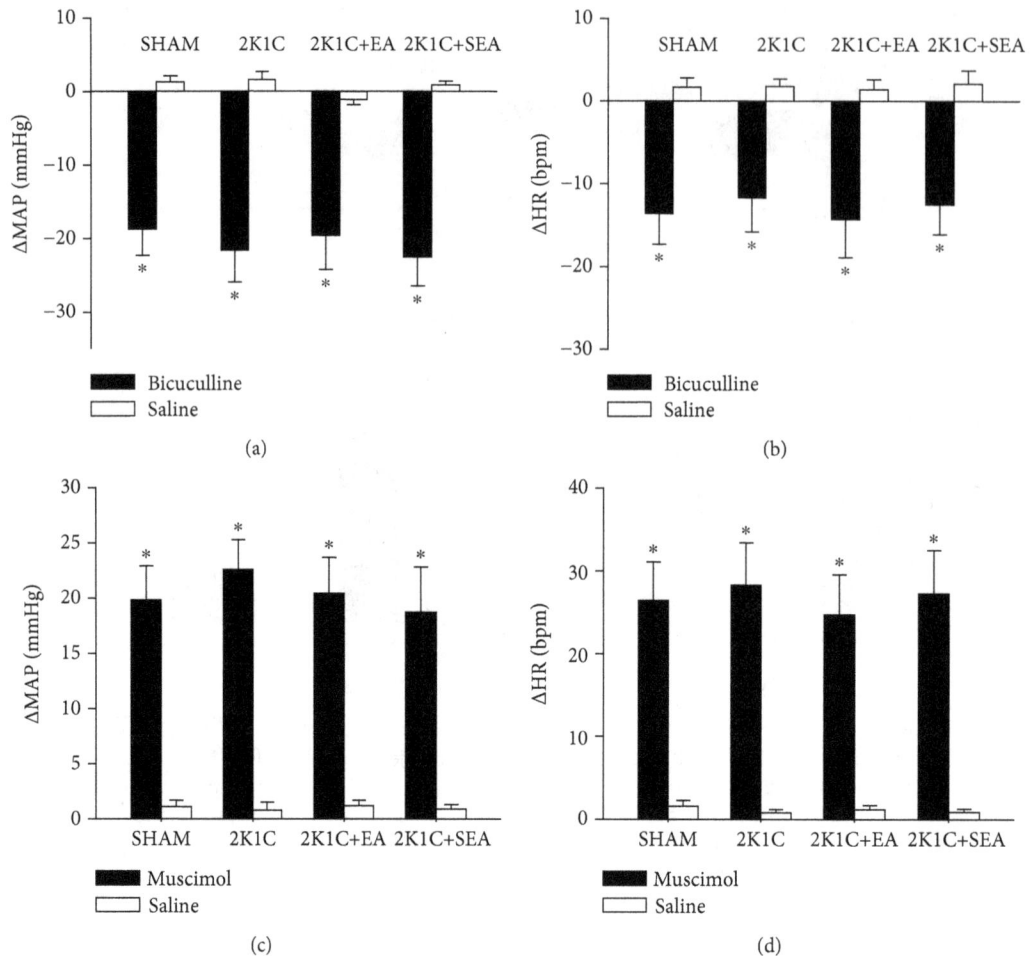

FIGURE 6: Effect of the GABA$_A$ receptor antagonist bicuculline and agonist muscimol on MAP and HR in the sham, 2K1C, 2K1C + EA, and 2K1C + SEA rats. MAP (a) and HR (b) changes evoked by microinjection of bicuculline (10 pmol in 50 nL) into the NTS. MAP (c) and HR (d) changes evoked by microinjection of muscimol (100 pmol in 50 nL) into the NTS. Values are means ± SE ($n = 7$ or 5 rats in each group). * $P < 0.05$ vs. saline control in each group.

NTS and that EA significantly decreased the function of GABA$_B$ receptors in the NTS in renovascular hypertensive rats. These results suggest that EA is capable of attenuating the increased GABAergic inhibition in the NTS, leading to restoring baroreflex central gain and sensitivity. However, the detailed mechanisms of EA on GABA$_B$ receptor function in the NTS of renovascular hypertensive rats have not been firmly established.

The GABA$_B$ receptor is a G protein-coupled receptor that mediates slow and prolonged inhibitory neurotransmission in the brain [15]. The pressor response to baclofen microinjected into the NTS is elevated in spontaneously hypertensive rats, deoxycorticosterone acetate salt-induced hypertensive rats, renal wrap hypertensive rats, and angiotensin II infusion-induced hypertensive rats [18–21]. Enhanced expression of the GABA$_B$ receptor in the NTS has also been reported in hypertensive rat models, such as Ang II-induced hypertensive rats and renal wrap hypertensive rats [18, 21, 39]. Consistent with these observations, the present study results indicated that the GABA$_B$ receptor, but not GABA$_A$ expression, was increased in the NTS of 2K1C

hypertensive rats. However, little is known about the cellular mechanisms of enhanced GABA$_B$ receptor expression in the NTS of hypertensive rats. One possibility is that enhanced GABA$_B$ receptor expression in the NTS is caused by high BP, because elevated peripheral arterial pressure may increase the central input signal, leading to altered gene expression in brain cardiovascular regulatory areas. This seems unlikely, however, because we have previously observed that GABA$_B$ receptor expression is unaltered in the NTS of rats made hypertensive by peripheral infusion of N (ω)-nitro-L-arginine methyl ester [21]. A second possibility is that enhanced GABA$_B$ receptor expression in 2K1C rats is caused by angiotensin II, because angiotensin II activity in the NTS is increased in 2K1C rats, and angiotensin II increases GABA$_B$ expression [21, 40, 41]. Therefore, identifying the exact signaling pathways controlling gene regulation that are altered and lead to elevated GABA$_B$ receptor expression in the NTS requires further investigation.

In summary, our data demonstrate that renovascular hypertension alters the function and expression of the

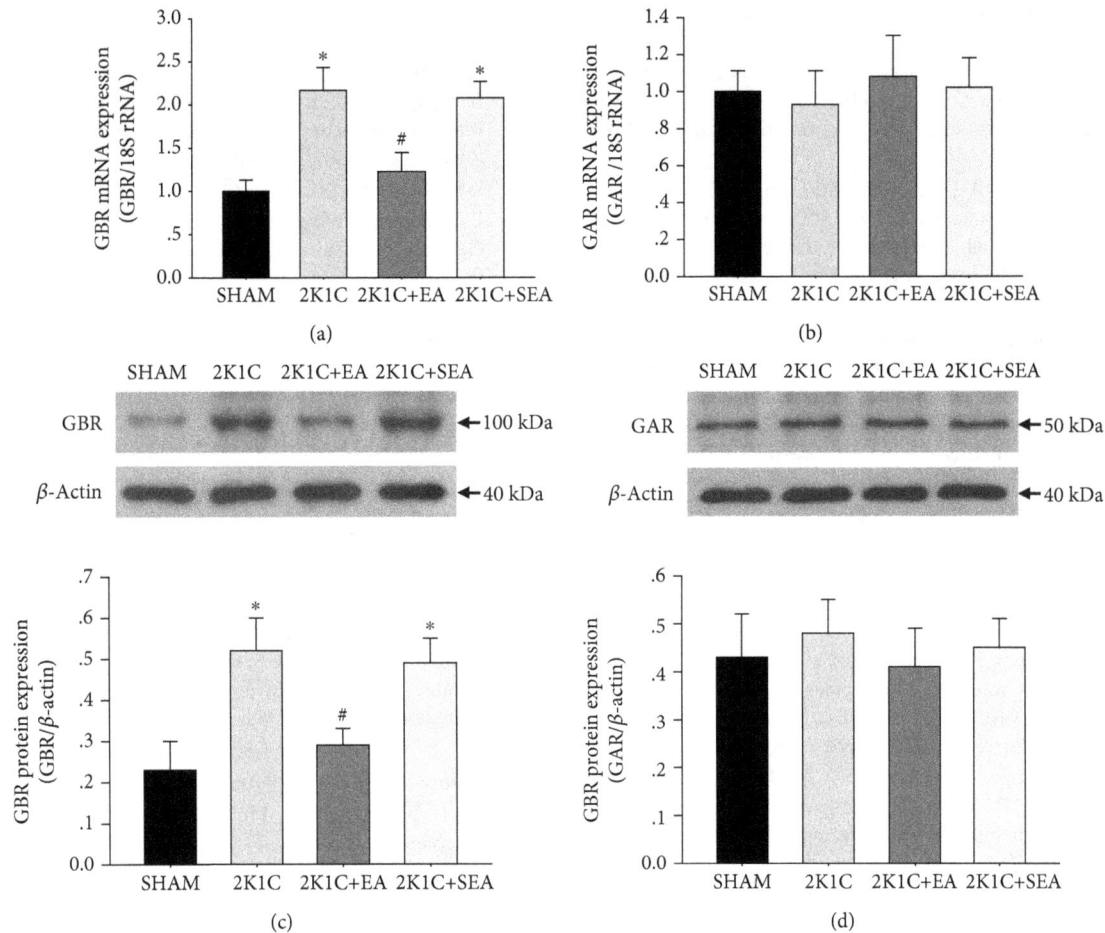

FIGURE 7: Effect of long-term EA treatment on GABA$_B$ and GABA$_A$ receptor expressions in the NTS of rats. (a, b) GABA$_B$ receptor (GBR) and GABA$_A$ receptor (GAR) mRNA levels within the NTS in the sham, 2K1C, 2K1C + EA, and 2K1C + SEA groups which were detected with real-time RT-PCR. Data were normalized with 18 S rRNA. (c, d) Quantitative analysis of GABA$_B$ receptor (GBR) and GABA$_A$ receptor (GAR) protein levels within the NTS in the sham, 2K1C, 2K1C + EA, and 2K1C + SEA groups. The upper panel shows the representative immunoblots of GABA$_B$ receptor (GBR) and GABA$_A$ receptor (GAR) protein levels within the NTS in each group. Values are normalized using β-actin. Values are means ± SE ($n = 6$ in each group). $^{*}P < 0.05$ vs. the sham group; $^{#}P < 0.05$ vs. the 2K1C group.

GABA$_B$ receptor in the NTS and increases GABAergic inhibition in the NTS, which partly leads to an increase in MAP and sympathetic activity. This indicates that EA attenuates hypertension partly through the GABA$_B$ receptor pathway in renovascular hypertensive rats. Our findings provide further evidence and insight into the beneficial effect of EA on renovascular hypertension.

Authors' Contributions

QZ and Y-YT designed the study. QZ and Y-YT performed the experiments and data collection. F-RY and D-YC provided critical technical assistance. QZ, Y-YT, F-RY, and D-YC analyzed the data and wrote the manuscript. All authors approved the manuscript. Qi Zhang and Ying-Ying Tan contributed equally to this work.

Acknowledgments

This work was supported by the National Natural Science Foundation of China (nos. 31171101, 81470543, and 81774295) and partly by the Key Laboratory Project of Educational Commission of Shaanxi Province of China (14JS026).

References

[1] L. Cheng, P. Li, S. C. Tjen-A-Looi, and J. C. Longhurst, "What do we understand from clinical and mechanistic studies on

acupuncture treatment for hypertension?," *Chinese Medicine*, vol. 10, no. 1, p. 36, 2015.

[2] J. C. Longhurst and S. C. Tjen-A-Looi, "Evidence-based blood pressure reducing actions of electroacupuncture: mechanisms and clinical application," *Acta Physiologica Sinica*, vol. 69, no. 5, pp. 587–597, 2017.

[3] M. Li, S. C. Tjen-A-Looi, Z. L. Guo, and J. C. Longhurst, "Repetitive electroacupuncture attenuates cold-induced hypertension through enkephalin in the rostral ventral lateral medulla," *Scientific Reports*, vol. 6, no. 1, p. 35791, 2016.

[4] P. Li, S. C. Tjen-A-Looi, L. Cheng et al., "Long-lasting reduction of blood pressure by electroacupuncture in patients with hypertension: randomized controlled trial," *Medical Acupuncture*, vol. 27, no. 4, pp. 253–266, 2015.

[5] C. R. Zhang, C. M. Xia, M. Y. Jiang et al., "Repeated electroacupuncture attenuating of apelin expression and function in the rostral ventrolateral medulla in stress-induced hypertensive rats," *Brain Research Bulletin*, vol. 97, pp. 53–62, 2013.

[6] S. X. Ma, J. Ma, G. Moise, and X. Y. Li, "Responses of neuronal nitric oxide synthase expression in the brainstem to electroacupuncture Zusanli (ST 36) in rats," *Brain Research*, vol. 1037, no. 1-2, pp. 70–77, 2005.

[7] S. C. Tjen-A-Looi, Z. L. Guo, and J. C. Longhurst, "GABA in nucleus tractus solitarius participates in electroacupuncture modulation of cardiopulmonary bradycardia reflex," *American Journal of Physiology Regulatory, Integrative and Comparative Physiology*, vol. 307, no. 11, pp. R1313–R1323, 2014.

[8] L. Y. Xiao, X. R. Wang, Y. Yang et al., "Applications of acupuncture therapy in modulating plasticity of central nervous system," *Neuromodulation*, 2017.

[9] T. E. Lohmeier and R. Iliescu, "The baroreflex as a long-term controller of arterial pressure," *Physiology*, vol. 30, no. 2, pp. 148–158, 2015.

[10] L. Ma, B. Cui, Y. Shao et al., "Electroacupuncture improves cardiac function and remodeling by inhibition of sympathoexcitation in chronic heart failure rats," *American Journal of Physiology. Heart and Circulatory Physiology*, vol. 306, no. 10, pp. H1464–H1471, 2014.

[11] Y. Y. Tan, Y. Y. Wang, and Q. Zhang, "Electroacupuncture of "Quchi" (LI 11) inhibits the elevation of arterial blood pressure and abnormal sympathetic nerve activity in hypertension rats," *Zhen Ci Yan Jiu*, vol. 41, no. 2, pp. 144–149, 2016.

[12] S. C. Tjen-A-Looi, Z. L. Guo, M. Li, and J. C. Longhurst, "Medullary GABAergic mechanisms contribute to electroacupuncture modulation of cardiovascular depressor responses during gastric distention in rats," *American Journal of Physiology. Regulatory, Integrative and Comparative Physiology*, vol. 304, no. 5, pp. R321–R332, 2013.

[13] G. M. Toney and S. W. Mifflin, "Sensory modalities conveyed in the hindlimb somatic afferent input to nucleus tractus solitarius," *Journal of Applied Physiology*, vol. 88, no. 6, pp. 2062–2073, 2000.

[14] J. T. Potts, "Inhibitory neurotransmission in the nucleus tractus solitarii: implications for baroreflex resetting during exercise," *Experimental Physiology*, vol. 91, no. 1, pp. 59–72, 2006.

[15] W. Zhang and S. Mifflin, "Plasticity of GABAergic mechanisms within the nucleus of the solitary tract in hypertension," *Hypertension*, vol. 55, no. 2, pp. 201–206, 2010.

[16] J. Zubcevic and J. T. Potts, "Role of GABAergic neurones in the nucleus tractus solitarii in modulation of cardiovascular activity," *Experimental Physiology*, vol. 95, no. 9, pp. 909–918, 2010.

[17] R. Luján, R. Shigemoto, and G. López-Bendito, "Glutamate and GABA receptor signalling in the developing brain," *Neuroscience*, vol. 130, no. 3, pp. 567–580, 2005.

[18] B. Li, Q. Liu, C. Xuan et al., "GABA$_B$ receptor gene transfer into the nucleus tractus solitarii induces chronic blood pressure elevation in normotensive rats," *Circulation Journal*, vol. 77, no. 10, pp. 2558–2566, 2013.

[19] E. J. Spary, A. Maqbool, S. Saha, and T. F. Batten, "Increased GABA$_B$ receptor subtype expression in the nucleus of the solitary tract of the spontaneously hypertensive rat," *Journal of Molecular Neuroscience*, vol. 35, no. 2, pp. 211–224, 2008.

[20] M. Vitela and S. W. Mifflin, "γ-Aminobutyric acid$_B$ receptor-mediated responses in the nucleus tractus solitarius are altered in acute and chronic hypertension," *Hypertension*, vol. 37, no. 2, pp. 619–622, 2001.

[21] Q. Zhang, F. Yao, S. T. O'Rourke, S. Y. Qian, and C. Sun, "Angiotensin II enhances GABA (B) receptor-mediated responses and expression in nucleus tractus solitarii of rats," *American Journal of Physiology Heart and Circulatory Physiology*, vol. 297, no. 5, pp. H1837–H1844, 2009.

[22] W. Pijacka, F. D. McBryde, P. J. Marvar, G. S. Lincevicius, A. P. Abdala, L. Woodward et al., "Carotid sinus denervation ameliorates renovascular hypertension in adult Wistar rats," *The Journal of Physiology*, vol. 594, no. 21, pp. 6255–6266, 2016.

[23] Z. R. Li, *Experimental Acupuncture*, China Press of Traditional Chinese Medicine, Beijing, China, 2003.

[24] G. T. Blanch, A. H. Freiria-Oliveira, G. F. Speretta et al., "Increased expression of angiotensin II type 2 receptors in the solitary–vagal complex blunts renovascular hypertension," *Hypertension*, vol. 64, no. 4, pp. 777–783, 2014.

[25] V. A. Braga, M. A. Burmeister, R. V. Sharma, and R. L. Davisson, "Cardiovascular responses to peripheral chemoreflex activation and comparison of different methods to evaluate baroreflex gain in conscious mice using telemetry," *American Journal of Physiology. Regulatory, Integrative and Comparative Physiology*, vol. 295, no. 4, pp. R1168–R1174, 2008.

[26] M. S. Johnson, V. G. DeMarco, C. M. Heesch et al., "Sex differences in baroreflex sensitivity, heart rate variability, and end organ damage in the TGR(mRen2)27 rat," *American Journal of Physiology Heart and Circulatory Physiology*, vol. 301, no. 4, pp. H1540–H1550, 2011.

[27] M. Milic, P. Sun, F. Liu et al., "A comparison of pharmacologic and spontaneous baroreflex methods in aging and hypertension," *Journal of Hypertension*, vol. 27, no. 6, pp. 1243–1251, 2009.

[28] S. C. Tjen-A-Looi, P. Li, and J. C. Longhurst, "Medullary substrate and differential cardiovascular responses during stimulation of specific acupoints," *American Journal of Physiology. Regulatory, Integrative and Comparative Physiology*, vol. 287, no. 4, pp. R852–R862, 2004.

[29] W. Zhou, L. W. Fu, S. C. Tjen-A-Looi, P. Li, and J. C. Longhurst, "Afferent mechanisms underlying stimulation modality-related modulation of acupuncture-related cardiovascular responses," *Journal of Applied Physiology*, vol. 98, no. 3, pp. 872–880, 2005.

[30] V. A. Tsyrlin, M. M. Galagudza, N. V. Kuzmenko, M. G. Pliss, N. S. Rubanova, and Y. I. Shcherbin, "Arterial baroreceptor reflex counteracts long-term blood pressure increase in the rat model of renovascular hypertension," *PLoS One*, vol. 8, no. 6, article e64788, 2013.

[31] H. H. Chen, P. W. Cheng, W. Y. Ho et al., "Renal denervation improves the baroreflex and GABA system in chronic kidney disease-induced hypertension," *Scientific Reports*, vol. 6, no. 1, p. 38447, 2016.

[32] T. N. Thrasher, "Arterial baroreceptor input contributes to long-term control of blood pressure," *Current Hypertension Reports*, vol. 8, no. 3, pp. 249–254, 2006.

[33] K. Heusser, J. Tank, F. C. Luft, and J. Jordan, "Baroreflex failure," *Hypertension*, vol. 45, no. 5, pp. 834–839, 2005.

[34] J. W. Lima, V. S. Hentschke, D. D. Rossato et al., "Chronic electroacupuncture of the ST36 point improves baroreflex function and haemodynamic parameters in heart failure rats," *Autonomic Neuroscience*, vol. 193, pp. 31–37, 2015.

[35] D. Michikami, A. Kamiya, T. Kawada et al., "Short-term electroacupuncture at Zusanli resets the arterial baroreflex neural arc toward lower sympathetic nerve activity," *American Journal of Physiology. Heart and Circulatory Physiology*, vol. 291, no. 1, pp. H318–H326, 2006.

[36] L. C. Michelini and J. E. Stern, "Exercise-induced neuronal plasticity in central autonomic networks: role in cardiovascular control," *Experimental Physiology*, vol. 94, no. 9, pp. 947–960, 2009.

[37] J. F. Paton, J. Deuchars, Z. Ahmad, L. F. Wong, D. Murphy, and S. Kasparov, "Adenoviral vector demonstrates that angiotensin II-induced depression of the cardiac baroreflex is mediated by endothelial nitric oxide synthase in the nucleus tractus solitarii of the rat," *The Journal of Physiology*, vol. 531, no. 2, pp. 445–458, 2001.

[38] J. F. Fang, J. Y. Du, X. M. Shao, J. Q. Fang, and Z. Liu, "Effect of electroacupuncture on the NTS is modulated primarily by acupuncture point selection and stimulation frequency in normal rats," *BMC Complementary and Alternative Medicine*, vol. 17, no. 1, p. 182, 2017.

[39] V. R. Durgam, M. Vitela, and S. W. Mifflin, "Enhanced γ-aminobutyric acid–B receptor agonist responses and mRNA within the nucleus of the solitary tract in hypertension," *Hypertension*, vol. 33, no. 1, pp. 530–536, 1999.

[40] E. B. Oliveira-Sales, M. A. Toward, R. R. Campos, and J. F. Paton, "Revealing the role of the autonomic nervous system in the development and maintenance of Goldblatt hypertension in rats," *Autonomic Neuroscience: Basic & Clinical*, vol. 183, pp. 23–29, 2014.

[41] F. Yao, C. Sumners, S. T. O'Rourke, and C. Sun, "Angiotensin II increases $GABA_B$ receptor expression in nucleus tractus solitarii of rats," *American Journal of Physiology Heart and Circulatory Physiology*, vol. 294, no. 6, pp. H2712–H2720, 2008.

10

N-Methyl-D-Aspartate Receptors Involvement in the Gentamicin-Induced Hearing Loss and Pathological Changes of Ribbon Synapse in the Mouse Cochlear Inner Hair Cells

Juan Hong,[1,2] Yan Chen,[1,3] Yanping Zhang,[1,3] Jieying Li,[1,3] Liujie Ren,[1,3] Lin Yang,[1,3] Lusen Shi,[4] Ao Li,[4] Tianyu Zhang,[1,3] Huawei Li◉,[1,3,5,6] and Peidong Dai◉[1,3]

[1]ENT Institute and Otorhinolaryngology Department of Affiliated Eye and ENT Hospital, State Key Laboratory of Medical Neurobiology, Fudan University, Shanghai 200031, China
[2]Department of Otorhinolaryngology-Head and Neck Surgery, Huashan Hospital, Fudan University, Shanghai 200040, China
[3]NHC Key Laboratory of Hearing Medicine, Fudan University, Shanghai 200031, China
[4]Department of Otolaryngology Head and Neck Surgery, Affiliated Drum Tower Hospital of Nanjing University Medical School, Jiangsu Provincial Key Medical Discipline (Laboratory), Nanjing 210008, China
[5]Institutes of Biomedical Sciences, The Institutes of Brain Science and the Collaborative Innovation Center for Brain Science, Fudan University, Shanghai 200032, China
[6]Shanghai Engineering Research Centre of Cochlear Implant, Shanghai 200031, China

Correspondence should be addressed to Huawei Li; hwli@shmu.edu.cn and Peidong Dai; daipeidongent@163.com

Academic Editor: Geng-lin Li

Cochlear inner hair cell (IHC) ribbon synapses play an important role in sound encoding and neurotransmitter release. Previous reports show that both noise and aminoglycoside exposures lead to reduced numbers and morphologic changes of synaptic ribbons. In this work, we determined the distribution of N-methyl-D-aspartate receptors (NMDARs) and their role in the gentamicin-induced pathological changes of cochlear IHC ribbon synaptic elements. In normal mature mouse cochleae, the majority of NMDARs were distributed on the modiolar side of IHCs and close to the IHC nuclei region, while most of synaptic ribbons and α-amino-3-hydroxy-5-methyl-4-isoxazolepropionic acid receptor (AMPAR) were located on neural terminals closer to the IHC basal poles. After gentamicin exposure, the NMDARs increased and moved towards the IHC basal poles. At the same time, synaptic ribbons and AMPARs moved toward the IHC bundle poles on the afferent dendrites. The number of ribbon synapse decreased, and this was accompanied by increased auditory brainstem response thresholds and reduced wave I amplitudes. NMDAR antagonist MK801 treatment reduced the gentamicin-induced hearing loss and the pathological changes of IHC ribbon synapse, suggesting that NMDARs were involved in gentamicin-induced ototoxicity by regulating the number and distribution of IHC ribbon synapses.

1. Introduction

Cochlear inner hair cell (IHC) ribbon synapses play an important role in sound encoding and glutamate release. The IHC ribbon synapses are the first afferent synaptic connection in the hearing pathway, and they are located between the IHCs and the terminals of spiral ganglion neurons (SGNs). Bursts of synaptic activity are induced through periodic excitation of IHCs by mechanisms that are intrinsic to the cochlea [1], resulting in IHC Ca^{2+} spikes, glutamate release, and ultimately bursts of action potentials in SGNs that are carried to the brain by auditory nerve fibers. Cochlear synaptic ribbon pairs consist of presynaptic ribbons, to which many synaptic vesicles are connected, and postsynaptic α-amino-3-hydroxy-5-methyl-4-isoxazolepropionic acid receptors (AMPARs), which are glutamate receptors that mediate the excitatory postsynaptic currents of the SGNs' afferent dendrites [2].

Cochlear ribbon synapses are very sensitive to aminoglycoside and noise-induced injury [3–6]. Liberman et al. reported the reorganization of synaptic ribbon locations, the loss of synaptic ribbons, and the downregulation of AMPAR expression in the peripheral terminals after noise exposure [7]. Liu et al. found that moderate ototoxicity in mice leads to reduced numbers and morphologic changes in the synaptic ribbons, which are accompanied by mild hearing loss but no significant loss of HCs or SGNs in the cochlea [8]. However, the mechanism behind these pathological changes in cochlear IHC ribbon synapse remains unclear.

In the mammalian inner ear, almost all SGNs express another glutamate receptor, N-methyl-D-aspartate receptor (NMDAR), in addition to AMPAR [9–12]. In the developing cochlea, NMDARs in the IHC-SGN synapses enhance the spontaneous activity and promote the survival of SGNs [13]. NMDARs have also been shown to be involved in regulating the number of surface AMPARs on the cell membrane of auditory neurons in cultured neurons and to be involved in the response to acoustic stimulation [14]. However, the function of NMDARs was not clear in the IHC-SGN synapses of the mature cochlea.

Several studies suggest that NMDARs play a role in ototoxicity in the cochlea [15–17]. Aminoglycosides generate excess free radicals in the cochlea that damage both sensory HCs and SGNs, resulting in permanent hearing loss [18]. By using a severe hearing loss model with a large dose of aminoglycoside, in which both HCs and SGNs were severely injured, Basile et al. demonstrated that the NMDA antagonist dizocilpine maleate (MK801) could attenuate aminoglycoside-induced damage to SGNs and IHCs [15]. However, in this severe hearing loss model, the detailed pathological changes in the afferent synaptic connection between the IHCs and SGNs could not be evaluated due to the extensive injury to the HCs and SGNs. In this study, we used a low dose of gentamicin (100 mg/kg bodyweight) [3, 8, 19] to obtain a mild hearing loss model in which most of the HCs survived. We systematically analyzed the detailed morphological configuration, distribution, and number of presynaptic ribbons, postsynaptic AMPARs, and NMDARs in the cochlear IHC-SGN synapses of adult mice. To determine the role of NMDARs in the IHC-SGN synaptic plasticity in response to ototoxicity, we used the NMDAR antagonist MK801, which prevented gentamicin-induced injury to the IHC ribbon synapse and thus prevented hearing loss *in vivo*.

2. Materials and Methods

2.1. Animals. In total, 30 female C57BL/6J mice with documented dates of birth (5 weeks old) were obtained from the Chinese Academy of Medical Sciences Animal Center (Shanghai, China). All mice were housed with free access to food and water at the Experimental Animal Center, Shanghai Medical College of Fudan University, China. No outer or middle ear pathologies were observed. The animals were divided randomly into three groups. The first group was injected daily with a low dose of gentamicin (100 mg/kg, Sigma-Aldrich, USA) in saline intraperitoneally (i.p.) for 4 or 7 consecutive days [3, 8, 19, 20]. The second group

of animals received daily i.p. injections of gentamicin (100 mg/kg in saline) and the NMDAR antagonist MK801 (0.2 mg/kg in saline, Sigma-Aldrich, USA) for 4 or 7 consecutive days [17, 21, 22]. The mice in the third group served as the control group and received daily injections of equivalent volumes of normal saline. This study was carried out in strict accordance with the "Guiding Directive for Humane Treatment of Laboratory Animals" issued by the Chinese National Ministry of Science and Technology in September 2006. We performed all animal procedures according to protocols that were approved by the Shanghai Medical Experimental Animal Administrative Committee and were consistent with the National Institute of Health's Guide for the Care and Use of Laboratory Animals. All efforts were made to minimize suffering and reduce the number of animals used [23].

2.2. Assessment of Auditory Function. Auditory brainstem response (ABR) tests were performed in a sound-attenuating chamber to determine auditory thresholds. Animals were anesthetized via i.p. injections with ketamine (100 mg/kg) and xylazine (25 mg/kg). Specific auditory stimuli (clicks and 4, 8, 16, and 24 kHz tone bursts) were measured using a Tucker-Davis Technology System 3 (Tucker-Davis Technologies, Gainesville, FL, USA) as described previously [23, 24]. ABR stimuli consisted of 5 ms tone pips with a 0.5 ms rise-fall time delivered at 30 stimuli. The ABR threshold was defined as the lowest stimulus level at which a repeatable morphology could be identified in the response waveform (at least two consistent peaks). The ABR wave I peak-to-peak amplitude was computed by off-line analysis of stored waveforms as previous studies [12, 25]. All ABR tests were performed on mice on the following day after the injections with gentamicin alone or in combination with MK-801 (i.e., ABR was performed on day 5 or day 8).

2.3. Cochlear Tissue Processing and Immunostaining. After the ABR recordings, the mice were sacrificed by cervical dislocation and then decapitated. The temporal bone was removed, and the cochlea was quickly separated. The round and oval windows were opened and perfused with 4% paraformaldehyde in phosphate-buffered saline (PBS) at pH 7.4 and postfixed in the same solution for 2 h at room temperature. All cochleae were decalcified in 10% ethylene diamine tetraacetic acid (EDTA) solution. As quickly as possible, the cochlear shell and spiral ligament were removed under a dissecting microscope in 0.01 mM PBS solution. The vestibular membrane and tectorial membrane were removed from the basal membrane. The apical, middle, and basal turns from the cochlear basilar membrane were processed for immunofluorescent staining with antibodies against myosin 7a. Considering the fact that ribbon synapses near the basal turn of the cochlea are most susceptible to ototoxicity exposure [3, 8, 19], in this paper, only the synaptic elements of the cochlear middle-basal turn (51%–75% of the cochlear length from the apex) were quantified to determine the gentamicin-induced synaptic pathology.

Specimens were blocked with 10% donkey serum in 10 mM PBS with 0.3% Triton X-100 for 1 h at room temperature and then incubated with primary antibody for 48 h at

4°C. The primary antibodies included mouse anti-C-terminal-binding protein-2 (CtBP2) (612044; BD Biosciences, USA) at 1 : 500 dilution; mouse anti-glutamate receptor 2, extracellular, clone 6C4 (GluA2) (MAB397; Millipore, Germany) at 1 : 2000 dilution; rabbit anti-NMDAR1 (GluN1) (AB9864R; Millipore, Germany) at 1 : 1000 dilution; chicken anti-200 kD neurofilament heavy chain (NF) (cat. number ab72996; Abcam, UK) at 1 : 1500 dilution; and rabbit anti-myosin 7a polyclonal (Proteus BioSciences, USA) at 1 : 500 dilution. On the following day, the appropriate Alexa Fluor-conjugated secondary antibodies were incubated overnight at 4°C. Nuclear staining was performed with DAPI (1 : 800 dilution; Sigma-Aldrich, USA). Negative controls were performed by omitting the primary antibodies [26–28].

2.4. Confocal Microscopy Imaging. For confocal microscopy imaging, a laser scanning confocal microscope was used (SP5; Leica Microsystems, Biberach, Germany) with a 63x oil immersion objective lens. Excitation wavelengths were 488, 568, and 647 nm, and local images were magnified digitally by 2.74-fold. In each region, 10 to 12 IHCs were typically assessed. Sequence scanning was performed at an interval of 0.50 μm [27]. The laser excitation power and microscope emission and detection settings were maintained across different observations. The resulting confocal image series (z-stack) contained a three-dimensional (3D) record of the imaged information in the entire volume of the explant. The 3D-reconstructed z-stack was viewed, rotated, and "sliced" to provide final images and movies as necessary using the software from a TCS SP8 confocal laser-scanning microscope (Leica, Heidelberg, Germany).

2.5. Synapse Counts and Positioning Analysis. The contrast and brightness of the images were processed using Adobe Photoshop CS6. Synapse counts from the confocal images were performed using ImageJ (NIH, USA). The ribbon pairs were identified by the positive colocalization for double staining with CtBP2 and GluA2. Immunofluorescently identified AMPAR patches and NMDAR patches were counted at afferent nerve fibers (ANFs). All IHCs observed in 2 or 3 image fields were counted [26, 27]. The total numbers of puncta and patches were divided by the total numbers of IHC nuclei to obtain the average number of ribbons and glutamate receptors for each IHC. To describe the distribution of ribbons in IHCs and glutamate receptors (AMPARs and NMDARs) in afferent dendritic terminals, the concepts of basal and bundle poles of IHCs were introduced [29]. To count the number of synaptic elements, we drew one line along the top of the IHC nuclei and another line along the bottom of the inner spiral bundles (ISBs). Then the field between these two lines was divided into two parts, the "IHC nuclei region" and "IHC basal pole region." As shown in Figure 1(d), the IHC nuclei region was defined as the half region proximal to the nuclei and the bundle poles of the IHCs, and the IHC basal pole region was defined as the half region proximal to the ISBs and the basal poles of IHCs. The synaptic elements located between the IHC nuclei region and IHC bundle pole were also counted within the IHC nuclei region for convenience.

2.6. Statistical Analysis. All data are shown as means ± SE. Statistical analyses were conducted using Microsoft Excel and GraphPad Prism® 6 software. In all experiments, n represents the number of replicates. Two-tailed, unpaired Student's t-tests were used to determine statistical significance when comparing two groups, and one-way ANOVA followed by Dunnett's multiple comparisons test was used when comparing more than two groups. A value of $p < 0.05$ was considered to indicate statistical significance.

3. Results

3.1. The Distributions of Ribbons, NMDARs, and AMPARs at the IHC-SGN Synaptic Connection in the Mature Cochlea under Physiological Conditions. We first evaluated the morphological features, distribution, and numbers of ribbons, NMDARs, and AMPARs in the IHC-SGN synaptic connection of the adult mouse cochlea. CtBP2 was used as a marker of presynaptic ribbons. GluN1 and GluA2 were used as markers of NMDARs and AMPARs, respectively. Consistent with a previous study [2], in normal mature cochleae, the CtBP2-positive IHC ribbons were distributed on the cell membrane at the basal poles of IHCs, close to the ISBs (Figures 2(a)–2(e)). The ISBs appeared as a dense meshwork of neuronal processes around the basal poles of the IHCs (Figures 2(b)–2(e)), and these mostly included radially directed dendritic terminals of afferent type I ANFs and the efferent fibers [27, 30].

We observed different distributions of NMDARs and AMPARs at the IHC-SGN synapses in normal mature cochleae. In order to quantify these synaptic elements, we defined the IHC nuclei region and IHC basal pole region (see Figures 1(a) and 1(d) and Materials and Methods). The majority of GluA2-positive AMPAR patches were observed in ISBs, which were found in the basal pole region of IHCs (Figures 1(a)–1(e)), while most of GluN1-positive NMDAR patches were distributed on the neural dendritic terminals that were closer to the IHC nuclei region (Figures 1(c) and 1(e)). In the IHC nuclei region, some NMDARs colocalized with GluA2-positive AMPAR puncta, which were smaller than the AMPAR patches in the IHC basal pole region. Counts of NMDARs in the mature mouse cochlear middle-basal turn yielded averages of 1.00 ± 0.22 and 5.40 ± 0.27 per IHC in the IHC basal pole region and the IHC nuclei region, respectively (Supplementary Table 2). The average numbers of AMPARs were 13.70 ± 0.42 and 1.20 ± 0.13 per IHC in the IHC basal pole region and the IHC nuclei region, respectively (Supplementary Table 1). The 3D-reconstructed images showed that in normal mature mouse cochleae, the majority of NMDARs were distributed on the modiolar side of IHCs and close to the IHC nuclei region, while the AMPARs were distributed at the IHC basal pole region, on the modiolar and pillar sides of IHCs (Figures 1(f) and 1(g) and Supplemental video 1).

3.2. A Low Dose of Gentamicin-Induced Moderate Hearing Loss and the Rearrangement of Cochlear IHC-SGN Synaptic Elements. In order to determine the mechanisms of synaptic pathology, the same dose of gentamicin (100 mg/kg) as

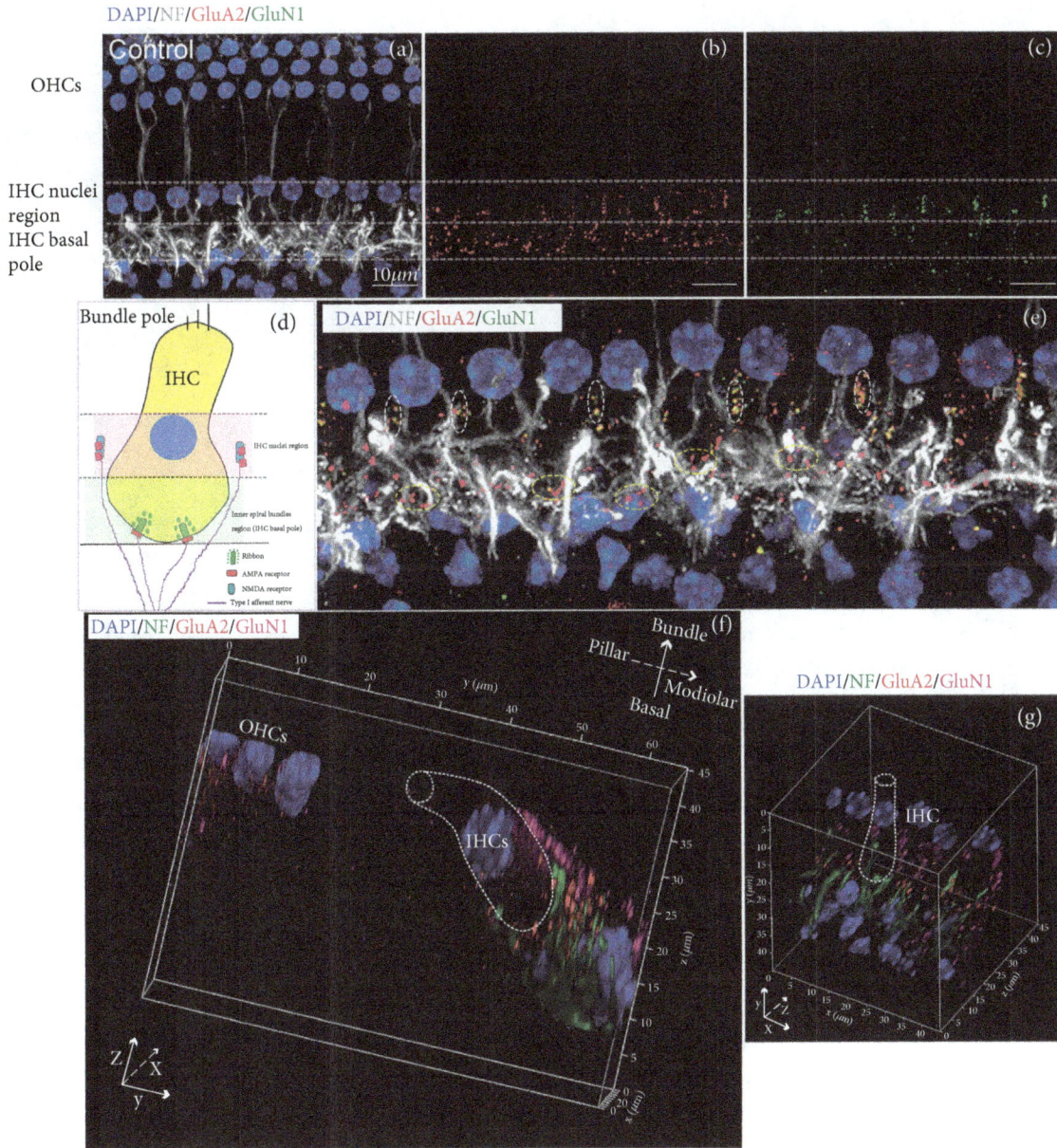

FIGURE 1: The different distributions of NMDARs and AMPARs at afferent dendritic terminals around IHCs in the normal mature cochlea. Postsynaptic AMPARs, NMDARs, and nerve fibers were identified by immunostaining for GluA2 (red), GluN1 (green), and neurofilament (NF) (grey), respectively. Nuclei were labeled with DAPI (blue). (a) The ISBs appeared as a dense meshwork of neuronal processes at the basal pole region of the IHCs. (b) AMPAR patches were mostly distributed among the ISBs around the basal poles of the IHCs. (c) Most of the NMDAR patches were distributed on the neural dendritic terminals, which were near the IHC nuclei region. (d) A diagram of the different locations of NMDARs and AMPARs at type I ANFs under physiological conditions. To count the number of synaptic elements, we drew one line along the top of the IHC nuclei and another line along the bottom of the ISBs. Then the field between these two lines was divided into two parts, the "IHC nuclei region" and the "IHC basal pole region." The IHC nuclei region was defined as the half region proximal to the nuclei and the bundle poles of the IHCs, and the IHC basal pole region was defined as the half region proximal to the ISBs and the basal poles of the IHCs. (e) Enlarged view of merged images (a), (b), and (c). Most of the NMDAR patches were distributed on the neural dendritic terminals between the adjoining IHCs and closer to the IHC nuclei region, while most of the AMPAR patches were observed among the ISBs around the basal poles of the IHCs. In the IHC nuclei region, some NMDARs colocalized with GluA2-positive AMPAR puncta (the dashed white circles), which were smaller than AMPAR patches in the IHC basal pole region (the dashed yellow circles). (f, g) The 3D-reconstructed images showing spatial distributions of AMPARs and NMDARs in SGN fibers around the IHCs. Postsynaptic AMPARs, NMDARs, and nerve fibers were identified by immunostaining for GluA2 (red), GluN1 (magenta), and NF (green), respectively. Nuclei were labeled with DAPI (blue). IHC: inner hair cell; OHC: outer hair cell; ISBs: inner spiral bundles; ANFs: afferent nerve fibers. Scale bar = 10 μm.

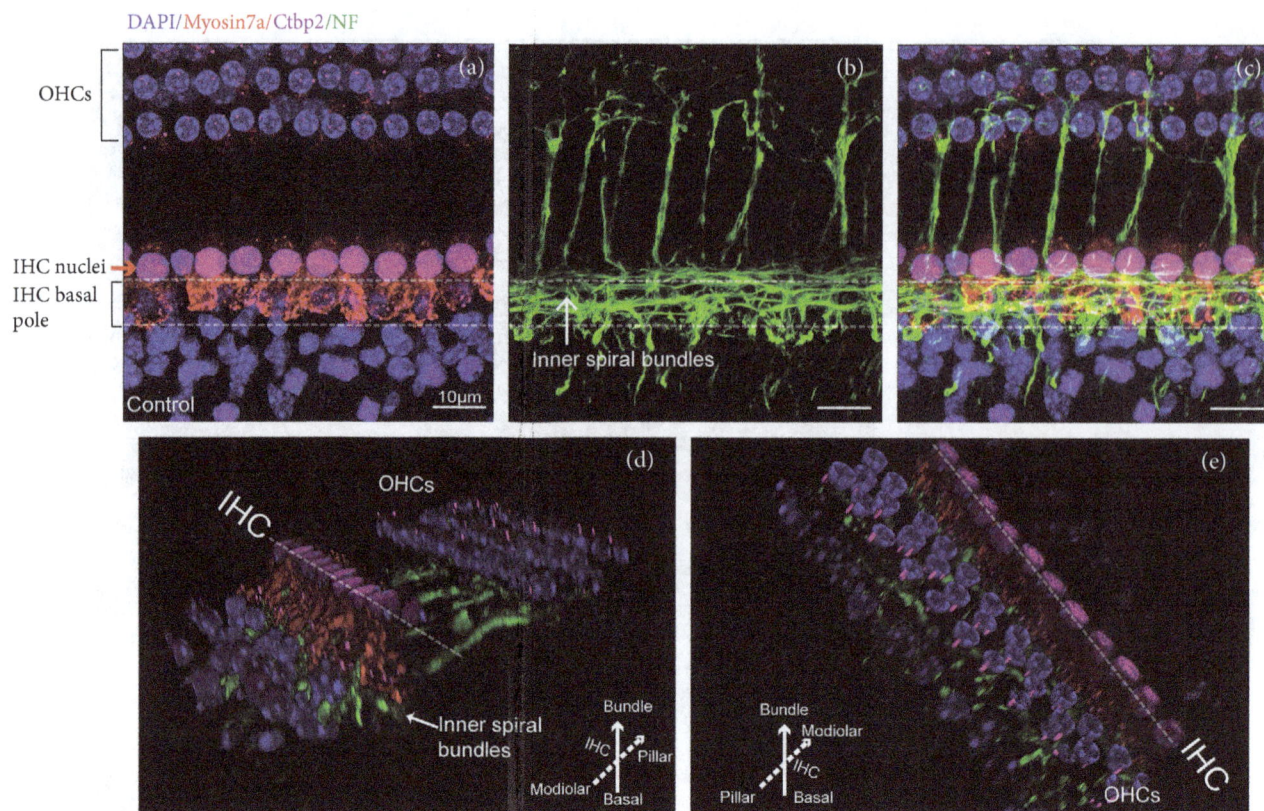

FIGURE 2: Spatial distribution of cochlear ribbons in IHCs and their relationship with inner spiral bundles in the normal mouse mature cochlea. The HCs, presynaptic ribbons, and nerve fibers were identified by immunostaining for myosin 7a (red), Ctbp2 (magenta), and neurofilament (NF) (green), respectively. Nuclei were labeled with DAPI (blue). (a) Ctbp2-positive ribbons (magenta puncta) were distributed at the basal poles of the IHCs and below the IHC nuclei. The IHC nuclei are marked with a red arrow. (b) NF staining showed that the ISBs appeared as nets of nerve fibers that include radially directed dendritic terminals of type I ANFs and efferent fibers of the olivocochlear system. (c) Merged images of (a) and (b). The IHC basal poles were surrounded by ISBs. (d, e) The 3D-reconstructed images showing the spatial relation among IHCs, presynaptic ribbons, and ISBs. (d) View from the modiolar side to the pillar side. (e) View from the pillar side to the modiolar side. IHC: inner hair cell; OHC: outer hair cell; ISBs: inner spiral bundles; ANFs: afferent nerve fibers. Scar bar = 10 μm.

used in previous studies was applied to the mice in this study [3, 8, 19]. Briefly, mice were injected daily with gentamicin (100 mg/kg) for 4 or 7 consecutive days, and mice receiving injections of normal saline served as controls. ABR tests were performed on the following day after gentamicin injections for 4 or 7 days. The mice were sacrificed, and the cochleae were isolated for immunostaining. Consistent with these previous reports [3, 8], we also found that a low dose of ototoxic gentamicin (100 mg/kg) led to moderate hearing loss and that this was associated with pathological changes in the presynaptic ribbons but with intact HCs and SGNs. Myosin 7a staining showed no obvious HC loss in any of the three turns after gentamicin treatment; however, moderate elevations in ABR thresholds for clicks and tone bursts at 4, 8, 16, and 24 kHz were found in the gentamicin-treated group ($p <$ 0.05, Figures 3(a)–3(f)). The amplitude of ABR wave I, reflecting the synchronous summated neural activity of the auditory nerve and functional level of IHC synapses between IHCs and terminals of SGNs [25, 31], was significantly reduced in gentamicin-treated mice (Figure 3(g), $p < 0.05$).

In normal mature cochleae, CtBP2-positive presynaptic ribbons were paired to GluA2-positive postsynaptic

AMPARs, and the paired CtBP2/GluA2 double-positive patches were defined as "ribbon synaptic pairs." In undamaged mouse cochleae, most of the ribbon synaptic pairs were distributed around the basal poles of the IHCs (Figure 4(a)). The average numbers of ribbon synaptic pairs were $13.30 \pm$ 0.37 and 0.80 ± 0.10 per IHC in the IHC basal pole region and the IHC nuclei region, respectively, in the control group (Supplementary Table 1). In the gentamicin-treated group, the number of ribbon synaptic pairs was significantly decreased. Moreover, presynaptic ribbons and postsynaptic AMPARs were relocated toward the IHC bundle poles, some of which reached to or across the IHC nuclei region (Figures 4(b) and 4(c) and Supplemental Videos 3 and 4).

In the IHC basal pole region, gentamicin treatment induced a significant decrease in the number of ribbons (13.30 ± 0.37, 6.40 ± 0.37, and 4.20 ± 0.23 in the control, 4-day gentamicin, and 7-day gentamicin groups, resp.) (Figure 4(e) and Supplementary Table 1). The average number of AMPARs was also significantly decreased in the IHC basal pole region in gentamicin-treated cochleae compared with the control group (13.70 ± 0.42, 7.20 ± 0.39, and 5.50 ± 0.37 in the control, 4-day gentamicin, and 7-day

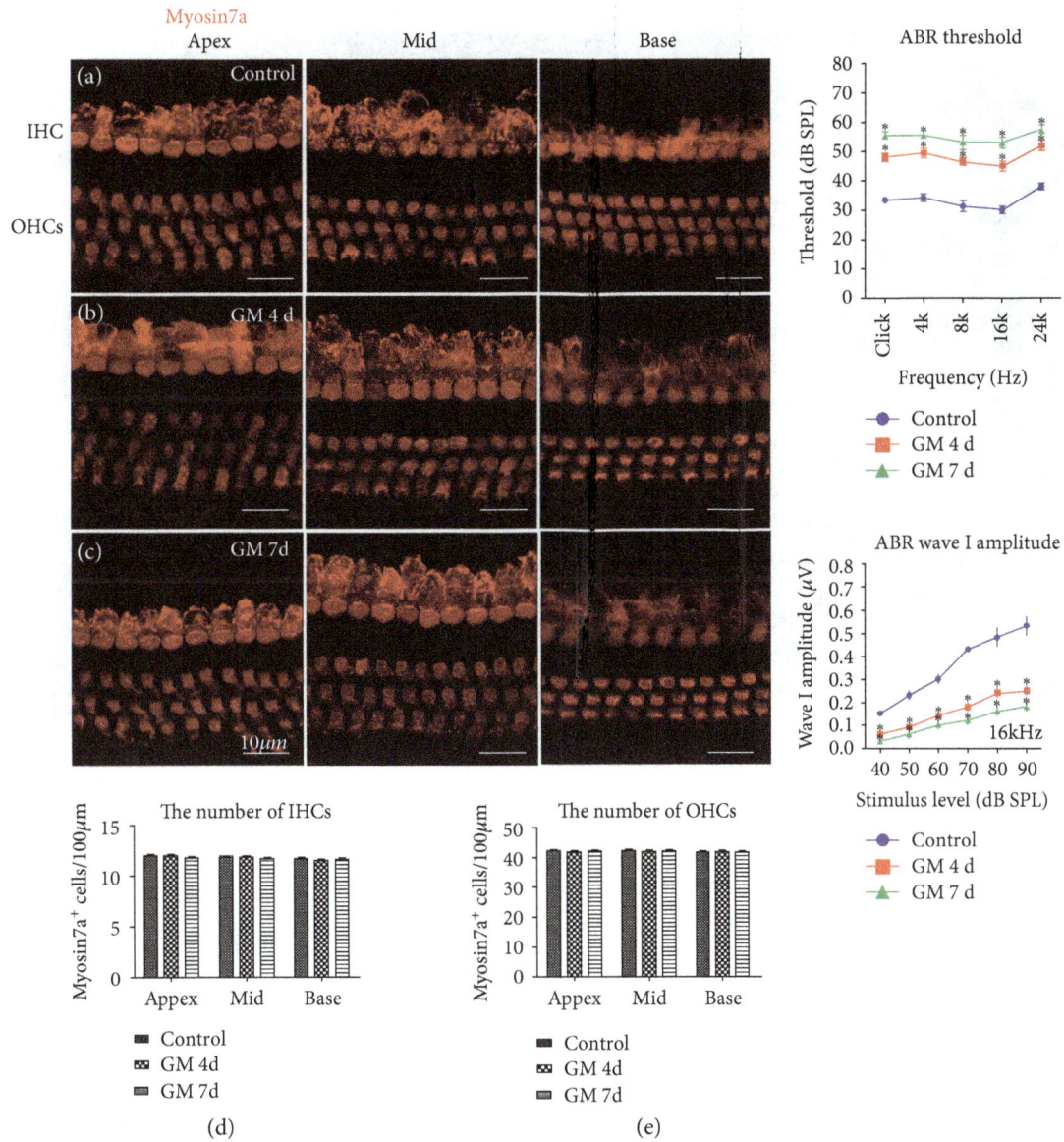

FIGURE 3: A low dose of gentamicin-induced moderate hearing loss with no obvious HC loss. The HCs were identified by immunostaining for myosin 7a (red) in the three turns of the cochlea. (a–c) After gentamicin treatment for 4 and 7 days, the morphology and arrangement of cochlear HCs were similar to the control group. (d-e) Quantitative data showed no HC loss in any of the three turns after gentamicin treatment. No significant difference was found in the number of IHCs or the three rows of OHCs among the control group and the gentamicin-treatment groups for 4 days or 7 days ($p > 0.05$). (f) A significant increase was observed in the ABR thresholds for clicks and for tone bursts at 4, 8, 16, and 24 kHz in the gentamicin-treated groups ($^*p < 0.05$, versus the control group). (g) A significant decline was observed in the ABR wave I amplitudes at 16 kHz in the gentamicin-treated groups ($^*p < 0.05$, *versus* the control group). GM 4 d, 7 d: gentamicin treatment for 4 days or 7 days; IHC: inner hair cell; OHC: outer hair cell. Scale bar = 10 μm. $^*p < 0.05$.

gentamicin groups, resp.) (Figure 4(f) and Supplementary Table 1). These results indicate that there was a significant decrease in the number of presynaptic ribbons and postsynaptic AMPARs at the basal poles of the IHCs (Figures 4(e)–4(g)), and thus the number of ribbon synaptic pairs significantly decreased at the basal poles of the IHCs in the gentamicin-treated group compared with the control group ($p < 0.05$) (Figure 4(g)). We also observed some anomalously aggregated ribbons and/or AMPARs at the IHC basal pole region in the gentamicin-treated cochleae (Figure 4(c)), which is consistent with a previous report [8].

In the IHC nuclei region in normal cochleae, the average number of AMPARs, ribbons, and ribbon synaptic pairs were 1.20 ± 0.13, 0.80 ± 0.10, and 0.80 ± 0.10 per IHC, respectively. After gentamicin treatment, there was a significant increase in the number of relocated AMPARs, ribbons, and ribbon synaptic pairs in the IHC nuclei region ($p < 0.05$). After gentamicin treatment for 4 days, the numbers of AMPARs, ribbons, and ribbon synaptic pairs were 3.80 ± 0.28, 2.20 ± 0.32, and 1.90 ± 0.32 per IHC in the IHC nuclei region, respectively. After gentamicin treatment for 7 days, the numbers of AMPARs, ribbons, and ribbon synaptic pairs

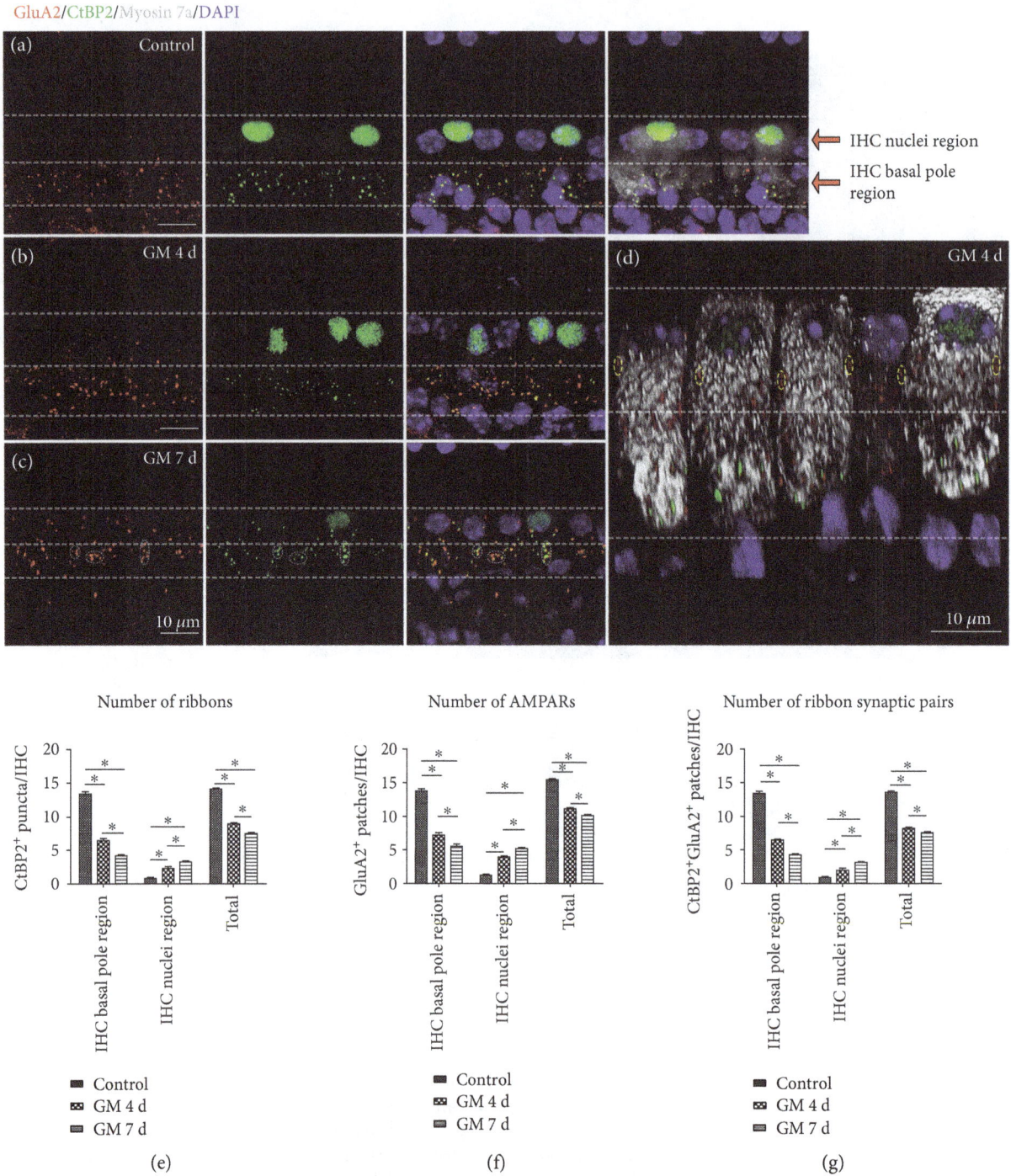

FIGURE 4: The number of cochlear ribbon synapses decreased and their locations changed from the basal pole region toward the nuclei region of the IHCs after gentamicin treatment. The IHCs were outlined by myosin 7a fluorescence in the cytoplasm (grey), and the nuclei were stained with DAPI (blue). The afferent synapses on the IHCs were labeled by immunostaining presynaptic ribbons with anti-CtBP2 (green) and the postsynaptic AMPARs with anti-GluA2 (red). (a) Ribbons and AMPARs were almost perfectly paired at the basal poles of the IHCs under physiological conditions. (b) After gentamicin treatment for 4 days, the ribbons and AMPARs moved towards the bundle poles of the IHCs. (c) After gentamicin treatment for 7 days, ribbons and AMPARs migrated towards the bundle poles of the IHCs, and some of them reached to or across the IHC nuclei region. The dashed white circles indicate some variegated ribbons and/or AMPARs at the IHC basal pole region. (d) The 3D-reconstructed image. The dashed yellow circles show orphan AMPARs near the bundle poles of the IHCs after 4 days of gentamicin treatment. (e) The numbers of CtBP2-positive ribbons. (f) The numbers of GluA2-positive AMPARs. (g) The numbers of CtBP2 and GluA2 double-positive ribbon synaptic pairs. GM 4 d, 7 d: gentamicin treatment for 4 days or 7 days; IHC: inner hair cell. Scale bar = 10 μm. $^{*}p < 0.05$.

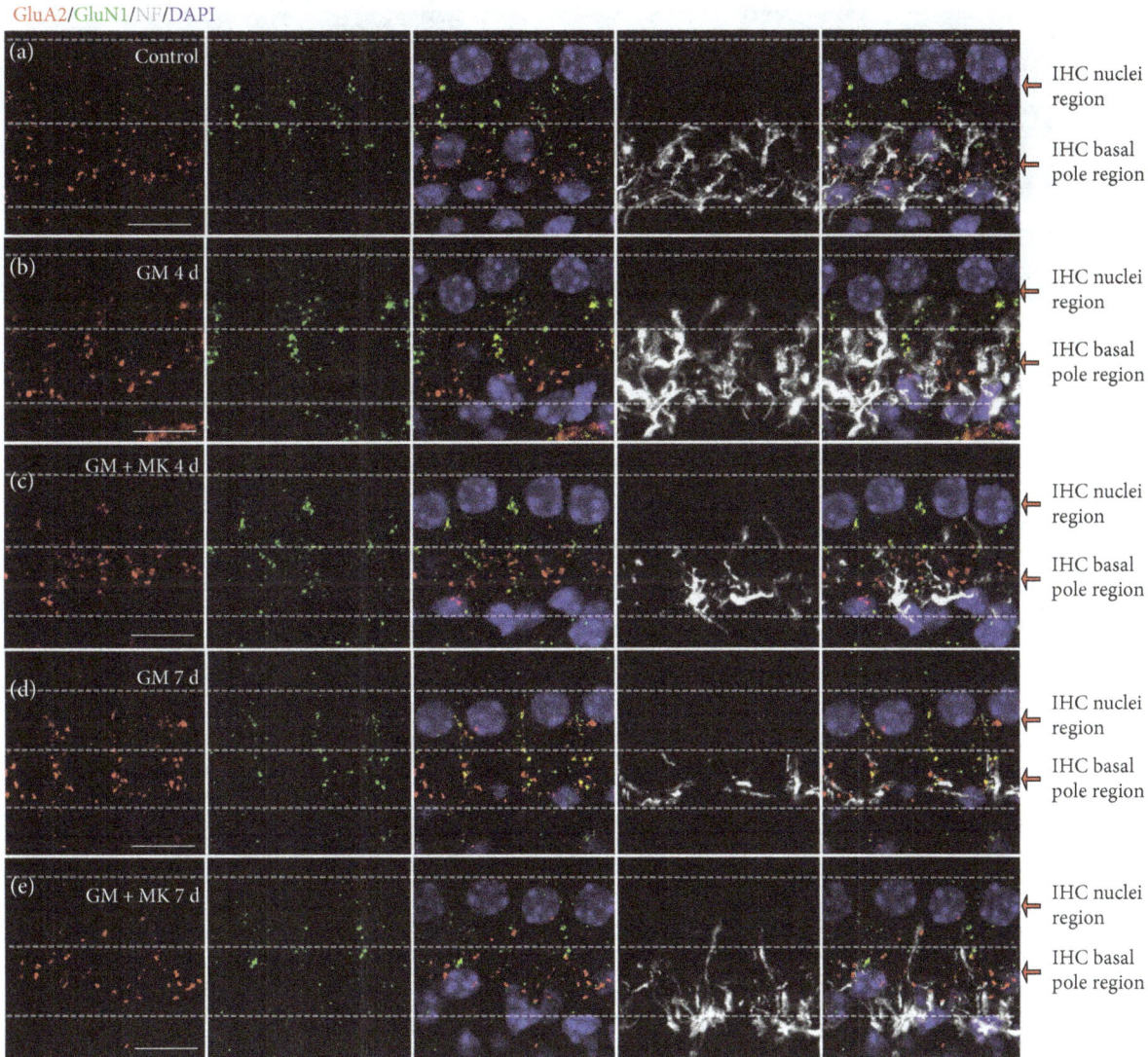

FIGURE 5: AMPARs and NMDARs were relocated on SGN dendrites after gentamicin exposure, and this was blocked by coinjection of the NMDAR antagonist MK801. Postsynaptic AMPARs, NMDARs, and nerve fibers were identified by immunostaining for GluA2 (red), GluN1 (green), and neurofilament (NF) (grey), respectively. Nuclei were labeled with DAPI (blue). (a) The different locations of NMDARs and AMPARs at afferent dendritic terminals in the normal mature cochlea. AMPAR patches were mostly observed on the ISBs around the basal poles of the IHCs, while NMDAR patches were almost all distributed on nerve terminals between the adjoining IHCs and closer to the IHC nuclei region. (b) After gentamicin treatment for 4 days, the AMPARs migrated upwards towards the bundle poles of the IHCs, while NMDARs migrated downwards towards the basal poles of the IHCs. (c) After the combined treatment with MK801 and gentamicin for 4 days, AMPARs and NMDARs were prevented from delocalizing to the dendritic terminals around the IHCs. (d) After gentamicin treatment for 7 days, the AMPARs and NMDARs had essentially switched locations along the dendritic terminals. Many colocalized AMPARs and NMDARs were observed laterally between the adjoining IHCs. (e) After the combined treatment with gentamicin and MK801 for 7 days, the gentamicin-induced rearrangements of AMPARs and NMDARs at the afferent dendritic terminals were partly blocked. GM 4 d, 7 d: gentamicin treatment for 4 days or 7 days; GM + MK 4d, 7d: combined treatment with gentamicin and MK801 for 4 days or 7 days; IHC: inner hair cell; ISBs: inner spiral bundles. Scale bar = 10 μm.

were 5.00 ± 0.31, 3.10 ± 0.28, and 3.00 ± 0.28 per IHC, respectively, in the IHC nuclei region (Figures 4(e)–4(g) and Supplementary Table 1). Moreover, many orphan AMPARs, which lack closely apposed presynaptic ribbons in the IHC, were observed in the IHC nuclei region after gentamicin treatment for 4 days (Figure 4(d)). More relocated ribbon synaptic pairs were found in the IHC nuclei region in the 7-day gentamicin group than the 4-day gentamicin group (Figure 4(g)), suggesting that the IHC ribbons matched up

again with the earlier relocated postsynaptic AMPARs in the 7-day gentamicin group.

3.3. A Low Dose of Gentamicin-Induced Rearrangement of NMDARs at Nerve Terminals Innervating the IHCs. We next explored the changes in NMDARs and its relationship with AMPARs after gentamicin injury. First, we found that the number of NMDARs was significantly increased in the SGN-IHC synapses after gentamicin treatment ($p < 0.05$)

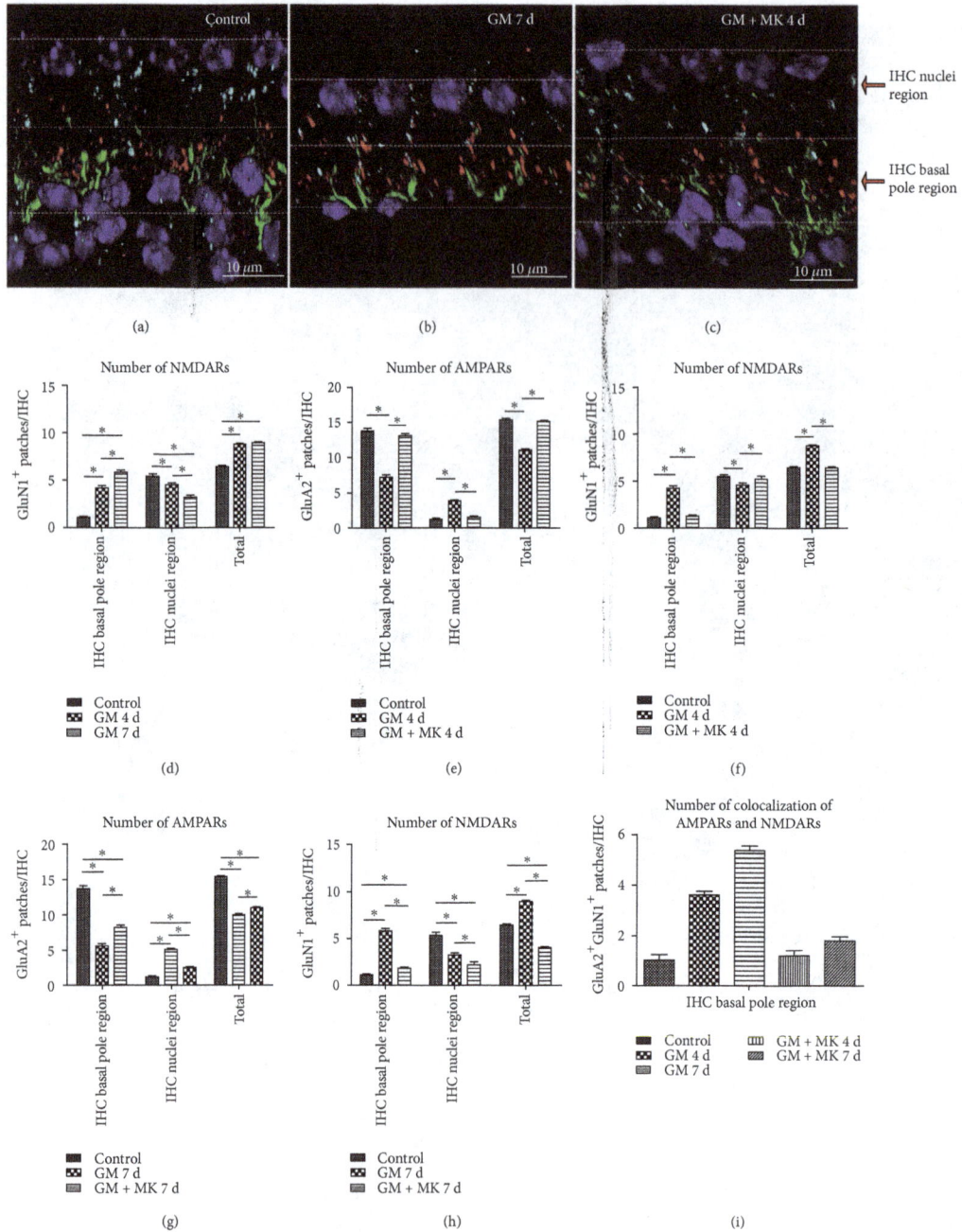

FIGURE 6: The 3D-reconstructed images and the numbers of NMDARs and AMPARs at the nerve fibers around the IHCs. Postsynaptic AMPARs, NMDARs, and nerve fibers around the IHCs were identified by immunostaining for GluA2 (red), GluN1 (cyan), and neurofilament (NF) (green). Nuclei were labeled with DAPI (blue). (a, b, c) In the study, we define the "IHC basal pole region" and the "IHC nuclei region" in every single IHC. The changed tendency in location of AMPARs and NMDARs was observed at the afferent dendrites around the adjacent IHC in the 3D-reconstructed images. (a) The locations of NMDARs and AMPARs at the afferent dendritic terminals in the normal cochlea. (b) AMPARs and NMDARs essentially switched locations on SGN dendrites after gentamicin treatment for 7 days. (c) The gentamicin-induced translocation of AMPARs and NMDARs was almost completely blocked after coinjection of MK801 and gentamicin for 4 days. (d, f, h) The numbers of GluN1-positive NMDARs. (e, g) The numbers of GluA2-positive AMPARs. (i) The numbers of colocalized AMPARs and NMDARs at the basal poles of the IHCs. GM 4 d, 7 d: gentamicin treatment for 4 days or 7 days; GM + MK 4d, 7d: combined treatment of gentamicin and MK801 for 4 days or 7 days; IHC: inner hair cell. $^{*}p < 0.05$.

(Figures 5(b), 5(d), 6(b), and 6(d)). Second, we observed the rearrangement of NMDARs at afferent dendritic terminals. NMDAR patches migrated towards the basal poles of the IHCs, closer to the ISBs. After gentamicin treatment, compared with the control group, the number of NMDAR patches significantly increased in the IHC basal pole region ($p < 0.05$) and significantly decreased in the IHC nuclei region ($p < 0.05$) (Figures 5(b), 5(d), 6(b), and 6(d) and 4 days, the numbers of NMDARs were 4.50 ± 0.30 and 4.20 ± 0.31 per IHC in the IHC nuclei region and the IHC basal

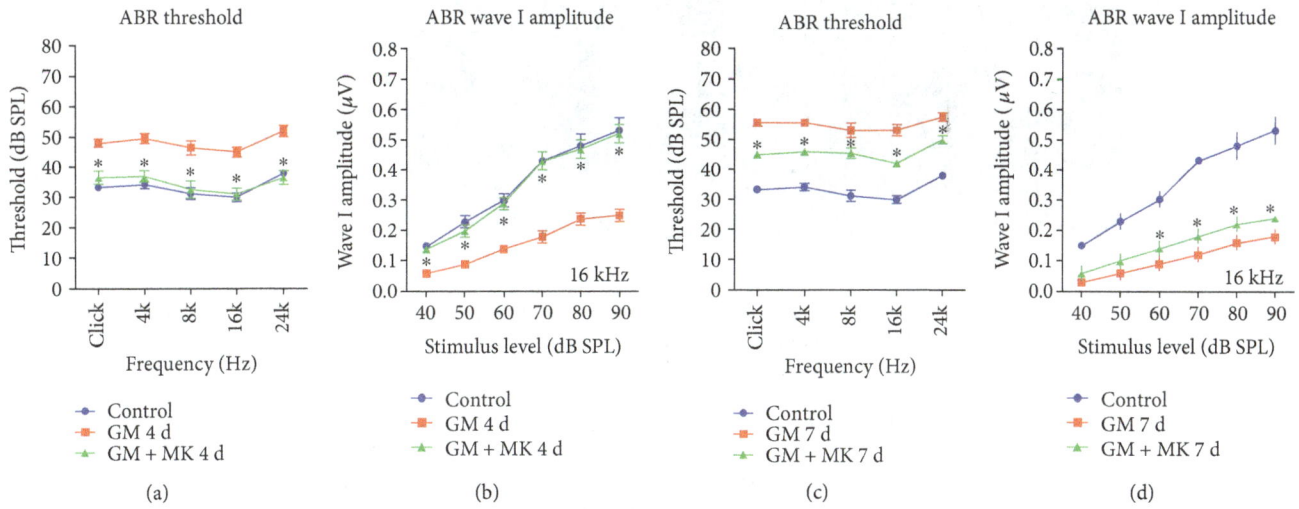

(a)

(b)

(c)

(d)

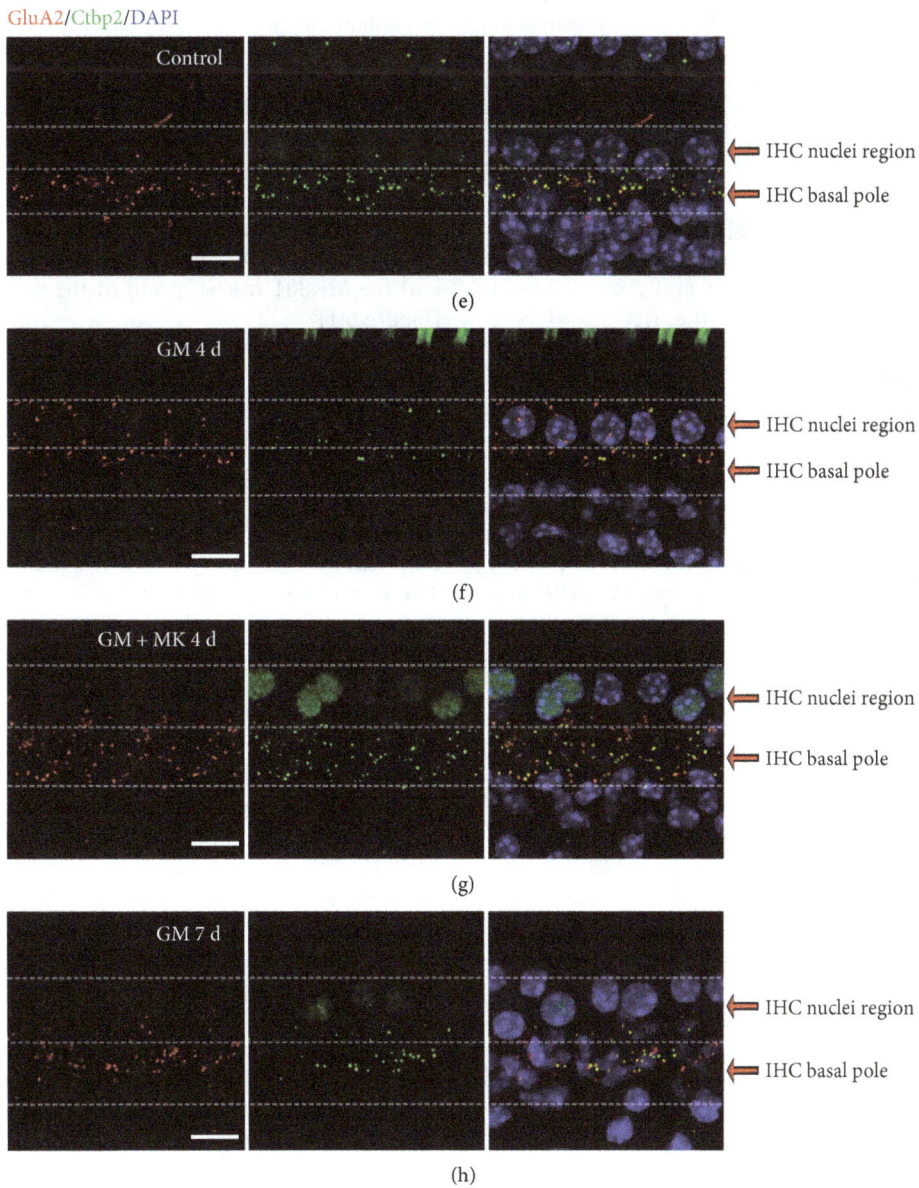

GluA2/Ctbp2/DAPI

(e)

(f)

(g)

(h)

FIGURE 7: Continued.

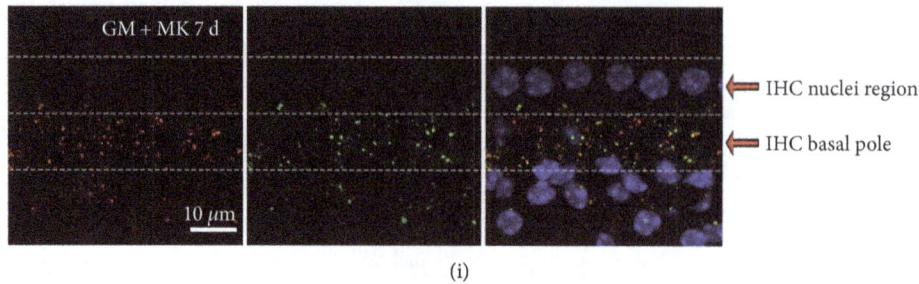

(i)

FIGURE 7: Cochlear ribbon synapses were maintained when MK801 was coinjected with gentamicin. (a-b) The elevation of ABR thresholds and the decline of ABR wave I amplitudes induced by gentamicin injury were successfully rescued by MK801 treatment in the 4-day treatment group ($^{*}p < 0.05$, *versus* gentamicin-only group). (c-d) The elevation of ABR thresholds and the decline of ABR wave I amplitudes induced by gentamicin injury were partly blocked by MK801 treatment in the 7-day treatment group ($^{*}p < 0.05$, *versus* gentamicin-only group). (e–i) Afferent ribbon synaptic pairs were observed by immunostaining presynaptic ribbons with anti-CtBP2 (green) and postsynaptic AMPARs with anti-GluA2 (red). Nuclei were labeled by DAPI (blue). (e) Ribbons and AMPARs were paired at the basal poles of the IHCs in the undamaged cochlea. (f) After gentamicin treatment for 4 days, AMPARs and ribbons moved upwards towards the bundle poles of the IHCs. The translocation of AMPARs occurred earlier than that of the presynaptic ribbons. (g) After the combined treatment with gentamicin and MK801 for 4 days, the ribbon synaptic pairs had similar location, morphology, and distribution as undamaged controls. (h) After gentamicin treatment for 7 days, AMPARs and ribbons were further relocated towards the bundle poles of the IHCs. Some large ribbons and/or AMPARs were also observed at the basal poles of the IHCs. (i) After the combined treatment with gentamicin and MK801 for 7 days, the quantity of the ribbon synaptic pairs was significantly increased in the IHC basal pole region compared with that in gentamicin-only treatment. GM 4 d, 7 d: gentamicin treatment for 4 days or 7 days; GM + MK 4d, 7d: combined treatment with gentamicin and MK801 for 4 or 7 days; IHC: inner hair cell. Scale bar = 10 μm. $^{*}p < 0.05$.

pole region, respectively (Figures 5(b) and 6(d), and Supplementary Table 2). After gentamicin treatment for 7 days, the numbers of NMDARs were 3.20 ± 0.25 and 5.80 ± 0.25 per IHC in the IHC nuclei region and the IHC basal pole region, respectively (Figures 5(d), 6(b), and 6(d) and Supplementary Table 2). Moreover, the number of colocalized AMPARs and NMDARs per IHC was also significantly increased in the IHC basal pole region after gentamicin treatment (Figure 6(i) and Supplementary Table 2).

3.4. Treatment with the NMDAR Antagonist MK801 Prevented the Gentamicin-Induced Rearrangement of AMPARs and NMDARs at the IHC-SGN Synaptic Connection. MK801 is a noncompetitive NMDA receptor antagonist that is thought to protect neurons in the brain against excitotoxicity induced by excessive glutamate activity [17, 32]. MK801 was used as a NMDAR antagonist with the dose range from 0.2 to 1.0 (mg/kg) in previous studies [17, 21, 22]. To explore the role of NMDARs in synaptic plasticity during ototoxicity, MK801 (0.2 mg/kg, i.p.) was used to rescue the gentamicin-induced damage. Briefly, mice were injected daily with MK801 and/ or gentamicin for 4 or 7 consecutive days, and mice receiving injections of normal saline served as controls. ABR tests were performed on the following day after injections for 4 or 7 days.

GluN1 staining showed that MK801 treatment clearly prevented the gentamicin-induced movement of NMDARs toward the IHC basal poles (Figures 5 and 6). The number, morphology, and distribution of GluN1-positive patches in MK801-treated cochleae were similar to normal cochleae (Figure 6). Compared with the gentamicin-only group, the number of NMDARs in the IHC nuclei region increased significantly in the MK801 rescue group in both the 4-day and 7-day treatment groups (Figures 6(f) and 6(h)). There was

no significant difference in the number of NMDARs in the IHC nuclei region between the undamaged control group and the MK801 rescue group in the 4-day treatment group (Figure 6(f)).

GluA2 staining showed that the gentamicin-induced movement toward the IHC bundle poles and the pathological changes of postsynaptic AMPARs were blocked by coinjection of MK801 (Figures 5–8). Moreover, compared with the gentamicin-only group, the number of colocalized AMPARs and NMDARs significantly decreased in the IHC basal pole region in the MK801 rescue group in both the 4-day and 7-day treatment groups ($p < 0.05$, Figures 6(f), 6(h), and 6(i)). These results suggested that MK801 treatment blocked the gentamicin-induced activation of NMDARs and the pathological changes of AMPARs in the SGN terminals.

3.5. NMDAR Antagonist MK801 Treatment Protects against Gentamicin-Induced Hearing Loss by Preventing the Disruption of Ribbon Synapses. We next explored whether gentamicin-induced hearing loss and disruption of ribbon synaptic pairs could be affected by the NMDAR antagonist MK801. In this experiment, we found that gentamicin-induced hearing loss was successfully rescued by MK801 treatment (Figures 7(a)–7(d)). Compared with the undamaged group, the ABR thresholds were significantly increased while ABR wave I amplitudes were significantly reduced after gentamicin injury. However, the elevation of ABR thresholds and reduction of wave I amplitudes induced by gentamicin injury was successfully rescued by MK801 treatment in both the 4-day and 7-day treatment groups. Indeed, no significant differences were seen in the ABR thresholds and wave I amplitude between the undamaged control group and the MK801 rescue group in the 4-day treatment group (Figures 7(a) and 7(b)), suggesting that MK801 treatment could attenuate the gentamicin-induced hearing loss.

GluA2/CtBP2/DAPI

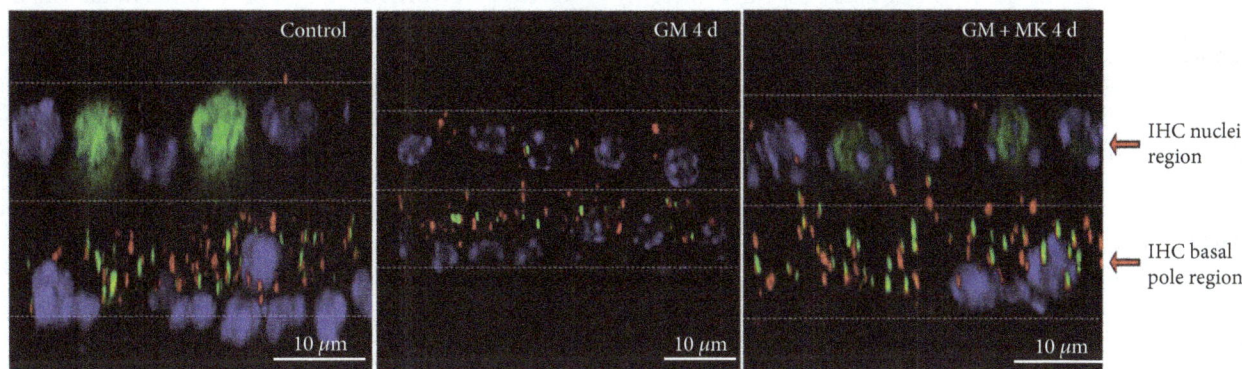

(a) (b) (c)

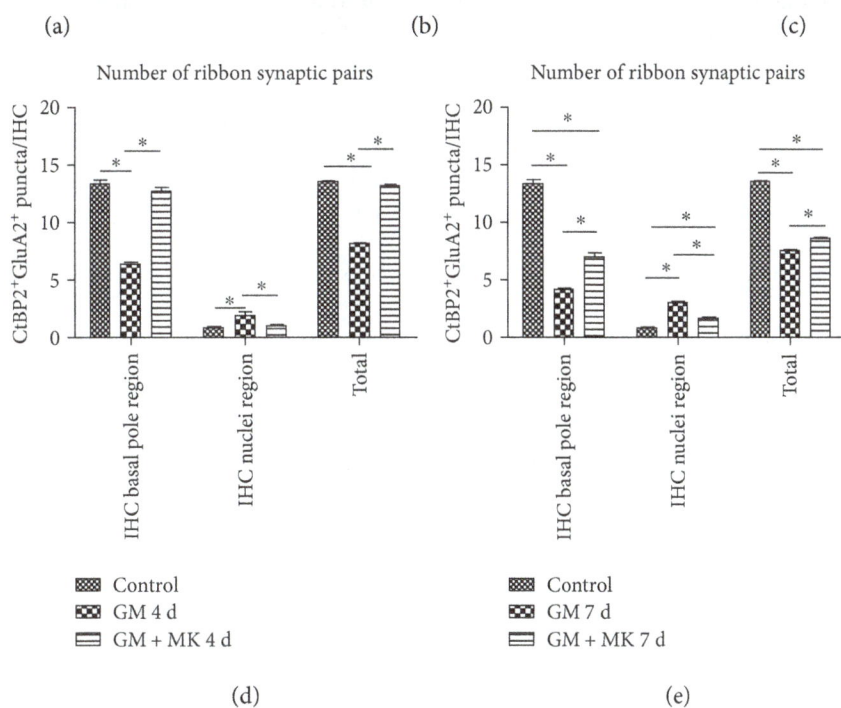

(d) (e)

FIGURE 8: The 3D-reconstructed images and numerical data for the ribbon pairs after different treatments. Afferent synapses on IHCs are seen by immunostaining presynaptic ribbons with anti-CtBP2 (green) and postsynaptic AMPARs with anti-GluA2 (red). Nuclei were labeled with DAPI (blue). (a, b, c) In the study, we define the "IHC basal pole region" and the "IHC nuclei region" in every single IHC. The changed tendency in location of AMPARs and ribbons was observed around the IHC in the 3D-reconstructed images. (a) Ribbons and AMPARs were paired at the basal poles of the IHCs in the control cochlea. (b) After gentamicin treatment for 4 days, the presynaptic ribbons and postsynaptic AMPARs were relocated towards the bundle poles of the IHCs. The number of ribbons and AMPARs was decreased at the basal pole of IHCs. (c) After combined treatment with gentamicin and MK801 for 4 days, most of the IHC ribbons and postsynaptic AMPARs remained at the basal poles of the IHCs, but a few AMPARs were still observed near the IHC nuclei region. (d) The number of ribbon synaptic pairs among the control group, gentamicin treatment group for 4 days, and combined treatment group with gentamicin and MK801 for 4 days. (e) The number of ribbon synaptic pairs among the control group, gentamicin treatment group for 7 days, and combined treatment group with gentamicin and MK801 for 7 days. GM 4 d, 7 d: gentamicin treatment for 4 days or 7 days; GM + MK 4d, 7d: combined treatment with gentamicin and MK801 for 4 days or 7 days; IHC: inner hair cell $^*p < 0.05$.

CtBP2 staining showed that the movement of presynaptic ribbons toward the IHC bundle poles in response to gentamicin was blocked by coinjection with MK801 (Figures 7 and 8). Not only the location but also the quantity, morphology, and distribution of presynaptic ribbons in the MK801-treated cochlea were comparable to normal undamaged cochleae (Figures 7(e)–7(i), and Supplemental Video 5). Compared with the gentamicin-only group, the numbers of ribbon synaptic pairs at the IHC basal pole region were significantly increased in the MK801 rescue groups at both 4 and 7 days (Figures 8(d) and 8(e)). There was no significant difference in the number of ribbon synaptic pairs in the IHC basal pole region between the control and the MK801 rescue group in the 4-day treatment group (Figure 8(d)). These results suggested that the rearrangement of NMDARs is a primary element of the injury in IHC-SGNs synapses induced by gentamicin and early interruption of NMDAR activation protected against gentamicin-induced pathological changes in the IHC synapses. Together, these results suggest that inhibition of NMDARs protected against gentamicin-induced hearing loss, likely by maintaining the integrity of the ribbon synapses.

4. Discussion

Transmission of nerve impulses at IHC-SGN synapses is mediated by the release of glutamate from ribbon terminals [2, 33]. Patch clamp recordings of the type I SGN afferent dendrite convincingly show that excitatory postsynaptic currents are AMPAR mediated and that NMDARs do not contribute to synaptic transmission at the type I SGN synapse under physiological conditions [34–37]. Although the role of NMDARs in ototoxicity was speculated to be through glutamate excitotoxicity [15–17], there was no direct morphological evidence for this or for the role of NMDARs in cochlear IHC-SGN synapses.

4.1. NMDARs and AMPARs Are Located in Different Regions of ANF Terminals under Physiological Conditions. GluA2, GluA3, and possibly GluA4 subunits of AMPAR are present in SGN afferent dendrites in the adult cochlea [38], and the GluA2 subunit determines the key biophysical properties of GluAs *in vivo* [39]. Under physiological conditions, GluA2-positive AMPAR patches were paired with CtBP2 positive IHC ribbons and were distributed in the ISBs around the basal poles of the IHCs (Figure 4), which was consistent with previous studies [2, 3, 8]. NMDARs are composed of the mandatory GluN1 subunit and a variety of GluN2A, B, C, and D subunits [38, 40]. In this paper, we found that the majority of NMDARs were distributed on the modiolar side and close to the nuclei region of IHCs. However, the AMPARs are mainly distributed at the IHC basal pole region, on the modiolar and pillar sides of IHCs. Some NMDARs were colocalized with small GluA2-positive puncta, which might be regarded as a "resting state" of small-puncta AMPARs in the central nervous system (Figure 1) [38, 41]. This study reported the different characteristics of the distribution of AMPARs and NMDARs at type I ANFs contacting IHCs in the adult mouse cochlea (Figures 1 and 5).

4.2. NMDARs Are Involved in AMPAR Rearrangement in the Cochlear IHC-SGN Synapse Connection as Part of the Ototoxic Mechanism of Gentamicin Treatment. Reorganization of postsynaptic AMPARs and NMDARs was observed after gentamicin treatment. Rows of NMDARs moved towards the IHC basal poles, while AMPAR patches moved towards the IHC bundle poles and reached to or across the IHC nuclei region on the afferent dendrites contacting the IHCs (Figures 5, 6, and 9). As a result, the spatial distribution AMPARs and NMDARs was different from the distribution under physiological conditions. The number of NMDARs in the ISBs was significantly increased in response to gentamicin treatment (Figures 5 and 6). In the central nervous system, calcium overload and cell death are mediated by NMDARs through glutamate excitotoxicity [40, 42–44], and our data suggest that rearrangement of

AMPARs and NMDARs might be involved in the glutamate excitotoxicity observed in cochlear IHC-SGN synapses after gentamicin treatment.

In the brain, NMDARs are required for the control of synaptic rearrangement and axonal remodeling [45]. Activation of synaptic NMDARs induces the membrane insertion of new AMPARs in cultured hippocampal neurons [46], and NMDAR agonists can regulate the expression of surface AMPARs on the cell membrane of cultured SGNs [14]. In the present study, coinjection of the NMDAR antagonist MK801 and gentamicin prevented the rearrangement of AMPARs and NMDARs at the dendritic terminals (Figures 5–8), suggesting that NMDAR activation is involved in the AMPAR rearrangement in IHC-SGN synapses in response to gentamicin. Furthermore, cotreatment with MK801 prevented gentamicin-induced damage of the IHC ribbon synapse (Figure 7) and reduced gentamicin-induced hearing loss (Figure 8), suggesting that NMDARs are involved in ototoxicity by regulating the number and distribution of ribbon synapses in the IHC-SGN afferent synapse connection.

4.3. Ribbons in IHCs Might Follow the Rearrangement of AMPARs at Afferent Dendritic Terminals in Response to Gentamicin Treatment. Studies of both noise-induced hearing loss and drug-induced hearing loss have shown reduced numbers and abnormal distributions of ribbons, which were found to be isolated in the cytoplasm and proximal to the IHC nuclei region [7, 8]. However, the mechanism and implications of this abnormal distribution of ribbons has remained unclear.

Under physiological conditions, presynaptic ribbons were paired to postsynaptic AMPARs. In gentamicin-induced ototoxicity, AMPARs on the SGN dendrites moved quickly toward the bundle poles of the IHCs, some of which reached to or across the IHC nuclei region. Orphan AMPARs lacking opposed ribbons were often observed in the IHC nuclei region of SGN afferent dendritic terminals in the 4-day gentamicin group. However, in the 7-day gentamicin group, the IHC ribbons were increasingly relocated and matched up again with postsynaptic AMPARs in the IHC nuclei region. These results suggest that the relocation of AMPARs takes place earlier than the relocation of the presynaptic ribbons and that the presynaptic ribbons in the IHC membrane might follow the movement of postsynaptic AMPARs at type I SGN afferent dendritic terminals in response to gentamicin treatment (Figure 4).

The expression of mature ribbons on the membrane of IHCs requires several intracellular processes, including the synthesis of glutamate vesicles, transportation, assembly, and final localization of ribbons at the membrane [2]. Sobkowicz et al. studied the distribution of synaptic ribbons in the developing organ of Corti and found that nerve fibers appear to be critical in influencing the location of the synaptic ribbon [47]. It has been suggested that nitric oxide, as a neuronal messenger, might be involved in transferring signals between presynaptic and postsynaptic elements and regulating the excitability at glutamatergic synapses. In the brain, neuronal nitric oxide synthase is broadly expressed

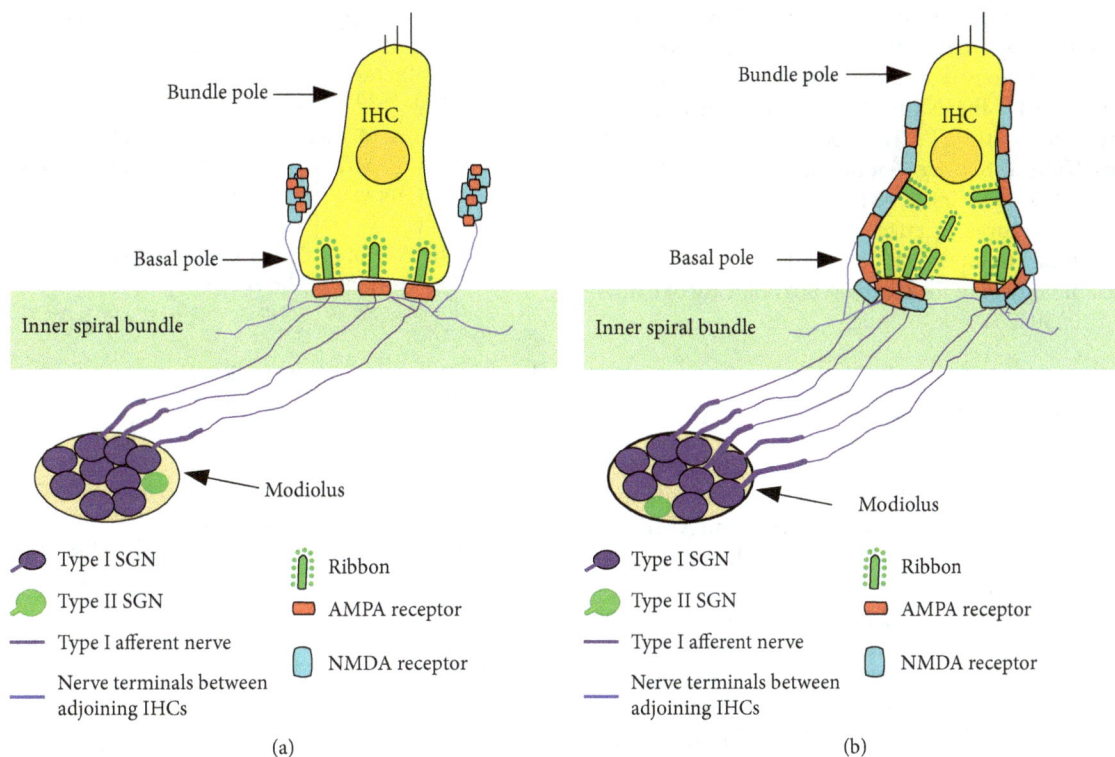

FIGURE 9: Diagrams illustrating the gentamicin-induced changes in ribbons, NMDARs, and AMPARs at the IHC-SGN synapse in the mouse cochlea. (a) In the normal mouse adult cochlea, presynaptic ribbons and postsynaptic AMPARs show a nearly one-to-one relationship. The ribbon synaptic pairs (double staining for CtBP2-positive puncta and GluA2-positive patches) are distributed around the basal poles of the IHCs. Most of the AMPARs are observed in the ISBs, but most NMDARs are distributed on the neural dendritic terminals between the adjoining IHCs and closer to the IHC nuclei region. In IHC nuclei region, some NMDARs colocalize with GluA2-positive AMPAR puncta, which are smaller than AMPAR patches in the IHC basal pole region. In the mouse cochlea, each IHC is contacted by roughly 10–20 ANFs depending on cochlear location. Each cochlear neuron is excited by a single ribbon synapse with a single IHC. (b) After gentamicin treatment, AMPARs and NMDARs are relocated at nerve fiber terminals around IHCs, and their locations are essentially reversed. AMPARs move upwards towards the bundle poles of the IHCs, and NMDARs migrate downwards towards the basal poles of the IHCs. The number of colocalized AMPARs and NMDARs gradually increases in the IHC basal pole region. Some anomalously aggregated ribbons and/or AMPARs in the IHC basal pole region are observed. IHC: inner hair cell; SGN: spiral ganglion neuron; ISBs: inner spiral bundles; ANFs: afferent nerve fibers.

and is associated with synaptic plasticity through NMDAR-mediated calcium influx [48]. The role of nitric oxide and synaptic plasticity in the progression of ototoxicity requires further study.

5. Conclusions

This study showed that NMDARs are involved in cochlear ribbon synaptic rearrangement in gentamicin-induced ototoxicity. The postsynaptic arrangement of AMPARs on the dendrites of SGNs might affect the number and location of presynaptic ribbons. Inhibition of NMDARs successfully prevented gentamicin-induced ototoxicity by preventing the relocation of AMPARs and NMDARs on the dendrites of the SGNs and thus maintaining the integrity of the ribbon synapses and preserving hearing function.

Authors' Contributions

Juan Hong, Peidong Dai, and Huawei Li conceived and designed the experiments. Juan Hong, Yan Chen, Yanping Zhang, Jieying Li, Liujie Ren, Lin Yang, Tianyu Zhang, Lusen Shi, and Ao Li performed the experiments. Juan Hong and Yan Chen analyzed the data. Juan Hong, Yan Chen, Huawei Li, and Peidong Dai drafted and revised the manuscript. Juan Hong and Yan Chen contributed equally to this work.

Acknowledgments

The authors wish to thank Dan You, Xiaoling Lu, Dongmei Tang, Wenli Ni, and Chenlong Li of the Eye and ENT Hospital of Fudan University for help in the experiment. The authors also thank Jin Li and Yalin Huang of the Institutes of Biomedical Sciences of Fudan University for providing technical support with the confocal microscope. This work was supported by grants from the National Science and Technology Support Program, China (Grant no. 2015BAK31B01), the National Key R&D Program of China (Grant nos. 2017YFA0103900, 2016YFC0905200), the National Natural Science Foundation of China (Grant nos. 81620108005, 81230019, 81570911, 81470687, and 81771010), the Natural Science Foundation of Zhejiang Province of China (Grant no. LY14H130002), and the Science and Technology Plan Project of Wenzhou City of China (Grant no. Y20130223).

Supplementary Materials

Supplementary Table 1: the number of presynaptic ribbons, postsynaptic AMPARs, and ribbon synaptic pairs in different groups. Supplementary Table 2: the number of the AMPARs and NMDARs at the IHC-SGN synapse in different groups. Legends of supplemental videos: Supplemental Video 1: spatial distribution of NMDARs and AMPARs in the IHC-SGN synapse of normal mouse mature cochlea. Supplemental Video 2: spatial distribution of NMDARs and AMPARs in the IHC-SGN synapse of gentamicin treated mouse cochlea (GM 7d). Supplemental Video 3: spatial distribution of ribbons and AMPARs in the IHC-SGN synapse of normal mouse mature cochlea. Supplemental Video 4: spatial distribution of ribbons and AMPARs in the IHC-SGN synapse of gentamicin-treated mouse cochlea (GM 4d). Supplemental Video 5: spatial distribution of ribbons and AMPARs in the IHC-SGN synapse of gentamicin and MK801-treated mouse cochlea (GM + MK 4d). (Supplementary Materials)

References

[1] S. L. Johnson, T. Eckrich, S. Kuhn et al., "Position-dependent patterning of spontaneous action potentials in immature cochlear inner hair cells," Nature Neuroscience, vol. 14, no. 6, pp. 711–717, 2011.

[2] R. Nouvian, D. Beutner, T. D. Parsons, and T. Moser, "Structure and function of the hair cell ribbon synapse," The Journal of Membrane Biology, vol. 209, no. 2-3, pp. 153–165, 2006.

[3] K. Liu, X. Jiang, C. Shi et al., "Cochlear inner hair cell ribbon synapse is the primary target of ototoxic aminoglycoside stimuli," Molecular Neurobiology, vol. 48, no. 3, pp. 647–654, 2013.

[4] S. G. Kujawa and M. C. Liberman, "Adding insult to injury: cochlear nerve degeneration after "temporary" noise-induced hearing loss," The Journal of Neuroscience, vol. 29, no. 45, pp. 14077–14085, 2009.

[5] S. G. Kujawa and M. C. Liberman, "Synaptopathy in the noise-exposed and aging cochlea: primary neural degeneration in acquired sensorineural hearing loss," Hearing Research, vol. 330, Part B, pp. 191–199, 2015.

[6] M. Lafon-Cazal, S. Pietri, M. Culcasi, and J. Bockaert, "NMDA-dependent superoxide production and neurotoxicity," Nature, vol. 364, no. 6437, pp. 535–537, 1993.

[7] L. D. Liberman, J. Suzuki, and M. C. Liberman, "Dynamics of cochlear synaptopathy after acoustic overexposure," Journal of the Association for Research in Otolaryngology, vol. 16, no. 2, pp. 205–219, 2015.

[8] K. Liu, D. Chen, W. Guo et al., "Spontaneous and partial repair of ribbon synapse in cochlear inner hair cells after ototoxic withdrawal," Molecular Neurobiology, vol. 52, no. 3, pp. 1680–1689, 2015.

[9] S. Usami, A. Matsubara, S. Fujita, H. Shinkawa, and M. Hayashi, "NMDA (NMDAR1) and AMPA-type (GluR2/3) receptor subunits are expressed in the inner ear," Neuroreport, vol. 6, no. 8, pp. 1161–1164, 1995.

[10] E. Soto, A. Flores, C. Ero´stegui, and R. Vega, "Evidence for NMDA receptor in the afferent synaptic transmission of the vestibular system," Brain Research, vol. 633, no. 1-2, pp. 289–296, 1994.

[11] J. Ruel, C. Chabbert, R. Nouvian et al., "Salicylate enables Cochlear arachidonic-acid-sensitive NMDA receptor responses," The Journal of Neuroscience, vol. 28, no. 29, pp. 7313–7323, 2008.

[12] M. Knipper, P. Van Dijk, I. Nunes, L. Ruttiger, and U. Zimmermann, "Advances in the neurobiology of hearing disorders: recent developments regarding the basis of tinnitus and hyperacusis," Progress in Neurobiology, vol. 111, pp. 17–33, 2013.

[13] Y. Zhang-Hooks, A. Agarwal, M. Mishina, and D. E. Bergles, "NMDA receptors enhance spontaneous activity and promote neuronal survival in the developing cochlea," Neuron, vol. 89, no. 2, pp. 337–350, 2016.

[14] Z. Chen, S. G. Kujawa, and W. F. Sewell, "Auditory sensitivity regulation via rapid changes in expression of surface AMPA receptors," Nature Neuroscience, vol. 10, no. 10, pp. 1238–1240, 2007.

[15] A. S. Basile, J. M. Huang, C. Xie, D. Webster, C. Berlin, and P. Skolnick, "N-methyl-D-aspartate antagonists limit aminoglycoside antibiotic-induced hearing loss," Nature Medicine, vol. 2, no. 12, pp. 1338–1343, 1996.

[16] J. A. Segal, B. D. Harris, Y. Kustova, A. Basile, and P. Skolnick, "Aminoglycoside neurotoxicity involves NMDA receptor activation," Brain Research, vol. 815, no. 2, pp. 270–277, 1999.

[17] M. Duan, K. Agerman, P. Ernfors, and B. Canlon, "Complementary roles of neurotrophin 3 and a N-methyl-D-aspartate antagonist in the protection of noise and aminoglycoside-induced ototoxicity," Proceedings of the National Academy of Sciences of the United States of America, vol. 97, no. 13, pp. 7597–7602, 2000.

[18] E. Selimoglu, "Aminoglycoside-induced ototoxicity," Current Pharmaceutical Design, vol. 13, no. 1, pp. 119–126, 2007.

[19] L. Chen, S. Xiong, Y. Liu, and X. Shang, "Effect of different gentamicin dose on the plasticity of the ribbon synapses in cochlear inner hair cells of C57BL/6J mice," Molecular Neurobiology, vol. 46, no. 2, pp. 487–494, 2012.

[20] H. Li and P. S. Steyger, "Systemic aminoglycosides are trafficked via endolymph into cochlear hair cells," Scientific Reports, vol. 1, no. 1, p. 159, 2011.

[21] P. Singer, D. Boison, H. Mohler, J. Feldon, and B. K. Yee, "Modulation of sensorimotor gating in prepulse inhibition by conditional brain glycine transporter 1 deletion in mice," European Neuropsychopharmacology, vol. 21, no. 5, pp. 401–413, 2011.

[22] A. S. de Miranda, F. Brant, L. B. Vieira et al., "A neuroprotective effect of the glutamate receptor antagonist MK801 on long-term cognitive and behavioral outcomes secondary to experimental cerebral malaria," Molecular Neurobiology, vol. 54, no. 9, pp. 7063–7082, 2017.

[23] L. Liu, Y. Chen, J. Qi et al., "Wnt activation protects against neomycin-induced hair cell damage in the mouse cochlea," *Cell Death & Disease*, vol. 7, no. 3, article e2136, 2016.

[24] S. Sun, H. Yu, H. Yu et al., "Inhibition of the activation and recruitment of microglia-like cells protects against neomycin-induced ototoxicity," *Molecular Neurobiology*, vol. 51, no. 1, pp. 252–267, 2015.

[25] E. Lobarinas, C. Spankovich, and C. G. le Prell, "Evidence of "hidden hearing loss" following noise exposures that produce robust TTS and ABR wave-I amplitude reductions," *Hearing Research*, vol. 349, pp. 155–163, 2017.

[26] W. Ni, C. Lin, L. Guo et al., "Extensive supporting cell proliferation and mitotic hair cell generation by *in vivo* genetic reprogramming in the neonatal mouse cochlea," *The Journal of Neuroscience*, vol. 36, no. 33, pp. 8734–8745, 2016.

[27] Y. Yuan, F. Shi, Y. Yin et al., "Ouabain-induced cochlear nerve degeneration: synaptic loss and plasticity in a mouse model of auditory neuropathy," *Journal of the Association for Research in Otolaryngology*, vol. 15, no. 1, pp. 31–43, 2014.

[28] X. Lu, S. Sun, J. Qi et al., "Bmi1 regulates the proliferation of cochlear supporting cells via the canonical Wnt signaling pathway," *Molecular Neurobiology*, vol. 54, no. 2, pp. 1326–1339, 2017.

[29] M. C. Liberman, "Noise-induced and age-related hearing loss: new perspectives and potential therapies," *F1000Res*, vol. 6, p. 927, 2017.

[30] D. O. J. Reijntjes and S. J. Pyott, "The afferent signaling complex: regulation of type I spiral ganglion neuron responses in the auditory periphery," *Hearing Research*, vol. 336, pp. 1–16, 2016.

[31] D. Bing, S. C. Lee, D. Campanelli et al., "Cochlear NMDA receptors as a therapeutic target of noise-induced tinnitus," *Cellular Physiology and Biochemistry*, vol. 35, no. 5, pp. 1905–1923, 2015.

[32] P. E. Schauwecker, "Neuroprotection by glutamate receptor antagonists against seizure-induced excitotoxic cell death in the aging brain," *Experimental Neurology*, vol. 224, no. 1, pp. 207–218, 2010.

[33] A. C. Meyer, T. Frank, D. Khimich et al., "Tuning of synapse number, structure and function in the cochlea," *Nature Neuroscience*, vol. 12, no. 4, pp. 444–453, 2009.

[34] J. Ruel, C. Chen, R. Pujol, R. P. Bobbin, and J. L. Puel, "AMPA-preferring glutamate receptors in cochlear physiology of adult guinea-pig," *The Journal of Physiology*, vol. 518, no. 3, pp. 667–680, 1999.

[35] E. Glowatzki and P. A. Fuchs, "Transmitter release at the hair cell ribbon synapse," *Nature Neuroscience*, vol. 5, no. 2, pp. 147–154, 2002.

[36] J. Ruel, J. Wang, G. Rebillard et al., "Physiology, pharmacology and plasticity at the inner hair cell synaptic complex," *Hearing Research*, vol. 227, no. 1-2, pp. 19–27, 2007.

[37] L. Grant, E. Yi, and E. Glowatzki, "Two modes of release shape the postsynaptic response at the inner hair cell ribbon synapse," *The Journal of Neuroscience*, vol. 30, no. 12, pp. 4210–4220, 2010.

[38] S. F. Traynelis, L. P. Wollmuth, C. J. McBain et al., "Glutamate receptor ion channels: structure, regulation, and function," *Pharmacological Reviews*, vol. 62, no. 3, pp. 405–496, 2010.

[39] J. T. R. Isaac, M. C. Ashby, and C. J. McBain, "The role of the GluR2 subunit in AMPA receptor function and synaptic plasticity," *Neuron*, vol. 54, no. 6, pp. 859–871, 2007.

[40] J. T. Sanchez, S. Ghelani, and S. Otto-Meyer, "From development to disease: diverse functions of NMDA-type glutamate receptors in the lower auditory pathway," *Neuroscience*, vol. 285, pp. 248–259, 2015.

[41] D. Liao, N. A. Hessler, and R. Malinow, "Activation of postsynaptically silent synapses during pairing-induced LTP in CA1 region of hippocampal slice," *Nature*, vol. 375, no. 6530, pp. 400–404, 1995.

[42] C. G. D'Aldin, J. Ruel, R. Assie, R. Pujol, and J. L. Puel, "Implication of NMDA type glutamate receptors in neural regeneration and neoformation of synapses after excitotoxic injury in the guinea pig cochlea," *International Journal of Developmental Neuroscience*, vol. 15, no. 4-5, pp. 619–629, 1997.

[43] I. J. Reynolds and T. G. Hastings, "Glutamate induces the production of reactive oxygen species in cultured forebrain neurons following NMDA receptor activation," *The Journal of Neuroscience*, vol. 15, no. 5, pp. 3318–3327, 1995.

[44] Y. Wang and Z. H. Qin, "Molecular and cellular mechanisms of excitotoxic neuronal death," *Apoptosis*, vol. 15, no. 11, pp. 1382–1402, 2010.

[45] R. C. Ewald and H. T. Cline, "NMDA receptors and brain development," in *Biology of the NMDA Receptor*, A. M. Dongen, Ed., pp. 1–29, CRC Press/Taylor & Francis, Boca Raton, FL, USA, 2009.

[46] W.-Y. Lu, H.-Y. Man, W. Ju, W. S. Trimble, J. F. MacDonald, and Y. T. Wang, "Activation of synaptic NMDA receptors induces membrane insertion of new AMPA receptors and LTP in cultured hippocampal neurons," *Neuron*, vol. 29, no. 1, pp. 243–254, 2001.

[47] H. M. Sobkowicz, J. E. Rose, G. L. Scott, and C. V. Levenick, "Distribution of synaptic ribbons in the developing organ of Corti," *Journal of Neurocytology*, vol. 15, no. 6, pp. 693–714, 1986.

[48] J. R. Steinert, C. Kopp-Scheinpflug, C. Baker et al., "Nitric oxide is a volume transmitter regulating postsynaptic excitability at a glutamatergic synapse," *Neuron*, vol. 60, no. 4, pp. 642–656, 2008.

11

Antidepressant Effects of Probucol on Early-Symptomatic YAC128 Transgenic Mice for Huntington's Disease

Cristine de Paula Nascimento-Castro [ID],[1] Ana Claudia Wink [ID],[1] Victor Silva da Fônseca [ID],[1] Claudia Daniele Bianco [ID],[1] Elisa C. Winkelmann-Duarte [ID],[1] Marcelo Farina [ID],[2] Ana Lúcia S. Rodrigues,[2] Joana Gil-Mohapel [ID],[3] Andreza Fabro de Bem [ID],[2,4] and Patricia S. Brocardo [ID][1]

[1]Department of Morphological Sciences, Center of Biological Sciences, Universidade Federal de Santa Catarina, 88040-900 Florianópolis, SC, Brazil
[2]Department of Biochemistry, Center of Biological Sciences, Universidade Federal de Santa Catarina, 88040-900 Florianópolis, SC, Brazil
[3]Division of Medical Sciences, UBC Island Medical Program, University of Victoria, Victoria, BC, Canada V8W 2Y2
[4]Department of Physiological Science, Institute of Biological Science, University of Brasilia, Brasília, DF, Brazil

Correspondence should be addressed to Patricia S. Brocardo; patricia.brocardo@ufsc.br

Academic Editor: Tara Walker

Huntington's disease (HD) is an autosomal dominant neurodegenerative disorder caused by a trinucleotide expansion in the HD gene, resulting in an extended polyglutamine tract in the protein huntingtin. HD is traditionally viewed as a movement disorder, but cognitive and neuropsychiatric symptoms also contribute to the clinical presentation. Depression is one of the most common psychiatric disturbances in HD, present even before manifestation of motor symptoms. Diagnosis and treatment of depression in HD-affected individuals are essential aspects of clinical management in this population, especially owing to the high risk of suicide. This study investigated whether chronic administration of the antioxidant probucol improved motor and affective symptoms as well as hippocampal neurogenic function in the YAC128 transgenic mouse model of HD during the early- to mild-symptomatic stages of disease progression. The motor performance and affective symptoms were monitored using well-validated behavioral tests in YAC128 mice and age-matched wild-type littermates at 2, 4, and 6 months of age, after 1, 3, or 5 months of treatment with probucol (30 mg/kg/day via water supplementation, starting on postnatal day 30). Endogenous markers were used to assess the effect of probucol on cell proliferation (Ki-67 and proliferation cell nuclear antigen (PCNA)) and neuronal differentiation (doublecortin (DCX)) in the hippocampal dentate gyrus (DG). Chronic treatment with probucol reduced the occurrence of depressive-like behaviors in early- and mild-symptomatic YAC128 mice. Functional improvements were not accompanied by increased progenitor cell proliferation and neuronal differentiation. Our findings provide evidence that administration of probucol may be of clinical benefit in the management of early- to mild-symptomatic HD.

1. Introduction

Huntington's disease (HD) is an autosomal dominant neurodegenerative disorder that affects 10.6–13.7 individuals per 100,000 in Western populations (for review, see [1]). HD results from an expansion of cytosine-adenine-guanine (CAG) trinucleotide repeats in exon 1 of the HD gene, leading to an extended polyglutamine tract in the N-terminal of the huntingtin protein [2]. The length of the CAG repeat is inversely correlated with the age of the onset of motor symptoms, which on average occurs in midlife, between 35–50 years of age [3]. The diagnosis of HD is based on the presence of motor symptoms and a positive family history [4, 5]; however, cognitive and behavioral symptoms are common comorbidities in HD [6–8].

Psychiatric manifestations are very common in HD patients, and these include depression, anxiety, and irritability [8]. Sadness and depression appear to be two of the earliest symptoms observed at the onset of the disease, as reported by first-degree relatives [9]. Indeed, major depression is the most common comorbidity in presymptomatic HD carriers [10, 11], while suicide risk is almost four times greater in HD patients than in the general population [12]. Of note, although the depressive phenotype observed in HD patients does not seem to be correlated with cognitive impairment, the development of motor symptoms, or CAG repeat length [13], a depressive phenotype appears to be associated with a more rapid decline in functional ability [14, 15].

Yeast artificial chromosome (YAC) 128 mice express the full-length human *HD* gene with 128 CAG repeats [16] and exhibit reproducible cognitive [17–19] and motor [16, 19, 20] deficits, as well as depressive-like behaviors [20–22] that mimic the disease progression in humans. While the mechanisms underlying the depressive phenotype observed in both HD patients and HD transgenic mice are not fully elucidated, deficits in hippocampal neuroplasticity, namely, hippocampal neurogenesis, are likely to contribute to these mood disturbances in HD. Indeed, a reduction in adult hippocampal neurogenesis has been reported in truncated transgenic HD mice, namely, the R6/1 [23–26], R6/2 [27–31], and N171-82Q [32] lines, as well as full-length transgenic HD YAC128 mice [21, 33]. In addition, treatment with selective serotonin reuptake inhibitors (SSRIs), which have been shown to potentiate neurogenic function in the hippocampus [34–36], has been shown to improve the phenotype and promote neurogenesis in R6/1, R6/2, and N171-82Q HD mice [25, 29, 32], while also attenuating the progression of brain atrophy both in R6/2 and N171-82Q HD mice [29, 32].

Antioxidants are able to positively modulate adult hippocampal neurogenesis [37–39], and recent studies describing the neuroprotective effect of antioxidants on several neurologic disorders have been published [40]. Probucol is a phenolic lipid-lowering compound with antioxidant properties that has been used in clinical treatment and prevention of cardiovascular diseases [41]. However, neuroprotective properties of this compound have been recently described. For instance, probucol has the ability to increase neuroplasticity [42, 43]. Moreover, probucol was shown to promote neuroprotective effects in toxin-induced models of neurodegenerative diseases, including Alzheimer's disease (AD) [42, 44, 45], Parkinson's disease (PD) [46], and HD [47]. In the present study, we investigated the potential beneficial effects of chronic treatment with probucol on the depressive-like behaviors and hippocampal neurogenesis in early- and mild-symptomatic YAC128 HD transgenic mice.

2. Material and Methods

2.1. Animals. The YAC128 (HD53 line) transgenic mouse colony was maintained on the FVB/N background strain (Charles River, Quebec, Canada). All animals were generated from our local colony with breeding couples generously provided by Dr. Brian Christie (University of Victoria, Canada). Animals were weaned and ear-punched at postnatal day 22 and group-housed according to their sex (maximum of five mice per cage). YAC128 and their WT counterparts were maintained at 20–22°C with free access to water and food, under a 12/12 h light–dark cycle (lights on at 0700 h). All manipulations were carried out between 0900 and 1600 h. For behavioral experiments, animals were placed in the experimental room 24 h before testing to ensure proper acclimatization to the environment. All animal procedures were performed in accordance with the National Institutes of Health Guide for the Care and Use of Laboratory Animals and were approved by the Committee on Ethics of Animal Experimentation of the Federal University of Santa Catarina (Florianópolis, Brazil; protocol number: PP00944). All efforts were made to minimize animal suffering and to reduce the number of animals used in these experiments.

DNA was extracted from mouse ear tissue, and genotyping was performed by polymerase chain reaction (PCR), using primers for detection of YAC LYA (left YAC arm) and RYA (right YAC arm), as recently described by us [21].

2.2. Drugs and Treatments. Probucol (Sigma, St. Louis, MO, USA; 30 mg/kg/day) was diluted in carboxymethylcellulose (CMC), 1 mg/mL. The probucol dose was chosen based on previous studies that reported neuroprotective effects of this compound [48–50]. YAC128 and wild-type (WT) mice were randomly divided into four experimental groups (with equal numbers of males and females included in each group, 10 mice/group): 1 (WT vehicle), 2 (YAC128 vehicle), 3 (WT probucol), and 4 (YAC128 probucol). Probucol-treated WT and YAC128 mice received probucol in drinking water for 5 months (from 1 to 6 months of age). Vehicle-treated WT and YAC128 mice received vehicle (CMC) in drinking water during the same period of time (Figure 1).

2.3. Behavioral Analyses. YAC128 and WT mice treated with either vehicle or probucol were submitted to the open field test followed by the tail suspension test (TST) at 2, 4, and 6 months of age. The forced swim test (FST) and the rotarod test were also performed at both 4 and 6 months (Figure 1). Mice tested at 2, 4, and 6 months of age were on vehicle or probucol treatment for 1, 3, and 5 months, respectively.

2.3.1. Open Field Test (OFT). To assess the effects of probucol on exploratory capacity, mice were evaluated in the OFT as previously described [51]. Mice were individually placed in a wooden box measuring $40 \times 60 \times 50$ cm. The distance traveled and the time spent in the center of the arena were measured during a 6 min period. Tests were recorded using a digital video camera (HD Pro webcam C920 Logitech, CA, USA) and analyzed using the ANY-maze video-tracking system (Stoelting Co., Wood Dale, IL, USA).

2.3.2. Rotarod Test. To evaluate the effects of probucol on the development of motor deficits, the rotarod test was used as previously described [52, 53]. The rotarod apparatus consisted of a rod 30 cm long and 3 cm in diameter that was

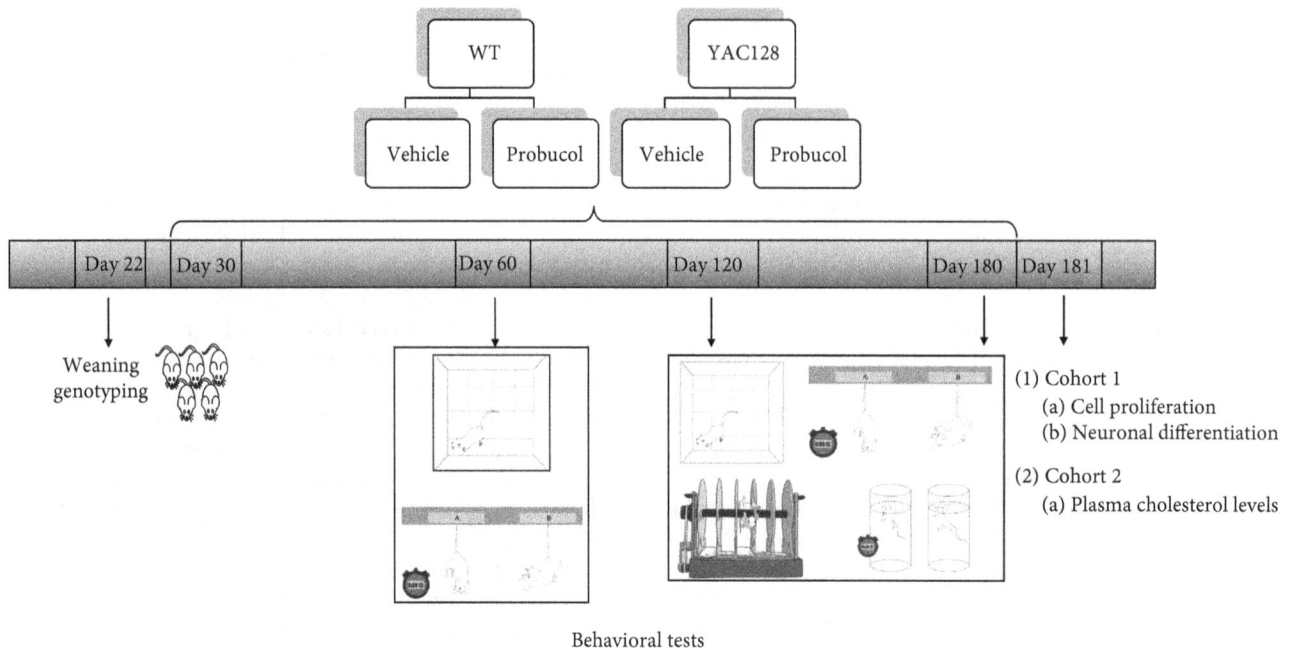

Behavioral tests

FIGURE 1: Experimental protocol. Thirty-day-old WT and YAC128 female and male mice received probucol (30 mg/kg/day) or vehicle (1% CMC) in drinking water for 5 months. Two distinct cohorts of animals were used. Animals from Cohort 1 were submitted to the tail suspension test (TST) and open field test (OFT) at 2, 4, and 6 months of age and to the forced swimming test (FST) and the rotarod test at 4 and 6 months. 24 h after the last behavioral test, mice were transcardially perfused; their brains were removed and processed for immunohistochemistry analyses of cell proliferation and neuronal differentiation. Animals from Cohort 2 were subjected to the same treatment regime and euthanized 24 hours after the last behavioral test to determine cholesterol plasma levels.

subdivided into four compartments (Insight®, São Paulo, Brazil). Before the test, mice were allowed to train for 60 s, at a constant speed of 5 rpm, for acclimation to the equipment. After a 2 h resting interval, each mouse was tested for four 5 min sessions on the rotarod, with a gradual acceleration rate from 5 to 37 rpm during each session and with a 30 min resting period between sessions. The latency to the first fall from the rotarod and the number of falls during each 5 min session were recorded.

2.3.3. Tail Suspension Test (TST).
The TST is useful in the screening of potential antidepressant drugs and other manipulations expected to affect depressive-like behaviors [54, 55]. In the TST, mice are placed in an inescapable and moderately stressful situation. In this test, immobility is interpreted as the absence of escape-related behaviors or helplessness. Briefly, acoustically and visually isolated mice were suspended 50 cm above the floor by adhesive tape placed approximately 1 cm from the tip of the tail for 6 minutes. Tests were recorded using a digital video camera (HD Pro webcam C920 Logitech, CA, USA) and analyzed by a highly trained observer blinded to the animals' identities. Animals were considered immobile when they hung passively and completely motionless. The total duration of immobility was measured according to the method described by [56].

2.3.4. Forced Swimming Test (FST).
Mice were individually forced to swim in an open cylindrical container (diameter, 10 cm; height, 25 cm) filled with water maintained at 25°C. The total duration of immobility during a 6 min period was

scored. Mice were judged to be immobile when they ceased struggling and remained floating motionless in the water, making only those movements necessary to keep their heads above the water [57].

2.4. Volumetric Analysis and Evaluation of Endogenous Hippocampal Cell Proliferation and Neuronal Differentiation

2.4.1. Tissue Processing.
Following behavioral analyses, one cohort of 6-month-old animals ($n = 5 - 6$ mice/group) was deeply anesthetized with an intraperitoneal (IP) injection of ketamine (100 mg/kg) and xylazine (8 mg/kg) and transcardially perfused with 0.9% sodium chloride followed by 4% paraformaldehyde (PFA). Brains were removed and left in 4% PFA overnight at 4°C and subsequently transferred to 30% sucrose. Following saturation in sucrose, serial coronal sections were obtained using a vibratome (Vibratome, Series 1000, St. Louis, MO, USA) at 30 μm thickness. Sections were collected into a 1/6 section-sampling fraction and stored in azide solution (0.5%) at 4°C.

2.4.2. Volumetric Analysis of the Total Hippocampus, the Dentate Gyrus Subregion, and the Striatum.
Nissl-stained coronal sections were used to estimate the total volume of the total hippocampal formation, the hippocampal dentate gyrus (DG) subregion, and the striatum. Images were captured with a ZEISS Axio Scan.Z1 scanner (Jena, Thuringia, Germany). Using the software ZEN Wildfield 2012 Blue Edition, the area of the whole hippocampus, the DG subregion, and the striatum was measured in each coronal section using

Cavalieri's principle. The volume was estimated using the following formula: $\sum A \times T \times I$, where $\sum A$ is the sum of the areas of each region of interest (whole hippocampus, DG subregion, or striatum), T is the section thickness (30 μm), and I is the number of section intervals (6).

2.4.3. Immunohistochemistry. Two adjacent series of sections were processed for detection of the endogenous proliferative markers Ki-67, a nuclear protein that is expressed during all active phases of the cell cycle, but is absent from cells at rest [58, 59], and proliferating cell nuclear antigen (PCNA), which is expressed during all active phases of the cell cycle and for a short period of time after cells become postmitotic [60]. Briefly, brain sections were incubated in citric acid (dissolved in 0.1 m TBS, pH = 6.0) for 5 min at 95°C. This process was repeated twice to ensure complete unmasking of the nuclear antigens. After quenching with 3% H_2O_2/10% methanol in 0.1 m PBS for 15 min and preincubation with 5% normal goat serum (NGS) for 1 h, sections were incubated for 48 h at 4°C with either a rabbit polyclonal anti-Ki-67 primary antibody (1 : 500; Vector Laboratories, Burlingame, CA, USA) or a rabbit polyclonal antibody against PCNA (1 : 100; Santa Cruz Biotechnology, Santa Cruz, CA, USA). After rinsing, sections were then incubated for 2 h with the secondary antibody (biotin-conjugated goat anti-rabbit IgG, 1 : 200; Vector Laboratories). Sections were incubated with the avidin–biotin–peroxidase complex (Vectastain ABC Elite Kit PK4000; Vector Laboratories) for 1 h, and the bound antibodies were visualized using 2,2-diaminobenzidine (DAB; DAB kit SK 4100; Vector Laboratories) as the chromogen. Sections were mounted onto 2% gelatin-coated microscope slides and dehydrated through a series of ethanol solutions of increasing concentrations (50, 70, and 95%) followed by a 5 min incubation in xylene (Synth, Diadema, SP, Brazil). Finally, slides were coverslipped with Entellan mounting medium (Merck, Darmstadt, Germany).

An additional series of brain sections containing the hippocampus was processed for immunohistochemistry against doublecortin (DCX), a microtubule-associated protein specifically expressed by newly differentiated and migrating neuroblasts (i.e., immature neurons) [61]. Briefly, after quenching with 3% H_2O_2/10% methanol in 0.1 m PBS for 15 min and preincubation with 5% normal horse serum (NHS) for 1 h, sections were incubated for 48 h at 4°C with a goat polyclonal anti-DCX primary antibody (1 : 400; C-18, Santa Cruz Biotechnology). Sections were then incubated for 2 h with the secondary antibody (biotin-conjugated horse anti-goat IgG, 1 : 200; Vector Laboratories). Bound antibodies were visualized as described above.

2.4.4. Morphological Quantification. All morphological analyses were performed on coded slides, with the experimenter blinded to the identity of the samples, using an Olympus IX83 microscope (Olympus, Hamburg, Germany) equipped with 10x, 20x, and 40x objectives (Olympus CellSens microscope imaging software (CellSens Dimension 1.2, Olympus)). A Peltier-cooled digital camera (Olympus DP73, Olympus) was used for image capturing. A modified stereological approach was used to estimate the total numbers of Ki-67-,

PCNA-, and DCX-positive cells present along the entire subgranular zone (SGZ) of the hippocampal DG as previously described [33]. All sections along the entire dorsal/ventral axis of the hippocampus that contained the DG subregion (i.e., from 1.34 mm posterior to the bregma to 3.52 mm posterior to the bregma [62]) were used for the analysis, resulting in 10–12 DG-containing sections per brain. All positive cells present along the entire SGZ of each DG section and located within two to three cell diameters below the granule cell layer (GCL) were counted. The results were expressed as the total number of labeled cells in the DG subregion of the hippocampus by multiplying the average number of labeled cells/ DG section by the total number of 30 μm thick-sections containing the DG (estimated to be 73 sections in the mouse brain), and these values were expressed by DG volume. Images were processed with Adobe Photoshop 4.0 (Adobe Systems, Mountain View, CA, USA). Only contrast enhancements and color level adjustments were made; otherwise, images were not digitally manipulated.

2.5. Total Plasma Cholesterol Levels. A separate cohort of 6-month-old animals ($n = 5$ mice/group) was euthanized by rapid decapitation for blood sample collection. The total plasma cholesterol levels were determined by an enzymatic colorimetric method, using commercial kit reagents (Labtest Diagnostica®, Lagoa Santa, MG, Brazil), according to the manufacturer's instructions. The total cholesterol levels were expressed in mg/dL.

2.6. Statistical Analyses. All statistical comparisons were performed using the Statistica 10 analytical software (StatSoft Inc., Tulsa, OK, USA). Results were expressed as mean ± standard error of the mean (SEM). Behavioral data were analyzed with repeated measures analysis of variance (ANOVA). Histological (i.e., volumetric) and immunohistochemical data were analyzed with two-way ANOVA for genotype and treatment followed by the Duncan post hoc test when appropriate. A P value of < 0.05 was considered to be statistically significant.

3. Results

3.1. Effects of Chronic Probucol Treatment on Depressive-Like Behavior in YAC128 Mice. To assess the occurrence of depressive-like behaviors, YAC128 and their age-matched WT counterparts were subjected to the TST at 2, 4, and 6 months of age and to the FST at 4 and 6 months of age. Repeated measures ANOVA indicated a significant main effect of genotype at 2, 4, and 6 months of age [$F(3, 34) = 8.21$, $P < 0.01$], with YAC128 mice showing an increase in immobility when compared to WT mice at all time points tested (2 months: $P < 0.05$ and 4 and 6 months: $P < 0.01$). In addition, a significant genotype versus probucol interaction was also noted [$F(3, 34) = 4.31$, $P \leq 0.01$]. Further post hoc analyses indicated that treatment with probucol was able to reverse the depressive-like behavior exhibited by YAC128 at 4 ($P \leq 0.01$) and 6 ($P < 0.01$) months of age, as demonstrated by a significant decrease in the immobility time in the TST (Figure 2(a)). With regard to the FST, repeated

(a)

(b)

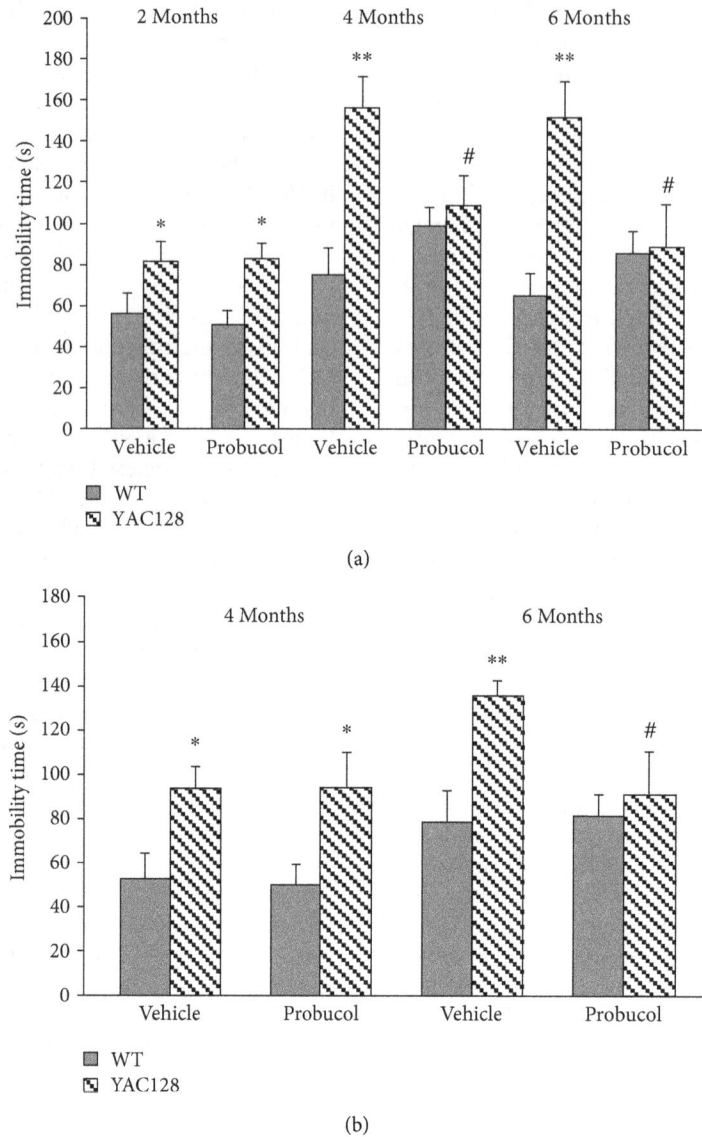

FIGURE 2: Antidepressant-like effects of chronic probucol treatment (30 mg/kg/day) on WT and YAC128 mice as assessed with the tail suspension test and forced swimming test. The total immobility time in the TST (a) and FST (b) was determined, and values are represented as mean ± SEM ($n = 10$ mice/group). Results were compared with repeated measures ANOVA followed by the Duncan post hoc test. $^*P < 0.05$ and $^{**}P < 0.01$ when compared to vehicle-treated WT animals, and $^\#P < 0.05$ when compared to vehicle-treated YAC128 mice.

measures ANOVA indicated a significant main effect of genotype $[F(2, 35) = 9.91, P < 0.01]$, with YAC128 mice showing an increase in immobility when compared to WT mice at both 4 and 6 months of age (4 months: $P < 0.05$ and 6 months: $P < 0.01$). Further post hoc analyses indicated that treatment with probucol was able to reverse the depressive-like behavior exhibited by YAC128 at 6 months of age ($P < 0.05$), as demonstrated by a significant decrease in the immobility time in the FST (Figure 2(b)).

3.2. Effects of Chronic Probucol Treatment on Motor Ability in YAC128 Mice. To discard any potential effects of probucol treatment on exploratory capacity and overall activity (which could potentially affect performance in the TST and FST), the distance traveled (in meters) and the time spent in the center

of the arena during a 6 min period were assessed by the OFT. A repeated measures ANOVA failed to detect any statistically significant effects of treatment $[F(3, 34) = 1.72, P = 0.18]$ and genotype $[F(3, 34) = 0.42, P = 0.73]$ and no significant genotype versus probucol interaction $[F(3, 34) = 0.40, P = 0.75]$ on this parameter. Thus, YAC128 mice at 2, 4, and 6 months of age showed similar exploratory behavior and overall activity as their age-matched WT controls, regardless of probucol treatment (Figure 3(a)). On the other hand, a repeated measures ANOVA revealed a significant effect of genotype with regard to the time spent in the center of the arena $[F(3, 34) = 4.06, P = 0.01]$, with 2-month-old mice spending significantly less time in the center when compared with their wild-type littermate controls ($P < 0.01$). However, no significant effect of treatment $[F(3, 34) = 0.25, P = 0.86]$ and no

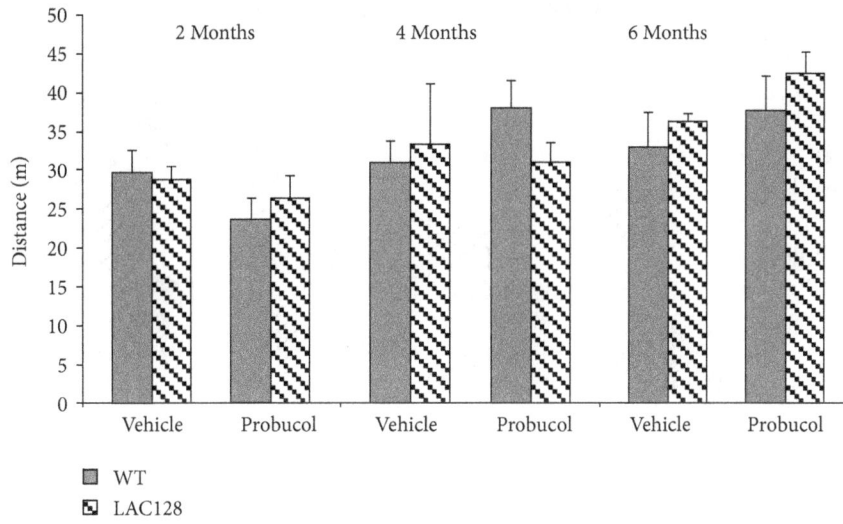

(a)

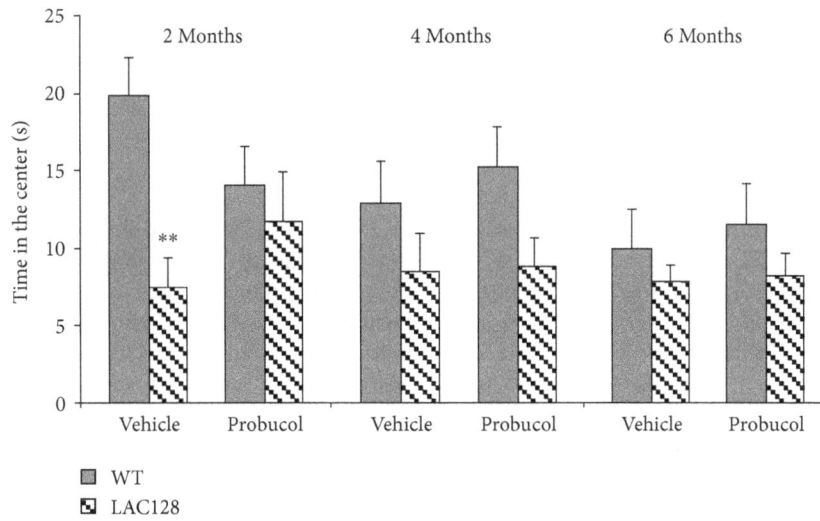

(b)

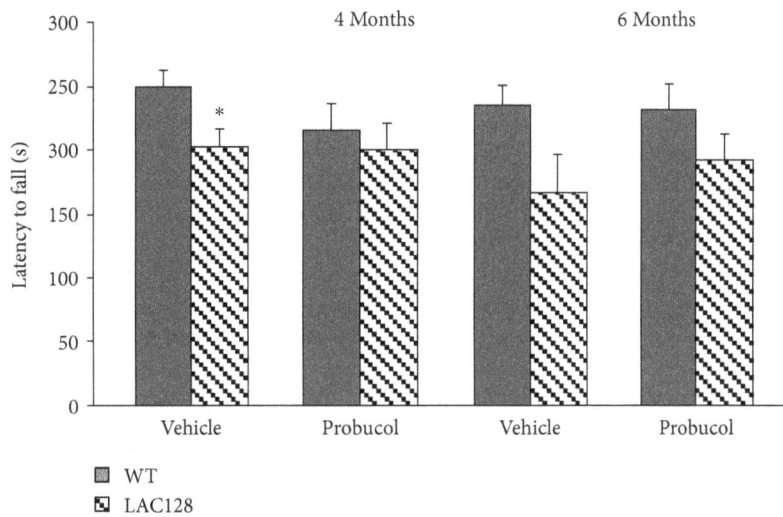

(c)

FIGURE 3: Continued.

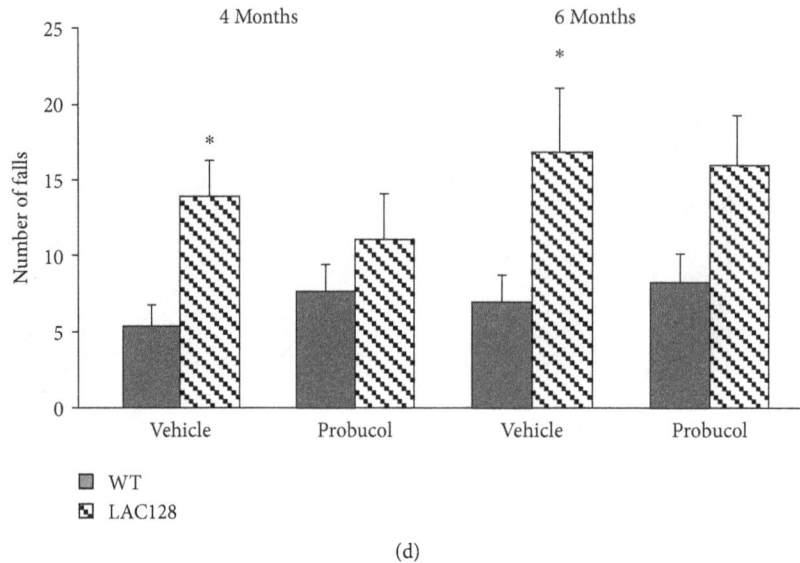

(d)

FIGURE 3: Effects of chronic treatment with probucol (30 mg/kg/day) on locomotion and motor balance in WT and YAC128 mice as assessed with the open field test (a and b) and the rotarod test (c and d). The distance traveled in the open field (a) and the time spent in the center of the open field (b) and the latency for the first fall (c) and the number of falls (d) in the rotarod were evaluated, and values are represented as mean ± SEM ($n = 8 - 10$ mice/group). Results were compared with repeated measures ANOVA followed by the Duncan post hoc test. $^*P < 0.05$ when compared with the WT group and $^{**}P < 0.01$.

significant genotype versus treatment interaction [$F(3, 34) = 1.84, P = 0.16$] were detected (Figure 3(b)).

To determine the effect of chronic probucol administration on motor coordination and balance, the performance of 4- and 6-month-old YAC128 and their age-matched WT controls was assessed in the rotarod. Repeated measures ANOVA revealed a significant main effect of genotype [$F(2, 27) = 3.85, P < 0.05$], but no significant main effect of treatment [$F(2, 27) = 0.80, P = 0.45$] nor a significant treatment versus genotype interaction [$F(2, 27) = 0.50, P = 0.60$] were detected with regard to the latency to the first fall (Figure 3(c)). Further post hoc analyses indicated a significant decrease in the latency to fall in 6-month-old YAC128 mice as compared with their WT littermates ($P < 0.05$). Similarly, a repeated measures ANOVA also revealed a significant main effect of genotype [$F(2, 27) = 5.18, P \leq 0.01$], but no significant main effect of treatment [$F(2, 27) = 0.01, P = 0.98$] nor a significant treatment versus genotype interaction [$F(2, 27) = 0.65, P = 0.52$] were detected with regard to the number of falls. Further post hoc analysis revealed an increase in the number of falls in both 4- and 6-month-old YAC128 mice as compared with their WT littermates ($P < 0.05$; Figure 3(d)).

3.3. Effects of Chronic Probucol Treatment on Hippocampal and Striatal Volume.
To determine whether gross changes in the hippocampus and striatum could be detected during the early stages of disease progression in the YAC128 mouse model and whether probucol treatment could reverse such alterations, we estimated the volume of the whole hippocampus, its DG subregion (given its relevance for neurogenesis), and the striatum. A two-way ANOVA revealed a significant effect of genotype [$F(1, 16) = 13.37, P < 0.01$] but no

significant effect of probucol treatment [$F(1, 16) = 0.04, P = 0.83$] nor an interaction between genotype and treatment [$F(1, 16) = 0.001, P = 0.97$] with regard to the volume of the whole hippocampus (Figure 4(a)). Further post hoc analyses indicated a significant decrease in hippocampal volume in 6-month-old YAC128 mice as compared with their WT littermates ($P < 0.05$). Similarly, a two-way ANOVA revealed a significant effect of genotype [$F(1, 16) = 6.62, P < 0.05$] but no significant effect of probucol treatment [$F(1, 16) = 1.26, P = 0.27$] nor an interaction between genotype and treatment [$F(1, 16) = 3.27, P = 0.09$] with regard to the volume of the hippocampal DG subregion (Figure 4(b)). Further post hoc analyses indicated a significant decrease in the volume of the DG subregion in 6-month-old YAC128 mice as compared with their WT littermates ($P < 0.05$). Moreover, a two-way ANOVA revealed a significant effect of genotype [$F(1, 12) = 39.98, P < 0.01$] but no significant effect of probucol treatment [$F(1, 12) = 0.06, P = 0.81$] nor an interaction between genotype and treatment [$F(1, 12) = 0.35, P = 0.56$] with regard to striatal volume (Figure 4(c)). Further post hoc analyses indicated a significant decrease in striatal volume in 6-month-old YAC128 mice as compared with their WT littermates ($P < 0.01$).

3.4. Effects of Chronic Probucol Treatment on Hippocampal Cell Proliferation on 6-Month-Old YAC128 Mice.
To analyze the potential effects of probucol on DG cell proliferation in YAC128 mice, we used the endogenous proliferation markers Ki-67 and PCNA [58–60]. A two-way ANOVA revealed no significant effects of genotype [$F(1, 20) = 2.79, P < 0.11$] and treatment [$F(1, 20) = 0.14, P = 0.70$] and no significant interaction between genotype and treatment [$F(1, 20) = 0.34, P = 0.56$] with regard to the density of Ki-67-positive

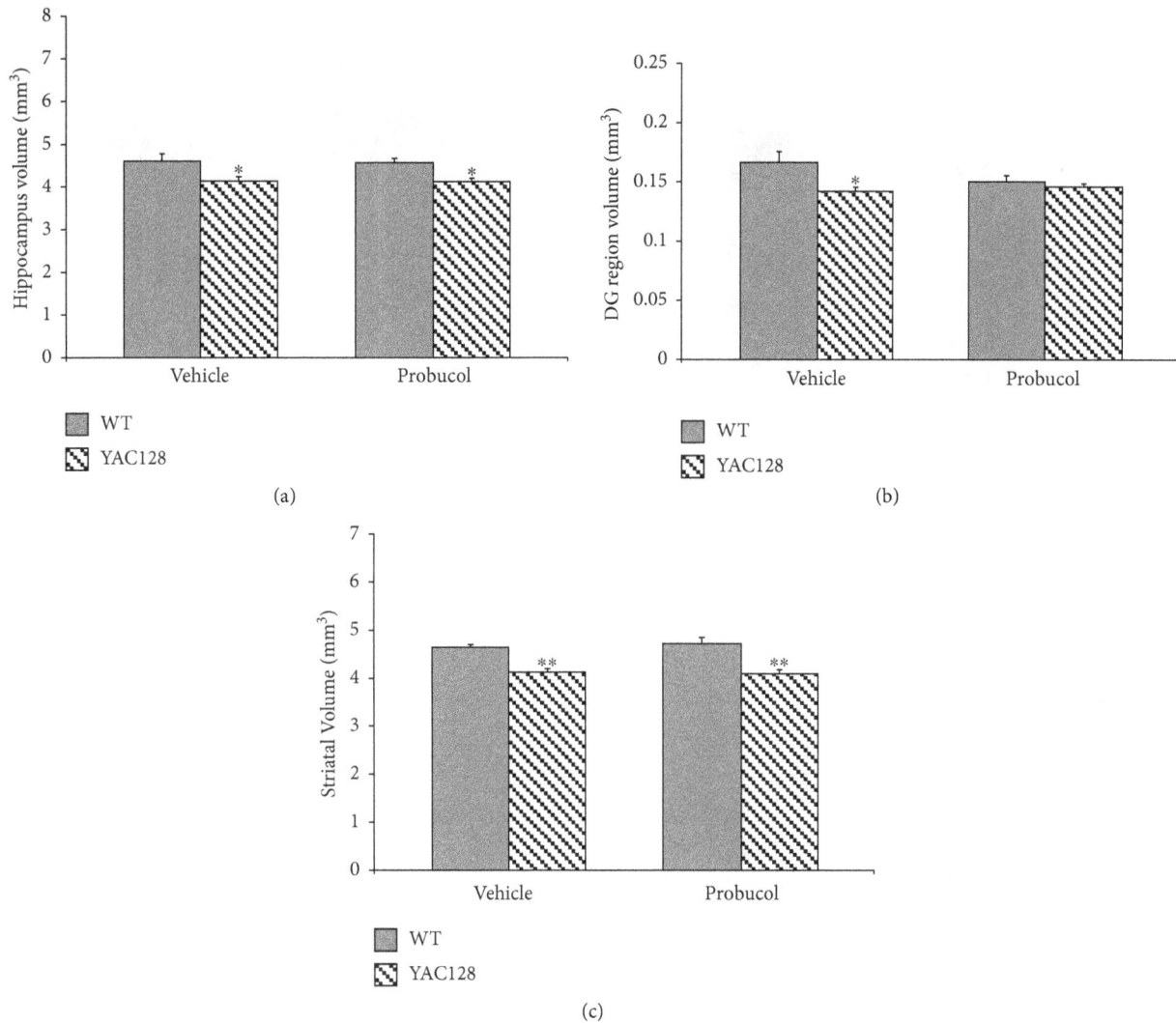

(a)

(b)

(c)

Figure 4: Volumetric analysis of the total hippocampus (a), the hippocampal DG subregion (b), and the striatum (c) in 6-month-old WT and YAC128 mice. Data are presented as mean ± SEM (4-5 mice/group), and results were analyzed with two-way ANOVA followed by the Duncan post hoc test. $^*P < 0.05$ and $^{**}P < 0.01$ when compared with the WT group.

cells present along the entire SGZ of the hippocampal DG (Figures 5(a) and 5(b)). Similarly, no significant effects of genotype $[F(1, 20) = 0.37, P = 0.54]$ and treatment $[F(1, 20) = 0.77, P = 0.39]$ and no significant interaction between genotype and treatment $[F(1, 20) = 0.02, P = 0.87]$ were observed with regard to the density of PCNA-positive mitotic cells present with the hippocampal DG of 6-month-old YAC128 and WT mice (Figures 5(c) and 5(d)).

3.5. Effects of Chronic Probucol Treatment on Hippocampal Neuronal Differentiation in 6-Month-Old YAC128 Mice. To analyze the potential effects of probucol on DG neuronal differentiation in YAC128 mice, we used the endogenous marker DCX, a microtubule-binding protein that is expressed in newly differentiated and migrating neuroblasts [61]. A two-way ANOVA revealed a significant effect of genotype on the density of DCX-positive cells present along the entire SGZ of the hippocampal DG $[F(1, 16) = 11.48, P < 0.01]$. However, there was no significant effect of treatment $[F(1, 16) = 0.18, P = 0.66]$ and no significant interaction between genotype and treatment $[F(1, 16) = 0.33, P = 0.56]$ with regard to the density of DCX-positive neuroblasts. Further post hoc analyses revealed a significant decrease in the number of DCX-positive neuroblasts in 6-month-old YAC128 mice when compared to their WT littermates ($P \leq 0.01$). However, probucol treatment during 5 months did not significantly affect the decline in DCX-positive cells observed in the YAC128 DG (Figure 6).

3.6. Effects of Chronic Treatment with Probucol on Total Plasma Cholesterol Levels in YAC128 Mice. Plasma cholesterol levels in both WT and YAC128 (treated with either probucol or vehicle) are shown in Supplementary Figure 1. Two-way ANOVA revealed no significant effects of genotype $[F(1, 16) = 1.88, P = 0.18]$ and treatment $[F(1, 16) = 0.64, P = 0.43]$ and no significant genotype versus treatment interaction $[F(1, 16) = 0.30, P = 0.58]$ with regard to plasma cholesterol levels.

(a)

(b)

(c)

(d)

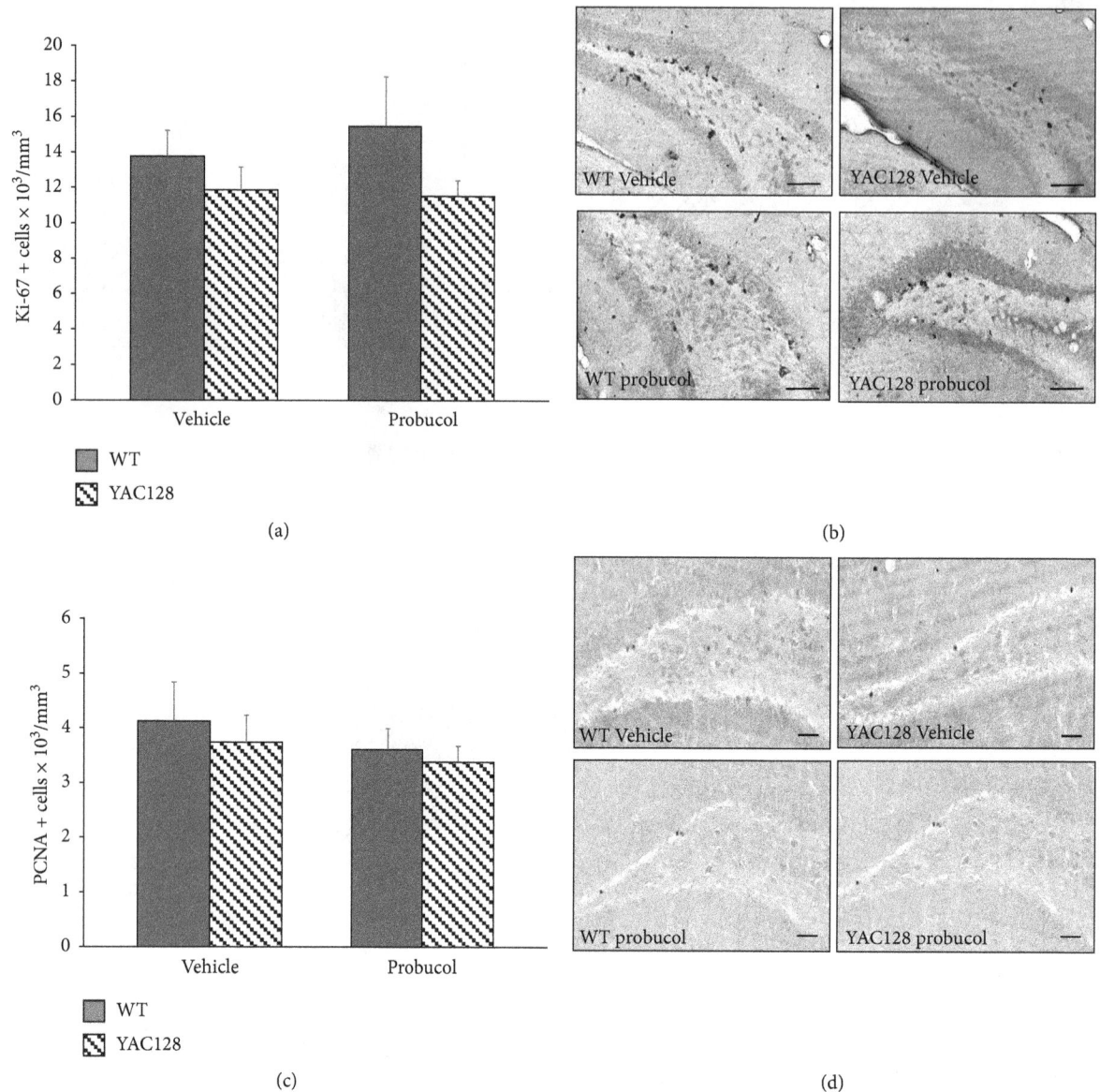

FIGURE 5: Evaluation of cell proliferation in the dentate gyrus of 6-month-old WT and YAC128 mice treated with probucol using endogenous cell cycle markers. Cell proliferation in the SGZ of the hippocampal DG was assessed by Ki-67- (a and b) and PCNA- (c and d) immunohistochemistry. Data are presented as mean ± SEM ($n = 6$ mice/group), and results were analyzed with two-way ANOVA followed by the Duncan post hoc test. Representative photomicrographs of Ki-67 (b) and PCNA (d) expression in the hippocampal DG of YAC128 and WT mice treated with either vehicle or probucol (scale bar = 50 μm).

4. Discussion

In the present study, YAC128 HD mice exhibited a depressive-like behavior as early as 2 months of age and this phenotype was maintained at least until animals reached 6 months of age, observed as a significant increase in the immobility time in the TST (at 2, 4, and 6 months of age) and FST (at 4 and 6 months of age). Previous studies have also observed the occurrence of depressive-like behaviors in this transgenic HD model starting at 3 months of age and progressing into later stages of the disease [18, 20, 22], and a recent study of our group has recapitulated this depressive phenotype in 3-month-old YAC128 mice [21]. In addition, several studies have reported the presence of depressive-like

behaviors during the early stages of disease progression in other HD transgenic mouse models such as the R6/1, N171-82Q, Hdh$^{Q111/Q11}$, and the bacterial artificial chromosome (BACH) models [22, 63–71]. Thus, the results reported in the present study corroborate these studies and further demonstrate that depressive-like behavior can be observed during the initial phase of the disease progression and as early as 2 months of age in the YAC128 HD transgenic mouse model. Of note, these results are in line with the symptoms observed in HD patients, highlighting the relevance of this transgenic mouse model in elucidating mechanisms concerned to the human disease.

The potential neuroprotective effect of chronic probucol treatment on mitigating the occurrence of depressive-like

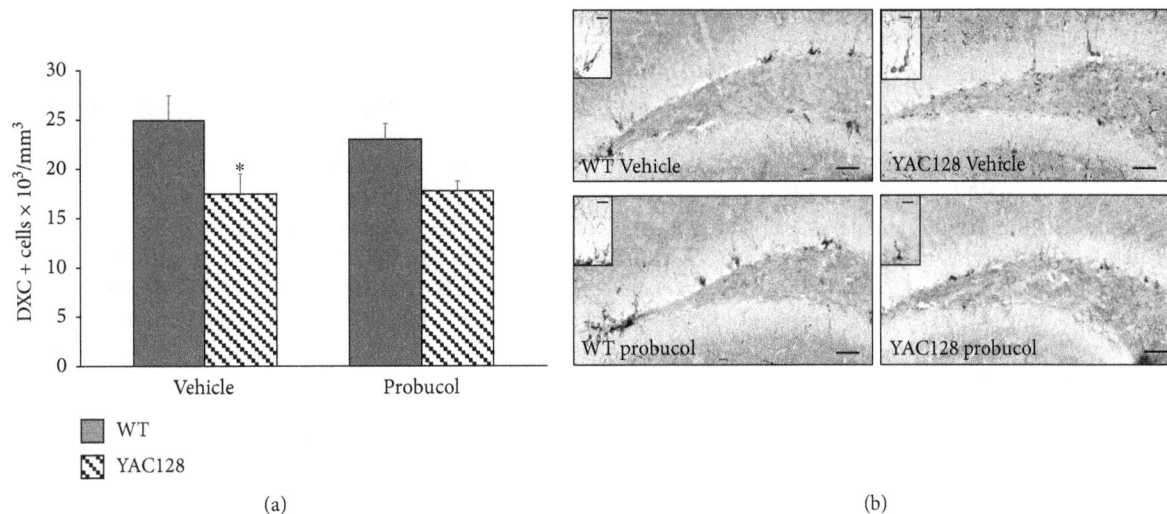

FIGURE 6: Evaluation of neuronal differentiation in the dentate gyrus of 6-month-old WT and YAC128 mice treated with vehicle or probucol using endogenous cell cycle markers. Neuronal differentiation in the SGZ of the hippocampal DG was assessed by DCX immunohistochemistry (a and b). Data are presented as mean ± SEM (5 mice/group), and results were analyzed with two-way ANOVA followed by the Duncan post hoc test. $^*P < 0.05$ when compared with the WT group. Representative photomicrographs of expression of DCX-positive cells (b) in the hippocampal DG of YAC128 and WT mice treated with either vehicle or probucol (scale bar = 50 μm or 20 μm, in detail).

behaviors in YAC128 mice was also investigated. Both WT and YAC128 mice received probucol in drinking water between 1 (i.e., before overt behavioral symptoms began) and 6 months of age. Our results show that chronic treatment (3 and 5 months, resp.) with probucol was able to prevent the occurrence of depressive-like behaviors in this HD transgenic mouse model at both 4 and 6 months of age. This is the first study showing a positive effect of probucol on regulating affective behaviors in a transgenic HD mouse model. The reduction in the immobility time elicited by probucol cannot be attributable to a psychostimulant action of this compound. This conclusion derives from the fact that in our study, probucol treatment produced a significant decrease in the immobility time in the FST or TST and did not alter the locomotor activity in animals as compared to control animals. However, a possible limitation of our study is the fact that repeating the open field test in the same animals can affect the performance in the test. For example, a significantly decreased time in the central area was only observed in the YAC128 mice at two months of age but not at later time points when animals are reexposed to the open field arena.

In this study, YAC128 mice presented motor deficits at 4 and 6 months of age, as shown by a significant reduction in rotarod latency time as well as a significant increase in the number of falls. Previous studies have demonstrated the presence of motor deficits in this HD transgenic mouse model at 3, 4 [18–20], and 6 [16] months of age. Pouladi et al. assessed motor dysfunction in these animals at 3 and 12 months of age and observed a significant worsening of motor performance at more advanced ages, demonstrating the progressive nature of this motor deficit [20]. Studies with other HD transgenic mouse models have demonstrated the presence of motor deficits in the BACH mice at 4 months of age [18], in the R6/1 at 2–5 months of age [25, 72], and

as early as 1 month in R6/2 mice [27]. Although probucol demonstrated a significant antidepressant-like effect, this compound was unable to reverse the motor deficits exhibited by YAC128 HD mice at both 4 and 6 months of age. Even though the reasons for this lack of effect are not currently understood, this confirms that distinct neuronal pathways and mechanisms mediate the depressive-like behaviors and motor deficits observed in YAC128 HD mice. Indeed, motor deficits are mainly a consequence of neuronal dysfunction in the striatum whereas the affective behaviors are likely the result of limbic system (i.e., hippocampal) dysfunction, and it is possible that probucol might act mainly by preventing hippocampal dysfunction (see discussion below). Nevertheless, probucol has been shown to attenuate motor impairment in a 3-nitropropionic (3-NP) lesion model of HD [47] and decrease hyperlocomotion induced by 6-hydroxydopamine (6-OHDA) in a mouse model of PD [46], showing that this compound might also be effective in improving motor deficits in models associated with more overt cell dysfunction and death (such as that observed in the 3-NP HD and 6-OHDA PD toxin-induced lesion models, which are characterized by a more acute damage).

Of note, the beneficial effects of probucol (a lipid-lowering compound) [73] were not associated with hypocholesterolemic effects, as no significant differences in the plasma levels of cholesterol were observed following 5 months of probucol treatment. Similar to various other studies [47, 74, 75], we did not find a significant effect of probucol treatment with regard to plasma cholesterol levels. There is a vast literature showing that the hypocholesterolemic effects of probucol are greatly dependent on the dose used, as well as on the animal species and/or strain employed. In fact, although probucol has been reported to display hypocholesterolemic effects in both humans and different animal species [73, 76], a significant number of studies were not able to replicate such effect. For example, [75] was unable to detect a significant effect of probucol treatment on serum cholesterol levels in rabbits following a 4-month treatment regimen (500 mg/kg/day). In line with this, in a key review article on the long-term use of probucol as a hypocholesterolemic drug, [77] reported that the results from different experimental and clinical studies with probucol were at times confusing and suggested that such discrepancies may be due, at least partly, to different experimental conditions, including type of subjects being studied (different animal species and/or strains and presence of diverse health conditions in humans), different diets, and varying treatment periods and drug doses. With respect to clinical studies, these same authors highlighted the fact that the hypocholesterolemic action of probucol is not equally observed in every patient [77].

The cardinal neuropathological characteristic of HD is striatal atrophy, with selective loss of striatal medium-sized gamma-aminobutiric acid (GABA)-ergic spiny neurons [78] with striatal neuronal atrophy and loss being strongly correlated with the development of the classic HD motor symptoms. Here, we found a significant decrease in striatal volume in 6-month-old YAC128 mice, a result that is in agreement with previous studies showing striatal atrophy in the YAC128 HD mouse model [16, 79–82]. However, as discussed earlier, other brain regions such as the hippocampus are also affected in HD [83–85], suggesting a role for this structure in affective disturbances, which are seen both in HD patients and transgenic mouse models for this disease. Indeed, we have also observed a decrease in the volume of the total hippocampus as well as of its DG subregion in 6-month-old YAC128 mice. Our results are in accordance with studies in diverse HD transgenic mouse models that have documented reduced cortical, globus pallidus, and hippocampal volumes [80, 86–89]. Moreover, in humans, Rosas et al. observed atrophy in several brain regions, including the hippocampus [85].

Furthermore, the hippocampus is one of the few regions of the brain that retains the ability to generate new neurons during adulthood. Several studies suggest that adult hippocampal neurogenesis plays a key role in psychiatric and neurological disorders, such as depression [90, 91]. Indeed, neuroimaging and meta-analysis studies have consistently demonstrated a reduction in hippocampal volume in individuals with depression [92–96]. In rodents, depression has been correlated with reduced adult hippocampal neurogenesis [97]. In addition, the fact that antidepressant treatment attenuates symptoms of depression while also positively regulating hippocampal neurogenesis [34, 35, 98] suggests a strong link between a reduction in adult hippocampal neurogenesis and the occurrence of depressive-like behaviors [99].

Given that YAC128 mice have decreased hippocampal cell proliferation and neuronal differentiation [21, 33] and that a deficit in neurogenesis has been postulated as an underlying cause of depression [97], in the present study, the effects of probucol treatment on adult hippocampal cell proliferation and neuronal differentiation in the YAC128 transgenic mouse model were also assessed. However, in the present study, no deficits in hippocampal cell proliferation (assessed with the Ki-67 and PCNA endogenous cell cycle markers) were observed in YAC128 mice at 6 months of age. This result is inconsistent with the work of Simpson et al., who observed a significant (albeit small) reduction in the number of Ki-67 positive cells but not of PCNA-positive cells in the hippocampal DG of YAC128 mice [33]. Other studies using truncated transgenic HD mice (R6/1 or R6/2) with ages between 2 and 5 months have also reported impairments in hippocampal cell proliferation using the endogenous cell cycle markers Ki-67 and PCNA [28], as well as the exogenous marker 5-bromo-2'-deoxyuridine (BrdU) [23, 26–28]. These discrepancies are likely due to differences between the transgenic mouse model used (the R6/2 model has a much faster and more severe disease progression [100], whereas the YAC128 model better replicates the slower disease progression observed in human HD patients [16, 38]) and how results are expressed in different studies (total cell numbers as in the case of the study by Simpson et al. [33] or cell densities as in the present study).

In addition, a significant decrease in the number of neuroblasts (DCX-positive immature neurons) in the YAC128 hippocampal DG was observed at 6 months of age. Again, these results are similar to those reported by Simpson et al., showing a significant decrease in hippocampal neuronal differentiation in this HD transgenic mouse model [33]. Other studies using truncated transgenic (R6/1 or R6/2) HD mice with ages between 1-2 months have also reported impairment in neuronal differentiation using the endogenous DCX marker [24, 28, 30, 31]. In contrast, Orvoen et al. failed to detect significant differences in the number of DCX-positive cells in the hippocampal DG of the truncated Hdh$^{Q111/Q111}$ mouse model. Nevertheless, these authors observed a deficit in dendritogenesis in the hippocampus of Hdh$^{Q111/Q111}$ mice [63], further supporting a compromised neuronal differentiation process in the HD brain. However, [64] observed no changes in neuronal differentiation (as assessed with DCX immunohistochemistry) in 3-month-old BACHD mice. Again, differences among the various transgenic mouse models and the genetic constructs they express are likely to account for these discrepancies. Moreover, we cannot exclude the fact that sex differences and/or estrous phase effects may have impacted the results reported here.

Probucol treatment for 5 months was unable to stimulate cell proliferation and hippocampal neuronal differentiation in 6-month-old YAC128 HD mice. Although probucol had no effect during these stages of the neurogenic process on the YAC128 mouse model, multiple mechanisms of action have been described for this compound, and therefore, it is likely that the beneficial effects reported in this study were mediated by an alternative mechanism. Indeed, probucol is a molecule with well-established anti-inflammatory and antioxidant properties [43–45, 47, 101–105], which is able to modulate the activity of endogenous antioxidant enzymes [44, 45, 47, 106], promote synaptic plasticity [42, 44], and increase the levels of brain-derived neurotrophic factor (BDNF) [43]. Of note, the antioxidant effect of probucol has been documented both in humans [102] and in animal models [44, 46]. Indeed, both *in vitro* and *in vivo* studies have demonstrated beneficial effects of probucol on models of neurodegenerative diseases such as AD [42, 44, 45], PD [46], and HD [47, 105], as well as cerebral endothelial dysfunction [43] and brain ischemia [48].

The etiology of neuronal loss in HD has not been fully elucidated, and therefore, several mechanisms have been proposed to contribute to neuronal dysfunction and death in the HD brain, including oxidative stress, synaptic dysfunction, and neurotransmitter dysregulation (e.g., glutamate-mediated excitotoxicity and dopamine-mediated toxicity), as well as a decrease in trophic support (namely, a reduction in BDNF levels; for review, see [107]). Previous studies have suggested that oxidative stress might not play a major role during the early and mild stages of disease progression in the YAC128 HD mouse model [108], and therefore, it is unlikely that the beneficial effects of probucol observed on the present study are mediated by a decrease in oxidative stress. Nevertheless, it is worth mentioning that probucol was able to counteract motor impairments and oxidative stress in a 3-NP lesion model of HD [47] as well as a 6-OHDA-lesion model of PD [46]. Again, this might be related to the fact that toxin-induced lesion models (such as the 3-NP HD and the 6-OHDA PD models) are associated with more acute and overt neuronal dysfunction and death as well as a marked increase in oxidative stress.

Synaptic dysfunction has been demonstrated in several animal models of HD [84, 109, 110], including early to mildly symptomatic YAC128 mice [111], and therefore, it is possible that the beneficial effects of probucol were the result of improved hippocampal synaptic plasticity. Of note, Santos et al. reported a significant decrease in the levels of synaptophysin in the hippocampus of a mouse model of AD ($A\beta 1$–40), a deficit that was reversed by probucol treatment [44]. In addition, this compound was also able to increase hippocampal levels of synaptosomal-associated protein 25 (SNAP-25) in 26-month-old rats [42]. SNAP-25 and synaptophysin are synaptic markers closely associated with synaptic vesicles and crucial for the processes of neurotransmission, synaptogenesis, and dendritic remodeling [112]. Whether such processes are impaired in the hippocampus of mildly symptomatic YAC128 mice is not currently known, and future studies are thus warranted to further elucidate this.

Stress, impaired neurogenesis, and defects in synaptic plasticity represent three interconnected factors that are associated with depression [113–115]. As a matter of fact, early-symptomatic YAC128 mice show alterations in short-term synaptic plasticity [111], and it is possible that probucol might have ameliorated these alterations, thus contributing to the antidepressant-like behavior observed. On the other hand, alterations in monoaminergic metabolism and neurotransmission (which are thought to contribute to the etiology of depression) have been extensively reported in human HD brains [116–120], and various preclinical studies have found a correlation between altered monoaminergic neurotransmission and the occurrence of depressive-like symptoms in transgenic mouse models of HD [67, 121]. Whether probucol can modulate monoaminergic neurotransmission is currently unknown, and future studies are warranted to test this hypothesis. Finally, although the hippocampus is a major

brain region in depression, other regions such as the prefrontal cortex, the cingulate cortex, the striatum, the amygdala, and the thalamus [122] have also been implicated in this mood disorder. All these regions are highly interconnected through complex neuronal circuits, and mood disorders are thought to alter these circuits. Thus, it seems reasonable to speculate that depression associated with HD may independently affect several of these circuits. Indeed, it is possible that the antidepressant-like effect of probucol may be related, at least in part, to the structural and functional preservation of these neuronal networks.

5. Conclusion

The results presented here demonstrate, for the first time, the beneficial effects of chronic probucol treatment on the occurrence of depressive-like behaviors in the YAC128 transgenic mouse model of HD. These beneficial effects of probucol were not related to an increase in hippocampal progenitor cell proliferation and neuronal differentiation. While future studies will further elucidate the underlying neuroprotective mechanisms of this compound, the present study indicates that probucol may be an effective modulator of depressive-like behaviors commonly observed during the early stages of HD.

Acknowledgments

The authors would like to thank Ruth Liliám Quispe Gaspar for her help with the genotyping process. Cristine de Paula Nascimento-Castro is supported by grants from Coordenação de Aperfeiçoamento de Pessoal de Nível Superior (CAPES). Ana Lúcia S. Rodrigues and Joana Gil-Mohapel acknowledge funding from the Science Without Borders funding program [Programa Ciência Sem Fronteiras/Conselho Nacional de Desenvolvimento Científico e Tecnológico (CNPq), Project no. 403120/2012-8] of the Brazilian Federal Government. Patricia S. Brocardo acknowledges funding from CNPq Project no. 480176/2013-2.

Supplementary Materials

Supplementary Figure 1: effects of chronic probucol treatment on cholesterol plasma levels in 6-month-old YAC128 mice and their WT littermate controls. Cholesterol levels are expressed as mg/dL. Values represent means ± SEM ($n = 5$ mice/group). No significant main effects of genotype and treatment and no significant interaction between genotype and treatment were found with regard to plasma cholesterol levels. *(Supplementary Materials)*

References

[1] G. P. Bates, R. Dorsey, J. F. Gusella et al., "Huntington disease," *Nature Reviews Disease Primers*, vol. 1, article 15005, 2015.

[2] M. Macdonald, "A novel gene containing a trinucleotide repeat that is expanded and unstable on Huntington's disease chromosomes," *Cell*, vol. 72, no. 6, pp. 971–983, 1993.

[3] L. W. Ho, J. Carmichael, J. Swartz, A. Wyttenbach, J. Rankin, and D. C. Rubinsztein, "The molecular biology of Huntington's disease," *Psychological Medicine*, vol. 31, no. 1, pp. 3–14, 2001.

[4] J. B. Penney, A. B. Young, I. Shoulson et al., "Huntington's disease in Venezuela: 7 years of follow-up on symptomatic and asymptomatic individuals," *Movement Disorders*, vol. 5, no. 2, pp. 93–99, 1990.

[5] S. E. Folstein, G. A. Chase, W. E. Wahl, A. M. McDonnell, and M. F. Folstein, "Huntington disease in Maryland: clinical aspects of racial variation," *American Journal of Human Genetics*, vol. 41, no. 2, pp. 168–179, 1987.

[6] K. Duff, J. S. Paulsen, L. J. Beglinger, D. R. Langbehn, J. C. Stout, and Predict-HD Investigators of the Huntington Study Group, "Psychiatric symptoms in Huntington's disease before diagnosis: the predict-HD study," *Biological Psychiatry*, vol. 62, no. 12, pp. 1341–1346, 2007.

[7] E. van Duijn, E. M. Kingma, R. Timman et al., "Cross-sectional study on prevalences of psychiatric disorders in mutation carriers of Huntington's disease compared with mutation-negative first-degree relatives," *The Journal of Clinical Psychiatry*, vol. 69, no. 11, pp. 1804–1810, 2008.

[8] S. Martinez-Horta, J. Perez-Perez, E. van Duijn et al., "Neuropsychiatric symptoms are very common in premanifest and early stage Huntington's disease," *Parkinsonism & Related Disorders*, vol. 25, pp. 58–64, 2016.

[9] S. C. Kirkwood, J. L. Su, P. M. Conneally, and T. Foroud, "Progression of symptoms in the early and middle stages of Huntington disease," *Archives of Neurology*, vol. 58, no. 2, pp. 273–278, 2001.

[10] E. A. Epping and J. S. Paulsen, "Depression in the early stages of Huntington disease," *Neurodegenerative Disease Management*, vol. 1, no. 5, pp. 407–414, 2011.

[11] W. Reedeker, R. C. van der Mast, E. J. Giltay, T. A. D. Kooistra, R. A. C. Roos, and E. van Duijn, "Psychiatric disorders in Huntington's disease: a 2-year follow-up study," *Psychosomatics*, vol. 53, no. 3, pp. 220–229, 2012.

[12] L. A. Farrer, J. M. Opitz, and J. F. Reynolds, "Suicide and attempted suicide in Huntington disease: implications for preclinical testing of persons at risk," *American Journal of Medical Genetics*, vol. 24, no. 2, pp. 305–311, 1986.

[13] B. Zappacosta, D. Monza, C. Meoni et al., "Psychiatric symptoms do not correlate with cognitive decline, motor symptoms, or CAG repeat length in Huntington's disease," *Archives of Neurology*, vol. 53, no. 6, pp. 493–497, 1996.

[14] L. J. Beglinger, J. J. O'Rourke, C. Wang et al., "Earliest functional declines in Huntington disease," *Psychiatry Research*, vol. 178, no. 2, pp. 414–418, 2010.

[15] J. M. Hamilton, D. P. Salmon, J. Corey-Bloom et al., "Behavioural abnormalities contribute to functional decline in Huntington's disease," *Journal of Neurology, Neurosurgery, and Psychiatry*, vol. 74, no. 1, pp. 120–122, 2003.

[16] E. J. Slow, J. van Raamsdonk, D. Rogers et al., "Selective striatal neuronal loss in a YAC128 mouse model of Huntington disease," *Human Molecular Genetics*, vol. 12, no. 13, pp. 1555–1567, 2003.

[17] J. M. Van Raamsdonk, J. Pearson, E. J. Slow, S. M. Hossain, B. R. Leavitt, and M. R. Hayden, "Cognitive dysfunction precedes neuropathology and motor abnormalities in the YAC128 mouse model of Huntington's disease," *The Journal of Neuroscience*, vol. 25, no. 16, pp. 4169–4180, 2005.

[18] M. A. Pouladi, L. M. Stanek, Y. Xie et al., "Marked differences in neurochemistry and aggregates despite similar behavioural and neuropathological features of Huntington disease in the full-length BACHD and YAC128 mice," *Human Molecular Genetics*, vol. 21, no. 10, pp. 2219–2232, 2012.

[19] A. L. Southwell, S. Franciosi, E. B. Villanueva et al., "Anti-semaphorin 4D immunotherapy ameliorates neuropathology and some cognitive impairment in the YAC128 mouse model of Huntington disease," *Neurobiology of Disease*, vol. 76, pp. 46–56, 2015.

[20] M. A. Pouladi, R. K. Graham, J. M. Karasinska et al., "Prevention of depressive behaviour in the YAC128 mouse model of Huntington disease by mutation at residue 586 of huntingtin," *Brain*, vol. 132, no. 4, pp. 919–932, 2009.

[21] V. S. da Fonsêca, A. R. da Silva Colla, C. de Paula Nascimento-Castro et al., "Brain-derived neurotrophic factor prevents depressive-like behaviors in early-symptomatic YAC128 Huntington's disease mice," *Molecular Neurobiology*, vol. 55, no. 9, pp. 7201–7215, 2018.

[22] C. T. Chiu, G. Liu, P. Leeds, and D. M. Chuang, "Combined treatment with the mood stabilizers lithium and valproate produces multiple beneficial effects in transgenic mouse models of Huntington's disease," *Neuropsychopharmacology*, vol. 36, no. 12, pp. 2406–2421, 2011.

[23] S. E. Lazic, H. Grote, R. J. E. Armstrong et al., "Decreased hippocampal cell proliferation in R6/1 Huntington's mice," *NeuroReport*, vol. 15, no. 5, pp. 811–813, 2004.

[24] S. E. Lazic, H. E. Grote, C. Blakemore et al., "Neurogenesis in the R6/1 transgenic mouse model of Huntington's disease: effects of environmental enrichment," *European Journal of Neuroscience*, vol. 23, no. 7, pp. 1829–1838, 2006.

[25] H. E. Grote, N. D. Bull, M. L. Howard et al., "Cognitive disorders and neurogenesis deficits in Huntington's disease mice are rescued by fluoxetine," *European Journal of Neuroscience*, vol. 22, no. 8, pp. 2081–2088, 2005.

[26] T. Renoir, T. Y. C. Pang, M. S. Zajac et al., "Treatment of depressive-like behaviour in Huntington's disease mice by chronic sertraline and exercise," *British Journal of Pharmacology*, vol. 165, no. 5, pp. 1375–1389, 2012.

[27] J. M. A. C. Gil, M. Leist, N. Popovic, P. Brundin, and Å. Petersén, "Asialoerythropoetin is not effective in the R6/2 line of Huntington's disease mice," *BMC Neuroscience*, vol. 5, no. 1, p. 17, 2004.

[28] J. M. A. C. Gil, P. Mohapel, I. M. Araújo et al., "Reduced hippocampal neurogenesis in R6/2 transgenic Huntington's disease mice," *Neurobiology of Disease*, vol. 20, no. 3, pp. 744–751, 2005.

[29] Q. Peng, N. Masuda, M. Jiang et al., "The antidepressant sertraline improves the phenotype, promotes neurogenesis and increases BDNF levels in the R6/2 Huntington's disease mouse model," *Experimental Neurology*, vol. 210, no. 1, pp. 154–163, 2008.

[30] Z. Kohl, M. Kandasamy, B. Winner et al., "Physical activity fails to rescue hippocampal neurogenesis deficits in the R6/2 mouse model of Huntington's disease," *Brain Research*, vol. 1155, pp. 24–33, 2007.

[31] V. Fedele, L. Roybon, U. Nordstrom, J. Y. Li, and P. Brundin, "Neurogenesis in the R6/2 mouse model of Huntington's disease is impaired at the level of NeuroD1," *Neuroscience*, vol. 173, pp. 76–81, 2011.

[32] W. Duan, Q. Peng, N. Masuda et al., "Sertraline slows disease progression and increases neurogenesis in N171-82Q mouse model of Huntington's disease," *Neurobiology of Disease*, vol. 30, no. 3, pp. 312–322, 2008.

[33] J. M. Simpson, J. Gil-Mohapel, M. A. Pouladi et al., "Altered adult hippocampal neurogenesis in the YAC128 transgenic mouse model of Huntington disease," *Neurobiology of Disease*, vol. 41, no. 2, pp. 249–260, 2011.

[34] J. E. Malberg, A. J. Eisch, E. J. Nestler, and R. S. Duman, "Chronic antidepressant treatment increases neurogenesis in adult rat hippocampus," *The Journal of Neuroscience*, vol. 20, no. 24, pp. 9104–9110, 2000.

[35] H. Manev, T. Uz, N. R. Smalheiser, and R. Manev, "Antidepressants alter cell proliferation in the adult brain in vivo and in neural cultures in vitro," *European Journal of Pharmacology*, vol. 411, no. 1-2, pp. 67–70, 2001.

[36] L. Santarelli, M. Saxe, C. Gross et al., "Requirement of hippocampal neurogenesis for the behavioral effects of antidepressants," *Science*, vol. 301, no. 5634, pp. 805–809, 2003.

[37] J. M. Gil and A. C. Rego, "The R6 lines of transgenic mice: a model for screening new therapies for Huntington's disease," *Brain Research Reviews*, vol. 59, no. 2, pp. 410–431, 2009.

[38] J. M. Gil-Mohapel, "Screening of therapeutic strategies for Huntington's disease in YAC128 transgenic mice," *CNS Neuroscience & Therapeutics*, vol. 18, no. 1, pp. 77–86, 2012.

[39] P. S. Brocardo and J. M. Gil-Mohapel, "Therapeutic strategies for Huntington's disease: from the bench to the clinic," *Current Psychopharmacology*, vol. 1, no. 2, pp. 137–154, 2012.

[40] T. Velusamy, A. S. Panneerselvam, M. Purushottam et al., "Protective effect of antioxidants on neuronal dysfunction and plasticity in Huntington's disease," *Oxidative Medicine and Cellular Longevity*, vol. 2017, Article ID 3279061, 15 pages, 2017.

[41] S. Yamashita, H. HBujo, H. Arai et al., "Long-term probucol treatment prevents secondary cardiovascular events: a cohort study of patients with heterozygous familial hypercholesterolemia in Japan," *Journal of Atherosclerosis and Thrombosis*, vol. 15, no. 6, pp. 292–303, 2008.

[42] D. Champagne, D. Pearson, D. Dea, J. Rochford, and J. Poirier, "The cholesterol-lowering drug probucol increases apolipoprotein E production in the hippocampus of aged rats: implications for Alzheimer's disease," *Neuroscience*, vol. 121, no. 1, pp. 99–110, 2003.

[43] J. Ma, S. Zhao, G. Gao, H. Chang, P. Ma, and B. Jin, "Probucol protects against asymmetric dimethylarginine-induced apoptosis in the cultured human brain microvascular endothelial cells," *Journal of Molecular Neuroscience*, vol. 57, no. 4, pp. 546–553, 2015.

[44] D. B. Santos, K. C. Peres, R. P. Ribeiro et al., "Probucol, a lipid-lowering drug, prevents cognitive and hippocampal synaptic impairments induced by amyloid β peptide in mice," *Experimental Neurology*, vol. 233, no. 2, pp. 767–775, 2012.

[45] D. B. Santos, D. Colle, E. L. G. Moreira et al., "Probucol mitigates streptozotocin-induced cognitive and biochemical changes in mice," *Neuroscience*, vol. 284, pp. 590–600, 2015.

[46] R. P. Ribeiro, E. L. G. Moreira, D. B. Santos et al., "Probucol affords neuroprotection in a 6-OHDA mouse model of Parkinson's disease," *Neurochemical Research*, vol. 38, no. 3, pp. 660–668, 2013.

[47] D. Colle, D. B. Santos, E. L. G. Moreira et al., "Probucol increases striatal glutathione peroxidase activity and protects against 3-nitropropionic acid-induced pro-oxidative damage in rats," *PLoS One*, vol. 8, no. 6, article e67658, 2013.

[48] S. Y. Park, J. H. Lee, C. D. Kim, B. Y. Rhim, K. W. Hong, and W. S. Lee, "Beneficial synergistic effects of concurrent treatment with cilostazol and probucol against focal cerebral ischemic injury in rats," *Brain Research*, vol. 1157, pp. 112–120, 2007.

[49] Y. S. Jung, J. H. Park, H. Kim et al., "Probucol inhibits LPS-induced microglia activation and ameliorates brain ischemic injury in normal and hyperlipidemic mice," *Acta Pharmacologica Sinica*, vol. 37, no. 8, pp. 1031–1044, 2016.

[50] A. Z. Zucoloto, M. F. Manchope, L. Staurengo-Ferrari et al., "Probucol attenuates lipopolysaccharide-induced leukocyte recruitment and inflammatory hyperalgesia: effect on NF-κB activation and cytokine production," *European Journal of Pharmacology*, vol. 809, pp. 52–63, 2017.

[51] J. N. Crawley, "Exploratory behavior models of anxiety in mice," *Neuroscience & Biobehavioral Reviews*, vol. 9, no. 1, pp. 37–44, 1985.

[52] C. Lopes, M. Ribeiro, A. I. Duarte et al., "IGF-1 intranasal administration rescues Huntington's disease phenotypes in YAC128 mice," *Molecular Neurobiology*, vol. 49, no. 3, pp. 1126–1142, 2014.

[53] R. J. Carter, J. Morton, and S. B. Dunnett, "Motor coordination and balance in rodents," *Current Protocols in Neuroscience*, vol. 15, no. 1, pp. 8.12.1–8.12.14, 2001.

[54] X. Liu and H. K. Gershenfeld, "Genetic differences in the tail-suspension test and its relationship to imipramine response among 11 inbred strains of mice," *Biological Psychiatry*, vol. 49, no. 7, pp. 575–581, 2001.

[55] N. Ripoll, D. J. P. David, E. Dailly, M. Hascoët, and M. Bourin, "Antidepressant-like effects in various mice strains in the tail suspension test," *Behavioural Brain Research*, vol. 143, no. 2, pp. 193–200, 2003.

[56] L. Steru, R. Chermat, B. Thierry, and P. Simon, "The tail suspension test: a new method for screening antidepressants in mice," *Psychopharmacology*, vol. 85, no. 3, pp. 367–370, 1985.

[57] R. D. Porsolt, A. Bertin, and M. Jalfre, "Behavioral despair in mice: a primary screening test for antidepressants," *Archives Internationales de Pharmacodynamie et de Thérapie*, vol. 229, no. 2, pp. 327–336, 1977.

[58] N. Kee, S. Sivalingam, R. Boonstra, and J. M. Wojtowicz, "The utility of Ki-67 and BrdU as proliferative markers of adult neurogenesis," *Journal of Neuroscience Methods*, vol. 115, no. 1, pp. 97–105, 2002.

[59] O. von Bohlen und Halbach, "Immunohistological markers for proliferative events, gliogenesis, and neurogenesis within the adult hippocampus," *Cell and Tissue Research*, vol. 345, no. 1, pp. 1–19, 2011.

[60] B. R. Christie and H. A. Cameron, "Neurogenesis in the adult hippocampus," *Hippocampus*, vol. 16, no. 3, pp. 199–207, 2006.

[61] J. P. Brown, S. Couillard-Despres, C. M. Cooper-Kuhn, J. Winkler, L. Aigner, and H. G. Kuhn, "Transient expression of doublecortin during adult neurogenesis," *The Journal of Comparative Neurology*, vol. 467, no. 1, pp. 1–10, 2003.

[62] K. B. Franklin and G. Paxinos, *Atlas the Mouse Brain in Stereotaxic Coordinates*, Elsevier, 2008.

[63] S. Orvoen, P. Pla, A. M. Gardier, F. Saudou, and D. J. David, "Huntington's disease knock-in male mice show specific anxiety-like behaviour and altered neuronal maturation," *Neuroscience Letters*, vol. 507, no. 2, pp. 127–132, 2012.

[64] S. Hult Lundh, N. Nilsson, R. Soylu, D. Kirik, and A. Petersen, "Hypothalamic expression of mutant huntingtin contributes to the development of depressive-like behavior in the BAC transgenic mouse model of Huntington's disease," *Human Molecular Genetics*, vol. 22, no. 17, pp. 3485–3497, 2013.

[65] B. Baldo, R. Y. Cheong, and A. Petersen, "Effects of deletion of mutant huntingtin in steroidogenic factor 1 neurons on the psychiatric and metabolic phenotype in the BACHD mouse model of Huntington disease," *PLoS One*, vol. 9, no. 10, article e107691, 2014.

[66] T. Renoir, T. Y. C. Pang, C. Mo et al., "Differential effects of early environmental enrichment on emotionality related behaviours in Huntington's disease transgenic mice," *The Journal of Physiology*, vol. 591, no. 1, pp. 41–55, 2013.

[67] T. Y. C. Pang, X. du, M. S. Zajac, M. L. Howard, and A. J. Hannan, "Altered serotonin receptor expression is associated with depression-related behavior in the R6/1 transgenic mouse model of Huntington's disease," *Human Molecular Genetics*, vol. 18, no. 4, pp. 753–766, 2009.

[68] T. Renoir, M. S. Zajac, X. du et al., "Sexually dimorphic serotonergic dysfunction in a mouse model of Huntington's disease and depression," *PLoS One*, vol. 6, no. 7, article e22133, 2011.

[69] T. Renoir, A. Argyropoulos, and A. J. Hannan, "Antidepressant-like effect of the norepinephrine-dopamine reuptake inhibitor bupropion in a mouse model of Huntington's disease with dopaminergic dysfunction," *Journal of Huntington's Disease*, vol. 1, no. 2, pp. 261–266, 2012.

[70] X. Du, T. Y. Pang, C. Mo, T. Renoir, D. J. Wright, and A. J. Hannan, "The influence of the HPG axis on stress response and depressive-like behaviour in a transgenic mouse model of Huntington's disease," *Experimental Neurology*, vol. 263, pp. 63–71, 2015.

[71] D. J. Wright, L. J. Gray, D. I. Finkelstein et al., "N-acetylcysteine modulates glutamatergic dysfunction and depressive behavior in Huntington's disease," *Human Molecular Genetics*, vol. 25, no. 14, pp. 2923–2933, 2016.

[72] A. J. Hannan and M. I. Ransome, "Deficits in spermatogenesis but not neurogenesis are alleviated by chronic testosterone therapy in R6/1 Huntington's disease mice," *Journal of Neuroendocrinology*, vol. 24, no. 2, pp. 341–356, 2012.

[73] J. W. Barnhart, J. A. Sefranka, and D. D. Mcintosh, "Hypocholesterolemic effect of 4,4'-(isopropylidenedithio)-bis(2,6-di-t-butylphenol) (probucol)," *The American Journal of Clinical Nutrition*, vol. 23, no. 9, pp. 1229–1233, 1970.

[74] E. L. Moreira, J. de Oliveira, M. F. Dutra et al., "Does methylmercury-induced hypercholesterolemia play a causal role in its neurotoxicity and cardiovascular disease?," *Toxicological Sciences*, vol. 130, no. 2, pp. 373–382, 2012.

[75] K. Prasad, J. Kalra, and P. Lee, "Oxygen free radicals as a mechanism of hypercholesterolemic atherosclerosis: effects of probucol," *International Journal of Angiology*, vol. 3, no. 1, pp. 100–112, 1994.

[76] S. Yamashita, D. Masuda, and Y. Matsuzawa, "Did we abandon probucol too soon?," *Current Opinion in Lipidology*, vol. 26, no. 4, pp. 304–316, 2015.

[77] T. E. Strandberg, H. Vanhanen, and T. A. Miettinen, "Probucol in long-term treatment of hypercholesterolemia," *General Pharmacology*, vol. 19, no. 3, pp. 317–320, 1988.

[78] J. P. Vonsattel, R. H. Myers, T. J. Stevens, R. J. Ferrante, E. D. Bird, and E. P. Richardson Jr., "Neuropathological classification of Huntington's disease," *Journal of Neuropathology and Experimental Neurology*, vol. 44, no. 6, pp. 559–577, 1985.

[79] Z. Bayram-Weston, L. Jones, S. B. Dunnett, and S. P. Brooks, "Light and electron microscopic characterization of the evolution of cellular pathology in YAC128 Huntington's disease transgenic mice," *Brain Research Bulletin*, vol. 88, no. 2-3, pp. 137–147, 2012.

[80] L. I. Petrella, J. M. Castelhano, M. Ribeiro et al., "A whole brain longitudinal study in the YAC128 mouse model of Huntington's disease shows distinct trajectories of neurochemical, structural connectivity and volumetric changes," *Human Molecular Genetics*, vol. 27, no. 12, pp. 2125–2137, 2018.

[81] J. M. Van Raamsdonk, Z. Murphy, E. J. Slow, B. R. Leavitt, and M. R. Hayden, "Selective degeneration and nuclear localization of mutant huntingtin in the YAC128 mouse model of Huntington disease," *Human Molecular Genetics*, vol. 14, no. 24, pp. 3823–3835, 2005.

[82] J. M. Van Raamsdonk, S. C. Warby, and M. R. Hayden, "Selective degeneration in YAC mouse models of Huntington disease," *Brain Research Bulletin*, vol. 72, no. 2-3, pp. 124–131, 2007.

[83] E. Spargo, I. P. Everall, and P. L. Lantos, "Neuronal loss in the hippocampus in Huntington's disease: a comparison with HIV infection," *Journal of Neurology, Neurosurgery, and Psychiatry*, vol. 56, no. 5, pp. 487–491, 1993.

[84] K. P. S. J. Murphy, R. J. Carter, L. A. Lione et al., "Abnormal synaptic plasticity and impaired spatial cognition in mice transgenic for exon 1 of the human Huntington's disease mutation," *The Journal of Neuroscience*, vol. 20, no. 13, pp. 5115–5123, 2000.

[85] H. D. Rosas, W. J. Koroshetz, Y. I. Chen et al., "Evidence for more widespread cerebral pathology in early HD: an MRI-based morphometric analysis," *Neurology*, vol. 60, no. 10, pp. 1615–1620, 2003.

[86] S. J. Sawiak, N. I. Wood, G. B. Williams, A. J. Morton, and T. A. Carpenter, "Use of magnetic resonance imaging for anatomical phenotyping of the R6/2 mouse model of Huntington's disease," *Neurobiology of Disease*, vol. 33, no. 1, pp. 12–19, 2009.

[87] Y. Cheng, Q. Peng, Z. Hou et al., "Structural MRI detects progressive regional brain atrophy and neuroprotective effects in N171-82Q Huntington's disease mouse model," *NeuroImage*, vol. 56, no. 3, pp. 1027–1034, 2011.

[88] J. J. Steventon, R. C. Trueman, D. Ma et al., "Longitudinal in vivo MRI in a Huntington's disease mouse model: global atrophy in the absence of white matter microstructural damage," *Scientific Reports*, vol. 6, no. 1, p. 32423, 2016.

[89] I. Rattray, E. J. Smith, W. R. Crum et al., "Correlations of behavioral deficits with brain pathology assessed through longitudinal MRI and histopathology in the Hdh$^{Q150/Q150}$

mouse model of Huntington's disease," *PLoS One*, vol. 12, no. 1, article e0168556, 2017.

[90] A. J. Eisch, H. A. Cameron, J. M. Encinas, L. A. Meltzer, G. L. Ming, and L. S. Overstreet-Wadiche, "Adult neurogenesis, mental health, and mental illness: hope or hype?," *The Journal of Neuroscience*, vol. 28, no. 46, pp. 11785–11791, 2008.

[91] W. Deng, J. B. Aimone, and F. H. Gage, "New neurons and new memories: how does adult hippocampal neurogenesis affect learning and memory?," *Nature Reviews Neuroscience*, vol. 11, no. 5, pp. 339–350, 2010.

[92] H. S. Mayberg, "Positron emission tomography imaging in depression: a neural systems perspective," *Neuroimaging Clinics of North America*, vol. 13, no. 4, pp. 805–815, 2003.

[93] P. Videbech and B. Ravnkilde, "Hippocampal volume and depression: a meta-analysis of MRI studies," *The American Journal of Psychiatry*, vol. 161, no. 11, pp. 1957–1966, 2004.

[94] Y. I. Sheline, P. W. Wang, M. H. Gado, J. G. Csernansky, and M. W. Vannier, "Hippocampal atrophy in recurrent major depression," *Proceedings of the National Academy of Sciences of the United States of America*, vol. 93, no. 9, pp. 3908–3913, 1996.

[95] Y. I. Sheline, M. Sanghavi, M. A. Mintun, and M. H. Gado, "Depression duration but not age predicts hippocampal volume loss in medically healthy women with recurrent major depression," *The Journal of Neuroscience*, vol. 19, no. 12, pp. 5034–5043, 1999.

[96] R. M. Sapolsky, "Why stress is bad for your brain," *Science*, vol. 273, no. 5276, pp. 749–750, 1996.

[97] B. R. Miller and R. Hen, "The current state of the neurogenic theory of depression and anxiety," *Current Opinion in Neurobiology*, vol. 30, pp. 51–58, 2015.

[98] M. R. Drew and R. Hen, "Adult hippocampal neurogenesis as target for the treatment of depression," *CNS & Neurological Disorders Drug Targets*, vol. 6, no. 3, pp. 205–218, 2007.

[99] B. L. Jacobs, H. van Praag, and F. H. Gage, "Adult brain neurogenesis and psychiatry: a novel theory of depression," *Molecular Psychiatry*, vol. 5, no. 3, pp. 262–269, 2000.

[100] L. Mangiarini, K. Sathasivam, M. Seller et al., "Exon 1 of the HD gene with an expanded CAG repeat is sufficient to cause a progressive neurological phenotype in transgenic mice," *Cell*, vol. 87, no. 3, pp. 493–506, 1996.

[101] S. Parthasarathy, S. G. Young, J. L. Witztum, R. C. Pittman, and D. Steinberg, "Probucol inhibits oxidative modification of low density lipoprotein," *The Journal of Clinical Investigation*, vol. 77, no. 2, pp. 641–644, 1986.

[102] K. D. Pfuetze and C. A. Dujovne, "Probucol," *Current Atherosclerosis Reports*, vol. 2, no. 1, pp. 47–57, 2000.

[103] S. Yamashita and Y. Matsuzawa, "Where are we with probucol: a new life for an old drug?," *Atherosclerosis*, vol. 207, no. 1, pp. 16–23, 2009.

[104] J. R. Paterson, A. G. Rumley, K. G. Oldroyd et al., "Probucol reduces plasma lipid peroxides in man," *Atherosclerosis*, vol. 97, no. 1, pp. 63–66, 1992.

[105] D. Colle, J. M. Hartwig, F. A. Antunes Soares, and M. Farina, "Probucol modulates oxidative stress and excitotoxicity in Huntington's disease models in vitro," *Brain Research Bulletin*, vol. 87, no. 4-5, pp. 397–405, 2012.

[106] M. Farina, F. Campos, I. Vendrell et al., "Probucol increases glutathione peroxidase-1 activity and displays long-lasting protection against methylmercury toxicity in cerebellar granule cells," *Toxicological Sciences*, vol. 112, no. 2, pp. 416–426, 2009.

[107] J. M. Gil and A. C. Rego, "Mechanisms of neurodegeneration in Huntington's disease," *The European Journal of Neuroscience*, vol. 27, no. 11, pp. 2803–2820, 2008.

[108] P. S. Brocardo, E. McGinnis, B. R. Christie, and J. Gil-Mohapel, "Time-course analysis of protein and lipid oxidation in the brains of YAC128 Huntington's disease transgenic mice," *Rejuvenation Research*, vol. 19, no. 2, pp. 140–148, 2016.

[109] R. Smith, P. Brundin, and J. Y. Li, "Synaptic dysfunction in Huntington's disease: a new perspective," *Cellular and Molecular Life Sciences*, vol. 62, no. 17, pp. 1901–1912, 2005.

[110] J. Y. Li, M. Plomann, and P. Brundin, "Huntington's disease: a synaptopathy?," *Trends in Molecular Medicine*, vol. 9, no. 10, pp. 414–420, 2003.

[111] M. Ghilan, C. A. Bostrom, B. N. Hryciw, J. M. Simpson, B. R. Christie, and J. Gil-Mohapel, "YAC128 Huntington's disease transgenic mice show enhanced short-term hippocampal synaptic plasticity early in the course of the disease," *Brain Research*, vol. 1581, pp. 117–128, 2014.

[112] T. Lang and R. Jahn, "Core proteins of the secretory machinery," in *Pharmacology of Neurotransmitter Release*, T. C. Südhof and K. Starke, Eds., pp. 107–127, Springer, Berlin, Heidelberg, 2008.

[113] I. Mahar, F. R. Bambico, N. Mechawar, and J. N. Nobrega, "Stress, serotonin, and hippocampal neurogenesis in relation to depression and antidepressant effects," *Neuroscience and Biobehavioral Reviews*, vol. 38, pp. 173–192, 2014.

[114] G. Serafini, S. Hayley, M. Pompili et al., "Hippocampal neurogenesis, neurotrophic factors and depression: possible therapeutic targets?," *CNS & Neurological Disorders Drug Targets*, vol. 13, no. 10, pp. 1708–1721, 2014.

[115] A. S. Hill, A. Sahay, and R. Hen, "Increasing adult hippocampal neurogenesis is sufficient to reduce anxiety and depression-like behaviors," *Neuropsychopharmacology*, vol. 40, no. 10, pp. 2368–2378, 2015.

[116] M. E. Castro, J. Pascual, T. Romon, J. Berciano, J. Figols, and A. Pazos, "5-HT1B receptor binding in degenerative movement disorders," *Brain Research*, vol. 790, no. 1-2, pp. 323–328, 1998.

[117] G. Richards, J. Messer, H. J. Waldvogel et al., "Up-regulation of the isoenzymes MAO-A and MAO-B in the human basal ganglia and pons in Huntington's disease revealed by quantitative enzyme radioautography," *Brain Research*, vol. 1370, pp. 204–214, 2011.

[118] L. J. Steward, K. E. Bufton, P. C. Hopkins, W. Ewart Davies, and N. M. Barnes, "Reduced levels of 5-HT3 receptor recognition sites in the putamen of patients with Huntington's disease," *European Journal of Pharmacology*, vol. 242, no. 2, pp. 137–143, 1993.

[119] C. Waeber and J. M. Palacios, "Serotonin-1 receptor binding sites in the human basal ganglia are decreased in Huntington's chorea but not in Parkinson's disease: a quantitative in vitro autoradiography study," *Neuroscience*, vol. 32, no. 2, pp. 337–347, 1989.

[120] E. H. Wong, G. P. Reynolds, D. W. Bonhaus, S. Hsu, and R. M. Eglen, "Characterization of [^{3}H]GR 113808 binding to 5-HT$_4$ receptors in brain tissues from patients with neurodegenerative disorders," *Behavioural Brain Research*, vol. 73, no. 1-2, pp. 249–252, 1996.

12

No Modulatory Effects when Stimulating the Right Inferior Frontal Gyrus with Continuous 6Hz tACS and tRNS on Response Inhibition: A Behavioral Study

Hannah Brauer [ID],[1,2] Navah Ester Kadish,[1] Anya Pedersen,[3] Michael Siniatchkin,[1] and Vera Moliadze [ID][1]

[1]Institute of Medical Psychology and Medical Sociology, University Hospital of Schleswig-Holstein (UKSH), Campus Kiel, Christian Albrechts University, Kiel, Germany
[2]Department of Child and Adolescent Psychiatry and Psychotherapy, School of Medicine, Christian Albrechts University, Kiel, Germany
[3]Clinical Psychology and Psychotherapy, Christian Albrechts University, Kiel, Germany

Correspondence should be addressed to Hannah Brauer; hannah.brauer@uksh.de

Academic Editor: Grzegorz Hess

Response inhibition is the cognitive process required to cancel an intended action. During that process, a "go" reaction is intercepted particularly by the right inferior frontal gyrus (rIFG) and presupplementary motor area (pre-SMA). After the commission of inhibition errors, theta activity (4–8 Hz) is related to the adaption processes. In this study, we intend to examine whether the boosting of theta activity by electrical stimulation over rIFG reduces the number of errors and the reaction times in a response inhibition task (Go/NoGo paradigm) during and after stimulation. 23 healthy right-handed adults participated in the study. In three separate sessions, theta tACS at 6 Hz, transcranial random noise (tRNS) as a second stimulation condition, and sham stimulation were applied for 20 minutes. Based on behavioral data, this study could not show any effects of 6 Hz tACS as well as full spectrum tRNS on response inhibition in any of the conditions. Since many findings support the relevance of the rIFG for response inhibition, this could mean that 6 Hz activity is not important for response inhibition in that structure. Reasons for our null findings could also lie in the stimulation parameters, such as the electrode montage or the stimulation frequency, which are discussed in this article in more detail. Sharing negative findings will have (1) positive impact on future research questions and study design and will improve (2) knowledge acquisition of noninvasive transcranial brain stimulation techniques.

1. Introduction

Response inhibition, as an important process of executive control, refers to the suppression of actions that are no longer required or that are inappropriate. It allows flexible and goal-directed behavior in ever-changing environments. The computational routine during response inhibition is well described [1, 2]. It is related to a dynamic information flow between the right inferior frontal cortex (rIFC) and the presupplementary motor area (pre-SMA) through basal ganglia to the primary motor cortex (M1) (for review, see [2–4]). In this network, pre-SMA and IFC seem to play a driving function regulating performance monitoring, continuous preparation of actions, and attentional control. Especially the rIFG (right inferior frontal gyrus) is an important structure for motor response inhibition. Lesion studies with transcranial magnetic stimulation (TMS) show that deactivation of the pars opercularis of the rIFG leads to more inhibition errors in a Go/NoGo task (e.g., [5]). Using the Go/NoGo task, Mazaheri and colleagues [6] demonstrated that errors during response inhibition can be predicted by theta-alpha coupling in healthy adults: after an error, there is a significant increase in theta power in pre-SMA and IFC and decrease of alpha power in the parieto-occipital cortex (POC) following an error and preceding a successful response. In children with ADHD, lower theta-alpha coupling was seen in comparison to healthy children [7]. It may be hypothesized that the increase in theta activity in pre-SMA and IFC would reduce the number of errors and improve inhibitory control.

Noninvasive transcranial brain stimulation (NTBS) techniques such as TMS and transcranial electrical stimulation (tES) are important tools in human systems and cognitive neuroscience which are able to modulate activity in the neural tissue underlying the stimulating area. To date, the majority of studies in humans use transcranial direct current stimulation (tDCS) to modulate cortical function. It is thought that tDCS is capable of inducing polarity-dependent, relatively long-lasting changes in the human brain (for recent reviews, see [8–11]). The most relevant for our study is that Jacobson and colleagues [12] and Cunillera and colleagues [13] described that anodal tDCS to the rIFG improves behavioral inhibition, suggesting that tDCS modulates cognitive control in healthy individuals. However, tDCS does not allow to investigate whether this modulation is related to specific frequencies.

Numerous studies have demonstrated that transcranial alternating current stimulation (tACS) provides the unique possibility of noninvasively modulating ongoing oscillatory activity in a frequency-specific way, which has been attributed to oscillatory entrainment by the specific stimulation frequency [14–17] (for review, see Antal and Herrmann [18]). Besides changing the frequency of oscillations, tACS is also able to enhance the power of a certain frequency band. Zaehle and colleagues [14] elevated endogenous alpha power in parieto-central regions with individual alpha frequency stimulation.

Recent studies on cognitive processes in both young and older healthy subjects indicate successful modulation of brain oscillations and behavioral outcome through frontal or parietal tAC stimulation. The majority of the studies suggest a particularly beneficial effect of tACS in the theta frequency [19–21]. Polania and colleagues [16] demonstrated that the tACS with 6 Hz frequency over the prefrontal cortex (DLPFC) can boost not only activity in the DLPFC but also in the parietal cortex, increasing working memory capacity. The authors provide evidence that tACS in the theta frequency range applied to the prefrontal cortex is able to increase frontoparietal connectivity and improve neuropsychological function. Further study confirmed the beneficial effect of theta tACS on accuracy in verbal working memory [22]. Pahor and Jausovec [23] observed reduced alpha power in posterior areas after theta tACS in resting EEG while theta power in frontal areas was enhanced.

Based on the findings reviewed above, the present study examines whether the boosting of theta activity by 6 Hz electrical stimulation over the rIFG reduces the number of errors as well as the reaction time in a response inhibition task during and after stimulation. For this purpose, 6 Hz tACS was applied over right IFG during a motor response inhibition task (Go/NoGo). To examine whether the effects of the 6 Hz tACS was specific for the applied frequency, a full spectrum random noise stimulation (tRNS) was added as a second stimulation condition. In contrast to tACS, tRNS applies alternating electrical currents of different frequencies

TABLE 1: Subject characteristics.

	Mean ± standard deviation	Exclusion criteria
Sex	16 females, 7 males	
Age	22.91 years ± 3.44	18 < age > 30
Edinburgh Handedness Inventory laterality quotient (HQ)	80.99 ± 22.46	HQ < 50
BDI II total score	4.52 ± 3.36	BDI > 13
ADHS-E percentile rank	58.48 ± 23.13	PR > 98
SCL-90-R T value GSI	45.78 ± 7.89	$T > 65$
SCL-90-R T value PST	47.17 ± 6.86	$T > 65$
SCL-90-R T value PSDI	46.70 ± 11.65	$T > 65$

Data are presented in M ± SD. No subject had to be excluded because of these exclusion criteria.

and amplitudes (for an overview, see [18, 24] and might hence be implemented as a control condition.

We hypothesized that the tACS at theta (6 Hz) during the task might reduce errors and reaction times in comparison to sham and tRNS stimulation.

2. Materials and Methods

The study was carried out in accordance with the latest revision of the Declaration of Helsinki. Experimental procedures were approved by the local ethics committee of the Christian Albrechts University, Kiel, Germany. Prior to the experiment, subjects gave their written informed consent.

2.1. Subjects. With G*Power [25], a sample size of 20 subjects was calculated for a 2×3 way ANOVA with repeated measures. Used parameters were an effect size of $f = 0.3$ (estimated based on Polania and colleagues [16], Iuculano and Cohen Kadosh [26], and van Driel and colleagues [27]), correlation of the repeated measures of $r = 0.5$, $\alpha = 0.05$, and a power of 0.80. Twenty-three healthy right-handed adults (age mean 22.91 years, range 18–30; 16 females) with normal or corrected to normal vision participated after giving informed consent. All participants were university students and were recruited via social media and flyers at the Kiel University. Exclusion criteria were (1) history or family history of epileptic seizures, (2) history of migraine, (3) unexplained loss of consciousness or brain related injury, (4) history of other neurological or psychiatric disorders, (5) cardiac pacemaker or intracranial metal implantation, and (6) intake of central nervous system-effective medication.

To exclude persons with psychological problems, the self-report questionnaire Symptom-Checklist-90-R/SCL-90-R [28] was used. Additionally the degree of ADHD symptoms was assessed with the screening questionnaire ADHS-E [29] and the severity of a depression with the revised version of the Beck Depression Inventory (BDI) II [30]. To assess the handedness of the subjects, the Edinburgh Inventory was used [31]. All these questionnaires were completed according to manual and at the end of the first session (see Table 1 for subject characteristics). Additionally, for each of the sessions, smoking and caffeine were assessed and protocolled.

After finishing each experimental session, the participants were asked to complete a questionnaire on the side effects of the stimulation, adapted from Poreisz and colleagues [32].

The questionnaire contains items pertaining to the presence and severity of headaches, change or difficulties in concentration, mood, visual perception, presence of fatigue, and discomforting sensations like pain, tingling, itching, or burning. The participants received one cinema voucher per session for their participation.

2.2. The Go/NoGo Task.
Subjects performed a Go/NoGo task and responded by pressing a mouse button with their right forefinger. During the paradigm, single white digits between 1 and 9 were presented on a black background. The task was presented in two blocks of 600 trials each, of which 120 (20%) were NoGo trials. Subjects were asked to respond to stimuli as quickly as possible by pressing a button as soon as a digit between 1 to 4 and 6 to 9 appeared ("Go" stimuli) and were told to withhold a button press when a "5" appeared ("NoGo" stimuli). Participants were instructed to keep their eyes focused on the fixation cross and to avoid any movement during the acquisition. Each stimulus was displayed for 0.2 s with an average interstimulus interval of 1.45 s (randomly jittered between 1.3 and 1.6 s). The fixation cross at the center of the screen was constantly visible during the interstimulus interval. The term "hit" will subsequently be used to refer to button presses during a Go trial, while the term "false alarm" will refer to commission errors, i.e., button presses during a NoGo trial. The term "correct withhold" will be used to describe correctly withholding button press in NoGo trials, and "miss" describes when the button is not pressed during a Go trial. The subjects were seated 63 cm away from the monitor (37.6 cm × 30 cm; 19 Zoll); stimuli were controlled via the presentation software version 19.0, Neurobehavioral Systems Inc., Berkeley, CA, http://www.neurobs.com).

2.3. Brain Stimulation.
Stimulation was performed with the NeuroConn DC-Stimulator (NeuroConn GmbH, Ilmenau, Germany) using 5 × 5 cm sponge electrodes. The active electrode was placed at the crossing point of T4-Fz and F8-Cz according to EEG 10–20 System [12]. The return electrode was placed over the left supraorbital cortex. Theta tACS was performed at a frequency of 6 Hz; in the tRNS condition, full spectrum tRNS (0.1–640 Hz) was used. Current intensity was 1 mA and stimulation lasted 20 min. Ramping at the beginning and the end of the stimulation was 10 s in all conditions. In the sham condition, 30 s of 6 Hz tACs was applied at the beginning.

2.4. Experimental Design.
In these two factorial repeated measures designs, subjects took part in all the conditions, each one week apart. Conditions were randomized, and subjects were blinded to the stimulation condition.

In order to keep the performance of the subjects as comparable as possible, the experimental sessions were performed at the same time of the day. In each of the sessions, the subjects completed a 2 min practice and afterwards two blocks of 15 min each of a Go/NoGo paradigm. Stimulation took place during the first block of the paradigm, followed by a resting period of 5 min and the second block without stimulation. So, the task was first performed online stimulation and afterwards offline. To avoid an influence of negative sensations during the ramping of the stimulation on the task performance, the task started 4.5 min after the beginning of the stimulation (see Figure 1).

3. Data Analysis and Statistics

3.1. Behavioral Data.
Statistical analysis was done with R [33] and visualization with prism (GraphPad Prism version 5.00 for Windows, GraphPad Software, San Diego, California, USA).

Errors were analyzed by calculating the relative frequency of reactions on NoGo stimuli (false alarms). Number of errors and the relative frequency of errors were not normally distributed and therefore logarithmized for parametric analyses [34]. To avoid nondefined values, relative frequencies of a value of 0 were replaced by 0.001 and of the value 1 by 0.999 [35]. Accuracy was calculated as the quotient of all correct responses (hits and rejections) and to every response. Reaction times were analyzed based on the median. For the relation of reaction times and numbers of errors, the "Inverse Efficiency Score" (IES) was calculated [36]. The IES is the quotient of the median of the reaction times of hits of a subject and the accuracy. This score is especially useful for tasks with very low error rates of up to 10% [37], which applies for the Go/NoGo task. To analyze the effects of stimulation and the time point of it on reaction times, errors and the IES 2 × 3 repeated measures ANOVAs with the within factor stimulation (6 Hz tACS vs. tRNS vs. sham) and time of testing (during stimulation vs. after stimulation) were calculated. Normal distribution was inspected with histograms. Sphericity was tested with the Mauchly's sphericity test. If sphericity was not fulfilled for a Greenhouse-Geisser epsilon < 0.75, p was corrected; according to Greenhouse-Geisser ($p_{(GG)}$), if Greenhouse-Geisser epsilon was >0.75, p was corrected according to Huynh-Feldt ($p_{(HF)}$). This correction was necessary in all three ANOVAs. In case of significant interaction effects (stimulation × time) or main effects of stimulation, additional exploratory t tests were performed and p values were compared to Bonferroni-adjusted alpha levels $\alpha/3 = 0.0167$ for three comparisons (global alpha level for the t tests was $\alpha = 0.05$). Additionally, Bayes factors (BFs) were calculated to obtain more precise evidence on the hypothesis H0 [38, 39].

3.2. Adverse Event Questionnaire.
For each side effect, the occurrence (yes/no) and severity (Likert scale: 1 mild–5 extremely high intensity) were checked. The number of adverse effects as well as the severity of each adverse effect were not normally distributed (Kolmogoroff-Smirnoff test) and therefore compared using the Mann–Whitney U tests.

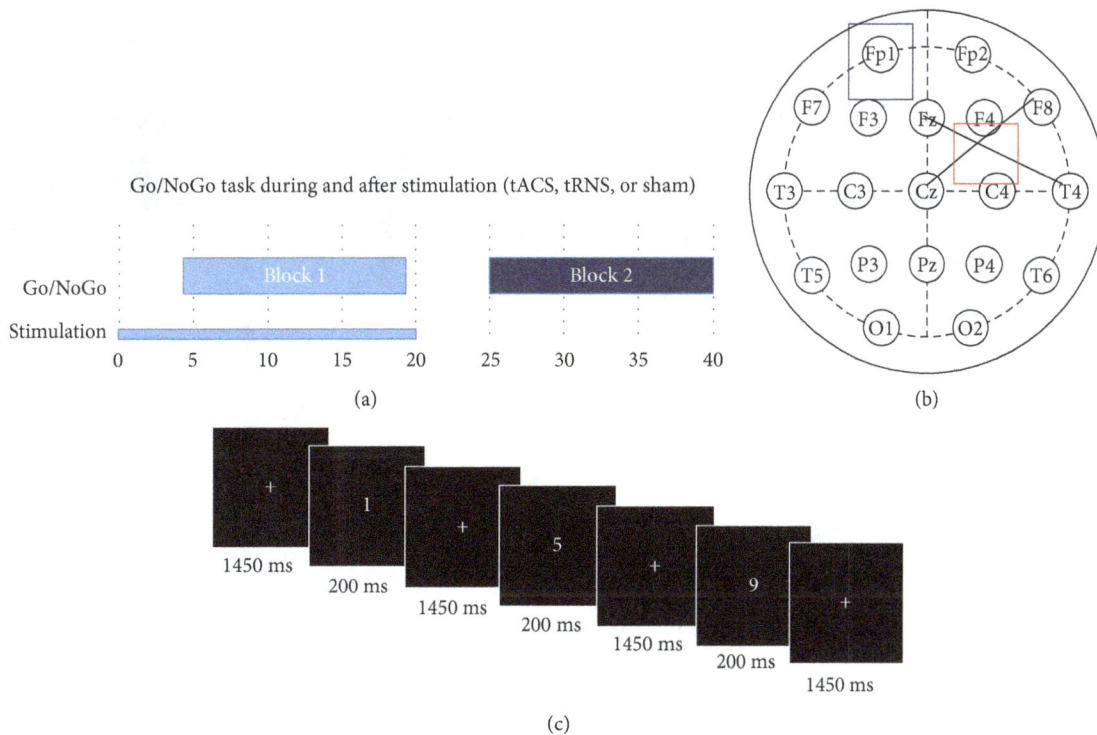

FIGURE 1: Experimental design. (a) Time course of the experiment: in each of the sessions, the subjects completed a 2 min practice and afterwards two blocks of 15 min each of a Go/NoGo paradigm. Stimulation took place during the first block of the paradigm, followed by a resting period of 5 min and the second block without stimulation. The task started 4.5 min after the beginning of the stimulation. (b) Electrode setup: active stimulation (5 × 5 cm) electrode was placed above rIFG, which was identified as the crossing point between T4-Fz and F8-Cz. The return electrode (5 × 7 cm) was placed above Fp1 following the international 10–20 system. (c) Go/NoGo task: subjects were asked to respond to stimuli as quickly as possible by pressing a button as soon as a digit between 1 to 4 or 6 to 9 appeared ("Go" stimuli) and were told to withhold a button press when a "5" appeared ("NoGo" stimuli). Participants were instructed to keep their eyes focused on the fixation cross and to avoid any movement during the acquisition. Each stimulus was displayed for 0.2 s with an average interstimulus interval of 1.45 s (randomly jittered between 1.3 and 1.6 s).

Statistical significance was defined as a two-tailed p value of less than 0.05.

4. Results

None of the subjects requested to terminate stimulation or asked for any medical intervention during or after the end of stimulation.

4.1. Behavioral Data. In a 2 × 3 ANOVA with repeated measures, there was no significant interaction effect between stimulation and time of testing on the numbers of committed inhibition errors ($F_{(2,44)} = 1.05$, $p_{(HF)} = 0.345$, $\eta^2 = 0.05$, and $BF_{01} = 7.90$). There was no main effect of stimulation ($p = 0.136$ and $BF_{01} = 5.12$), but an effect of time of testing ($p = 0.006$ and $BF_{01} = 0.44$) (Figure 2(a)). There is no significant interaction effect of stimulation and time of testing ($F_{(2,44)} = 0.70$, $p_{(HF)} = 0.472$, $\eta^2 = 0.03$, and $BF_{01} = 18.75$) on reaction time (Figure 2(b)). Also for the IES, there were no significant interaction effects between stimulation condition and time of testing ($F_{(2,44)} = 0.84$, $p_{(GG)} = 0.408$, $\eta^2 = 0.04$, and $BF_{01} = 13.38$). There was weak evidence for H0 for the effect of stimulation on IES ($BF_{01} = 2.64$). Evidence for H0 for the effect of stimulation on errors ($BF_{01} = 5.12$) and

reaction time ($BF_{01} = 6.9$) as well as for time of testing on reaction time ($BF_{01} = 3.48$) and IES ($BF_{01} = 17.93$) was positive to strong (Figure 2(c)).

4.2. Adverse Event Questionnaire. Figure 3 summarizes the adverse events during and after stimulation. Generally, it can be said that Mann–Whitney U tests showed a significantly higher incidence of tingling during 6 Hz tACS compared to tRNS ($p = 0.039$ and $U = 184.0$) and sham stimulation ($p = 0.007$ and $U = 161.0$). However, concerning the intensities (NAS 1–5) of the observed side effects, there was no significant difference between the stimulation conditions.

None of the subjects could distinguish between active and sham stimulations. The order of sessions had no effect on guess rate concerning the experimental condition. Sham stimulation as well as 6 Hz tACS and full spectrum tRNS were indistinguishable regarding side effects. Thus, the blinding procedure was judged as being successful.

4.3. Comparisons between the Side Effects during and after Stimulation. Mann–Whitney U tests showed a significantly higher incidence of tingling ($p = 0.0023$ and $U = 149.5$) during stimulation compared to the data obtained after for 6 Hz tACS. However, concerning the intensities (NAS 1–5) of the

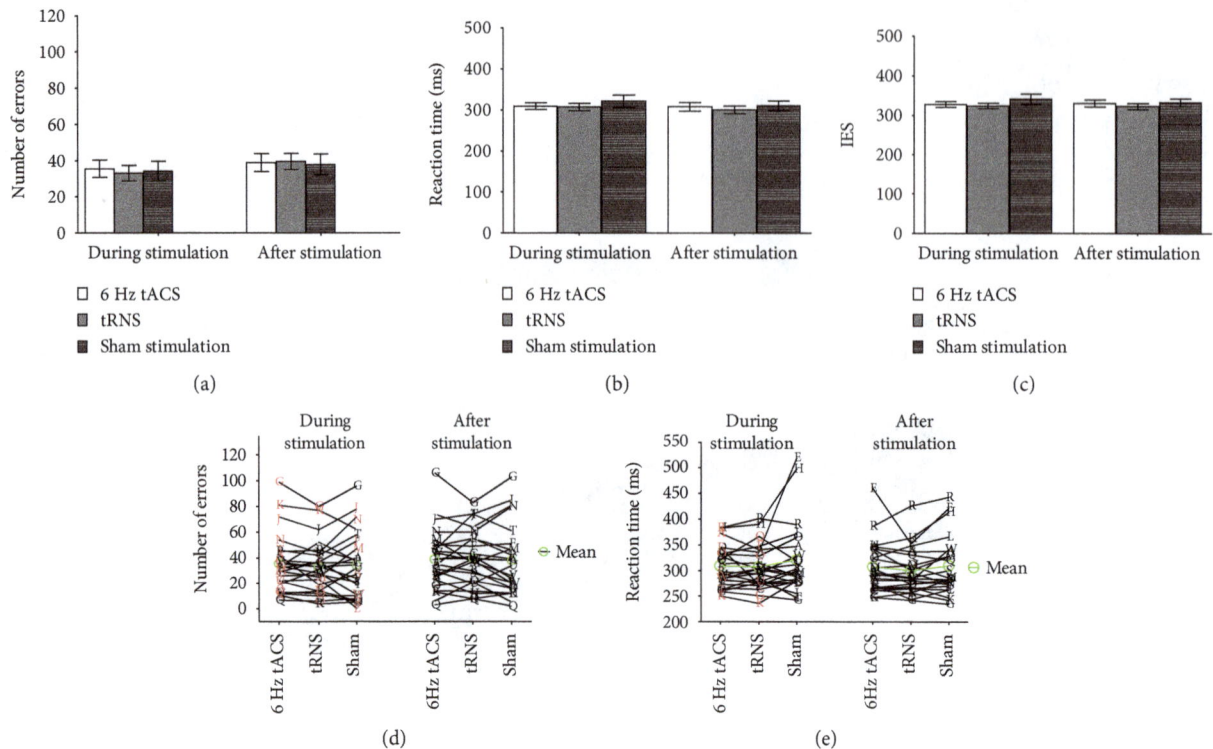

FIGURE 2: Behavioral data. In an 2×3 ANOVA with repeated measures, there was no significant interaction effect between stimulation and time of testing for number of false alarm trials (a) as well as reaction time for hit (b). (c) Inverse Efficiency Score. Also for the IES, there were no significant interaction effects between stimulation condition and time point. In (a), (b), and (c), means and standard deviations are reported. (d) and (e) Variability of stimulation. Each letter corresponds to one subject. The red color signifies that subjects identified the stimulation correctly.

observed side effects, there was no significant difference between the two time points.

5. Discussion

In the present study, we investigated the effect of transcranial alternating current stimulation on response inhibition in healthy young adults hypothesizing that tACS at theta (6 Hz) during the task will improve performance (errors and reaction times) in comparison to sham and transcranial random noise stimulation. As some studies report an improvement of performance not during stimulation but afterwards [40], we measured participants' Go/NoGo performance both while receiving stimulation ("online") and following the stimulation ("offline").

Based on the behavioral data in this study, we could not show effects of 6 Hz tACS and tRNS on response inhibition in healthy adults: both kinds of stimulation did not result in an improvement of performance such as less errors or faster reaction times compared to the tRNS and sham condition either during stimulation or after it.

Previous studies support the relevance of the rIFG for response inhibition [2, 41, 42]. However, by stimulating that structure with 6 Hz tACS, we were not able to modulate response inhibition. Therefore, our findings indicate the importance of region and frequency specific stimulation. It would be interesting to identify external and internal factors that might account for the negative results. Below, we discuss possible underlying mechanisms behind our negative findings in light of previous studies in the field.

5.1. Stimulation Parameters and Differences to Previous tES Studies. As mentioned above, anodal tDCS to the right inferior frontal gyrus (rIFG) improves behavioral inhibition [12, 13]. Compared to tDCS, a different mechanism is at work during tACS, requiring a different rationale for designing an experiment. It is especially crucial to identify a cognitive process that is characterized by a specific brain oscillation or combination of oscillations [18].

Even though behavioral outcomes of tACS have been demonstrated successfully, the underlying mechanisms have not been fully explored. While it is often hypothesized that tACS can phase-align neural oscillations, it is still relatively unclear whether it is able to modulate oscillatory power (for review, see [40, 43]). Only few studies have proven to enhance the power of a certain frequency band [14, 44]. Therefore, the applied tACS in our study might have affected only the oscillatory phase but not power, thus leading to our lack of significant effects.

Theta activity frequency used in this study ranges from 4 to 8 Hz and the tACS with 6 Hz frequency might not be suited to modulate theta activity in rIFG. Therefore, the exact parameters of the stimulation play an important role and still need to be optimized. However, it was shown that 6 Hz tACS over tempo parietal cortex can enhance cognition in older adults [21].

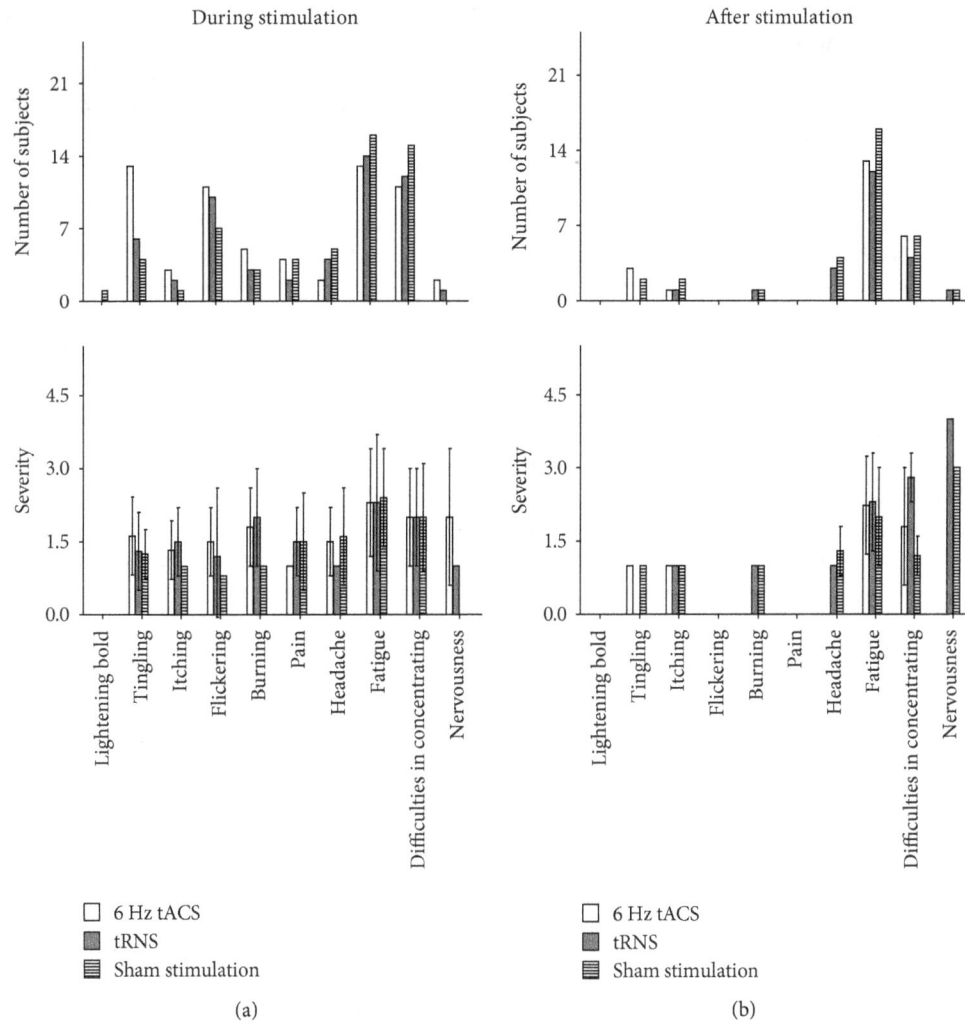

FIGURE 3: Adverse events during and after stimulation. (a) Mann–Whitney U tests showed a significantly higher incidence of tingling during 6 Hz tACS compared to tRNS ($p = 0.039$ and $U = 184.0$) and sham stimulation ($p = 0.007$ and $U = 161.0$). (b) There was a significantly higher incidence of tingling during compared to after stimulation for 6 Hz tACS ($p = 0.0023$ and $U = 149.5$).

We applied continuous theta tACS, even though the target theta activity occurred only after an error. During a Go/NoGo task, different attentional processes are relevant, including not only response inhibition but also other processes such as error monitoring. The task also requires sustained attention, which has been proven to be accompanied by a decrease of theta activity in medial frontal cortex [45, 46]. So therefore, the ongoing theta tACS might have enhanced theta activity where it was counterproductive to the performance in the Go/NoGo task. Chander and colleagues [47] showed that theta band tACS during a working memory task disrupted the task performance; this was associated with decreased frontal midline theta amplitude.

tACS is assumed to entrain spontaneous oscillations but the effect of theta power during response inhibition involves induced oscillations (for review, see [18, 48]). If spontaneous and induced oscillations involve two different mechanisms, tACS might only be a promising technique to manipulate spontaneous oscillations.

Previous studies indicate that state-triggered and closed loop stimulation boosts effects of noninvasive transcranial brain stimulation (for review, see Karabanov et al. [49]); e.g., in patients with Parkinson's disease, tACS applied to the motor cortex in their individual tremor frequency was able to suppress tremor amplitude. To maintain the optimal phase delay between tACS and the endogenous tremor rhythm, the phase of tACS was constantly adjusted, informed by the ongoing tremor activity [50]. In contrast, in our study, the phase of the 6 Hz tACS signal was not adjusted to the phase of the endogenous brain oscillations and was therefore independent. Therefore, closed loop stimulation might be more effective for specific modulation of brain function.

Another interesting finding is the negative effect of tRNS; as mentioned above, we use full spectrum tRNS (from 0.1 to 640 Hz) as a second condition to examine whether the effects of the 6 Hz tACS are specific for this frequency. tRNS is a relatively new form of brain stimulation, and studies have already shown how it can promote and sustain perceptual learning [51–53] besides its clear modulatory effects on the motor cortex [54]. However, higher frequencies (100–640 Hz) and not frequencies less than 100 Hz were responsible for this excitability increase (for review, see Antal and Paulus [55]).

Furthermore, different methodological factors (i.e., stimulation montage, intensity, and frequency of current) affecting specific brain networks interact with ongoing neural processes and transcranial brain stimulation effects also depend on the specifics of the experimental design [10, 17, 56] (for review, see Antal and Herrmann [18]).

Another possible explanation for the negative finding in our study could be the size of the electrodes (5×5 cm); the behavioral effects of transcranial electrical stimulation appear to be also critically dependent on the position of the return electrode. Changing the locations of the electrodes has been shown to alter the electric field in the brain [57–63]. Effects of tDCS and tACS also depend on the orientation of both the stimulating and reference/return electrodes altering the electric field in the brain; electrode size determines the extent of the stimulated area under the electrodes [64]. Our study used smaller active electrodes with a noncircular surface compared to many previous studies that stimulated the same area of interest using tACS/tRNS with larger or circular stimulation electrodes [21, 65, 66].

5.2. Individual Differences. Our negative results could also reflect in part the substantial individual variation in response to tES. Previous studies point out that the effectiveness of stimulation depends on initial brain state, for which baseline performance is a crude yet valuable indicator [67, 68] Morphological and anatomical characteristics determine the field amplitude of applied current by using the same electrode montages as demonstrated by tDCS study of Parazzini and colleagues, who compared the effects of four different electrode montages on three different head models [69]. Besides individual's anatomical features, there are much more determinants, like age, sex circadian rhythm, and hormonal levels to take into account [68, 70–72].

So far, most studies on physiological effects of tACS rely on aftereffects of the stimulation and resting-state measurements while research on behavioral effects of tACS mainly focused on online effects of the stimulation [14, 44, 73, 74].

Despite there being no behavioral online or offline effects of 6 Hz tACS as well as tRNS in our study, on a descriptive level, there was a tendency towards a change in the response behavior both in the control conditions (higher number of errors in the tRNS and shorter reaction times in the sham and tRNS condition) (Figures 2(d) and 2(e)). Yet, this effect did not yield statistical significance. Analysis of the behavioral response showed that 18 of the 23 subjects (72%) were either faster or produced less errors in the 6 Hz condition compared to sham, but did not improve on both. The reason of this result could lie in individual response strategies. Also, it is possible that the stimulation over rIFG reached different regions of rIFG in the different subjects. Hampshire and colleagues [75] suggest that two functionally distinct subregions of the rIFG might exist, one region being involved in attention while another region being involved in inhibition. Since the anatomy of rIFG is very complex, the

stimulation could have led to an improvement of reaction times or committing less inhibition errors, depending on the region reached by the stimulation. This is supported by the findings in previous tDCS research, where different montages have resulted in an improvement of either reaction times or errors [12, 13, 76–78].

It is possible that tACS will not increase theta activity upon a certain level and therefore will not lead to behavioral benefits in people who do not lack theta activity, whereas it might induce improvement in people with a deficit of theta activity. A comparable effect was shown by Herrman and colleagues [43] for alpha activity: alpha activity was only increased by stimulation with the individual alpha frequency (IAF) of the subject, when the IAF power had been low beforehand. If the IAF power had been high before stimulation, no additional increase was found. So even though our hypothesis in this study could not be proved in healthy young adults, it should be further investigated in persons with ADHD as the power of their individual theta frequency is expected to be lower [7]. Also, it is possible that, while being absent on a behavioral level, changes were induced on a neurophysiological level.

Additionally, the brain-derived neurotrophic factor (BDNF) polymorphism is suggested to have an impact on transcranial stimulation-induced plasticity in humans, which differs according to the mechanism of plasticity induction [79].

5.3. Suitability of the Paradigm. Van Boxtel and colleagues have discussed whether "there is a centrally located inhibitory mechanism" [80], which "suppresses irrelevant responses" and whether "inhibition is localized to right IFG alone" [3]. rIFG is known to be important in different inhibition paradigms besides the Go/NoGo, e.g., the "stop after go" paradigm. Depending on the paradigm, different networks are activated during motor inhibition. Comparing the activation in a stop signal, Go/NoGo, and antisaccade paradigm, pre-SMA and different regions of IFC are activated, but still they are related to an activation of rIFG [2]. We decided to use the Go/NoGo paradigm to be able to compare our results to those of previous studies [6].

Early findings by Menon and colleagues [81] have provided evidence for a distributed error processing system in the human brain that overlaps partially with brain regions involved in response inhibition and competition. The authors found that the IFC is activated both during response inhibition and error processing. Since in the study of Mazaheri et al. [6], response inhibition and error monitoring are combined, possibly stimulating the IFC, rather than the rIFG would lead to an improvement in the Go/NoGo task.

Task difficulty is also another contributor to the state-dependent nature of the effects of tES [82]. For healthy students, our Go/NoGo task is a relatively easy and simple task. Therefore, ceiling effects may have masked any change in performance. Yet, subjects made relatively high number of errors, possibly due to the comparatively short and jittered response window and the long duration of the task, leaving sufficient room for improvement in most subjects.

6. Conclusion Suggestions for Improvements

Based on behavioral data, we could not show effects of 6 Hz tACS and tRNS on response inhibition in healthy adults. The lack of the well-described effect supports the notion that the setup of our montage and paradigm might not have been effective in showing improved performance during and after 6 Hz tACS.

A behavioral baseline would be an additional possibility to control for intraindividual differences. Yet, the lack of a baseline measure in our study poses a clear limitation. However, our within-subject design enables the comparison to a sham condition as a control condition with sessions at the same time of the day.

To determine whether the negative results translate to a larger population, a higher number of participants is required. The results derived from our study could contribute to the exploration of effects of noninvasive transcranial brain stimulation in a healthy population and should help to optimize existing stimulation protocols. Further studies should include simultaneous EEG recordings to investigate the underlying neurophysiological processes. Sharing negative findings will have (1) positive impact on future research questions and study design and (2) will improve knowledge acquisition of noninvasive transcranial brain stimulation techniques.

Acknowledgments

We acknowledge the financial support by Land Schleswig-Holstein within the funding program Open Access Publications funds and by STIPED funding from the European Union's Horizon 2020 research and innovation programme (no. 731827).

References

[1] A. R. Aron, T. E. Behrens, S. Smith, M. J. Frank, and R. A. Poldrack, "Triangulating a cognitive control network using diffusion-weighted magnetic resonance imaging (MRI) and functional MRI," *The Journal of Neuroscience*, vol. 27, no. 14, pp. 3743–3752, 2007.

[2] A. R. Aron, "From reactive to proactive and selective control: developing a richer model for stopping inappropriate responses," *Biological Psychiatry*, vol. 69, no. 12, pp. e55–e68, 2011.

[3] A. R. Aron, T. W. Robbins, and R. A. Poldrack, "Inhibition and the right inferior frontal cortex," *Trends in Cognitive Sciences*, vol. 8, no. 4, pp. 170–177, 2004.

[4] J. Duque, I. Greenhouse, L. Labruna, and R. B. Ivry, "Physiological markers of motor inhibition during human behavior," *Trends in Neurosciences*, vol. 40, no. 4, pp. 219–236, 2017.

[5] C. D. Chambers, M. A. Bellgrove, M. G. Stokes et al., "Executive "brake failure" following deactivation of human frontal lobe," *Journal of Cognitive Neuroscience*, vol. 18, no. 3, pp. 444–455, 2006.

[6] A. Mazaheri, I. L. C. Nieuwenhuis, H. van Dijk, and O. Jensen, "Prestimulus alpha and mu activity predicts failure to inhibit motor responses," *Human Brain Mapping*, vol. 30, no. 6, pp. 1791–1800, 2009.

[7] A. Mazaheri, C. Fassbender, S. Coffey-Corina, T. A. Hartanto, J. B. Schweitzer, and G. R. Mangun, "Differential oscillatory electroencephalogram between attention-deficit/hyperactivity disorder subtypes and typically developing adolescents," *Biological Psychiatry*, vol. 76, no. 5, pp. 422–429, 2014.

[8] G. Hartwigsen, T. O. Bergmann, D. M. Herz et al., "Modeling the effects of noninvasive transcranial brain stimulation at the biophysical, network, and cognitive level," *Progress in Brain Research*, vol. 222, pp. 261–287, 2015.

[9] A. J. Woods, A. Antal, M. Bikson et al., "A technical guide to tDCS, and related non-invasive brain stimulation tools," *Clinical Neurophysiology*, vol. 127, no. 2, pp. 1031–1048, 2016.

[10] A. Fertonani and C. Miniussi, "Transcranial electrical stimulation: what we know and do not know about mechanisms," *The Neuroscientist*, vol. 23, no. 2, pp. 109–123, 2017.

[11] T. O. Bergmann, A. Karabanov, G. Hartwigsen, A. Thielscher, and H. R. Siebner, "Combining non-invasive transcranial brain stimulation with neuroimaging and electrophysiology: current approaches and future perspectives," *Neuro Image*, vol. 140, pp. 4–19, 2016.

[12] L. Jacobson, D. C. Javitt, and M. Lavidor, "Activation of inhibition: diminishing impulsive behavior by direct current stimulation over the inferior frontal gyrus," *Journal of Cognitive Neuroscience*, vol. 23, no. 11, pp. 3380–3387, 2011.

[13] T. Cunillera, D. Brignani, D. Cucurell, L. Fuentemilla, and C. Miniussi, "The right inferior frontal cortex in response inhibition: a tDCS-ERP co-registration study," *Neuro Image*, vol. 140, pp. 66–75, 2016.

[14] T. Zaehle, S. Rach, and C. S. Herrmann, "Transcranial alternating current stimulation enhances individual alpha activity in human EEG," *PLoS One*, vol. 5, no. 11, article e13766, 2010.

[15] A. Pogosyan, L. D. Gaynor, A. Eusebio, and P. Brown, "Boosting cortical activity at beta-band frequencies slows movement in humans," *Current Biology*, vol. 19, no. 19, pp. 1637–1641, 2009.

[16] R. Polania, M. A. Nitsche, C. Korman, G. Batsikadze, and W. Paulus, "The importance of timing in segregated theta phase-coupling for cognitive performance," *Current Biology*, vol. 22, no. 14, pp. 1314–1318, 2012.

[17] V. Moliadze, A. Antal, and W. Paulus, "Boosting brain excitability by transcranial high frequency stimulation in the ripple range," *The Journal of Physiology*, vol. 588, no. 24, pp. 4891–4904, 2010.

[18] A. Antal and C. S. Herrmann, "Transcranial alternating current and random noise stimulation: possible mechanisms," *Neural Plasticity*, vol. 2016, Article ID 3616807, 12 pages, 2016.

[19] N. Jausovec and K. Jausovec, "Increasing working memory capacity with theta transcranial alternating current stimulation (tACS)," *Biological Psychology*, vol. 96, pp. 42–47, 2014.

[20] N. Jausovec, K. Jausovec, and A. Pahor, "The influence of theta transcranial alternating current stimulation (tACS) on working memory storage and processing functions," *Acta Psychologica*, vol. 146, pp. 1–6, 2014.

[21] D. Antonenko, M. Faxel, U. Grittner, M. Lavidor, and A. Floel, "Effects of transcranial alternating current stimulation on cognitive functions in healthy young and older adults," *Neural Plasticity*, vol. 2016, Article ID 4274127, 13 pages, 2016.

[22] O. Meiron and M. Lavidor, "Prefrontal oscillatory stimulation modulates access to cognitive control references in retrospective metacognitive commentary," *Clinical Neurophysiology*, vol. 125, no. 1, pp. 77–82, 2014.

[23] A. Pahor and N. Jausovec, "The effects of theta transcranial alternating current stimulation (tACS) on fluid intelligence," *International Journal of Psychophysiology*, vol. 93, no. 3, pp. 322–331, 2014.

[24] K. Heimrath, M. Fiene, K. S. Rufener, and T. Zaehle, "Modulating human auditory processing by transcranial electrical stimulation," *Frontiers in Cellular Neuroscience*, vol. 10, p. 53, 2016.

[25] E. Erdfelder, F. Faul, and A. Buchner, "GPOWER: a general power analysis program," *Behavior Research Methods, Instruments, & Computers*, vol. 28, no. 1, pp. 1–11, 1996.

[26] T. Iuculano and R. Cohen Kadosh, "The mental cost of cognitive enhancement," *The Journal of Neuroscience*, vol. 33, no. 10, pp. 4482–4486, 2013.

[27] J. van Driel, I. G. Sligte, J. Linders, D. Elport, and M. X. Cohen, "Frequency band-specific electrical brain stimulation modulates cognitive control processes," *PloS One*, vol. 10, no. 9, article e0138984, 2015.

[28] G. H. Franke, *Die Symptom-Checkliste von Derogatis (SCL-90-R) - Deutsche Version-Manual*, Beltz, 2nd edition, 2002.

[29] S. Schmidt and F. Petermann, *ADHS-Screening für Erwachsene (ADHS-E): Ein Verfahren zur Erfassung von Symptomen einer ADHS im Erwachsenenalter*, Pearson Assessment, Frankfurt/Main, 2009.

[30] M. Hautzinger, F. Keller, and C. Kühner, "Beck depressionsinventar (BDI-II)," *Revision*, Harcourt Test Services, Frankfurt/Main, Deutsche Bearbeitung von Beck, A. T., Steer, R. A., & Brown, G. K. (1996). Beck Depression Inventory-II (BDI-II). San Antonio, TX: Harcourt Assessment Inc, 2006.

[31] R. C. Oldfield, "The assessment and analysis of handedness: the Edinburgh inventory," *Neuropsychologia*, vol. 9, no. 1, pp. 97–113, 1971.

[32] C. Poreisz, K. Boros, A. Antal, and W. Paulus, "Safety aspects of transcranial direct current stimulation concerning healthy subjects and patients," *Brain Research Bulletin*, vol. 72, no. 4-6, pp. 208–214, 2007.

[33] R Core Team, *R: a Language and Environment for Statistical Computing*, R Foundation for Statistical Computing, Wien, Österreich, 2015.

[34] D. Stroux, A. Shushakova, A. J. Geburek-Höfer, P. Ohrmann, F. Rist, and A. Pedersen, "Deficient interference control during working memory updating in adults with ADHD: an event-related potential study," *Clinical Neurophysiology*, vol. 127, no. 1, pp. 452–463, 2016.

[35] M. J. Kane, A. R. A. Conway, T. K. Miura, and G. J. H. Colflesh, "Working memory, attention control, and the N-back task: a question of construct validity," *Journal of Experimental Psychology Learning, Memory, and Cognition*, vol. 33, no. 3, pp. 615–622, 2007.

[36] J. T. Townsend and F. G. Ashby, *The Stochastic Modeling of Elementary Psychological Processes*, Cambridge University Press, Cambridge, 1983.

[37] I. M. Zielinski, B. Steenbergen, C. M. Baas, P. Aarts, and M. L. A. Jongsma, "Event-related potentials during target-response tasks to study cognitive processes of upper limb use in children with unilateral cerebral palsy," *Journal of Visualized Experiments*, no. 107, article e53420, 2016.

[38] M. E. J. Masson, "A tutorial on a practical Bayesian alternative to null-hypothesis significance testing," *Behavior Research Methods*, vol. 43, no. 3, pp. 679–690, 2011.

[39] A. E. Raftery, "Bayesian model selection in social research," *Sociological Methodology*, vol. 25, p. 111, 1995.

[40] D. Veniero, A. Vossen, J. Gross, and G. Thut, "Lasting EEG/MEG aftereffects of rhythmic transcranial brain stimulation: level of control over oscillatory network activity," *Frontiers in Cellular Neuroscience*, vol. 9, p. 477, 2015.

[41] A. R. Aron, P. C. Fletcher, E. T. Bullmore, B. J. Sahakian, and T. W. Robbins, "Stop-signal inhibition disrupted by damage to right inferior frontal gyrus in humans," *Nature Neuroscience*, vol. 6, no. 2, pp. 115-116, 2003.

[42] N. C. Swann, W. Cai, C. R. Conner et al., "Roles for the presupplementary motor area and the right inferior frontal gyrus in stopping action: electrophysiological responses and functional and structural connectivity," *Neuro Image*, vol. 59, no. 3, pp. 2860–2870, 2012.

[43] C. S. Herrmann, S. Rach, T. Neuling, and D. Struber, "Transcranial alternating current stimulation: a review of the underlying mechanisms and modulation of cognitive processes," *Frontiers in Human Neuroscience*, vol. 7, p. 279, 2013.

[44] T. Neuling, S. Rach, and C. S. Herrmann, "Orchestrating neuronal networks: sustained after-effects of transcranial alternating current stimulation depend upon brain states," *Frontiers in Human Neuroscience*, vol. 7, p. 161, 2013.

[45] J. van Driel, K. R. Ridderinkhof, and M. X. Cohen, "Not all errors are alike: theta and alpha EEG dynamics relate to differences in error-processing dynamics," *The Journal of Neuroscience*, vol. 32, no. 47, pp. 16795–16806, 2012.

[46] M. S. Clayton, N. Yeung, and R. Cohen Kadosh, "The roles of cortical oscillations in sustained attention," *Trends in Cognitive Sciences*, vol. 19, no. 4, pp. 188–195, 2015.

[47] B. S. Chander, M. Witkowski, C. Braun et al., "tACS phase locking of frontal midline theta oscillations disrupts working memory performance," *Frontiers in Cellular Neuroscience*, vol. 10, p. 120, 2016.

[48] G. Thut, P. G. Schyns, and J. Gross, "Entrainment of perceptually relevant brain oscillations by non-invasive rhythmic stimulation of the human brain," *Frontiers in Psychology*, vol. 2, p. 170, 2011.

[49] A. Karabanov, A. Thielscher, and H. R. Siebner, "Transcranial brain stimulation: closing the loop between brain and stimulation," *Current Opinion in Neurology*, vol. 29, no. 4, pp. 397–404, 2016.

[50] J.-S. Brittain, P. Probert-Smith, T. Z. Aziz, and P. Brown, "Tremor suppression by rhythmic transcranial current stimulation," *Current Biology*, vol. 23, no. 5, pp. 436–440, 2013.

[51] A. Fertonani, C. Pirulli, and C. Miniussi, "Random noise stimulation improves neuroplasticity in perceptual learning,"

The Journal of Neuroscience, vol. 31, no. 43, pp. 15416–15423, 2011.

[52] M. Cappelletti, E. Gessaroli, R. Hithersay et al., "Transfer of cognitive training across magnitude dimensions achieved with concurrent brain stimulation of the parietal lobe," *The Journal of Neuroscience*, vol. 33, no. 37, pp. 14899–14907, 2013.

[53] R. Camilleri, A. Pavan, F. Ghin, L. Battaglini, and G. Campana, "Improvement of uncorrected visual acuity and contrast sensitivity with perceptual learning and transcranial random noise stimulation in individuals with mild myopia," *Frontiers in Psychology*, vol. 5, p. 1234, 2014.

[54] D. Terney, L. Chaieb, V. Moliadze, A. Antal, and W. Paulus, "Increasing human brain excitability by transcranial high-frequency random noise stimulation," *Journal of Neuroscience*, vol. 28, no. 52, pp. 14147–14155, 2008.

[55] A. Antal and W. Paulus, "Transcranial alternating current stimulation (tACS)," *Frontiers in Human Neuroscience*, vol. 7, p. 317, 2013.

[56] V. Moliadze, D. Atalay, A. Antal, and W. Paulus, "Close to threshold transcranial electrical stimulation preferentially activates inhibitory networks before switching to excitation with higher intensities," *Brain Stimulation*, vol. 5, no. 4, pp. 505–511, 2012.

[57] M. A. Nitsche and W. Paulus, "Excitability changes induced in the human motor cortex by weak transcranial direct current stimulation," *The Journal of Physiology*, vol. 527, no. 3, pp. 633–639, 2000.

[58] M. A. Nitsche, S. Doemkes, T. Karaköse et al., "Shaping the effects of transcranial direct current stimulation of the human motor cortex," *Journal of Neurophysiology*, vol. 97, no. 4, pp. 3109–3117, 2007.

[59] M. Bikson, A. Datta, A. Rahman, and J. Scaturro, "Electrode montages for tDCS and weak transcranial electrical stimulation: role of "return" electrode's position and size," *Clinical Neurophysiology*, vol. 121, no. 12, pp. 1976–1978, 2010.

[60] V. Moliadze, A. Antal, and W. Paulus, "Electrode-distance dependent after-effects of transcranial direct and random noise stimulation with extracephalic reference electrodes," *Clinical Neurophysiology*, vol. 121, no. 12, pp. 2165–2171, 2010.

[61] A. R. Mehta, A. Pogosyan, P. Brown, and J.-S. Brittain, "Montage matters: the influence of transcranial alternating current stimulation on human physiological tremor," *Brain Stimulation*, vol. 8, no. 2, pp. 260–268, 2015.

[62] P. C. Miranda, A. Mekonnen, R. Salvador, and G. Ruffini, "The electric field in the cortex during transcranial current stimulation," *Neuro Image*, vol. 70, pp. 48–58, 2013.

[63] A. Opitz, W. Paulus, S. Will, A. Antunes, and A. Thielscher, "Determinants of the electric field during transcranial direct current stimulation," *Neuro Image*, vol. 109, pp. 140–150, 2015.

[64] K.-A. Ho, J. L. Taylor, T. Chew et al., "The effect of transcranial direct current stimulation (tDCS) electrode size and current intensity on motor cortical excitability: evidence from single and repeated sessions," *Brain Stimulation*, vol. 9, no. 1, pp. 1–7, 2016.

[65] K. S. Rufener, P. Ruhnau, H.-J. Heinze, and T. Zaehle, "Transcranial random noise stimulation (tRNS) shapes the processing of rapidly changing auditory information," *Frontiers in Cellular Neuroscience*, vol. 11, p. 162, 2017.

[66] C. Y. Looi, J. Lim, F. Sella et al., "Transcranial random noise stimulation and cognitive training to improve learning and cognition of the atypically developing brain: a pilot study," *Scientific Reports*, vol. 7, no. 1, p. 4633, 2017.

[67] J. C. Horvath, J. D. Forte, and O. Carter, "Evidence that transcranial direct current stimulation (tDCS) generates little-to-no reliable neurophysiologic effect beyond MEP amplitude modulation in healthy human subjects: a systematic review," *Neuropsychologia*, vol. 66, pp. 213–236, 2015.

[68] B. Krause and R. Cohen Kadosh, "Not all brains are created equal: the relevance of individual differences in responsiveness to transcranial electrical stimulation," *Frontiers in Systems Neuroscience*, vol. 8, p. 25, 2014.

[69] M. Parazzini, S. Fiocchi, I. Liorni, and P. Ravazzani, "Effect of the interindividual variability on computational modeling of transcranial direct current stimulation," *Computational Intelligence and Neuroscience*, vol. 2015, Article ID 963293, 9 pages, 2015.

[70] I. Laakso, S. Tanaka, S. Koyama, V. de Santis, and A. Hirata, "Inter-subject variability in electric fields of motor cortical tDCS," *Brain Stimulation*, vol. 8, no. 5, pp. 906–913, 2015.

[71] V. Moliadze, T. Schmanke, S. Andreas, E. Lyzhko, C. M. Freitag, and M. Siniatchkin, "Stimulation intensities of transcranial direct current stimulation have to be adjusted in children and adolescents," *Clinical Neurophysiology*, vol. 126, no. 7, pp. 1392–1399, 2015.

[72] V. Moliadze, E. Lyzhko, T. Schmanke, S. Andreas, C. M. Freitag, and M. Siniatchkin, "1 mA cathodal tDCS shows excitatory effects in children and adolescents: insights from TMS evoked N100 potential," *Brain Research Bulletin*, vol. 140, pp. 43–51, 2018.

[73] A. Vossen, J. Gross, and G. Thut, "Alpha power increase after transcranial alternating current stimulation at alpha frequency (α-tACS) reflects plastic changes rather than entrainment," *Brain Stimulation*, vol. 8, no. 3, pp. 499–508, 2015.

[74] F. H. Kasten, J. Dowsett, and C. S. Herrmann, "Sustained after-effect of α-tACS lasts up to 70 min after stimulation," *Frontiers in Human Neuroscience*, vol. 10, p. 245, 2016.

[75] A. Hampshire, S. R. Chamberlain, M. M. Monti, J. Duncan, and A. M. Owen, "The role of the right inferior frontal gyrus: inhibition and attentional control," *Neuro Image*, vol. 50, no. 3, pp. 1313–1319, 2010.

[76] F. Dambacher, T. Schuhmann, J. Lobbestael, A. Arntz, S. Brugman, and A. T. Sack, "No effects of bilateral tDCS over inferior frontal gyrus on response inhibition and aggression," *PLoS One*, vol. 10, no. 7, p. e0132170, 2015.

[77] T. Ditye, L. Jacobson, V. Walsh, and M. Lavidor, "Modulating behavioral inhibition by tDCS combined with cognitive training," *Experimental Brain Research*, vol. 219, no. 3, pp. 363–368, 2012.

[78] D. F. Stramaccia, B. Penolazzi, G. Sartori, M. Braga, S. Mondini, and G. Galfano, "Assessing the effects of tDCS over a delayed response inhibition task by targeting the right inferior frontal gyrus and right dorsolateral prefrontal cortex," *Experimental Brain Research*, vol. 233, no. 8, pp. 2283–2290, 2015.

[79] A. Antal, L. Chaieb, V. Moliadze et al., "Brain-derived neurotrophic factor (BDNF) gene polymorphisms shape cortical plasticity in humans," *Brain Stimulation*, vol. 3, no. 4, pp. 230–237, 2010.

[80] G. J. M. van Boxtel, M. W. van der Molen, J. R. Jennings, and C. H. M. Brunia, "A psychophysiological analysis of inhibitory motor control in the stop-signal paradigm," *Biological Psychology*, vol. 58, no. 3, pp. 229–262, 2001.

[81] V. Menon, N. E. Adleman, C. D. White, G. H. Glover, and A. L. Reiss, "Error-related brain activation during a Go/NoGo response inhibition task," *Human Brain Mapping*, vol. 12, no. 3, pp. 131–143, 2001.

[82] K. T. Jones and M. E. Berryhill, "Parietal contributions to visual working memory depend on task difficulty," *Frontiers in Psychiatry*, vol. 3, p. 81, 2012.

13

Low-Frequency Repetitive Transcranial Magnetic Stimulation for Stroke-Induced Upper Limb Motor Deficit: A Meta-Analysis

Lan Zhang,[1,2] **Guoqiang Xing,**[1,3] **Shiquan Shuai,**[1] **Zhiwei Guo,**[1] **Huaping Chen,**[1] **Morgan A. McClure,**[1] **Xiaojuan Chen,**[4] **and Qiwen Mu**[1,5]

[1]*Department of Imaging & Imaging Institute of Rehabilitation and Development of Brain Function,*
The Second Clinical Medical College of North Sichuan Medical College, Nanchong Central Hospital, Nanchong 637000, China
[2]*Department of Radiology, Langzhong People's Hospital, Nanchong 637000, China*
[3]*Lotus Biotech.com LLC., John Hopkins University-MCC, Rockville, MD 20850, USA*
[4]*North Sichuan Medical College, Nanchong 637000, China*
[5]*Peking University Third Hospital, Beijing 100080, China*

Correspondence should be addressed to Qiwen Mu; muqiwen99@yahoo.com

Academic Editor: Andrea Turolla

Background and Purpose. This meta-analysis aimed to evaluate the therapeutic potential of low-frequency repetitive transcranial magnetic stimulation (LF-rTMS) over the contralesional hemisphere on upper limb motor recovery and cortex plasticity after stroke. *Methods.* Databases of PubMed, Medline, ScienceDirect, Cochrane, and Embase were searched for randomized controlled trials published before Jun 31, 2017. The effect size was evaluated by using the standardized mean difference (SMD) and a 95% confidence interval (CI). Resting motor threshold (rMT) and motor-evoked potential (MEP) were also examined. *Results.* Twenty-two studies of 1 Hz LF-rTMS over the contralesional hemisphere were included. Significant efficacy was found on finger flexibility (SMD = 0.75), hand strength (SMD = 0.49), and activity dexterity (SMD = 0.32), but not on body function (SMD = 0.29). The positive changes of rMT (SMD = 0.38 for the affected hemisphere and SMD = −0.83 for the unaffected hemisphere) and MEP (SMD = −1.00 for the affected hemisphere and SMD = 0.57 for the unaffected hemisphere) were also significant. *Conclusions.* LF-rTMS as an add-on therapy significantly improved upper limb functional recovery especially the hand after stroke, probably through rebalanced cortical excitability of both hemispheres. Future studies should determine if LF-rTMS alone or in conjunction with practice/training would be more effective. *Clinical Trial Registration Information.* This trial is registered with unique identifier CRD42016042181.

1. Introduction

Stroke is a global disease with high rates of long-term disability [1]. Around the world, 25%–74% of stroke survivors require different levels of assistance for daily living mainly due to upper limb hemiplegia [2]. In search for better therapies, scientists have been trying to understand the relationship between stroke motor recovery and cortical reorganization [3]. The equilibrium of cortical excitability between the two hemispheres is often disrupted after stroke. In the affected hemisphere, both the cortical excitability and the homonymous motor representation of the affected hemisphere decrease; whereas the excitability in the unaffected hemisphere increases [4].

Repetitive transcranial magnetic stimulation (rTMS) is a noninvasive stimulation to induce electrical currents in the brain tissues. Currently, rTMS is being explored as a novel therapy in modulating cortical excitability to improve motor functions in stroke patients [5]. Of the two forms of rTMS, high-frequency rTMS (HF-rTMS > 1.0 Hz), applied over the ipsilesional hemisphere, facilitates cortical excitability [6], whereas, low-frequency rTMS (LF-rTMS ≤ 1.0 Hz), applied over the contralesional hemisphere, decreases cortical excitability [7].

The effect of rTMS is primarily determined by the stimulation frequency [8] and targeted region [3]. Although both LF-rTMS and HF-rTMS could treat motor dysfunction in poststroke patients, LF-rTMS is considered safer and superior to HF-rTMS in motor function recovery [9–12]. Lomarev et al. [13] reported increased risk for seizures by HF-rTMS of 20–25 Hz. To date, the majority of rTMS trials on motor recovery after stroke used the protocol of LF-rTMS with 1 Hz. In comparison, the HF-rTMS studies involved only a small number of trials and applied varied frequency protocols (3 Hz to 25 Hz). According to Cho et al. [14], the primary motor cortex (M1) forms a main part of the motor cortices and contributes to the high order control of motor behaviors. Until now, most studies about the efficacy of LF-rTMS on functional rehabilitation have focused on the M1. In healthy subjects, LF-rTMS applied over the M1 increased the resting motor threshold (rMT) and decreased the motor-evoked potential (MEP) size of the ipsilateral hemisphere, suggesting a suppressive effect of LF-rTMS in the intact M1 [15].

Multiple studies have investigated the therapeutic effect of LF-rTMS after stroke [8, 16–19], with the outcomes of pinch force [19–22], grip force [10, 22–25], finger tapping [8, 9, 26–29], and overall function [15, 30–34]. Other studies also explored the impact of rTMS on cortical excitability [10, 18, 19, 26]. However, inconsistent reports exist regarding the benefits of LF-rTMS: Some studies showed no beneficial effect of LF-rTMS [16, 23, 29] and one study reported worsening effects of LF-rTMS such as decreased finger-tapping speed; [35] other investigators proposed that inhibition of the contralesional motor areas may lead to deterioration of the function of the unaffected hand [24, 26]. Although a few previous meta-analyses had investigated the therapeutic effect of rTMS after stroke [11, 36–38], they focused on the mixed effect of combined LF-rTMS and HF-rTMS interventions or on the combined outcomes of varying motor measurements. So far, there is a lack of in-depth systematic meta-analysis about the efficacy of LF-rTMS on upper limb function recovery.

The primary objective of this study was to evaluate the effects of LF-rTMS on upper limb motor recovery after stroke in several aspects: "finger flexibility," "hand strength," "activity dexterity," and "body function level." The effects of LF-rTMS on motor cortex excitability which were represented by MEP and rMTin poststroke patients were also evaluated.

2. Methods

2.1. Protocol. Our meta-analysis followed the PRISMA statement.

2.2. Search Strategy. The databases of PubMed, ScienceDirect, Embase, and the Cochrane Library were searched for randomized controlled trials published before June 31, 2017. The search terms were "stroke/cerebrovascular accident, repetitive transcranial magnetic stimulation/rTMS, and upper limb/hand." The search was limited to human studies. Manual searches of the reference lists of the pertinent articles were also conducted to identify relevant articles [11, 36].

2.3. Study Selection. The preliminary screening was based on the title and abstract. As there were several separate aims of the paper, the articles with either any motor function assessment or MEP/rMT outcomes were all considered. Two reviewers independently assessed the eligibility of the literature. If there was a disagreement, the two reviewers checked the full text of the article and discussed with each other to reach an agreement. The selected articles were then assessed in their entirety. Studies were included if they met the following criteria: (1) they were randomized controlled trials; (2) they have ≥five patients in a trial; (3) the patients were adults (≥18 yrs); (4) the focus was on the effects on the upper limb in poststroke patients; (5) the types of intervention were LF-rTMS over the contralesional M1; (6) the outcomes were on continuous scales that evaluated the motor function of upper limb or cortical excitability; and (7) they were published in peer-reviewed English journals.

2.4. Quality Appraisal. Each included study was individually assessed by two reviewers according to a modified checklist of Moher et al. [39] that provided the following criteria: (1) blinding procedure (0 indicated a nonblind or no-mention procedure, 1 or 2 represented single blind or double blind, resp.); (2) dropout number; (3) description of baseline demographic data (was recorded as 1 if described, if not as 0); (4) point estimate and variability (was denoted as 1 if provided); and (5) description of adverse events (was recorded as the number and type of adverse event).

2.5. Data Extraction. A standard form was jointly designed by two reviewers for collecting the relevant data from each study for the following information: (1) patient characteristics; (2) trial design; (3) rTMS protocol; (4) outcome measures; (5) the duration of follow-up; and (6) mean difference and standard deviation (SD) of the scores immediately (short term) and chronically (long term) after the interventions (assessment within one day after the last rTMS session was considered as short-term outcome; assessment at one month or longer after the last rTMS session was considered long-term outcome [40]). Statistical analysis used the data of between different interventions. If the changes in scores of both groups were not clearly defined, the mean and SD of the scores after intervention for both groups were extracted on the premise of no statistical differences in baseline between the two groups. If the outcome was expressed only as a graph, the software GetData Graph Digitizer 2.25 (http://getdata-graph-digitizer.com/) was used to extract the required data.

2.6. Data Synthesis and Analysis. To elaborate the therapeutic effect of LF-rTMS on upper extremity recovery after stroke, the motor measures were categorized into four subclasses according to a previous study [41] of upper limb outcome measures in stroke rehabilitation: "finger flexibility," "hand strength," "activity dexterity," and "body function level." The results of the finger tapping were pooled to evaluate finger flexibility. The results of pinch force and grip force were pooled to evaluate hand strength. The results of action research arm test (ARAT), Wolf motor function test (WMFT), Jebsen-Taylor test (JTT), and nine-hole peg test

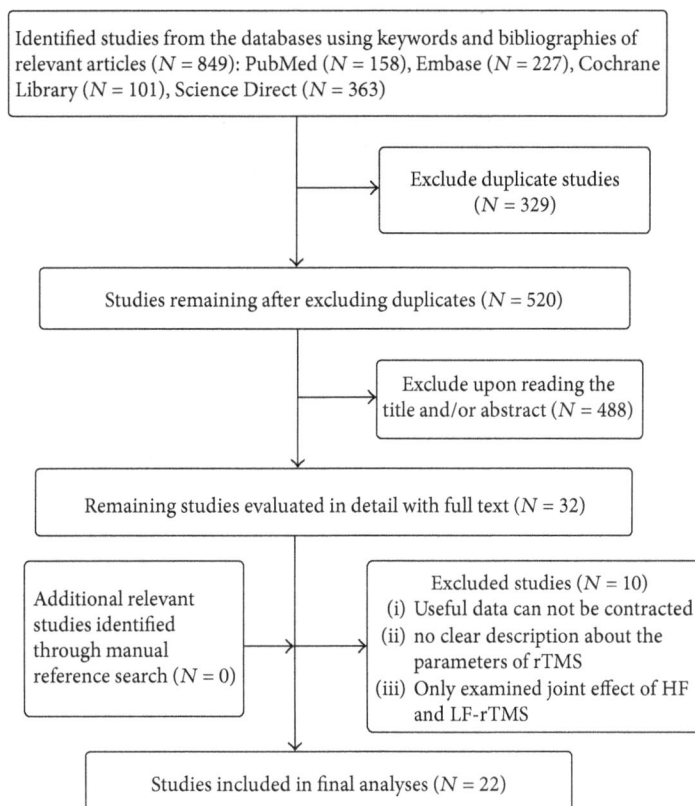

Figure 1: Selection process flow diagram.

(NHPT) were pooled to evaluate activity dexterity. The results of upper extremity Fugl-Meyer Assessment (FMA) were pooled to evaluate body function. For evaluating cortical excitability, the results of the rMT and MEP in both hemispheres were extracted [42, 43].

The meta-analysis was performed by using the Review Manager Software version 5.2 (Cochrane Collaboration, Oxford, England) with the formulation Hedges' g [44]. Data were described as mean $\pm$ SD. For the outcomes using different scales, we refer to the Cochrane Hand Book (Cochrane Collaboration, Oxford, England). The effect size of LF-rTMS was expressed by the standardized mean difference (SMD) with a 95% confidence interval (CI). The heterogeneity was tested by using the I^2 test [45]. If a significant heterogeneity was found ($I^2 \geq 50\%$), the random effect model was applied; otherwise, a fixed model was used. In addition, the trim and fill method [46] was constructed by using STATA/SE version 11.0 (STATA Corporation, Texas, USA) to test publication bias. The value of statistical significance was set at $P < 0.05$. Finally, effect sizes were classified as small (<0.2), medium (0.2–0.8), or large (>0.8) [47]. Sensitivity analysis was conducted to investigate the impact of lesion site, timing of stimulation from stroke onset, and other characteristics on the results.

3. Results

3.1. Study Identification. Of the total 849 studies found after the initial database search, 22 studies were identified

($N = 619$) finally. The flow diagram of the selection process is shown in Figure 1.

All of the included studies applied 1 Hz rTMS over the contralesional M1. Except one study [15] that included patients with severe motor deficits and one study [21] that included patients with mild to severe deficit, all the others recruited patients with mild to moderate motor deficits. Most studies excluded the patients with other neuropsychiatric comorbidities such as aphasia, spatial neglect, or visual field deficit. Five studies [20, 24–27] used LF-rTMS as monotherapy and gained significant effect size; the others used LF-rTMS as cotherapy of active training, that is, in most of the studies, patients were also undergoing other treatments and training in both the rTMS and control groups. The details of the included studies and the results of quality assessment are shown in Tables 1 and 2 separately.

3.2. Motor Function Measurement

3.2.1. Finger Flexibility. Six studies ($N = 176$) [8–10, 27–29] assessed the short-term finger flexibility. LF-rTMS had a high medium mean effect size of 0.75 (95% CI = 0.44–1.06; $P < 0.001$) without heterogeneity ($I^2 = 0\%$) (fixed-effect model) (Figure 2(a)). The SMD for long term was 0.53 (95% CI, 0.12–0.94; $P = 0.01$) without heterogeneity ($I^2 = 0\%$).

3.2.2. Hand Strength. Eleven studies ($N = 227$) [9, 10, 17–25] evaluated short-term hand strength that showed a medium effect size of LF-rTMS therapy (SMD = 0.49; 95% CI = 0.22–0.76; $P < 0.001$; and $I^2 = 12\%$) in the fixed-effect model

TABLE 1: Characteristics of the selected studies.

Study	N (Exp/Ctr)	Mean age	Time poststroke	Lesion site	Trial design	rTMS protocol	Outcome measurement Motor function	Neurophysiology	Follow-up	Combined training/practice
Takeuchi et al. [19]	10/10	59 Y	6–60 m	Subcortical	P	1.0 Hz, 90% rMT, 1500 pulses × 1 days	Pinch force	rMT, MEP		Motor training
Fregni et al. [26]	10/5	56 Y	6–120 m	(13/15) Subcortical	P	1.0 Hz, 100% rMT, 1500 pulses × 5 days	PPT, JTT	rMT		
Liepert et al. [24]	12/12	63 Y	<2 wks	Subcortical	C	1.0 Hz, 90% rMT, 1200 pulses × 1 days	NHPT, grip force			
Takeuchi et al. [18]	10/10	62.3 Y	7–121 m	Subcortical	P	1.0 Hz, 90% rMT, 1500 pulses × 1 days	Pinch force	rMT, MEP		Motor training
Dafotakis et al. [20]	12/12	45.5 Y	1–4 m	Subcortical	C	1.0 Hz, 100% rMT, 600 pulses × 1 days	Pinch force			
Nowak et al. [27]	15/15	46 Y	1–4 m	Subcortical	C	1.0 Hz, 100% rMT, 600 pulses × 1 days	Finger tapping,			
Khedr et al. [10]	12/12	57.9 Y	1–2 wks	Nonspecified	P	1.0 Hz, 100% rMT, 900 pulses × 5 days	Finger tapping, grip force	MEP	3 m	Passive movement
Emara et al. [8]	20/20	54 Y	2–13.5 m	Nonspecified	P	1.0 Hz, 110%–120% rMT, 1500 pulses × 10 days	Finger tapping		3 m	Physical therapy
Theilig et al. [15]	12/12	61 Y	2 wks–58 m	Nonspecified	P	1.0 Hz, 100% rMT, 900 pulses × 10 days	WMFT	MEP		Extensor activity
Takeuchi et al. [17]	9/9	61.5 Y	62–71.9 m	Subcortical	P	1.0 Hz, 90% rMT, 1200 pulses × 1 days	Pinch force	MEP		Motor training
Conforto et al. [21]	15/15	55.8 Y	5–45 days	Nonspecified	P	1.0 Hz, 90% rMT, 1500 pulses × 10 days	Pinch force, JTT		1 m	Rehabilitation treatment
Seniow et al. [30]	20/20	63.4 Y	12–129 days	Nonspecified	P	1.0 Hz, 90% rMT, 1800 pulses × 15 days	FMA		3 m	Motor training
Sasaki et al. [9]	11/9	65 Y	6–29 days	Nonspecified	P	1.0 Hz, 90% rMT, 1800 pulses × 5 days	Finger tapping, grip force			Motor training
Higgins et al. [22]	6/5	66.2 Y	18–315 m	Not reported	P	1.0 Hz, 110% rMT, 1.200 pulses × 8 days	Pinch force		1 m	Task-oriented training
Sung et al. [28]	15/12	63.2 Y	3–12 m	Nonspecified	P	1.0 Hz, 90% rMT, 600 pulses × 10 days	Finger tapping, WMFT	rMT, MEP		Occupational therapy
Wang et al. [32]	17/15	62.6 Y	2–6 m	Nonspecified	P	1.0 Hz, 90% rMT, 600 pulses × 10 days	WMFT	rMT, MEP		Task-oriented training
Rose et al. [23]	11/10	64.6 Y	7–150 m	Not reported	P	1.0 Hz, 100% rMT, 1200 pulses × 16 days	Grip force, FMA	rMT, MEP	1 m	Functional task practice
Galvão et al. [31]	10/10	61 Y	>6 m	Not reported	P	1.0 Hz, 90% rMT, 1500 pulses × 10 days	FMA		1 m	Physical therapy

TABLE 1: Continued.

Study	N (Exp/ Ctr)	Mean age	Time poststroke	Lesion site	Trial design	rTMS protocol	Outcome measurement Motor function	Outcome measurement Neurophysiology	Follow-up	Combined training/ practice
Ludemann-Podubecka et al. [29]	20/20	67 Y	0.25–4 m	Nonspecified	P	1.0 Hz, 100% rMT, 900 pulses × 15 days	Finger tapping, WMFT	MEP	6 m	Task-oriented training
Zheng et al. [33]	55/53	66 Y	<1 m	Nonspecified	P	1.0 Hz, 90% rMT, 1800 pulses × 24 days	FMA, WMFT			Occupational therapy
Matsuura et al. [25]	10/10	73. Y	<1 m	Subcortical	P	1.0 Hz, 100% rMT, 1200 pulses × 5 days	Grip force, FMA			
Du et al. [34]	23/23		3 days–1 m	Nonspecified	P	1.0 Hz, 110–120% rMT, 1200 pulses × 20 days	FMA		6 m	Motor exercises

Ctr: control group; Exp: experimental group; P: parallel sham control; C: crossover sham control; FMA: Fugl-Meyer assessment; ARAT: action research arm test; JTT: Jebsen-Taylor test; m: month; MEP: motor-evoked potential; NHPT: nine-hole peg test; PPT: purdue pegboard test; rMT: resting motor threshold; wk: week; Y: years; WMFT: Wolf motor function test.

TABLE 2: Quality appraisal of the selected articles.

Study	Blind process	Description of baseline data	Dropout	Point estimate and variability	Overall quality appraisal score
Takeuchi et al. [19]	2	1	0	0	3
Fregni et al. [26]	2	1	0	1	4
Liepert et al. [24]	2	0	0	1	3
Takeuchi et al. [18]	2	1	0	0	3
Dafotakis et al. [20]	0	1	0	1	2
Nowak et al. [27]	0	1	0	1	2
Khedr et al. [10]	2	1	0	1	4
Emara et al. [8]	2	1	0	1	4
Theilig et al. [15]	2	1	0	0	3
Takeuchi et al. [17]	1	1	0	1	3
Conforto et al. [21]	2	1	1	0	2
Seniow et al. [30]	2	1	7	0	2
Sasaki et al. [9]	0	1	0	0	1
Higgins et al. [22]	1	1	2	0	1
Sung et al. [28]	2	1	0	1	4
Wang et al. [32]	2	1	0	1	4
Rose et al. [23]	2	1	3	0	2
Galvão et al. [31]	2	1	0	0	3
Ludemann-Podubecka et al. [29]	2	1	0	0	3
Zheng et al. [33]	2	1	4	0	2
Matsuura et al. [25]	2	1	0	1	4
Du et al. [34]	2	1	0	1	4

In the case of any dropout, the total score will be subtracted by 1.

(Figure 2(b)). No significant treatment effect was found for long-term effect: SMD = 0.38; 95% CI = −0.36 to 1.13; $P = 0.31$; and $I^2 = 58\%$.

3.2.3. Upper Limb Activity Dexterity.
The pooled outcomes of ten trials ($N = 299$) [15, 21, 23, 24, 26, 28, 29, 32, 33] were used to evaluate the short-term upper limb activity dexterity. The result of the fixed-effect model showed a medium effect size of 0.32 (95% CI = 0.09–0.55; $P = 0.006$) without heterogeneity ($I^2 = 0\%$) (Figure 2(c)). No significant long-term treatment effect was found: SMD = 0.14; 95% CI = −0.22 to 0.49; $P = 0.45$; and $I^2 = 0\%$.

3.2.4. Body Function Level.
The pooled results from seven studies ($N = 313$) [23, 25, 28, 30–34] for short-term effect of LF-rTMS on body function level showed a nonsignificant mean effect size of 0.29 (95% CI = −0.06–0.64; $P = 0.10$) (random effect model) due to the presence of heterogeneity ($I^2 = 52\%$) (Figure 2(d)). No significant long-term effect of LF-rTMS was found on body function [23, 30, 31]: SMD = 0.10; 95% CI = −0.70 to 0.90; $P = 0.80$; and $I^2 = 77\%$.

3.2.5. Comparison of the Motor Effect Sizes.
The short-term effectiveness of LF-rTMS appears to follow this descending order: finger ability is greater than hand strength which is greater than the activity dexterity and greater than body function. A similar long-term therapeutic effect of LF-rTMS was observed (Figure 3).

3.3. Neurophysiologic Measurement

3.3.1. MEPs in Both Hemispheres.
Four studies ($N = 122$) [10, 28, 32, 34] were pooled to explore the effects of LF-rTMS on MEPs in the affected hemisphere; and eight studies ($N = 200$) [10, 15, 17–19, 23, 29, 34] were pooled for MEPs in the unaffected hemisphere, by using the fixed effect model with the amplitude of the MEPs. The results showed a significant enhancing effect of MEP in the affected hemisphere (SMD = 0.38, 95% CI = 0.02–0.74; $P = 0.04$) without heterogeneity ($I^2 = 0\%$) (Figure 4(a)) and a highly significant suppressing effect of MEP in the unaffected hemisphere (SMD = −0.83, 95% CI = −1.13 to −0.54; $P < 0.0001$), without significant heterogeneity ($I^2 = 18\%$) (Figure 4(b)).

3.3.2. rMTs in Both Hemispheres.
Four studies ($N = 121$) [26, 28, 32, 34] assessed the effect of LF-rTMS on rMT of the affected hemisphere by using the fixed-effect model that showed a large suppressing effect size (SMD = −1.00, 95% CI = −1.90 to −0.11; $P = 0.03$; $I^2 = 79\%$) (Figure 4(c)). LF-rTMS, however, induced an enhancing effect on rMT at a trend level in the unaffected hemisphere (SMD = 0.57; 95% CI = 0.04–1.10; $P = 0.03$; and $I^2 = 56\%$) (Figure 4(d)).

3.4. Publication Bias.
Funnel plots conducted with the trim and fill method for the included studies were illustrated in Figure 2. The trim and fill analyses showed that only the

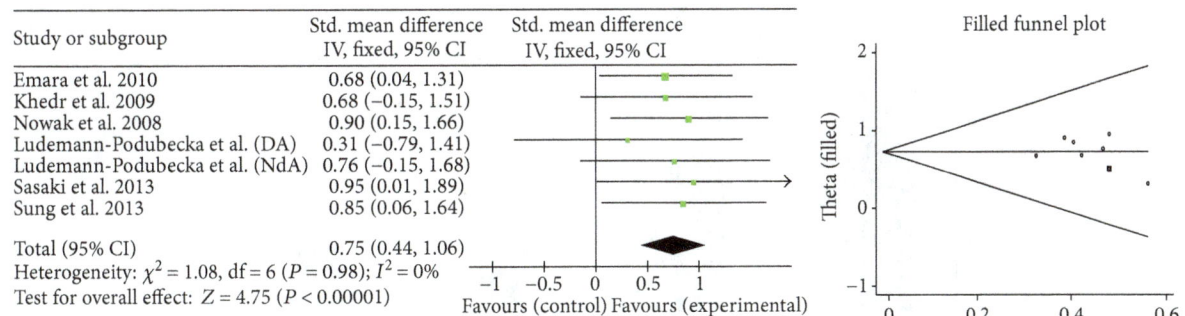

(a) Finger flexibility

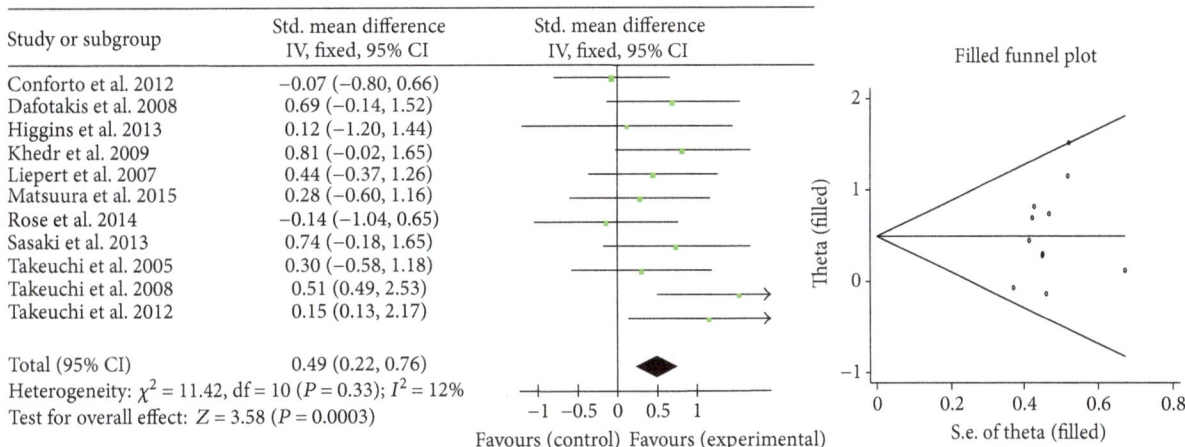

(b) Hard strength

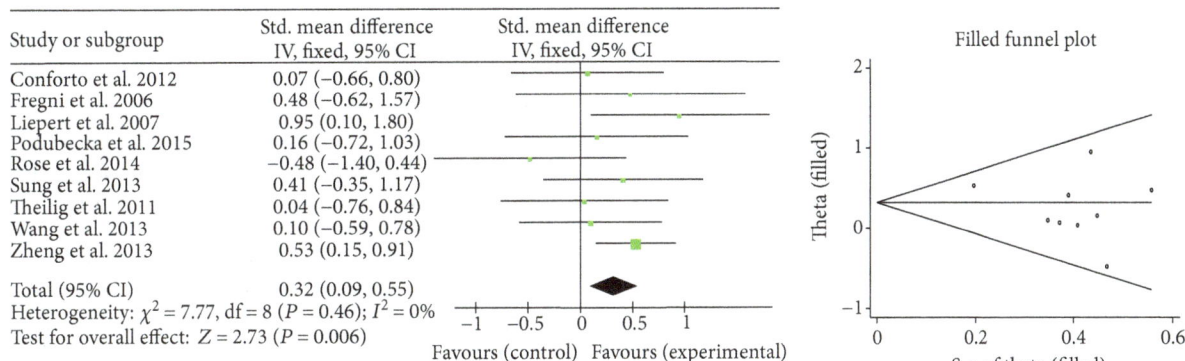

(c) Activity dexterity

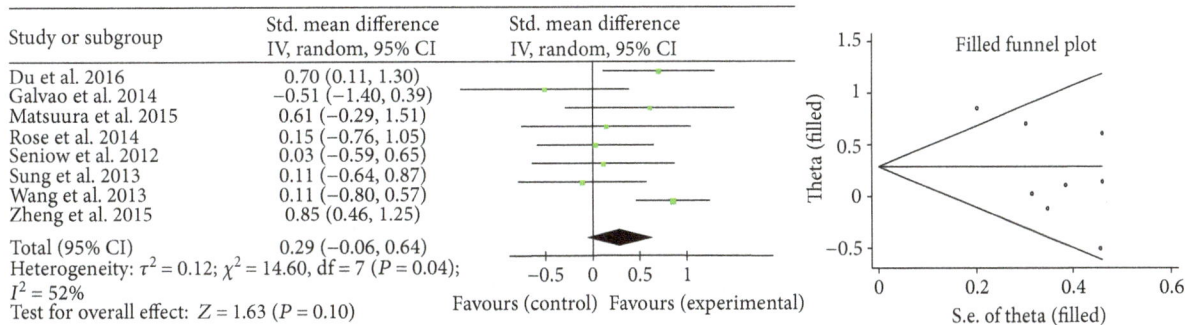

(d) Body function level

FIGURE 2: Forest plots of the short-term effect and the funnel plot analyses using the trim and fill method.

Short- and long-term effect size of different upper limb outcome measure

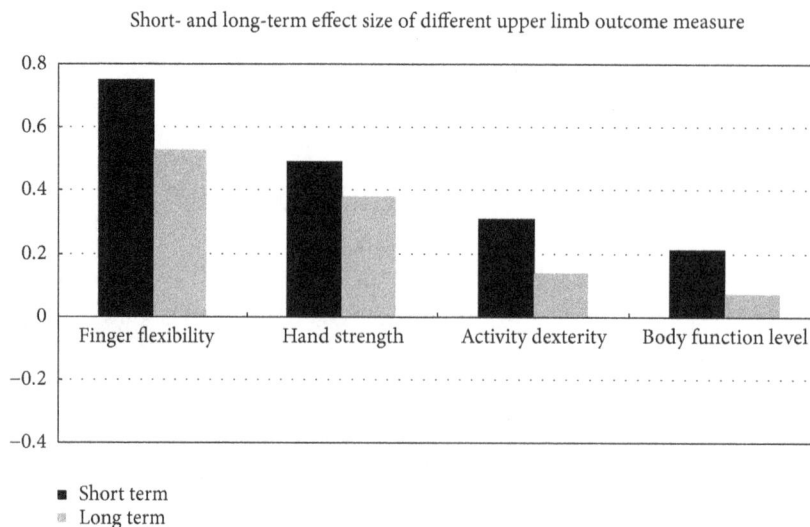

FIGURE 3: The bars show the pooled effect sizes of various upper extremity measure outcomes.

"finger flexibility" subclass had one study trimmed and the effect size was only slightly affected (adjusted effect size = 0.73, 0.43–1.02); no deletion or trimming occurred to other three subclasses and the effect sizes were unchanged.

3.5. Sensitivity Analyses. The lesion site and poststroke duration were matched between the four subgroups in two sensitivity analyses. One of the sensitivity analyses excluded eight trials that only involved subcortical stroke [17–20, 24–27] (based on the above four categories of motor function, SMD were 0.72, 0.28, 0.26, and 0.15) and the other excluded nine trials [10, 17–19, 22–24, 26, 31] that only involved acute/chronic stroke (<two weeks/>six months) [11] (SMD were 0.76, 0.36, 0.32, and 0.33), whereas the third sensitivity analysis only included rTMS plus motor training cotherapy after excluding five trials [20, 24–27] that did not specify potential cotherapy. The results were SMD = 0.72, 0.50, 0.26, and 0.15 (online-only data Supplement Figures I, II, and III).

4. Discussion

The present analysis provides the evidence that LF-rTMS applied over the contralesional M1 was effective for upper limb motor recovery, probably through modulating cortical excitability in poststroke patients. Although most of the trial participants were also undergoing other trainings, the trainings were carried out in both groups (rTMS group and control group) which could partially offset the impact of training on results. However, it is still not clear if the efficacy of LF-rTMS was due to its own function or its synergistic effect with other trainings. And more researches are needed in this direction.

These upper limb motor recoveries follow the previously reported four different effects of LF-rTMS on finger dexterity, hand strength, activity dexterity, and body function level [41]. Based on this classification, the short-term effectiveness of LF-rTMS appears to follow this descending order: finger ability is greater than hand strength and is greater than

activity dexterity. The improvement in body function did not reach a significant level. A similar long-term therapeutic effect of LF-rTMS was observed, that is, rTMS not only produced short-term acute clinical effects but also maintained such motor improvement at the distal of the affected upper limb than at the proximal end (Figure 3).

Long-term efficacy is more important than short-term efficacy, because long-lasting beneficial effect of rTMS on upper limb motor function is a more reliable indicator for a successful clinic intervention. It is noted that although the descending trends of the various motor classifications were consistent between short term and long term—the effect size was larger at short term than at long term. Based on the follow-up data and because of the difference between the short-term and long-term effect size of LF-rTMS, it was inferred that LF-rTMS can not only produce better functional improvements but also accelerate this process in stroke patients. In other words, at short term, LF-rTMS stimulates the speed and degree of the motor recovery; whereas, at long term, LF-rTMS further maintains and improves the degree of recovery. Further research is required to test this hypothesis.

Different motor scales measured the domains differently. A better understanding of the different outcome measures and accurate interpretation of the results can help guide more efficient rehabilitation of the patient under different clinical conditions. For example, finger tapping and grip force could inform more about fine finger manipulation tasks and grasping abilities, respectively, whereas the FMA represents mixed measures, with most items (87%) related to the body structure domain [41]. Discrepancy exists in the literature. One early study showed no significant effect of LF-rTMS on upper limb coordination in motor outcomes [30]. Another study found no significant effect of LF-rTMS on the whole arm movements except for grip force [23]. Other studies, however, reported marked motor improvements of the finger and hand after LF-rTMS therapy [10, 17–20].

Although the mechanism is unknown, the results of this analysis may provide some explanations. It is known that the adaptive reorganization of stroke-induced motor deficit

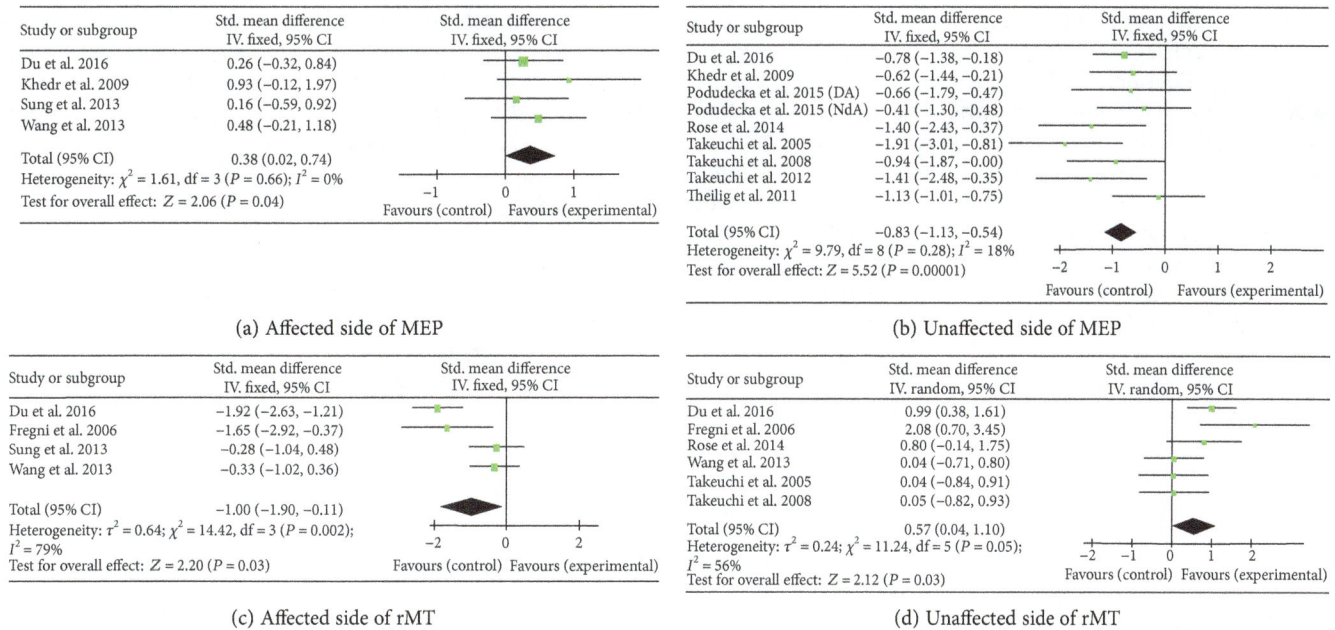

(a) Affected side of MEP

(b) Unaffected side of MEP

(c) Affected side of rMT

(d) Unaffected side of rMT

FIGURE 4: Forest plots of the mean effect sizes for MEP and rMT between the affected hand and unaffected hand. MEP: motor-evoked potential; rMT: resting motor threshold.

follows the patterns of from-the-proximal-to-distal limb and the distal limb especially the upper limb which is the most difficult to rehabilitate after stroke according to the neurodevelopment treatment [48]. The results of this meta-analysis indicate that LF-rTMS may be more effective in targeting the distal limb. One explanation for the discrepancy is that the LF-rTMS of our included trials was directed at the M1 which contributes to the high order control of motor behaviors [3]. It is known that the hand movement representation of the cortex coordinates upper limb movements through forearm muscle-controlled wrist, elbow, and shoulder [10]. Another possibility is that the speed and dexterity of finger movement are controlled primarily by corticospinal projections that are often damaged after stroke [10], but they are more readily targeted and influenced by rTMS application on the corticospinal projections. In contrast, combined activities that depend on both corticospinal and brain stem spinal pathways are less influenced by rTMS [10].

To avoid the possibility that some significant outcomes might be due to a high initial motor control, only the data of intergroup differences were analyzed. In our analysis, except one study [15] that recruited patients with severe motor deficits, all other studies recruited patients with mild-to-moderate motor deficits who did not show substantial functional disparity in both hand and arm motor outcomes. As such, our current findings may only apply to those patients of mild-to-moderate stroke. Besides, the sensitivity analysis of the trials which involved only the active training plus LF-rTMS versus those LF-rTMS without training produced similar results as the original combined results. Therefore, rTMS could indeed make further improvement on the hand flexibility which is considered the most difficult part of upper limb motor rehabilitation and which has

limited success using the traditional training rehabilitation techniques alone [48].

There is evidence that cortical reorganization occurs during motor recovery of stroke [49]. The shift of balance in cortical activation between the two hemispheres has been vigorously investigated in stroke patients [3]. Compared with most other therapies, the curative effect of rTMS on stroke is based upon the activity changes of the cortex. Decreasing the excitability of corticospinal neurons, as reflected in the cumulative increase of rMT and decrease of MEP in the unaffected hemisphere, has been found associated with motor recovery [50]. However, a previous meta-analysis [36] did not show significant motor cortex improvements though a trend of positive changes in the MEP and MT groups was found. This may be due to the fact that both the LF-rTMS and HF-rTMS studies were included in the meta-analysis which included only very limited number of studies. In this current study, the LF-rTMS induced a highly significant suppressing effect on MEP in the contralesional hemisphere and a significant enhancing effect on MEP in the ipsilesional hemisphere. However, because only three trials evaluated MEP of the ipsilesional hemisphere, more studies are required to reach a reliable conclusion. A similar regulatory effect of cortical excitation exists for the results of rMT, but enhanced rMT only at a trend level in the contralesional hemisphere. These pooled effects were in agreement with the previous reports of the positive effect of LF-rTMS in modulating cortical excitability after stroke [26, 28, 32].

It is known that rTMS could enhance the motor function recovery of paretic upper limbs [51]. Increasing factors are shown to influence the effects that should be investigated in order to optimize the therapeutic effect of rTMS. A number of studies have been done in this regard. It is recognized that valid comparable measurement across studies is required to compare the effect of different interventions. So far, however, there is no consensus yet regarding the best outcome measures for evaluating hand function rehabilitation. FMA is one of the most common outcome measures used by 36% of the studies that reported hand motor rehabilitation. Santisteban et al. [41] suggested that homogenous outcome measures were critical for across study efficacy evaluation of different rehabilitation techniques and feasibility of meta-analyses that were missing in earlier assessments for upper limb motor function. This present study demonstrates that it is possible to evaluate the motor outcomes at four different levels that can specify different motor recoveries of the various parts of the upper limb following LF-rTMS.

A recent study showed that differences in patients' characters and stimulation parameters such as age, gender, lesion location, and timing from stroke onset as well as frequency of rTMS could influence the effects of rTMS on upper extremity motor recovery [51]. However, the exact stimulation parameter for different patients remains to be experimentally determined. For example, one recent study demonstrated age-dependent motor cortical plasticity in LF-rTMS-treated patients, but not in HF-rTMS-treated stroke patients [51]. Another study showed that HF-rTMS was more beneficial for motor improvement than LF-rTMS in the early phase [52], but not in the late phase of stroke [10]. Thus, the optimal protocols of rTMS for different types of upper limb rehabilitation still need to be elucidated by large cohort studies and big data analysis.

Recently, Meyer et al. [53] reported that somatosensory impairments are negatively associated with motor recovery in the upper limb. This suggests that the level of the remaining sensorimotor control may play a role in neurorehabilitation. To date, most of the published rTMS studies on motor recovery in stroke patients have not reported on sensorimotor coimpairments and most of the studies excluded patients with neuropsychiatric comorbidities such as aphasia, spatial neglect, or visual field deficit which are positively correlated with the severity of somatosensory deficits [53]. Accordingly, it may be inferred that the present results would hardly be affected by mild to moderate sensorimotor impairment, but for the more severe sensorimotor impairment, proof-of-principle studies would be necessary. In addition, consensus in outcome measurement, validation of rTMS frequency, treatment timing and duration, and lesion sites in different age groups of male and female patients could refine the current findings.

Some limitations exist in this study. First, several uncontrollable variables of the patients such as age, gender, side of onset, severity of motor deficit, and sensorimotor impairment may confound the results. Second, variations in the number of trial days (i.e., session numbers) and stimulus intensity of rTMS interventions may affect the results. Especially, the more number of rTMS trial days and increased number of pulses could be more effective [54]. Of the four functional outcome categories of this study, the "hand strength" measurement group received the least numbers of rTMS sessions and pulses. This was followed by the "finger flexibility" group. "Activity dexterity" and "body function level" groups shared similar more numbers of rTMS sessions

and pulses. It is possible that the outcome differences among the four outcome groups could still exist if each group had received equal numbers of rTMS sessions and pulses. Moreover, studies published in non-English journals were not included in this analysis.

5. Conclusion

This meta-analysis indicates that LF-rTMS applied over the contralesional M1 has significant add-on therapeutic effect on upper limb motor dysfunction especially the functional recovery of the hand in patients with mild-moderate stroke. Future studies should verify whether cotherapy of LF-rTMS plus training will induce better hand motor rehabilitation than that of rTMS or training monotherapy.

Acknowledgments

This work was supported by the National Natural Science Foundation of China (no. 81271559) and the State Administration of Foreign Experts Affairs, China (no. SZD201516, no. SZD201606).

Supplementary Materials

Supplementary Figure I: sensitivity analysis examining whether the result was influenced by lesion site. Supplementary Figure II: sensitivity analysis examining whether the result was influenced by combining training. Supplementary Figure III: sensitivity analysis examining whether the result was influenced by time post stroke. (*Supplementary Materials*)

References

[1] R. Bonita, N. Solomon, and J. B. Broad, "Prevalence of stroke and stroke-related disability. Estimates from the Auckland stroke studies," *Stroke*, vol. 28, no. 10, pp. 1898–1902, 1997.

[2] J. M. Veerbeek, G. Kwakkel, E. E. Van Wegen, J. C. Ket, and M. W. Heymans, "Early prediction of outcome of activities of daily living after stroke: a systematic review," *Stroke*, vol. 42, no. 5, pp. 1482–1488, 2011.

[3] Q. Tang, G. Li, T. Liu et al., "Modulation of inter hemispheric activation balance in motor-related areas of stroke patients with motor recovery: systematic review and meta-analysis of fMRI studies," *Neuroscience & Biobehavioral Reviews*, vol. 57, pp. 392–400, 2015.

[4] N. S. Ward and L. G. Cohen, "Mechanisms underlying recovery of motor function after stroke," *Archives of Neurology*, vol. 61, no. 12, pp. 1844–1848, 2004.

[5] P. M. Rossini and S. Rossi, "Transcranial magnetic stimulation: diagnostic, therapeutic, and research potential," *Neurology*, vol. 68, no. 7, pp. 484–488, 2007.

[6] A. Pascual-Leone, A. Amedi, F. Fregni, and L. B. Merabet, "The plastic human brain cortex," *Annual Review of Neuroscience*, vol. 28, no. 1, pp. 377–401, 2005.

[7] F. Maeda, J. P. Keenan, J. M. Tormos, H. Topka, and A. Pascual-Leone, "Modulation of corticospinal excitability by repetitive transcranial magnetic stimulation," *Clinical Neurophysiology*, vol. 111, no. 5, pp. 800–805, 2000.

[8] T. Emara, R. Moustafa, N. Elnahas et al., "Repetitive transcranial magnetic stimulation at 1 Hz and 5 Hz produces sustained improvement in motor function and disability after ischemic stroke," *European Journal of Neurology*, vol. 17, no. 9, pp. 1203–1209, 2010.

[9] N. Sasaki, S. Mizutani, W. Kakuda, and M. Abo, "Comparison of the effects of high- and low-frequency repetitive transcranial magnetic stimulation on upper limb hemiparesis in the early phase of stroke," *Journal of Stroke and Cerebrovascular Diseases*, vol. 22, no. 4, pp. 413–418, 2013.

[10] E. M. Khedr, M. R. Abdel-Fadeil, A. Farghali, and M. Qaid, "Role of 1 and 3 Hz repetitive transcranial magnetic stimulation on motor function recovery after acute ischemic stroke," *European Journal of Neurology*, vol. 16, no. 12, pp. 1323–1330, 2009.

[11] W. Y. Hsu, C. H. Cheng, K. K. Liao, I. H. Lee, and Y. Y. Lin, "Effects of repetitive transcranial magnetic stimulation on motor functions in patients with stroke a meta-analysis," *Stroke*, vol. 43, no. 7, pp. 1849–1857, 2012.

[12] N. Takeuchi, T. Tada, M. Toshima, Y. Matsuo, and K. Ikoma, "Repetitive transcranial magnetic stimulation over bilateral hemispheres enhances motor function and training effect of paretic hand in patients after stroke," *Journal of Rehabilitation Medicine*, vol. 41, no. 13, pp. 1049–1054, 2009.

[13] M. P. Lomarev, D. Y. Kim, S. P. Richardson, B. Voller, and M. Hallett, "Safety study of high-frequency transcranial magnetic stimulation in patients with chronic stroke," *Clinical Neurophysiology*, vol. 118, no. 9, pp. 2072–2075, 2007.

[14] S. H. Cho, H. K. Shin, Y. H. Kwon et al., "Cortical activation changes induced by visual biofeedback tracking training in chronic stroke patients," *NeuroRehabilitation*, vol. 22, pp. 77–84, 2007.

[15] S. Theilig, J. Podubecka, K. Bosl, R. Wiederer, and D. A. Nowak, "Functional neuromuscular stimulation to improve severe hand dysfunction after stroke: does inhibitory rTMS enhance therapeutic efficiency?," *Experimental Neurology*, vol. 230, no. 1, pp. 149–155, 2011.

[16] M. B. Iyer, N. Schleper, and E. M. Wassermann, "Priming stimulation enhances the depressant effect of low-frequency repetitive transcranial magnetic stimulation," *Journal of Neuroscience*, vol. 23, no. 34, pp. 10867–10872, 2003.

[17] N. Takeuchi, T. Tada, Y. Matsuo, and K. Ikoma, "Low-frequency repetitive TMS plus anodal transcranial DCS prevents transient decline in bimanual movement induced by contralesional inhibitory rTMS after stroke," *Neurorehabilitation and Neural Repair*, vol. 26, no. 8, pp. 988–998, 2012.

[18] N. Takeuchi, T. Tada, M. Toshima, T. Chuma, Y. Matsuo, and K. Ikoma, "Inhibition of the unaffected motor cortex by 1 Hz repetitive transcranial magnetic stimulation enhances motor performance and training effect of the paretic hand in patients with chronic stroke," *Journal of Rehabilitation Medicine*, vol. 40, no. 4, pp. 298–303, 2008.

[19] N. Takeuchi, T. Chuma, Y. Matsuo, I. Watanabe, and K. Ikoma, "Repetitive transcranial magnetic stimulation of contralesional primary motor cortex improves hand function after stroke," *Stroke*, vol. 36, no. 12, pp. 2681–2686, 2005.

[20] M. Dafotakis, C. Grefkes, S. B. Eickhoff, H. Karbe, G. R. Fink, and D. A. Nowak, "Effects of rTMS on grip force control following subcortical stroke," *Experimental Neurology*, vol. 211, no. 2, pp. 407–412, 2008.

[21] A. B. Conforto, S. M. Anjos, G. Saposnik et al., "Transcranial magnetic stimulation in mild to severe hemiparesis early after stroke: a proof of principle and novel approach to improve motor function," *Journal of Neurology*, vol. 259, no. 7, pp. 1399–1405, 2012.

[22] J. Higgins, L. Koski, and H. Xie, "Combining rTMS and task-oriented training in the rehabilitation of the arm after stroke: a pilot randomized controlled trial," *Stroke Research and Treatment*, vol. 2013, Article ID 539146, 8 pages, 2013.

[23] D. K. Rose and C. Patten, "Does inhibitory repetitive transcranial magnetic stimulation augment functional task practice to improve arm recovery in chronic stroke?," *Stroke Research and Treatment*, vol. 2014, Article ID 305236, 10 pages, 2014.

[24] J. Liepert, S. Zittel, and C. Weiller, "Improvement of dexterity by single session low-frequency repetitive transcranial magnetic stimulation over the contralesional motor cortex in acute stroke: a double-blind placebo-controlled crossover trial," *Restorative Neurology and Neuroscience*, vol. 25, no. 5-6, pp. 461–465, 2007.

[25] A. Matsuura, K. Onoda, H. Oguro, and S. Yamaguchi, "Magnetic stimulation and movement-related cortical activity for acute stroke with hemiparesis," *European Journal of Neurology*, vol. 22, no. 12, pp. 1526–1532, 2015.

[26] F. Fregni, P. S. Boggio, A. C. Valle et al., "A sham-controlled trial of a 5-day course of repetitive transcranial magnetic stimulation of the unaffected hemisphere in stroke patients," *Stroke*, vol. 37, no. 8, pp. 2115–2122, 2006.

[27] D. A. Nowak, C. Grefkes, M. Dafotakis et al., "Effects of low-frequency repetitive transcranial magnetic stimulation of the contralesional primary motor cortex on movement kinematics and neural activity in subcortical stroke," *Archives of Neurology*, vol. 65, no. 6, pp. 741–747, 2008.

[28] W. H. Sung, C. P. Wang, C. L. Chou, Y. C. Chen, Y. C. Chang, and P. Y. Tsai, "Efficacy of coupling inhibitory and facilitatory repetitive transcranial magnetic stimulation to enhance motor recovery in hemiplegic stroke patients," *Stroke*, vol. 44, no. 5, pp. 1375–1382, 2013.

[29] J. Ludemann-Podubecka, K. Bosl, S. Theilig, R. Wiederer, and D. A. Nowak, "The effectiveness of 1 Hz rTMS over the primary motor area of the unaffected hemisphere to improve hand function after stroke depends on hemispheric dominance," *Brain Stimulation*, vol. 8, no. 4, pp. 823–830, 2015.

[30] J. Seniow, M. Bilik, M. Lesniak, K. Waldowski, S. Iwanski, and A. Czlonkowska, "Transcranial magnetic stimulation combined with physiotherapy in rehabilitation of poststroke hemiparesis: a randomized, double-blind, placebo-controlled study," *Neurorehabilitation and Neural Repair*, vol. 26, no. 9, pp. 1072–1079, 2012.

[31] S. C. B. Galvão, R. B. C. Dos Santos, P. B. Dos Santos, M. E. Cabral, and K. Monte-Silva, "Efficacy of coupling repetitive transcranial magnetic stimulation and physical therapy to reduce upper-limb spasticity in patients with stroke: a randomized controlled trial," *Archives of Physical Medicine and Rehabilitation*, vol. 95, no. 2, pp. 222–229, 2014.

[32] C. P. Wang, P. Y. Tsai, T. F. Yang, K. Y. Yang, and C. C. Wang, "Differential effect of conditioning sequences in coupling inhibitory/facilitatory repetitive transcranial magnetic stimulation for post-stroke motor recovery," *CNS Neuroscience & Therapeutics*, vol. 20, no. 4, pp. 355–363, 2014.

[33] C. J. Zheng, W. J. Liao, and W. G. Xia, "Effect of combined low-frequency repetitive transcranial magnetic stimulation and virtual reality training on upper limb function in subacute stroke: a double-blind randomized controlled trail," *Journal of Huazhong University of Science and Technology [Medical Sciences]*, vol. 35, pp. 248–254, 2015.

[34] J. Du, L. Tian, W. Liu et al., "Effects of repetitive transcranial magnetic stimulation on motor recovery and motor cortex excitability in patients with stroke: a randomized controlled trial," *European Journal of Neurology*, vol. 23, no. 11, pp. 1666–1672, 2016.

[35] L. Jancke, H. Steinmetz, S. Benilow, and U. Ziemann, "Slowing fastest finger movements of the dominant hand with low-frequency rTMS of the hand area of the primary motor cortex," *Experimental Brain Research*, vol. 155, no. 2, pp. 196–203, 2004.

[36] Q. Le, Y. Qu, Y. Tao, and S. Zhu, "Effects of repetitive transcranial magnetic stimulation on hand function recovery and excitability of the motor cortex after stroke: a meta-analysis," *American Journal of Physical Medicine & Rehabilitation*, vol. 93, no. 5, pp. 422–430, 2014.

[37] E. M. Khedr and N. A. Fetoh, "Short- and long-term effect of rTMS on motor function recovery after ischemic stroke," *Restorative Neurology and Neuroscience*, vol. 28, no. 4, pp. 545–559, 2010.

[38] Z. Hao, D. Wang, Y. Zeng, and M. Liu, "Repetitive transcranial magnetic stimulation for improving function after stroke," *Cochrane Database of Systematic Reviews*, vol. 31, article CD008862, 2013.

[39] D. Moher, K. F. Schulz, and D. Altman, "The consort statement: revised recommendations for improving the quality of reports of parallel-group randomized trials," *Journal of the American Medical Association*, vol. 285, no. 15, pp. 1987–1991, 2001.

[40] C. L. Chung and M. K. Mak, "Effect of repetitive transcranial magnetic stimulation on physical function and motor signs in Parkinson's disease: a systematic review and meta-analysis," *Brain Stimulation*, vol. 9, no. 4, pp. 475–487, 2016.

[41] L. Santisteban, M. Teremetz, J. P. Bleton, J. C. Baron, M. A. Maier, and P. G. Lindberg, "Upper limb outcome measures used in stroke rehabilitation studies: a systematic literature review," *PLoS One*, vol. 11, no. 5, article e0154792, 2016.

[42] M. V. Sale, N. C. Rogasch, and M. A. Nordstrom, "Different stimulation frequencies alter synchronous fluctuations in motor evoked potential amplitude of intrinsic hand muscles—a TMS study," *Frontiers in Human Neuroscience*, vol. 10, p. 100, 2016.

[43] K. Funase, T. S. Miles, and B. R. Gooden, "Trial-to-trial fluctuations in h-reflexes and motor evoked potentials in human wrist flexor," *Neuroscience Letters*, vol. 271, no. 1, pp. 25–28, 1999.

[44] R. J. Grissom and J. J. Kim, *Effect Sizes for Research: A Broad Practical Approach*, Lawrence Erlbaum Associates Publishers, Mahwah, NJ, USA, 2005.

[45] J. P. Higgins and S. G. Thompson, "Quantifying heterogeneity in a meta-analysis," *Statistics in Medicine*, vol. 21, no. 11, pp. 1539–1558, 2002.

[46] S. J. Duval and R. L. Tweedie, "Trim and fill: a simple funnel-plot based method of accounting for publication bias in meta-analysis," *Biometrics*, vol. 56, no. 2, pp. 455–463, 2000.

[47] J. Cohen, *Statistical Power Analysis for the Behavioral Sciences*, Academic Press, New York NY, USA, 1977.

[48] B. Bobath and FCSP, Cofounder, Centre, *Adult Hemiplegia: Evaluation and Treatment*, William Heinemann, London, England, 2nd edition, 1978.

[49] T. L. Sutcliffe, W. C. Gaetz, W. J. Logan, D. O. Cheyne, and D. L. Fehlings, "Cortical reorganization after modified constraint-induced movement therapy in pediatric hemiplegic cerebral palsy," *Journal of Child Neurology*, vol. 22, no. 11, pp. 1281–1287, 2007.

[50] M. Hallett, "Transcranial magnetic stimulation: a primer," *Neuron*, vol. 55, no. 2, pp. 187–199, 2007.

[51] S. Y. Kim and S. B. Shin, "Factors associated with upper extremity functional recovery following low-frequency repetitive transcranial magnetic stimulation in stroke patients," *Annals of Rehabilitation Medicine*, vol. 40, no. 3, pp. 373–382, 2016.

[52] C. Kim, H. E. Choi, H. Jung, B. J. Lee, K. H. Lee, and Y. J. Lim, "Comparison of the effects of 1 Hz and 20 Hz rTMS on motor recovery in subacute stroke patients," *Annals of Rehabilitation Medicine*, vol. 38, no. 5, pp. 585–591, 2014.

[53] S. Meyer, N. D. Bruyn, C. Lafosse et al., "Somatosensory impairments in the upper limb poststroke: distribution and association with motor function and visuospatial neglect," *Neurorehabilitation and Neural Repair*, vol. 30, no. 8, pp. 731–742, 2016.

[54] D. R. De Jesus, G. P. Favalli, S. S. Hoppenbrouwers et al., "Determining optimal rTMS parameters through changes in cortical inhibition," *Clinical Neurophysiology*, vol. 125, no. 4, pp. 755–762, 2014.

14

Adult Gross Motor Learning and Sleep: Is There a Mutual Benefit?

Monica Christova [ID],[1,2] **Hannes Aftenberger,**[1] **Raffaele Nardone** [ID],[3,4] **and Eugen Gallasch**[2]

[1]*Institute of Physiotherapy, University of Applied Sciences FH-Joanneum, Graz, Austria*
[2]*Otto Loewi Research Center, Physiology Section, Medical University of Graz, Graz, Austria*
[3]*Department of Neurology, Franz Tappeiner Hospital, Merano, Italy*
[4]*Department of Neurology, Christian Doppler Clinic, Paracelsus Medical University, Salzburg, Austria*

Correspondence should be addressed to Monica Christova; monica.christova@medunigraz.at

Academic Editor: Sergio Bagnato

Posttraining consolidation, also known as offline learning, refers to neuroplastic processes and systemic reorganization by which newly acquired skills are converted from an initially transient state into a more permanent state. An extensive amount of research on cognitive and fine motor tasks has shown that sleep is able to enhance these processes, resulting in more stable declarative and procedural memory traces. On the other hand, limited evidence exists concerning the relationship between sleep and learning of gross motor skills. We are particularly interested in this relationship with the learning of gross motor skills in adulthood, such as in the case of sports, performing arts, devised experimental tasks, and rehabilitation practice. Thus, the present review focuses on sleep and gross motor learning (GML) in adults. The literature on the impact of sleep on GML, the consequences of sleep deprivation, and the influence of GML on sleep architecture were evaluated for this review. While sleep has proven to be beneficial for most gross motor tasks, sleep deprivation in turn has not always resulted in performance decay. Furthermore, correlations between motor performance and sleep parameters have been found. These results are of potential importance for integrating sleep in physiotherapeutic interventions, especially for patients with impaired gross motor functions.

1. Introduction

Several human behaviors such as playing sports, playing music, and handcrafting are composed of unique combinations of gross and fine motor skills. Perfect execution of such highly coordinated tasks involves complex operations within the sensory and motor control structures [1, 2] including learning over a long period of time [3]. Learning commonly starts with initial task acquisition and results in reaching proficiency and stabilization of the learned information for further recall. Within the learning process, two phases can commonly be discriminated: encoding and consolidation. While encoding refers to the initial performance improvement occurring during practice (online learning), consolidation refers to the stabilization of memories during a period after practice [4, 5]. After consolidation, an additional performance improvement may occur even in the absence of further practice, an effect denoted as offline gain or offline learning [6]. Depending on the specificity of the task, such offline gains can occur during wakefulness but can also occur during diurnal or nocturnal sleep [7–9].

An extensive amount of literature has provided evidence that sleep plays an active role in the consolidation of memories [10–12]. The majority of the studies have addressed explicit memory and the role of the hippocampus in the formation of long-term memory. For example, by using a word list remembering task, consolidation was shown to take place during slow-wave sleep (SWS) rather than during rapid eye movement (REM) sleep [13]. In the case of consolidation of implicit memory, most studies focus on fine motor skills, such as serial reaction time tasks and sequential finger tapping tasks [8, 14–16]. Conclusions derived from research on cognitive or fine motor tasks do not generalize to gross and more complex motor skills [17]. The literature addressing gross motor skills primarily focuses on motor development in childhood and infancy, and to date, there is little knowledge about the role of sleep in adult gross motor learning (GML).

This review focuses on sleep and learning of novel gross motor skills in adults. Acquiring gross motor skills (e.g., dancing, playing a musical instrument, and golfing) often requires stepwise learning under the supervision of a demonstrator and, therefore, is less comparable to the learning of repetitive tasks such as finger tapping in front of a computer screen. Gross movements involve larger body segments and require more complex muscle synergies including postural stabilization and anticipatory adjustment [18]. Therefore, cortical and subcortical structures are likely involved in the encoding and consolidation of such skills [19]. Furthermore, training of gross motor skills often involves large muscle groups, which may lead to muscle fatigue and physical exhaustion [20]. It is therefore conceivable that GML also influences sleep duration and sleep architecture similarly to athletic exercise [21], and the question arises whether there is a mutual relationship between sleep and GML. More detailed knowledge on the relationship between sleep and GLM could be of relevance for physical therapy, as well as for the treatment of motor disabilities after stroke or brain tumor surgery.

Thus, in the present review, three aspects are highlighted to reveal possible relationships between GML and sleep. The first aspect focuses on the impact of sleep on skill consolidation compared to wakefulness. Here, bimanual tasks, dancing, inverse steering bicycling, or cascade juggling in combination with diurnal/nocturnal sleep are addressed. The second aspect focuses on the opposite direction, namely, whether GML can affect sleep architecture. Specifically, the effect of sports (trampoline, snakeboard) on REM and SWS is described in order to examine a possible correlation between the learning process and sleep parameters. Finally, the third aspect focuses on the impact of sleep deprivation on GML and memory consolidation. To this end, we review studies with a stepwise decrease in sleep duration as an experimental approach, mainly in the field of sports and virtual reality training.

2. Methods

The present work is a comprehensive review of computerized medical literature databases and searches. The MEDLINE database, accessed by PubMed electronic databases, was searched using the following free terms and medical subject headings combined in multiple search strategies: "gross motor learning/memory/skill," "complex motor skill," "motor adaptation," "sleep," "offline learning," "consolidation," and "deprivation." The search was limited to studies written in English. Studies including infants and children (up 14 years old) were excluded. No other exclusion criteria were applied, in particular regarding the number of participants, presence of a placebo group, or outcome measures. Full-text articles were retrieved for the selected titles, and reference lists of the retrieved articles were screened for additional publications. Only original articles (excluding single case reports) reporting data on studies examining the relationship between GML and sleep were considered eligible for inclusion. Gross motor tasks are defined here as tasks involving at least three joints, uni- or bimanual, as well as whole-body movements. In advance of this review, an introductory chapter on memory formation and sleep as identified by research on cognitive and fine motor tasks, is provided.

3. Common Mechanisms in Memory Formation and Sleep

The process of memory formation involves two main phases: encoding and consolidation. The encoding phase is associated with hippocampal long-term potentiation (LTP) plasticity [22], which involves the formation of a new memory trace that is initially fragile and vulnerable to external influences. Second, in the consolidation phase, a fragile memory trace is transferred to more permanent long-term storage throughout the neocortex [23] for further recall during retrieval. Thus, the consolidation phase is also associated with systemic reorganization. The significance of the consolidation phase has been explored by means of pharmacological and electrophysiological interventions administered at different time windows after learning [24, 25].

The perception and processing of information during encoding and retrieval requires the awake and active state of the brain. In contrast, skill consolidation takes place in the absence of attention and during sleep. There is assumed to be less interference from other stimuli during sleep, which protects the stabilization of a newly created memory trace [26–28]. In addition to this protective role of sleep in a passive manner, a reactivation of memory representations in hippocampal and nonhippocampal areas via synaptic plasticity mechanisms has been demonstrated in animal models [29] and in human studies [30, 31] during the different sleep phases, predominantly in SWS (for a review, see also [10]).

Two theoretical models have been proposed for these interactions between memory formation and sleep: the active system consolidation hypothesis and the synaptic homeostasis hypothesis. The first model refers to the dialog between the hippocampus and the neocortex, which is associated with learning during wakefulness and reactivation during non-REM (NREM) sleep [32]. This reactivation ensures the redistribution of new information within cortical networks via strengthening of synaptic connections [33]. According to the synaptic homeostasis hypothesis [34], strengthening of synaptic connections occurs during encoding in wakefulness. During subsequent SWS, synaptic strengthening becomes renormalized, thus removing irrelevant and less integrated information and restoring the synaptic capacity for new learning.

Increased protein synthesis, as required for synaptic strengthening, was first found during NREM sleep [35]. Specifically, the stage of NREM sleep is proposed as the period in which short-lasting LTP is converted to longer-lasting LTP involving new protein synthesis [36]. In the absence of protein synthesis, short-lasting LTP will fade out after some hours [37]. To this end, sleep has been reported to elevate cortical messenger RNA levels of genes associated with protein synthesis [38, 39], which are critical for strengthening existing synapses and building new ones (for a review, see [24]). In addition, different processes of synaptic reorganization occur during NREM and REM sleep, as summarized in the review by Gorgoni et al. [40]. Finally, electrophysiological markers within sleep stages NREM2, SWS (stages NREM3 and NREM4 according to the classification of Kales and Rechtschaffen [41]), and REM have also been related to the induction of LTP-like plasticity in the context of memory consolidation.

Sleep stage NREM2 is characterized by the presence of sleep spindles and K-complexes, and here the sleep spindles play a functional role in memory consolidation. Sleep spindles, defined as bursts at the sigma frequency range between 11 and 16 Hz and lasting up to 3 sec [42–44], are generated within the thalamic reticular nucleus. Spindle activity causes Ca^2 influx at the dendrites of pyramidal neurons and triggers a cascade of molecular processes, which lead to gene expression and protein synthesis necessary for LTP of the postsynaptic membrane of neocortical synapses [45, 46]. Furthermore, LTP at excitatory synapses is linked to a growth of synaptic spines [47]. An increase in dendritic spines after motor learning in mice was shown to be promoted by NREM2 sleep [29]. Positive correlations have been found between spindle duration and density with offline learning [48, 49] but not with nonspecific motor activity [50]. Specifically, increased spindle activity was found after visuomotor tasks [51] and after finger motor sequences [52]. Also using a motor finger sequence task but with experimental cuing with odor during NREM2 sleep, Laventure et al. [53] demonstrated that sleep spindles in particular contribute to the consolidation of motor sequence memories. These findings suggest the importance of sleep spindle activity for the strengthening of motor memory traces, promoted by functional and structural plasticity.

The SWS stage is characterized by the prevalence of slow oscillations, which represent the neuronal membrane potential oscillations that are expressed in the electroencephalogram (EEG) as slow-wave activity (SWA) within the 0.5–4 Hz frequency band [54, 55]. The slow oscillations are of thalamocortical origin and comprise periods of membrane depolarization (sustained firing) alternated with periods of membrane hyperpolarization (neuronal silence). While the activity during the depolarization phases has been attributed to corticocortical glutamatergic synaptic connections [56], which reflect an excitatory/inhibitory balance, the hyperpolarization phases have been related to intracellular mechanisms suppressing neuronal excitability [57]. The significance of slow oscillations in the formation of motor memory was demonstrated during training of a visuomotor adaptation task [58] that increased the SWA, which was correlated with improved task performance after sleep. On the other hand, slow-wave deprivation impaired the sleep-related consolidation of a visuomotor adaptation task [59], whereas boosting the slow oscillations with low-frequency transcranial alternating current stimulation facilitated the consolidation of declarative memory [60]. The role of slow waves in memory consolidation has been attributed both to synaptic depression and synaptic potentiation mechanisms (for a review, see [61]).

The REM sleep stage, characterized by desynchronized EEG activity, is sensitive to the induction of synaptic plasticity changes. The waves of excitation (ponto-geniculo-

occipital, PGO waves) during REM sleep were first described in the rat brainstem [62]. These waves project to the hippocampus and the amygdala [63] and show increased intensity and density after intensive learning, which correlates with task improvement [64]. These waves have also been proposed as regulators of synaptic plasticity, since they are comprised of waves of glutamate terminating on forebrain areas [65]. In addition to PGO waves, factors such as theta activity, increased acetylcholine levels, and increased transcription of plasticity-related genes during REM sleep [66] contribute to the induction of bidirectional plasticity (LTP/LTD). Bidirectional plasticity supports memory-associated synaptic remodeling in the hippocampus [67]. In addition, REM sleep has been demonstrated to selectively eliminate and maintain the postsynaptic dendritic spines of layer 5 pyramidal neurons in the mouse motor cortex during motor learning and memory consolidation [68]. Human imaging studies [69] have shown increased post training activation during REM sleep in the brain areas involved in task acquisition.

4. Effects of Sleep on Gross Motor Learning

The effect of day/night sleep on GML was examined with uni- and bimanual motor tasks, as well as with whole-body movements in healthy volunteers. In the study of Kempler and Richmond [70], the task consisted of bimanual movements, involving sequential combinations of three positions with both arms simultaneously. This task, performed by 70 adults, was initially practiced for 6 min with video assistance and then retested, whereby the number of accurate cycles was calculated. Participants showed a higher number of accurate cycles of the task at retest after nocturnal sleep but did not exhibit a significant change after wakefulness. Another study, implementing bimanual movements [71], examined the influence of night sleep in adaptive skill learning. Right-handed university students played a shooter video game, which requires fast responses to changing visual and auditory stimuli. In this task, the players simultaneously manipulated the keyboard with the left hand and the mouse with the right hand. A training period of 28 min, preceded by a baseline score evaluation, was performed in the morning or in the evening. Posttraining tests were carried out immediately after training, or 12 or 24 hours after training in separate groups. Performance improved along with training and then deteriorated after 12 hours wakefulness. However, performance recovered and stabilized after night sleep. Sleep-dependent learning gains were also reported by Kuriyama et al. [72] who demonstrated not only that performance on a complex nine-element bimanual finger taping task could benefit from night sleep (28.9% improvement) but also that these gains correlated with task complexity and coordination. The results were compared to more simple tasks, which showed 17–20% overnight improvement. Interestingly, the maximum benefit was observed for the most difficult skills, which were unable to be mastered prior to sleep.

Performance gains after nocturnal sleep have also been demonstrated at unimanual tasks. Malangre and Blischke [73] and Malangre et al. [74] employed a pegboard task on an electronic board where a sequence of gross reaching movements including the joints of the wrist, elbow, and shoulder were performed with the nondominant hand in the horizontal plane. One group practiced in the morning, the second in the evening. Retests were carried out 15 min after acquisition in order to control the early retention as well as after 12 and 24 hours [73]. Mean execution time along all retests was reduced after nocturnal sleep but not after the wake periods.

Sleep-related effects were also examined with coordination movements involving the whole body. Long complex dance choreography was implemented on a PlayStation 2 Game Dance Stage [75]. Using constant visual feedback, young male volunteers learned a dance consisting of a set of sequential movements in the evening or in the morning. Twelve and 24 hours later, they were retested on the same choreography in order to assess sequence-specific learning but were also tested on a new set of movements in order to examine the transfer from a newly acquired skill to a novel similar task. Sleep resulted in improved performance when the same dance was retested; however, the performance of the new set of dance movements was not improved by sleep.

In addition to nocturnal sleep the effectiveness of diurnal sleep on GML has also been examined. Before and after a 2-hour day nap, during which NREM and REM sleep were controlled with polysomnographic recordings, young female subjects performed a highly coordinated three-ball cascade juggling for 15 min [76]. Juggling performance significantly improved at retest in the nap group but not in the awake group. Moreover, these performance gains were further retained on the following day [77]. The effect of a 2-hour midday nap on a complex posturolocomotor task (learning to ride an inverse steering bicycle) was investigated in another recent study [78]. The authors implemented straight-line or slalom bike riding and, in contrast to the previous studies, there was no benefit from the midday nap. Moreover, a significant decrease in accuracy at slalom and at straight-line riding was found after the nap but also after wakefulness. The performance decrease was negatively related to the sleep parameters (REM duration and spindle activity). These findings were attributed to the need to forget more recently acquired interfering tasks in order to protect more relevant skills that are needed daily.

A "multitask research strategy" was used by Blischke et al. [79] to investigate the effect of nocturnal sleep on learning a set of different task domains, including finger tapping tasks, pursuit tracking and countermovement jump, where subjects were required to produce a vertical force impulse of 60% of the individual maximum. Whereas performance of small finger movements (sequential finger tapping) was improved after sleep, gross body movements (vertical jump) remained stable across the sleeping period. These results indicate a differential effect of nocturnal sleep on small and gross motor learning.

In contrast, a beneficial effect of overnight sleep on learning a novel walking task was found by Al-Sharman and Siengsukon [80]. This task consisted of walking along an irregular elliptical path approximately 30 m long and 0.5 m wide while performing a mental cognitive task (counting backwards) in order to approximate walking in a natural environment. The task required whole-body coordination and adaptation to environmental stimuli. Improved step length and reduced time were found at retest after 12 hours including 7 hours of sleep but not after 12 hours awake. Importantly, a correlation between sleep quality and offline learning was reported.

5. Factors Influencing the Effect of Sleep on GML

While in the majority of these studies sleep enhanced gross motor performance [72–74, 76, 77, 80], others have reported stabilization without further improvement [71, 79] or even performance deterioration [78]. Factors such as type of motor task, training specificity, presleep performance level and complexity can be causes for such inconsistencies. Complex explicit tasks with high cognitive demands such as sequential bilateral arm or manual movements, cascade juggling, or walking with counting generally benefit from sleep. Moreover, performance gains correlate positively with task complexity [72]. One reason could be that less complex skills, being easier to master, reach a ceiling effect before sleep. Another reason could be that greater cognitive efforts induce fatigue, which can be successfully restored in sleep. The importance of task complexity was emphasized in a recent study [81] wherein the sleep-related improvements were absent with shorter sequences and more regular movement patterns.

Studies employing whole-body postural tasks, which mainly involve implicit learning strategies (vertical jump, inverse bicycling), have reported an absence of effects or even decreased performance accuracy at retest. Broadly, implicitly acquired movements such as vertical jump and inverse bicycling [78], which predominantly involve procedural memory, do not appear to benefit from sleep for memory consolidation. A similar differential effect of sleep, whether a task is explicit or implicit, was reported by Robertson et al. [6] for nongross motor sequence learning. In addition, at such whole-body postural tasks, participants are unlikely to reach asymptotic performance after a short training period, which can limit the postsleep performance gains, as shown by Hauptmann et al. [82]. Finally, the possibility that irrelevant movement patterns, such as riding a bicycle in an inverse direction, tend to be removed during sleep in order to selectively enhance the memories for activities pertinent to daily life cannot be excluded, which is in accordance to the synaptic homeostasis hypothesis [34]. Additionally, transfer of new dance choreography movements was not promoted by sleep [75], which suggests that adaptation to new settings might occur independently of sleep. Perhaps representations that were not particularly engaged in the learning preceding sleep and therefore not involved in the formation of the movement schemata [83], cannot be influenced by the SWS downscaling and therefore remain unaffected by sleep.

Further important factors concerning sleep-related learning are the time-of-day effect, sleep duration, and sleep environment. Performing the trainings/retests at opposite times of day (morning/evening for the wake group versus evening/morning for the sleep group) as in the study of Al-Sharman and Siengsukon [80] may account for different offline gains because of endogenous circadian influences [84]. An equitable testing can be achieved by using a study design with 24-hour delay as done in other studies [70, 73]. In most of the GML studies, the sleeping duration was between 6 and 8 hours at night. Commonly, the participants did not spend the night in a sleep lab; therefore, recording of sleep quality was carried out using sleepiness scales and questionnaires [70, 74], actigraphy [80], or self-report [75]. Only sleeping overnight in a sleep lab ensures objective assessment of sleep architecture, which enables the determination of possible correlations between the sleep parameters and learning scores. On the other hand, an overnight stay in an unfamiliar environment may influence sleep quality, a problem that can be solved by providing a baseline night for familiarization. In some studies, the quality of diurnal sleep has been controlled with polysomnography [76–78], which enables comparisons between the sleep and learning parameters. Despite the fact that a daytime nap and a full night's sleep have different physiological characteristics, they are both able to induce behavioral gains in GML. This observation was also demonstrated using the same task (juggling) in the studies of Morita et al. [76, 77].

Similar results, in which improvements occurred after a whole night's sleep [15, 75] but also after a short nap [8, 85], have been reported for simple motor sequence tasks. A direct comparison between diurnal and nocturnal sleep [86] revealed lower spindle density but higher spindle activity and amplitude in daytime naps compared to those in night sleep. Furthermore, the same study showed that daytime naps protected procedural memories (mirror tracing task) from deterioration, whereas a full night's sleep improved performance. Since the presence of both REM and SWS phases are crucial for evolving LTP changes and memory consolidation, it is of interest to examine whether longer sleep is associated with higher GML gains. Additionally, defining the minimum/effective duration of diurnal sleep could be of importance when scheduling practice-rest in rehabilitation sessions, for example.

Age can influence sleep-related motor learning gains, as shown with simple motor tasks. For example, postsleep consolidation in older adults was found to be dependent on the movement kinematic [87]: while a finger sequence task failed to show sleep-related gains, a kinematically adapted gross motor whole-hand task showed sleep-dependent consolidation. In addition, studies using less complex tasks such as finger sequences [88] and mirror tracking [89] also reported lack of sleep-dependent consolidation (for a review, see also [90]). The majority of the studies on GML have focused on sleep-induced performance gains in young adults. Only the study of Al-Sharman and Siengsukon [91] verified these effects in the elderly, showing decreased walking time and increased accuracy after sleep in middle-aged and older individuals.

Older individuals also show a changed sleep architecture characterized by a reduction in total sleep time, REM, SWS [92–94], and sleep spindles [95], which have been shown to be important for memory consolidation and performance

improvement [48]. However, such aging-related changes cannot explain why older adults can benefit from sleep after GML but not after learning fine motor tasks, as shown by Gudberg et al. [87]. Apparently, gross motor movements are more complex, thus requiring activation of larger brain networks, which appears to be a higher demand on motor-controlling structures in the elderly than in young individuals. This higher demand could still be accomplished by sleep even at reduced sleep efficiency. Alternatively, improvement in fine motor tasks could be limited in older adults as a result of aging [96]. Future research, including analysis of resting state networks, could be helpful to examine and compare sleep-related gross and fine ML consolidation in different age groups.

6. Effect of Sleep Deprivation on GML

Sleep is a state of reduced energy demands at the cellular and network level and is thus essential for maintaining behavioral and cognitive capabilities [97]. Sleep deficiency causes deterioration of motor and neurocognitive performance and involves changes at several systematic levels, for example, decreased physical performance, increased mental fatigue, changes in metabolism and endocrine functions, pain perception, and cognitive and emotional changes (for a review, see [98, 99]). In the brain, lack of sleep has an impact on neurotransmitter release [100, 101], which results in a decreased capacity to learn, store, and retrieve the learned material. Such decreased learning capacity might be partially explained by alterations in use-dependent synaptic plasticity.

Molecular and electrophysiological studies show that sleep loss inhibits hippocampal LTP and facilitates LTD induction [102, 103]. Additionally, prolonged wakefulness has been associated with net synaptic potentiation, whereas sleep preserves the overall balance of synaptic strength [104]. In support of these findings, transcranial magnetic stimulation (TMS) studies on humans have demonstrated that sleep deprivation increases cortical excitability [105] and decreases intracortical inhibition [106]. If LTP and cortical excitability are increased after sleep deprivation, then further learning-induced LTP would be less effective, which might be a reason for the observed learning and memory decline. Furthermore, sleep deprivation may impair memory consolidation by reducing the synthesis of proteins needed to support synaptic plasticity [107].

The effect of sleep loss on motor learning has been studied in healthy subjects using experimentally induced sleep deprivation. Sleep deprivation is commonly defined as a sleep time of less than 4 hours per 24 hours [108], although different durations have been reported. In one of the first works dedicated to the impact of sleep deprivation on gross motor performance, Holland [109] investigated the effect of one night of wakefulness on a jump and manipulation task in male college students. The experimentally imposed sleeplessness did not affect speed or accuracy of both discrete short-term tasks but did decrease long-term physical performance, as measured by a bicycle work test. Performance decline after sleep deprivation has been demonstrated in athletes in a variety of exercises (for a review, see [110]).

While psychomotor tasks such as reaction time were diminished after sleep loss, gross motor functions remained unaffected [111]. Tasks involving longer-lasting physical efforts or higher cognitive demands tend to be more sensitive to sleep deficits.

Further evidence for the impact of sleep deprivation on GM training comes from studies examining bimanual dexterity in medical residents. Lehmann et al. [108] used a virtual surgery stimulator task, which involved both arms. Surgical residents and medical students were initially trained in tasks lasting between 20 and 30 min for 5 days in order to reach comparable skill levels. The subsequently reduced sleep duration (1.6–3.8 hours) did not influence motor or cognitive performance. Comparable findings were reported by DeMaria et al. [112] after learning of laparoscopic skills. In contrast, Eastridge et al. [113] and Taffinder et al. [114] found an increased number of errors and time to complete all tasks on simulated laparoscopy after sleep deprivation. The heterogeneity of these findings can be explained by the variability in sleep and task duration and the different proficiency levels of the residents in the different studies. Furthermore, the participants in these studies were to some extent acquainted with the laparoscopic tasks but also with the limited and irregular amount of sleep, thus being less vulnerable to both task acquisition and sleep loss. Therefore, these results cannot be directly considered for naive subjects or patients.

The effect of sleep deprivation on motor learning has also been studied in patients with sleep disorders. Sleep disorders such as insomnia, narcolepsy, or obstructive sleep apnea (OSA), which are characterized by elevated arousal and abnormal sleep architecture, result in a reduced capacity for consolidating explicit motor sequences and motor adaptation skills (for a review, see Cellini [115]).

7. Effect of GML on Sleep Architecture

Sleep following learning of gross motor skills not only facilitates memory consolidation but may also influence sleep homeostasis. For example, motor learning in rats induced a local increase in SWA in the cortical region directly involved in the motor task [116], and the SWA increase correlated positively with performance improvement. In humans, evidence from earlier studies has demonstrated the influence of aerobic but not anaerobic exercise on sleep variables [117–119] with specific alterations in NREM2 and SWS stages, which reflect increased activity of the metabolic recovery processes after extensive motor activity. In later studies, the effect of GLM on sleep variables has been shown primarily with whole-body coordination movements.

The effect of learning a new complex sport activity (trampolining) on REM sleep was investigated by Buchegger et al. [120] and compared to the effect of learning other control anaerobic tasks in a 13-week program once a week for 2 hours. Only the trampoliners showed a significant increase in subsequent REM sleep, a result that probably reflects the motor complexity of the task. Implementing another procedural whole-body coordination task, Erlacher and Schredl [121] studied the effect of gross motor learning

on sleep in a balanced within-subject design. Subjects learned either snakeboard riding for 2 hours or took part in a control ergometry task for the same period. However, no difference was found between the experimental and control condition in sleep, REM parameters, or subjective sleep rating. Using a combination of simple procedural tasks (pursuit rotor, simple tracing, operation task, and ball and cup) Fogel and Smith [48] found that sleep spindle density at stage NREM2 was positively related to the overall task improvement without involvement of REM sleep mechanisms. Since gross motor learning was represented by only one of the tasks in this study (ball and cup), it cannot be concluded whether this task alone would have produced the same effect. However, in another study by Milner et al. [122], the effect of the "ball and cup" task solely on a 20 min daytime nap was investigated in habitual and nonhabitual nappers. Interestingly, the number of sleep spindles and sigma power (13.5–15 Hz) in stage NREM2 predicted the task performance following the nap but only in the habitual nappers.

Two studies, primarily investigating the effect of diurnal sleep on GML, also examined the influence of the task on REM/NREM sleep without, however, comparison to a control task. In the first study, cascade juggling for 15 min showed an effect on day nap [76], and alterations in EEG spectral power relative to that in a baseline nap were observed during NREM sleep. Specifically, there was an increase in spectral power in the band related to slow waves (0.5–1.5 Hz, "delta band") and in the band related to sleep spindles (11.5–15.5 Hz, "sigma band"). These increases were correlated with improved motor performance. Similarly, higher sleep spindle activity and longer REM durations were found in the second study, after learning a novel complex gross motor task (riding an inverse steering bicycle) by Hoedlmoser et al. [78], although the authors observed a negative correlation with task improvement.

The variable findings concerning the effect of GML on sleep parameters and the correlation between performance gains and sleep architecture could be due to the methodological differences and the level of task difficulty. A night prior to the study for adaptation and control of the first-night effect [123] was not provided in these studies. Apparently, individual sleep habits should also be considered, especially in studies where daytime sleep/nap is examined. Additionally, the tested participants in some studies had a background in sports, while in other studies, the participants did not, which could account for the differences in responsiveness to the task nature and complexity. Nagai et al. [124] demonstrated the importance of task complexity for sleep consolidation by using Fos expression to evaluate neuronal activation in mice. Their results showed that complex but not simple training engaged the motor cortex and the hippocampus to a greater extent and induced a longer sleep duration, which was correlated with greater performance.

Overall, NREM sleep variables were mostly influenced by GML, probably via synaptic potentiation mechanisms occurring after learning. This observation has also been supported by animal studies showing that changes in SWA are driven by synaptic potentiation [116] after learning a task involving an increase in dendritic branching at layers

II, III, and V [125] and an enhancement in the strength of horizontal intracortical connections [126]. An increase in SWA was also reported after application of other LTP induction interventions such as 5 Hz repetitive TMS of M1 [127] or paired associative stimulation [128].

8. Importance for Rehabilitation Practice

The motor rehabilitation process, particularly that for physio- and occupational therapy, involves relearning of lost skills or learning of compensatory/substitution tasks. These tasks are commonly gross motor actions, which consist of motor sequences, complex coordination patterns, and motor adaptations, for example walking with prosthesis, performing daily life activities with a paretic hand, or navigation of a wheelchair by patients with spinal cord injuries. The acquisition of such tasks is associated with the development of new motor strategies and large reorganizational map changes, which takes place over days and weeks. Thus, a proper scheduling of single therapy sessions along with rest/sleep periods is relevant for the success of the therapy. Furthermore, the effectiveness of multiple naps for motor recovery over a longer time is of interest. The optimal integration of sleep in rehabilitation practice and maximization of the effect of sleep is also of particular importance for neurological conditions, in which gross motor functions are affected, such as in patients with neurological and neuropsychological disorders like cerebral palsy, Parkinson's disease, autism, and motor apraxia or in children with developmental disorders.

Considering the results from studies on healthy individuals, it could be of potential clinical benefit to incorporate, for example, a diurnal sleep of at least 90–100 min in order to increase the likelihood of the REM and NREM phases. Furthermore, since current evidence has shown that acquiring a movement set related to the learned one but containing new elements was not promoted by sleep [75], it may be advantageous to introduce a task before sleep and practice it in the same form after sleep. Considering that most neurological disorders also involve specific structural or functional changes within the learning-related brain structures, often together with cognitive changes, direct evidence coming from studies on patients is critical. The effect of sleep on motor learning in a stroke population has already been examined and summarized in previous reviews [129, 130]. Stroke victims, in contrast to healthy age-matched controls, have been reported to benefit from sleep when learning both implicit and explicit versions of discrete and continuous tasks. However, small finger tasks, performed with the less affected hand, were commonly utilized; therefore, direct conclusions regarding the consolidation of activities relevant to daily life cannot be drawn. Studies on stroke patients addressing the effect of sleep on learning whole-body or bimanual tasks in relation to lesion localization and post-stroke time are warranted.

Sleep deficiency or changed sleep architecture is reported in several neurological conditions including multiple sclerosis [131, 132], Parkinson's disease [133], stroke [134], and traumatic brain injury [135, 136]. Further, associations between sleep characteristic and physical functions have been found in older veterans with different comorbidities [137]. Longer (>7.5 hours) or shorter (<6 hours) sleep time and fragmented sleep are significantly correlated with poor performance in daily life and instrumental daily life activities. Thus, defining sleep disorders, which may negatively influence motor performance in these risk groups, should be considered in physiotherapy. Improving sleep disturbances with pharmacological and nonpharmacological interventions may be assumed to in turn improve learning outcomes, as already demonstrated in patients with OSA [138]. Considering that learning complex GML tasks affects sleep architecture [76, 78], we anticipate a reciprocal effect: on one side, sleep disturbances might be normalized by motor performance; on the other side, normal sleep can stabilize and enhance GML gains.

9. Conclusions

GML and sleep interact via common synaptic plasticity mechanisms and, thus, can influence each other. Therefore, the question arises whether this influence is of a mutual benefit. In healthy adults, sleep can stabilize and improve the consolidation of more complex GM tasks, probably because of the higher cognitive/motor demands, which require more pronounced synaptic stabilization that takes place during sleep. The learning gains are demonstrated in both implicit and explicit tasks and predominantly in young adults. Only a few studies have addressed and shown these benefits in the elderly population as well. GML can be concluded to benefit from sleep. However, age- and gender-related sleep differences, as well as variability in individual sleep patterns, should be considered in future studies. In turn, training of GM tasks can influence sleep variables across all NREM sleep stages. Again, this effect is related to task complexity but also to sleep habits. Whether the performance-induced changes in sleep architecture can be interpreted as improved sleep quality remains speculative to conclude from the current findings. Moreover, a positive correlation between learning and sleep parameters was not shown in all studies.

Interestingly, some of the described effects are specific for GML and are thus in contrast to the findings on sleep and learning paradigms involving fine or simple motor skills. Therefore, further research, especially on neurological patients with impaired GM functions, is warranted. A better understanding of the interaction between sleep and GML may contribute to the optimization of therapeutic strategies by integrating sleep with physiotherapy for these patient groups.

Additional Points

Research Agenda. (1) Characterisation of age-dependent effects on sleep-related gains using more complex gross motor tasks (e.g., juggling and dance choreography); (2) investigation of whether sleep promotes equal consolidation of daily life-relevant versus daily life-irrelevant tasks; (3) effects of sleep deprivation on GML performance involving whole-body movements; (4) comparison of sleep-related gains following learning of explicit versus implicit gross motor tasks; (5) comparison of sleep-related effects of gross versus fine motor learning in stroke patients; (6) effectiveness of daytime naps after motor therapy in physiotherapy on functional improvement in stroke patients; (7) relevance of lesion location and poststroke stage on sleep-related GM training; (8) testing of sleep-stage-dependent noninvasive brain stimulation for enhancing memory consolidation; and (9) influences of stimulating factors (music, sonification of movements, and augmented reality) on learning and sleep performance.

References

[1] J. H. Kim, J. K. Han, B. N. Kim, and D. H. Han, "Brain networks governing the golf swing in professional golfers," *Journal of Sports Sciences*, vol. 33, no. 19, pp. 1980–1987, 2015.

[2] I. Wollman, V. Penhune, M. Segado, T. Carpentier, and R. J. Zatorre, "Neural network retuning and neural predictors of learning success associated with cello training," *Proceedings of the National Academy of Sciences of the United States of America*, vol. 115, no. 26, pp. E6056–E6064, 2018.

[3] F. J. Kottke, "From reflex to skill: the training of coordination," *Archives of Physical Medicine and Rehabilitation*, vol. 61, no. 12, pp. 551–561, 1980.

[4] A. Karni and D. Sagi, "The time course of learning a visual skill," *Nature*, vol. 365, no. 6443, pp. 250–252, 1993.

[5] R. Shadmehr and T. Brashers-Krug, "Functional stages in the formation of human long-term motor memory," *The Journal of Neuroscience*, vol. 17, no. 1, pp. 409–419, 1997.

[6] E. M. Robertson, A. Pascual-Leone, and R. C. Miall, "Current concepts in procedural consolidation," *Nature Reviews Neuroscience*, vol. 5, no. 7, pp. 576–582, 2004.

[7] J. Doyon, M. Korman, A. Morin et al., "Contribution of night and day sleep vs. simple passage of time to the consolidation of motor sequence and visuomotor adaptation learning," *Experimental Brain Research*, vol. 195, no. 1, pp. 15–26, 2009.

[8] M. Korman, J. Doyon, J. Doljansky, J. Carrier, Y. Dagan, and A. Karni, "Daytime sleep condenses the time course of motor memory consolidation," *Nature Neuroscience*, vol. 10, no. 9, pp. 1206–1213, 2007.

[9] M. P. Walker, T. Brakefield, J. Seidman, A. Morgan, J. A. Hobson, and R. Stickgold, "Sleep and the time course of motor skill learning," *Learning & Memory*, vol. 10, no. 4, pp. 275–284, 2003.

[10] B. Rasch and J. Born, "About sleep's role in memory," *Physiological Reviews*, vol. 93, no. 2, pp. 681–766, 2013.

[11] R. Stickgold, "Sleep-dependent memory consolidation," *Nature*, vol. 437, no. 7063, pp. 1272–1278, 2005.

[12] M. P. Walker and R. Stickgold, "Sleep, memory, and plasticity," *Annual Review of Psychology*, vol. 57, no. 1, pp. 139–166, 2006.

[13] L. Marshall and J. Born, "The contribution of sleep to hippocampus-dependent memory consolidation," *Trends in Cognitive Sciences*, vol. 11, no. 10, pp. 442–450, 2007.

[14] G. Albouy, V. Sterpenich, G. Vandewalle et al., "Interaction between hippocampal and striatal systems predicts subsequent consolidation of motor sequence memory," *PLoS One*, vol. 8, no. 3, article e59490, 2013.

[15] S. Fischer, M. Hallschmid, A. L. Elsner, and J. Born, "Sleep forms memory for finger skills," *Proceedings of the National Academy of Sciences of the United States of America*, vol. 99, no. 18, pp. 11987–11991, 2002.

[16] M. P. Walker, T. Brakefield, A. Morgan, J. A. Hobson, and R. Stickgold, "Practice with sleep makes perfect: sleep-dependent motor skill learning," *Neuron*, vol. 35, no. 1, pp. 205–211, 2002.

[17] G. Wulf and C. H. Shea, "Principles derived from the study of simple skills do not generalize to complex skill learning," *Psychonomic Bulletin & Review*, vol. 9, no. 2, pp. 185–211, 2002.

[18] N. Kanekar and A. S. Aruin, "Improvement of anticipatory postural adjustments for balance control: effect of a single training session," *Journal of Electromyography and Kinesiology*, vol. 25, no. 2, pp. 400–405, 2015.

[19] S. Y. Chiou, M. Hurry, T. Reed, J. X. Quek, and P. H. Strutton, "Cortical contributions to anticipatory postural adjustments in the trunk," *The Journal of Physiology*, vol. 596, no. 7, pp. 1295–1306, 2018.

[20] A. Zając, M. Chalimoniuk, A. Gołaś, J. Lngfort, and A. Maszczyk, "Central and peripheral fatigue during resistance exercise—a critical review," *Journal of Human Kinetics*, vol. 49, no. 1, pp. 159–169, 2015.

[21] K. A. Kubitz, D. M. Landers, S. J. Petruzzello, and M. Han, "The effects of acute and chronic exercise on sleep. A meta-analytic review," *Sports Medicine*, vol. 21, no. 4, pp. 277–291, 1996.

[22] T. V. P. Bliss and T. Lømo, "Long-lasting potentiation of synaptic transmission in the dentate area of the anaesthetized rabbit following stimulation of the perforant path," *The Journal of Physiology*, vol. 232, no. 2, pp. 331–356, 1973.

[23] J. N. Sanes, "Neocortical mechanisms in motor learning," *Current Opinion in Neurobiology*, vol. 13, no. 2, pp. 225–231, 2003.

[24] T. Abel, R. Havekes, J. M. Saletin, and M. P. Walker, "Sleep, plasticity and memory from molecules to whole-brain networks," *Current Biology*, vol. 23, no. 17, pp. R774–R788, 2013.

[25] J. L. McGaugh, "Memory—a century of consolidation," *Science*, vol. 287, no. 5451, pp. 248–251, 2000.

[26] S. Diekelmann, C. Buchel, J. Born, and B. Rasch, "Labile or stable: opposing consequences for memory when reactivated during waking and sleep," *Nature Neuroscience*, vol. 14, no. 3, pp. 381–386, 2011.

[27] A. R. Eugene and J. Masiak, "The neuroprotective aspects of sleep," *MEDtube Science*, vol. 3, no. 1, pp. 35–40, 2015.

[28] E. M. Robertson, "From creation to consolidation: a novel framework for memory processing," *PLoS Biology*, vol. 7, no. 1, article e19, 2009.

[29] G. Yang, C. S. W. Lai, J. Cichon, L. Ma, W. Li, and W. B. Gan, "Sleep promotes branch-specific formation of dendritic spines after learning," *Science*, vol. 344, no. 6188, pp. 1173–1178, 2014.

[30] T. O. Bergmann, M. Mölle, L. Marshall, L. Kaya-Yildiz, J. Born, and H. Roman Siebner, "A local signature of LTP- and LTD-like plasticity in human NREM sleep,"

European Journal of Neuroscience, vol. 27, no. 9, pp. 2241–2249, 2008.

[31] L. Mascetti, A. Foret, J. Schrouff et al., "Concurrent synaptic and systems memory consolidation during sleep," *The Journal of Neuroscience*, vol. 33, no. 24, pp. 10182–10190, 2013.

[32] S. Diekelmann, I. Wilhelm, and J. Born, "The whats and whens of sleep-dependent memory consolidation," *Sleep Medicine Reviews*, vol. 13, no. 5, pp. 309–321, 2009.

[33] G. B. Feld and S. Diekelmann, "Sleep smart—optimizing sleep for declarative learning and memory," *Frontiers in Psychology*, vol. 6, p. 622, 2015.

[34] G. Tononi and C. Cirelli, "Sleep and the price of plasticity: from synaptic and cellular homeostasis to memory consolidation and integration," *Neuron*, vol. 81, no. 1, pp. 12–34, 2014.

[35] P. Ramm and C. T. Smith, "Rates of cerebral protein synthesis are linked to slow wave sleep in the rat," *Physiology & Behavior*, vol. 48, no. 5, pp. 749–753, 1990.

[36] H. Nakanishi, Y. Sun, R. K. Nakamura et al., "Positive correlations between cerebral protein synthesis rates and deep sleep in *Macaca mulatta*," *European Journal of Neuroscience*, vol. 9, no. 2, pp. 271–279, 1997.

[37] K. G. Reymann and J. U. Frey, "The late maintenance of hippocampal LTP: requirements, phases, "synaptic tagging," "late-associativity" and implications," *Neuropharmacology*, vol. 52, no. 1, pp. 24–40, 2007.

[38] C. Cirelli, C. M. Gutierrez, and G. Tononi, "Extensive and divergent effects of sleep and wakefulness on brain gene expression," *Neuron*, vol. 41, no. 1, pp. 35–43, 2004.

[39] M. Mackiewicz, K. R. Shockley, M. A. Romer et al., "Macromolecule biosynthesis: a key function of sleep," *Physiological Genomics*, vol. 31, no. 3, pp. 441–457, 2007.

[40] M. Gorgoni, A. D'Atri, G. Lauri, P. M. Rossini, F. Ferlazzo, and L. de Gennaro, "Is sleep essential for neural plasticity in humans, and how does it affect motor and cognitive recovery?," *Neural Plasticity*, vol. 2013, Article ID 103949, 13 pages, 2013.

[41] A. Kales and A. Rechtschaffen, Eds., *A Manual of Standardized Terminology, Techniques and Scoring System for Sleep Stages of Human Subjects*, US National Institute of Neurological Diseases and Blindness, Neurological Information Network, Bethesda, MD, USA, 1968.

[42] A. Boutin, B. Pinsard, A. Bore, J. Carrier, S. M. Fogel, and J. Doyon, "Transient synchronization of hippocampo-striato-thalamo-cortical networks during sleep spindle oscillations induces motor memory consolidation," *NeuroImage*, vol. 169, pp. 419–430, 2018.

[43] S. M. Purcell, D. S. Manoach, C. Demanuele et al., "Characterizing sleep spindles in 11,630 individuals from the National Sleep Research Resource," *Nature Communications*, vol. 8, article 15930, 2017.

[44] S. C. Warby, S. L. Wendt, P. Welinder et al., "Sleep-spindle detection: crowdsourcing and evaluating performance of experts, non-experts and automated methods," *Nature Methods*, vol. 11, no. 4, pp. 385–392, 2014.

[45] M. Rosanova and D. Ulrich, "Pattern-specific associative long-term potentiation induced by a sleep spindle-related spike train," *The Journal of Neuroscience*, vol. 25, no. 41, pp. 9398–9405, 2005.

[46] T. J. Sejnowski and A. Destexhe, "Why do we sleep?," *Brain Research*, vol. 886, no. 1-2, pp. 208–223, 2000.

[47] F. Engert and T. Bonhoeffer, "Dendritic spine changes associated with hippocampal long-term synaptic plasticity," *Nature*, vol. 399, no. 6731, pp. 66–70, 1999.

[48] S. M. Fogel and C. T. Smith, "Learning-dependent changes in sleep spindles and stage 2 sleep," *Journal of Sleep Research*, vol. 15, no. 3, pp. 250–255, 2006.

[49] M. Molle, O. Yeshenko, L. Marshall, S. J. Sara, and J. Born, "Hippocampal sharp wave-ripples linked to slow oscillations in rat slow-wave sleep," *Journal of Neurophysiology*, vol. 96, no. 1, pp. 62–70, 2006.

[50] A. Morin, J. Doyon, V. Dostie et al., "Motor sequence learning increases sleep spindles and fast frequencies in post-training sleep," *Sleep*, vol. 31, no. 8, pp. 1149–1156, 2008.

[51] M. Tamaki, T. Matsuoka, H. Nittono, and T. Hori, "Fast sleep spindle (13–15 Hz) activity correlates with sleep-dependent improvement in visuomotor performance," *Sleep*, vol. 31, no. 2, pp. 204–211, 2008.

[52] M. Barakat, J. Doyon, K. Debas et al., "Fast and slow spindle involvement in the consolidation of a new motor sequence," *Behavioural Brain Research*, vol. 217, no. 1, pp. 117–121, 2011.

[53] S. Laventure, S. Fogel, O. Lungu et al., "NREM2 and sleep spindles are instrumental to the consolidation of motor sequence memories," *PLoS Biology*, vol. 14, no. 3, article e1002429, 2016.

[54] M. Molle, L. Marshall, S. Gais, and J. Born, "Grouping of spindle activity during slow oscillations in human non-rapid eye movement sleep," *The Journal of Neuroscience*, vol. 22, no. 24, pp. 10941–10947, 2002.

[55] M. Steriade, "Corticothalamic resonance, states of vigilance and mentation," *Neuroscience*, vol. 101, no. 2, pp. 243–276, 2000.

[56] S. K. Esser, S. L. Hill, and G. Tononi, "Sleep homeostasis and cortical synchronization: I. Modeling the effects of synaptic strength on sleep slow waves," *Sleep*, vol. 30, no. 12, pp. 1617–1630, 2007.

[57] M. Bazhenov, I. Timofeev, M. Steriade, and T. J. Sejnowski, "Model of thalamocortical slow-wave sleep oscillations and transitions to activated states," *The Journal of Neuroscience*, vol. 22, no. 19, pp. 8691–8704, 2002.

[58] R. Huber, M. Felice Ghilardi, M. Massimini, and G. Tononi, "Local sleep and learning," *Nature*, vol. 430, no. 6995, pp. 78–81, 2004.

[59] E. C. Landsness, D. Crupi, B. K. Hulse et al., "Sleep-dependent improvement in visuomotor learning: a causal role for slow waves," *Sleep*, vol. 32, no. 10, pp. 1273–1284, 2009.

[60] L. Marshall, H. Helgadottir, M. Molle, and J. Born, "Boosting slow oscillations during sleep potentiates memory," *Nature*, vol. 444, no. 7119, pp. 610–613, 2006.

[61] D. Miyamoto, D. Hirai, C. C. A. Fung et al., "Top-down cortical input during NREM sleep consolidates perceptual memory," *Science*, vol. 352, no. 6291, pp. 1315–1318, 2016.

[62] M. Jouvet and F. Michel, "Electromyographic correlations of sleep in the chronic decorticate & mesencephalic cat," *Comptes Rendus des Séances de la Société de Biologie et de Ses Filiales*, vol. 153, no. 3, pp. 422–425, 1959.

[63] S. Datta and D. F. Siwek, "Excitation of the brain stem pedunculopontine tegmentum cholinergic cells induces

wakefulness and REM sleep," *Journal of Neurophysiology*, vol. 77, no. 6, pp. 2975–2988, 1997.

[64] S. Datta, "Avoidance task training potentiates phasic pontine-wave density in the rat: a mechanism for sleep-dependent plasticity," *The Journal of Neuroscience*, vol. 20, no. 22, pp. 8607–8613, 2000.

[65] S. Datta, V. Mavanji, J. Ulloor, and E. H. Patterson, "Activation of phasic pontine-wave generator prevents rapid eye movement sleep deprivation-induced learning impairment in the rat: a mechanism for sleep-dependent plasticity," *The Journal of Neuroscience*, vol. 24, no. 6, pp. 1416–1427, 2004.

[66] G. R. Poe, C. M. Walsh, and T. E. Bjorness, "Cognitive neuroscience of sleep," *Progress in Brain Research*, vol. 185, pp. 1–19, 2010.

[67] G. Barmashenko, J. Buttgereit, N. Herring et al., "Regulation of hippocampal synaptic plasticity thresholds and changes in exploratory and learning behavior in dominant negative NPR-B mutant rats," *Frontiers in Molecular Neuroscience*, vol. 7, p. 95, 2014.

[68] W. Li, L. Ma, G. Yang, and W. B. Gan, "REM sleep selectively prunes and maintains new synapses in development and learning," *Nature Neuroscience*, vol. 20, no. 3, pp. 427–437, 2017.

[69] P. Maquet, S. Laureys, P. Peigneux et al., "Experience-dependent changes in cerebral activation during human REM sleep," *Nature Neuroscience*, vol. 3, no. 8, pp. 831–836, 2000.

[70] L. Kempler and J. L. Richmond, "Effect of sleep on gross motor memory," *Memory*, vol. 20, no. 8, pp. 907–914, 2012.

[71] T. P. Brawn, K. M. Fenn, H. C. Nusbaum, and D. Margoliash, "Consolidation of sensorimotor learning during sleep," *Learning & Memory*, vol. 15, no. 11, pp. 815–819, 2008.

[72] K. Kuriyama, R. Stickgold, and M. P. Walker, "Sleep-dependent learning and motor-skill complexity," *Learning & Memory*, vol. 11, no. 6, pp. 705–713, 2004.

[73] A. Malangre and K. Blischke, "Sleep-related offline improvements in gross motor task performance occur under free recall requirements," *Frontiers in Human Neuroscience*, vol. 10, p. 134, 2016.

[74] A. Malangre, P. Leinen, and K. Blischke, "Sleep-related offline learning in a complex arm movement sequence," *Journal of Human Kinetics*, vol. 40, no. 1, pp. 7–20, 2014.

[75] L. Genzel, A. Quack, E. Jäger, B. Konrad, A. Steiger, and M. Dresler, "Complex motor sequence skills profit from sleep," *Neuropsychobiology*, vol. 66, no. 4, pp. 237–243, 2012.

[76] Y. Morita, K. Ogawa, and S. Uchida, "The effect of a daytime 2-hour nap on complex motor skill learning," *Sleep and Biological Rhythms*, vol. 10, no. 4, pp. 302–309, 2012.

[77] Y. Morita, K. Ogawa, and S. Uchida, "Napping after complex motor learning enhances juggling performance," *Sleep Science*, vol. 9, no. 2, pp. 112–116, 2016.

[78] K. Hoedlmoser, J. Birklbauer, M. Schabus, P. Eibenberger, S. Rigler, and E. Mueller, "The impact of diurnal sleep on the consolidation of a complex gross motor adaptation task," *Journal of Sleep Research*, vol. 24, no. 1, pp. 100–109, 2015.

[79] K. Blischke, D. Erlacher, H. Kresin, S. Brueckner, and A. Malangré, "Benefits of sleep in motor learning—prospects and limitations," *Journal of Human Kinetics*, vol. 20, no. 1, pp. 23–35, 2008.

[80] A. Al-Sharman and C. F. Siengsukon, "Sleep enhances learning of a functional motor task in young adults," *Physical Therapy*, vol. 93, no. 12, pp. 1625–1635, 2013.

[81] K. Blischke and A. Malangre, "Task complexity modulates sleep-related offline learning in sequential motor skills," *Frontiers in Human Neuroscience*, vol. 11, p. 374, 2017.

[82] B. Hauptmann, E. Reinhart, S. A. Brandt, and A. Karni, "The predictive value of the leveling off of within session performance for procedural memory consolidation," *Cognitive Brain Research*, vol. 24, no. 2, pp. 181–189, 2005.

[83] P. A. Lewis and S. J. Durrant, "Overlapping memory replay during sleep builds cognitive schemata," *Trends in Cognitive Sciences*, vol. 15, no. 8, pp. 343–351, 2011.

[84] A. Keisler, J. Ashe, and D. T. Willingham, "Time of day accounts for overnight improvement in sequence learning," *Learning & Memory*, vol. 14, no. 10, pp. 669–672, 2007.

[85] S. Mednick, K. Nakayama, and R. Stickgold, "Sleep-dependent learning: a nap is as good as a night," *Nature Neuroscience*, vol. 6, no. 7, pp. 697–698, 2003.

[86] F. J. van Schalkwijk, C. Sauter, K. Hoedlmoser et al., "The effect of daytime napping and full-night sleep on the consolidation of declarative and procedural information," *Journal of Sleep Research*, 2017.

[87] C. Gudberg, K. Wulff, and H. Johansen-Berg, "Sleep-dependent motor memory consolidation in older adults depends on task demands," *Neurobiology of Aging*, vol. 36, no. 3, pp. 1409–1416, 2015.

[88] R. M. C. Spencer, A. M. Gouw, and R. B. Ivry, "Age-related decline of sleep-dependent consolidation," *Learning & Memory*, vol. 14, no. 7, pp. 480–484, 2007.

[89] C. F. Siengsukon and L. A. Boyd, "Sleep to learn after stroke: implicit and explicit off-line motor learning," *Neuroscience Letters*, vol. 451, no. 1, pp. 1–5, 2009.

[90] W. Backhaus, H. Braass, T. Renné, C. Gerloff, and F. C. Hummel, "Motor performance is not enhanced by daytime naps in older adults," *Frontiers in Aging Neuroscience*, vol. 8, p. 125, 2016.

[91] A. Al-Sharman and C. F. Siengsukon, "Performance on a functional motor task is enhanced by sleep in middle-aged and older adults," *Journal of Neurologic Physical Therapy*, vol. 38, no. 3, pp. 161–169, 2014.

[92] T. M. Buckley and A. F. Schatzberg, "Aging and the role of the HPA axis and rhythm in sleep and memory-consolidation," *The American Journal of Geriatric Psychiatry*, vol. 13, no. 5, pp. 344–352, 2005.

[93] S. Fogel, N. Martin, M. Lafortune et al., "NREM sleep oscillations and brain plasticity in aging," *Frontiers in Neurology*, vol. 3, p. 176, 2012.

[94] M. M. Ohayon, "Sleep and the elderly," *Journal of Psychosomatic Research*, vol. 56, no. 5, pp. 463–464, 2004.

[95] K. Crowley, J. Trinder, Y. Kim, M. Carrington, and I. M. Colrain, "The effects of normal aging on sleep spindle and K-complex production," *Clinical Neurophysiology*, vol. 113, no. 10, pp. 1615–1622, 2002.

[96] S. Dayanidhi and F. J. Valero-Cuevas, "Dexterous manipulation is poorer at older ages and is dissociated from decline of hand strength," *The Journals of Gerontology: Series A*, vol. 69, no. 9, pp. 1139–1145, 2014.

[97] H. H. K. Fullagar, S. Skorski, R. Duffield, D. Hammes, A. J. Coutts, and T. Meyer, "Sleep and athletic performance: the effects of sleep loss on exercise performance,

and physiological and cognitive responses to exercise," *Sports Medicine*, vol. 45, no. 2, pp. 161–186, 2015.

[98] A. J. Krause, E. B. Simon, B. A. Mander et al., "The sleep-deprived human brain," *Nature Reviews Neuroscience*, vol. 18, no. 7, pp. 404–418, 2017.

[99] R. V. Rial, M. C. Nicolau, A. Gamundi et al., "The trivial function of sleep," *Sleep Medicine Reviews*, vol. 11, no. 4, pp. 311–325, 2007.

[100] R. G. Peñalva, M. Lancel, C. Flachskamm, J. M. H. M. Reul, F. Holsboer, and A. C. E. Linthorst, "Effect of sleep and sleep deprivation on serotonergic neurotransmission in the hippocampus: a combined in vivo microdialysis/EEG study in rats," *European Journal of Neuroscience*, vol. 17, no. 9, pp. 1896–1906, 2003.

[101] N. D. Volkow, D. Tomasi, G. J. Wang et al., "Evidence that sleep deprivation downregulates dopamine D2R in ventral striatum in the human brain," *The Journal of Neuroscience*, vol. 32, no. 19, pp. 6711–6717, 2012.

[102] I. G. Campbell, M. J. Guinan, and J. M. Horowitz, "Sleep deprivation impairs long-term potentiation in rat hippocampal slices," *Journal of Neurophysiology*, vol. 88, no. 2, pp. 1073–1076, 2002.

[103] C. Kopp, F. Longordo, J. R. Nicholson, and A. Luthi, "Insufficient sleep reversibly alters bidirectional synaptic plasticity and NMDA receptor function," *The Journal of Neuroscience*, vol. 26, no. 48, pp. 12456–12465, 2006.

[104] V. V. Vyazovskiy, C. Cirelli, M. Pfister-Genskow, U. Faraguna, and G. Tononi, "Molecular and electrophysiological evidence for net synaptic potentiation in wake and depression in sleep," *Nature Neuroscience*, vol. 11, no. 2, pp. 200–208, 2008.

[105] R. Huber, H. Mäki, M. Rosanova et al., "Human cortical excitability increases with time awake," *Cerebral Cortex*, vol. 23, no. 2, pp. 332–338, 2013.

[106] P. Kreuzer, B. Langguth, R. Popp et al., "Reduced intracortical inhibition after sleep deprivation: a transcranial magnetic stimulation study," *Neuroscience Letters*, vol. 493, no. 3, pp. 63–66, 2011.

[107] R. Havekes, C. G. Vecsey, and T. Abel, "The impact of sleep deprivation on neuronal and glial signaling pathways important for memory and synaptic plasticity," *Cellular Signalling*, vol. 24, no. 6, pp. 1251–1260, 2012.

[108] K. S. Lehmann, P. Martus, S. Little-Elk et al., "Impact of sleep deprivation on medium-term psychomotor and cognitive performance of surgeons: prospective cross-over study with a virtual surgery simulator and psychometric tests," *Surgery*, vol. 147, no. 2, pp. 246–254, 2010.

[109] G. J. Holland, "Effects of limited sleep deprivation on performance of selected motor tasks," *Research Quarterly*, vol. 39, no. 2, pp. 285–294, 1968.

[110] S. L. Halson, "Sleep in elite athletes and nutritional interventions to enhance sleep," *Sports Medicine*, vol. 44, Supplement 1, pp. 13–23, 2014.

[111] T. Reilly and T. Deykin, "Effects of partial sleep loss on subjective states, psychomotor and physical performance tests," *Journal of Human Movement Studies*, vol. 9, pp. 157–170, 1983.

[112] E. J. DeMaria, C. L. McBride, T. J. Broderick, and B. J. Kaplan, "Night call does not impair learning of laparoscopic skills," *Surgical Innovation*, vol. 12, no. 2, pp. 145–149, 2005.

[113] B. J. Eastridge, E. C. Hamilton, G. E. O'Keefe et al., "Effect of sleep deprivation on the performance of simulated laparoscopic surgical skill," *American Journal of Surgery*, vol. 186, no. 2, pp. 169–174, 2003.

[114] N. J. Taffinder, I. McManus, Y. Gul, R. C. G. Russell, and A. Darzi, "Effect of sleep deprivation on surgeons' dexterity on laparoscopy simulator," *The Lancet*, vol. 352, no. 9135, p. 1191, 1998.

[115] N. Cellini, "Memory consolidation in sleep disorders," *Sleep Medicine Reviews*, vol. 35, pp. 101–112, 2017.

[116] E. C. Hanlon, U. Faraguna, V. V. Vyazovskiy, G. Tononi, and C. Cirelli, "Effects of skilled training on sleep slow wave activity and cortical gene expression in the rat," *Sleep*, vol. 32, no. 6, pp. 719–729, 2009.

[117] C. M. Shapiro, "Sleep and the athlete," *British Journal of Sports Medicine*, vol. 15, no. 1, pp. 51–55, 1981.

[118] L. Torsvall, T. Åkerstedt, and L. Göran, "Effects on sleep stages and EEG power density of different degrees of exercise in fit subjects," *Electroencephalography and Clinical Neurophysiology*, vol. 57, no. 4, pp. 347–353, 1984.

[119] J. Trinder, S. J. Paxton, J. Montgomery, and G. Fraser, "Endurance as opposed to power training: their effect on sleep," *Psychophysiology*, vol. 22, no. 6, pp. 668–673, 1985.

[120] J. Buchegger, R. Fritsch, A. Meier-Koll, and H. Riehle, "Does trampolining and anaerobic physical fitness affect sleep?," *Perceptual and Motor Skills*, vol. 73, no. 1, pp. 243–252, 1991.

[121] D. Erlacher and M. Schredl, "Effect of a motor learning task on REM sleep parameters," *Sleep and Hypnosis*, vol. 8, no. 2, pp. 41–46, 2006.

[122] C. E. Milner, S. M. Fogel, and K. A. Cote, "Habitual napping moderates motor performance improvements following a short daytime nap," *Biological Psychology*, vol. 73, no. 2, pp. 141–156, 2006.

[123] T. Agnew, "Common sense solutions for sleepless nights: night-time care in residential homes can be complicated for residents and staff, but as a new report shows, training and common sense pay off," *Nursing Older People*, vol. 20, no. 5, pp. 7-8, 2008.

[124] H. Nagai, L. De Vivo, M. Bellesi, M. F. Ghilardi, G. Tononi, and C. Cirelli, "Sleep consolidates motor learning of complex movement sequences in mice," *Sleep*, vol. 40, no. 2, 2017.

[125] G. S. Withers and W. T. Greenough, "Reach training selectively alters dendritic branching in subpopulations of layer II–III pyramids in rat motor-somatosensory forelimb cortex," *Neuropsychologia*, vol. 27, no. 1, pp. 61–69, 1989.

[126] M. S. Rioult-Pedotti, D. Friedman, G. Hess, and J. P. Donoghue, "Strengthening of horizontal cortical connections following skill learning," *Nature Neuroscience*, vol. 1, no. 3, pp. 230–234, 1998.

[127] R. Huber, S. K. Esser, F. Ferrarelli, M. Massimini, M. J. Peterson, and G. Tononi, "TMS-induced cortical potentiation during wakefulness locally increases slow wave activity during sleep," *PLoS One*, vol. 2, no. 3, article e276, 2007.

[128] R. Huber, S. Maatta, S. K. Esser et al., "Measures of cortical plasticity after transcranial paired associative stimulation predict changes in electroencephalogram slow-wave activity during subsequent sleep," *The Journal of Neuroscience*, vol. 28, no. 31, pp. 7911–7918, 2008.

[129] W. Backhaus, S. Kempe, and F. C. Hummel, "The effect of sleep on motor learning in the aging and stroke

population—a systematic review," *Restorative Neurology and Neuroscience*, vol. 34, no. 1, pp. 153–164, 2015.

[130] C. Gudberg and H. Johansen-Berg, "Sleep and motor learning: implications for physical rehabilitation after stroke," *Frontiers in Neurology*, vol. 6, p. 241, 2015.

[131] A. M. Bamer, K. Cetin, K. L. Johnson, L. E. Gibbons, and D. M. Ehde, "Validation study of prevalence and correlates of depressive symptomatology in multiple sclerosis," *General Hospital Psychiatry*, vol. 30, no. 4, pp. 311–317, 2008.

[132] G. Merlino, L. Fratticci, C. Lenchig et al., "Prevalence of "poor sleep" among patients with multiple sclerosis: an independent predictor of mental and physical status," *Sleep Medicine*, vol. 10, no. 1, pp. 26–34, 2009.

[133] S. Zoccolella, M. Savarese, P. Lamberti, R. Manni, C. Pacchetti, and G. Logroscino, "Sleep disorders and the natural history of Parkinson's disease: the contribution of epidemiological studies," *Sleep Medicine Reviews*, vol. 15, no. 1, pp. 41–50, 2011.

[134] C. L. Bassetti, "Sleep and stroke," *Seminars in Neurology*, vol. 25, no. 1, pp. 19–32, 2005.

[135] R. J. Castriotta, M. C. Wilde, J. M. Lai, S. Atanasov, B. E. Masel, and S. T. Kuna, "Prevalence and consequences of sleep disorders in traumatic brain injury," *Journal of Clinical Sleep Medicine*, vol. 3, no. 4, pp. 349–356, 2007.

[136] O. Mahmood, L. J. Rapport, R. A. Hanks, and N. L. Fichtenberg, "Neuropsychological performance and sleep disturbance following traumatic brain injury," *Journal of Head Trauma Rehabilitation*, vol. 19, no. 5, pp. 378–390, 2004.

[137] Y. Song, J. M. Dzierzewski, C. H. Fung et al., "Association between sleep and physical function in older veterans in an adult day healthcare program," *Journal of the American Geriatrics Society*, vol. 63, no. 8, pp. 1622–1627, 2015.

[138] S. Landry, D. M. O'Driscoll, G. S. Hamilton, and R. Conduit, "Overnight motor skill learning outcomes in obstructive sleep apnea: effect of continuous positive airway pressure," *Journal of Clinical Sleep Medicine*, vol. 12, no. 5, pp. 681–688, 2016.

15

Effects of Antipsychotic Drugs on the Epigenetic Modification of Brain-Derived Neurotrophic Factor Gene Expression in the Hippocampi of Chronic Restraint Stress Rats

Mi Kyoung Seo,[1] Young Hoon Kim,[2] Roger S. McIntyre,[3,4] Rodrigo B. Mansur,[3,4] Yena Lee,[3] Nicole E. Carmona,[3] Ah Jeong Choi,[1] Gyung-Mee Kim,[5] Jung Goo Lee ⓘ,[1,5,6] and Sung Woo Park ⓘ[1,6,7]

[1]Paik Institute for Clinical Research, Inje University, Busan, Republic of Korea
[2]Department of Psychiatry, Gongju National Hospital, Gongju, Republic of Korea
[3]Mood Disorders Psychopharmacology Unit, University Health Network, University of Toronto, Toronto, ON, Canada
[4]Department of Psychiatry, University of Toronto, Toronto, ON, Canada
[5]Department of Psychiatry, College of Medicine, Haeundae Paik Hospital, Inje University, Busan, Republic of Korea
[6]Department of Health Science and Technology, Graduate School, Inje University, Busan, Republic of Korea
[7]Department of Convergence Biomedical Science, College of Medicine, Inje University, Busan, Republic of Korea

Correspondence should be addressed to Jung Goo Lee; iybihwc@naver.com and Sung Woo Park; swpark@inje.ac.kr

Academic Editor: Malgorzata Kossut

Recent studies have shown that antipsychotic drugs have epigenetic effects. However, the effects of antipsychotic drugs on histone modification remain unclear. Therefore, we investigated the effects of antipsychotic drugs on the epigenetic modification of the BDNF gene in the rat hippocampus. Rats were subjected to chronic restraint stress (6 h/d for 21 d) and then were administered with either olanzapine (2 mg/kg) or haloperidol (1 mg/kg). The levels of histone H3 acetylation and MeCP2 binding at BDNF promoter IV were assessed with chromatin immunoprecipitation assays. The mRNA levels of total BDNF with exon IV, HDAC5, DNMT1, and DNMT3a were assessed with a quantitative RT-PCR procedure. Chronic restraint stress resulted in the downregulation of total and exon IV BDNF mRNA levels and a decrease in histone H3 acetylation and an increase in MeCP2 binding at BDNF promoter IV. Furthermore, there were robust increases in the expression of HDAC5 and DNMTs. Olanzapine administration largely prevented these changes. The administration of haloperidol had no effect. These findings suggest that the antipsychotic drug olanzapine induced histone modification of BDNF gene expression in the hippocampus and that these epigenetic alterations may represent one of the mechanisms underlying the actions of antipsychotic drugs.

1. Introduction

Schizophrenia is a complex and chronic mental illness with a lifetime prevalence of approximately 1% [1, 2]. It is a genetic disorder with a heritability of up to 80% [3], and the majority of patients with schizophrenia suffer from psychotic, affective, and cognitive symptoms as well as functional impairments [4–6]. Although advances have been made in the treatment of schizophrenia, its etiology and pathophysiology have yet to be fully elucidated. In fact, heterogeneous phenotypes and lack of clear pathological lesions in the brain have been major hurdles in the field of schizophrenia research [7].

Of the suggested models that describe the development of schizophrenia, neurodevelopmental and neurodegeneration models represent two nonmutually exclusive theories regarding the etiology and course of this disorder [7–10]. Furthermore, the roles of multiple epigenetic mechanisms in the development of schizophrenia are now becoming a primary focus of research [7, 10, 11]. Epigenetic modifications are most commonly regulated by DNA methylation and histone modification [12–14]. The entire length of DNA in a single somatic cell exists within the nucleus complex along with chromatin [15, 16]. The primary structural unit of chromatin is the nucleosome, which is composed of the standard length of DNA and four pairs of basic histone proteins (H2A, H2B, H3, and H4) [17, 18]. In vertebrates, methylation of the CpG dinucleotide within proximal promoters is frequently linked to transcriptional repression (i.e., gene silencing) [19]. The gene silencing effect of DNA methylation is mediated by methyl-CpG-binding protein 2 (MeCP2), which is one of several CpG-binding proteins [20, 21], which recruits histone deacetylases (HDACs) to remove active modifications and repress gene transcription [20, 21]. MeCP2 can also enhance the repressive chromatin state via the addition of repressive H3K9 methylation to histone methyltransferase [19, 22].

An increasing amount of evidence suggests that epigenetic modifications in certain brain regions and neural circuits may be important mechanisms underlying the development of schizophrenia [23–26]. The altered functioning of cortical pyramidal neurons and cortical parvalbumin- (PV-) positive GABAergic interneurons may be related to the psychotic and cognitive symptoms of schizophrenia [27–29]. Huang and Akbarian found an average 8-fold deficit in repressive chromatin-associated DNA methylation at GAD1 promoters in patients with schizophrenia [30] and it has been shown that histone 3 (H3), one of the histone proteins, was particularly dysregulated in schizophrenia patients [31]. Furthermore, the di- and trimethylation of H3K9 and H3K17, which are known to regulate GAD1 expression, were found to be elevated in cortical neurons in a postmortem study of patients with schizophrenia [31].

Following the introduction of chlorpromazine in 1952, antipsychotic drugs have been widely used for the treatment of schizophrenia [1, 32]. Subsequently, as research data have accumulated, it has been suggested that antipsychotic drugs may be involved in the regulation of epigenetic changes in the brain. An in vivo study by Dong et al. [33] demonstrated that the antipsychotic drugs clozapine and sulpiride increased the cortical and striatal demethylation of hypermethylated RELN and GAD1 promoters in the prefrontal cortex of mice after 7 d of methionine treatment. Clozapine attenuated the decrease in histone H3 acetylation at lysine 9 residues in the prefrontal cortex and ameliorated memory impairments and social deficits in mice treated with phencyclidine [34]. Additionally, Melka et al. [35] reported that olanzapine altered methylation in genes associated with dopamine neurotransmission in the hippocampus and cerebellum of rats. In humans, frontocortical DNA methylation of the BDNF gene was correlated with a genotype that was associated with major psychosis in a genome-wide epigenomic study of major psychosis [36]. Moreover, Abdolmaleky et al. [37] showed that antipsychotic drugs attenuated the aberrant DNA methylation of the dysbindin (BTNBP1) promoter in the saliva and postmortem brain samples of patients with schizophrenia and psychotic bipolar disorder.

BDNF is a neurotrophic factor and, as mentioned above, epigenetic changes of the BDNF gene are related to the pathophysiology of schizophrenia [7, 38, 39]. The reduced expression of BDNF and increases in the promoter

methylation of BDNF exons IV and IX have been identified in the frontal cortex and hippocampus of patients with schizophrenia [40, 41]. Although it may be postulated that antipsychotic drugs influence the epigenetic mechanisms associated with the BDNF gene, there is a relative lack of studies investigating the epigenetic effects of antipsychotic drugs on the BDNF gene in the brain. Therefore, the present study evaluated the manner in which antipsychotic drugs alter epigenetic changes in the BDNF gene in the rat hippocampus. To assess this, we used a chronic restraint stress model to induce morphological and functional changes in the hippocampus [42–44]. A recent study from our research group demonstrated that chronic restraint stress decreased the levels of BDNF expression and acetylated histone H3 at BDNF promoter IV in the rat hippocampus [45]. Epigenetic changes in the BDNF gene induced by antipsychotic drugs may be more apparent when measured under conditions of reduced BDNF or acetylated histone levels. Furthermore, certain atypical antipsychotic drugs, but not typical antipsychotic drug haloperidol, attenuated chronic restraint stress-induced decreases in BDNF expression level [46–48]. As a result, the primary aims of the present study were to investigate the levels of total and exon IV BDNF mRNA and the levels of histone H3 acetylation and MeCP2 binding at BDNF promoter IV. Additionally, the mRNA levels of HDAC5, DNMT1, and DNMT3a in the hippocampus were assessed following the chronic administration of olanzapine and haloperidol to rats that were either exposed or not exposed to 21 d of chronic restraint stress.

2. Materials and Methods

2.1. Animals and Drug Administration. All experiments involving animals were approved by the Committee for Animal Experimentation and the Institutional Animal Laboratory Review Board of Inje Medical College (approval number 2015-029). For the present study, male Sprague-Dawley rats (Orient Bio, Gyeonggi-Do, Korea) weighing 200–250 g were housed 2 or 3 per cage with ad libitum food and water and maintained at 21°C on a 12/12 h light/dark cycle. After 7 d of acclimatization, the rats were randomly divided into 6 groups of 6 rats each ($n = 6$ animals/group). All drugs were dissolved in vehicle (0.8% glacial acetic acid in 0.9% saline) and injected intraperitoneally (i.p.) into the animals. The first group (vehicle control) received vehicle (1 mL/kg, i.p.) without restraint stress; the second (olanzapine) and third (haloperidol) groups received olanzapine (2 mg/kg, i.p.) and haloperidol (1 mg/kg, i.p.), respectively, without restraint stress; the fourth group (vehicle + stress) received vehicle at 10:00 and was then completely restrained for 6 h from 11:00 to 17:00 in specially designed plastic restraint tubes (dimensions: 20 cm high, 7 cm in diameter); and the fifth (olanzapine + stress) and sixth (haloperidol + stress) groups received olanzapine (2 mg/kg, i.p.) and haloperidol (1 mg/kg, i.p.), respectively, and were then immobilized in the same way as the rats in the fourth group. All procedures were repeated once daily for 3 weeks. In our preliminary experiment, the expression patterns of BDNF according to time (2 and 6 h) and period

TABLE 1: Individual-level data for each group analyzed by qRT-PCR and ChIP.

	– Restraint stress			+ Restraint stress		
	VEH	OLA	HAL	VEH	OLA	HAL
Total BDNF mRNA	1.00 ± 0.07	1.38 ± 0.05	0.89 ± 0.09	0.54 ± 0.04	1.03 ± 0.10	0.65 ± 0.14
BDNF exon IV mRNA	1.00 ± 0.06	1.55 ± 0.05	0.99 ± 0.07	0.55 ± 0.06	1.10 ± 0.12	0.57 ± 0.26
Acetyl-H3	1.00 ± 0.20	1.44 ± 0.22	1.00 ± 0.37	0.37 ± 0.40	0.88 ± 0.39	0.36 ± 0.29
MeCP2	1.00 ± 0.37	0.64 ± 0.21	1.21 ± 0.27	1.51 ± 0.28	0.73 ± 0.28	1.25 ± 0.22
HDAC5 mRNA	1.00 ± 0.05	0.80 ± 0.06	1.06 ± 0.13	1.47 ± 0.06	0.72 ± 0.14	1.35 ± 0.07
DNMT1 mRNA	1.00 ± 0.09	0.73 ± 0.08	1.05 ± 0.09	1.44 ± 0.11	0.81 ± 0.14	1.20 ± 0.08
DNMT3a mRNA	1.00 ± 0.04	0.64 ± 0.05	1.09 ± 0.09	1.80 ± 0.12	1.21 ± 0.09	1.72 ± 0.13

(1, 7, and 21 d) of restraint stress were analyzed by Western blotting (Supplementary Materials; Figure S1). Six-hour-daily stress for 1, 7, and 21 d significantly reduced BDNF expression levels. To assess the chronic effects of antipsychotic drugs on restraint stress, a stress period of 21 d was used.

Olanzapine was supplied by Eli Lilly Research Laboratories (Indianapolis, IN, USA), and haloperidol was purchased from Sigma (St. Louis, MO, USA). The clinical effects of many antipsychotic drugs are reflected by a dopamine D2 receptor occupancy of 60–70% [49, 50]. All drug doses in the present study were calculated based on rat studies that investigated D2 receptor occupancy [51, 52] and produced plasma levels well within the therapeutic range of the doses used for the clinical treatment of patients with schizophrenia [53].

2.2. Measurement of mRNA Levels by Quantitative Real-Time Polymerase Chain Reaction (qRT-PCR).
Total RNA was isolated using TRIzol® (Invitrogen, Carlsbad, CA, USA) as previously described by Seo et al. [45]. RNA samples were reverse transcribed into cDNA using amfiRivertII™ cDNA Synthesis Master Mix (GenDepot, Baker, TX, USA), and a qRT-PCR procedure was performed using SYBR® Green Supermix (Bio-Rad, Hercules, CA, USA) and the CFX96™ Real-Time PCR Detection System (Bio-Rad). The specificity of amplification was verified by melting curves. The oligonucleotide sequences of the primers used in the present study were described previously [45], and the qRT-PCR procedure for DNMT1 and DNMT3a was performed with the following primers: DNMT1, forward 5′-GAGTGGGA TGGCTTCTT CAG-3′, reverse 5′-GTGTCTGTCCAGGATGTTG C-3′; DNMT3a, forward 5′-ACGCCAAAGAAGTGTCTGCT-3′, reverse 5′-CTTTGCCCTG CTTTATGCAG-3′; and glyceraldehyde 3-phosphate dehydrogenase (GAPDH), forward 5′-TCCCTCAAGATTGTCAGCAA-3′, reverse 5′-AGAT CCACAACGGA TACATT-3′. ΔCt, which represents the difference between GAPDH and the target gene samples, was calculated using the following formula: ΔCt = Ct$_{\text{target gene}}$ – Ct$_{\text{GAPDH}}$. Then, the fold difference was quantified using the $2^{-\Delta\Delta\text{ct}}$ method; the final value was expressed as a value relative to the vehicle control. All samples were assayed in twice.

2.3. Chromatin Immunoprecipitation (ChIP) Assays.
The ChIP assays in the present study were performed as described previously [45]. Hippocampal samples were cross-linked, homogenized, and sonicated to generate 200–500 bp chromatin fragments. Then, chromatin lysate (10 μg) was immunoprecipitated with an antibody (10 μg) directed against either acetyl-histone H3 (K9 + K14; 06–599; Millipore, Billerica, MA, USA) or MeCP2 (ab2828; Abcam, Cambridge, UK). Protein-associated chromatin was extracted in phenol/chloroform (Amresco, Solon, OH, USA) and precipitated in ethanol (Merck, Hunterdon, NJ, USA) prior to qRT-PCR analysis. The ChIP results were normalized to the input DNA. ΔCt, which represents the difference between the input and immunoprecipitated samples, was calculated using the following formula: ΔCt = Ct$_{\text{ip}}$ – Ct$_{\text{input}}$. Then, the fold difference was quantified using the $2^{-\Delta\Delta\text{ct}}$ method, and the final value was expressed as a value relative to the vehicle control. All samples were assayed in twice.

2.4. Statistical Analysis.
All statistical analyses were performed using GraphPad Prism version 7.01 (GraphPad Software, La Jolla, CA, USA). A two-way analysis of variance (ANOVA) was performed to determine whether the main effects of restraint stress and treatment and the interactive effect of restraint stress × treatment were significant. Tukey's multiple comparison tests were used for post hoc comparisons. p values ≤ 0.05 were considered to indicate statistical significance. All data are presented as a mean ± standard error of the mean (SEM).

3. Results

Individual-level data for each group analyzed by qRT-PCR and ChIP are shown in Table 1.

3.1. Effects on Hippocampal BDNF mRNA Levels.
A two-way ANOVA assessing total BDNF mRNA levels (Figure 1(a)) revealed significant main effects of restraint stress ($F_{[1,30]} = 66.370$, $p < 0.001$) and treatment ($F_{[2,30]} = 38.500$, $p < 0.001$) and a significant interaction effect of restraint stress × treatment ($F_{[2,30]} = 4.043$, $p = 0.028$). A post hoc analysis for the main effect of restraint stress revealed that stress decreased the level of total BDNF mRNA relative to the vehicle control ($p = 0.001$), while the post hoc analysis for the main effect of treatment revealed that chronic

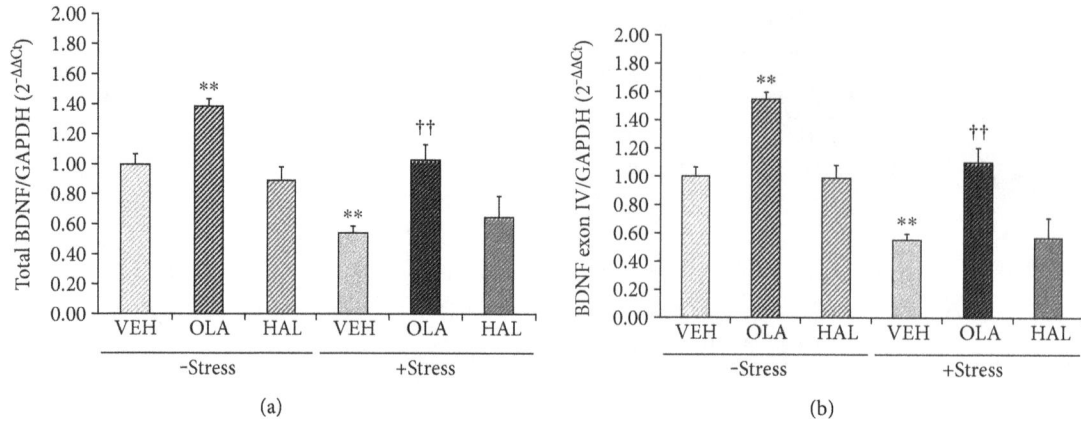

(a)

(b)

FIGURE 1: Effects of antipsychotic drugs on total and exon IV brain-derived neurotrophic factor (BDNF) mRNA levels in the rat hippocampus. Rats were given a daily injection of either vehicle (VEH), olanzapine (OLA), or haloperidol (HAL) for 21 d in conjunction with either exposure to (+ stress) or no exposure to (− stress) restraint stress. The mRNA levels of total BDNF (a) and exon IV BDNF (b) in the rat hippocampus were measured using a quantitative real-time polymerase chain reaction (qRT-PCR) procedure. The quantitative analysis was normalized to glyceraldehyde-3-phosphate dehydrogenase (GAPDH). $^{**}p < 0.01$ versus vehicle control; $^{\dagger\dagger}p < 0.01$ versus vehicle + stress.

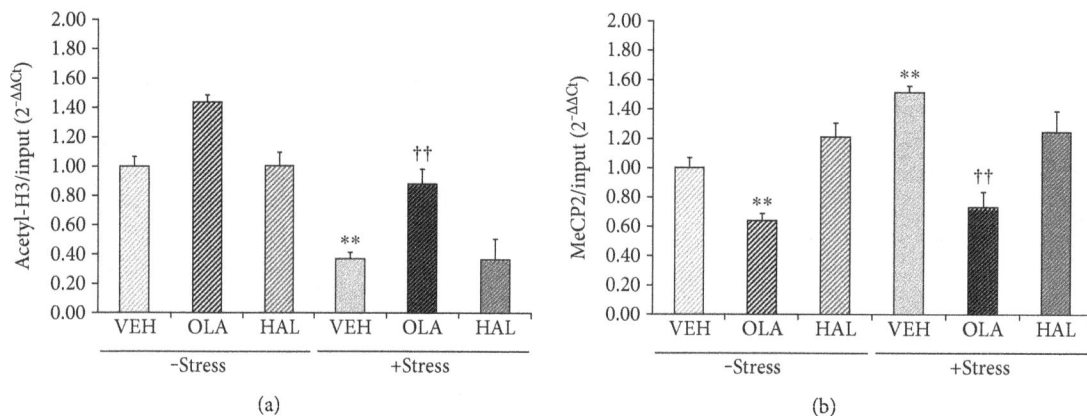

(a)

(b)

FIGURE 2: Effects of antipsychotic drugs on acetylated histone H3 and methyl CpG-binding protein 2 (MeCP2) levels at BDNF promoter IV in the rat hippocampus. Rats were given a daily injection of either VEH, OLA, or HAL for 21 d in conjunction with either + stress or − stress. Chromatin immunoprecipitation (ChIP) assays were performed to measure the levels of acetylated H3 (a) and MeCP2 (b) at BDNF promoter IV in the rat hippocampus using specific antibodies. These levels were quantified by a qRT-PCR procedure. $^{**}p < 0.01$ versus vehicle control; $^{\dagger\dagger}p < 0.01$ versus vehicle + stress.

olanzapine, but not chronic haloperidol, administration increased the expression of total BDNF mRNA compared with the vehicle control group in the stress-free condition ($p = 0.009$) and reversed the stress-induced decrease in BDNF levels ($p < 0.001$). The significant interaction effect of stress × treatment indicated that the positive effect of olanzapine on the level of BDNF expression was greater in the stress condition than in the stress-free condition.

The present study also investigated whether antipsychotic drugs influenced exon IV BDNF mRNA expression in the stress-free and stress conditions (Figure 1(b)). There were significant main effects of restraint stress ($F_{[1,30]} = 120.600$, $p < 0.001$) and treatment ($F_{[2,30]} = 67.790$, $p < 0.001$) and a trend for an interaction effect of restraint stress × treatment ($F_{[2,30]} = 3.091$, $p = 0.060$). The post hoc analyses for the main effects of restraint stress and treatment revealed that

chronic stress significantly reduced the levels of exon IV BDNF mRNA compared with the vehicle control group ($p < 0.001$). This reduction was reversed by chronic olanzapine, but not chronic haloperidol, treatment ($p < 0.001$). Additionally, chronic olanzapine, but not chronic haloperidol, treatment increased exon IV mRNA levels in the stress-free condition ($p < 0.001$).

3.2. Effects on the BDNF Promoter IV Epigenetic State in the Hippocampus. To determine whether the antipsychotic drugs affected histone modification at promoter IV of the BDNF gene, ChIP assays were performed to evaluate the levels of acetylated histones H3 and MeCP2 binding in BDNF promoter IV. When the levels of histone H3 acetylation (Figure 2(a)), a marker of transcriptional activation, were examined following chronic treatment with olanzapine and haloperidol in the stress-free and stress conditions, significant main effects of restraint stress ($F_{[1,30]} = 124.500$, $p < 0.001$) and treatment ($F_{[2,30]} = 30.500$, $p < 0.001$) and a significant interaction effect of restraint stress × treatment ($F_{[2,30]} = 5.363$, $p = 0.010$) were detected. Post hoc analyses revealed that stress significantly reduced the level of acetylated histone H3 ($p < 0.001$) and that chronic treatment with olanzapine reversed this reduction ($p < 0.001$). Olanzapine treatment did not significantly alter the level of acetylated histone H3 in the stress-free condition ($p = 0.086$), although it appeared to increase histone H3 levels. In contrast, chronic haloperidol treatment did not affect histone H3 levels irrespective of exposure to restraint stress.

MeCP2 binds to the cyclic adenosine monophosphate (AMP) response element (CRE) site within BDNF promoter IV [54]. MeCP2 can decrease BDNF expression and suppress the transcription of promoter IV by blocking the binding of CRE-binding protein (CREB), a transcription factor, to CRE [54, 55]. A two-way ANOVA revealed significant main effects of restraint stress ($F_{[1,30]} = 9.214$, $p = 0.005$) and treatment ($F_{[2,30]} = 38.120$, $p < 0.001$) and a significant interaction effect of restraint stress × treatment ($F_{[2,33]} = 3.280$, $p = 0.050$). The level of MeCP2 binding at promoter IV (Figure 2(b)) increased after chronic stress ($p = 0.009$), but this increase was reversed by chronic olanzapine ($p < 0.001$), but not chronic haloperidol, treatment. Additionally, treatment with olanzapine, but not haloperidol, decreased MeCP2 levels in the stress-free condition ($p = 0.004$) and this reduction was greater in the stress condition (2.07-fold decrease) than in the stress-free condition (1.56-fold decrease).

3.3. Effects on HDAC5 mRNA Level in the Hippocampus.
HDACs can participate in gene silencing due to their binding to MeCP2 along with other corepressors, such as mSin3A [20, 21, 55]. In particular, mechanistic evidence for the role of HDAC5, which is a class II HDAC, was identified in rodents that administered with antidepressant drugs and exposed to stressful environments [45, 56–58]. To investigate the mechanisms underlying histone modification induced by restraint stress and olanzapine treatment observed in the present study, HDAC5 expression levels were measured using qRT-PCR (Figure 3).

There were significant main effects of restraint stress ($F_{[1,30]} = 10.550$, $p = 0.003$) and treatment ($F_{[2,30]} = 34.110$, $p < 0.001$) on the HDAC5 expression level as well as a significant interaction effect of restraint stress × treatment ($F_{[2,30]} = 7.788$, $p = 0.002$). A post hoc analysis of all groups revealed that HDAC5 levels increased only in the restraint stress group ($p = 0.003$) and that this increase was blocked by olanzapine treatment ($p < 0.001$). In contrast, chronic treatment with haloperidol had no effect on the HDAC5 level in the hippocampi of rats in either the stress-free or stress condition.

3.4. Effects on DNMT1 and DNMT3a mRNA Levels in the Hippocampus.
DNA methylation is dependent on the enzymatic function of several DNA methyltransferases, including DNMT1, DNMT3a, and DNMT3b [59]. In particular, DNMT1 and DNMT3a are required for maintaining DNA

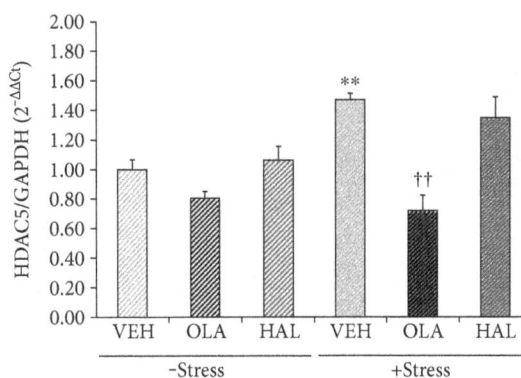

FIGURE 3: Effects of antipsychotic drugs on histone deacetylase 5 (HDAC5) mRNA levels in the rat hippocampus. Rats were given a daily injection of either VEH, OLA, or HAL for 21 d in conjunction with either + stress or − stress. HDAC5 mRNA levels in the rat hippocampus were assessed using a qRT-PCR procedure. The quantitative analysis was normalized to GAPDH. **$p < 0.01$ versus vehicle control; ††$p < 0.01$ versus vehicle + stress.

methylation in central nervous system neurons in adult mice [60]. Therefore, the influence of antipsychotic drugs on DNMT1 (Figure 4(a)) and DNMT3a (Figure 4(b)) mRNA levels in the stress-free and stress conditions was investigated in the present study.

A two-way ANOVA revealed significant main effects of restraint stress (DNMT1: $F_{[1,30]} = 12.380$, $p = 0.001$ and DNMT3a: $F_{(1,30)} = 115.900$, $p < 0.001$) and treatment (DNMT1: $F_{[2,30]} = 23.270$, $p < 0.001$ and DNMT3a: $F_{[2,30]} = 30.460$, $p < 0.001$) for these enzymes but not an interaction effect. A post hoc analysis revealed that restraint stress resulted in an overall upregulation of DNMT1 ($p = 0.010$) and DNMT3a ($p < 0.001$) levels; chronic olanzapine, but not chronic haloperidol, treatment induced a downregulation of these levels in both the stress-free (DNMT1: $p = 0.039$ and DNMT3a: $p < 0.001$) and stress (DNMT1: $p < 0.001$ and DNMT3a: $p = 0.002$) conditions.

4. Discussion

In the present study, the 21 d restraint stress procedure affected BDNF mRNA expression levels and the epigenetic regulation of BDNF promoter exon IV, HDAC5, DNMT1, and DNMT3a in the rat hippocampus. Chronic restraint stress also decreased the levels of total and exon IV BDNF mRNA, decreased acetylated histone H3 and increased MeCP2 at promoter IV of the BDNF gene, and increased the levels of HDAC5, DNMT1, and DNMT3a mRNA expression. Changes induced by 21 d restraint stress were attenuated by olanzapine administration, while haloperidol did not influence the total and exon IV BDNF levels or BDNF epigenetic regulation.

Similar changes have been reported in previous studies. For example, 21 d restraint stress significantly reduced BDNF expression in the rat hippocampus [61] and decreased BDNF exon IV levels in both the mouse and rat hippocampi [62, 63], which lends support to the present findings. It has also been reported that olanzapine increases total BDNF

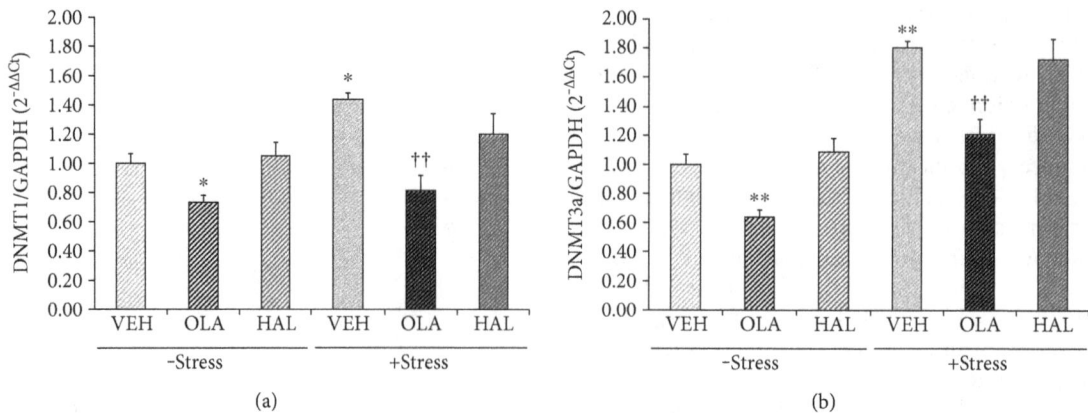

FIGURE 4: Effects of antipsychotic drugs on DNA methyltransferase (DNMT) 1 and DNMT3a mRNA levels in the rat hippocampus. Rats were given a daily injection of either VEH, OLA, or HAL for 21 d in conjunction with either + stress or − stress. The DNMT1 (a) and DNMT3a (b) mRNA levels in the rat hippocampus were assessed using a qRT-PCR procedure. The quantitative analysis was normalized to GAPDH. $^*p < 0.05$ versus vehicle control, $^{**}p < 0.01$ versus vehicle control, and $^{\dagger\dagger}p < 0.01$ versus vehicle + stress.

mRNA levels and normalizes MK-801-induced reductions of BDNF mRNA expression in the rat hippocampus [64, 65]. In the present study, the decreases in total and BDNF exon IV mRNA induced by restraint stress were rescued by treatment with olanzapine; however, the administration of haloperidol failed to show any effects.

The present study also demonstrated that 21 d restraint stress decreased the levels of acetylated histone H3 at promoter IV of the BDNF gene and that this decrease was reversed by olanzapine administration. Several studies have reported interactions between stress and the histone modification of the BDNF gene in the rat and mouse hippocampus. For example, Fuchikami et al. [62] reported that single immobilization stress resulted in a significant decrease in the levels of acetylated histone H3 at promoter IV of the BDNF gene at 2 and 24 h [62], while another study reported that 21 d restraint stress caused mild increases in the levels of H3K4me3 and reductions in H3K9me3 levels in the dentate gyrus [66]. The acetylation of lysine residues at the N-terminus of histone proteins reduces positive net charges which, in turn, results in a reduction in the affinity between histones and DNA. This exposure allows for the binding of transcription factors to the promoters of specific genes. The K9, K14, K18, K23, K27, and K36 regions of histone H3 are acetylated, and acetylation at K9 and K14 of histone H3 enhances transcription [67, 68]. Thus, the present study utilized antibodies that detected histone H3 acetylated at K9 and K14.

MeCP2 is a transcriptional regulator that plays a role in the structural stability of chromatin [69]. Thus, mutations that disrupt MeCP2 function can be expected to increase gene expression, disturb neuronal function, and give rise to behavioral disorders, such as Rett syndrome [69, 70]. In the present study, the administration of olanzapine decreased MeCP2 levels at BDNF promoter IV in rats exposed to 21 d restraint stress, which is similar to previous studies showing increased MeCP2 following exposure to stress. For example, Seo et al. [45] reported that 21 d restraint stress and maternal separation independently increased MeCP2 levels at BDNF

promoter IV in the rat hippocampus. However, it has also been shown that prolonged prenatal stress (PNS) did not significantly change MeCP2 levels in either the prefrontal cortex or hippocampus of PNS mouse offspring [71]. The present finding that olanzapine administration decreased MeCP2 occupancy in the BDNF promoter IV region of rats exposed to 21 d restraint stress suggests that olanzapine may regulate MeCP2-dependent transcription of the BDNF gene.

DNA methylation is associated with common and critical processes in mammals, including transposon silencing and genomic imprinting [72]. The DNMT3a, DNMT3b, and DNMT1 proteins are primarily responsible for the establishment of genomic DNA methylation patterns and play important roles in human development, reproduction, and mental health [73]. Boersma et al. [74] found that PNS decreased total BDNF expression and increased DNMT1 and DNMT-3a expression in the amygdala and hippocampus of PNS-exposed offspring. Another study showed that clozapine reduced stress-induced elevations in DNMT1 binding to BDNF promoters in the frontal cortex of PNS-exposed offspring [71]. Although the method of stress induction used in the present study differed from those used in these previous studies, 21 d restraint stress also elevated the levels of DNMT1 and DNMT3a mRNA expression in the rat hippocampus; however, these increases were subsequently reversed by olanzapine. In contrast, haloperidol, a typical antipsychotic drug, did not alter these levels.

Histone acetylation and deacetylation remodel chromatin structures and regulate gene expression [75]. The functions of HDACs include the removal of acetyl groups from the N-terminus of the lysine tail; this modification of chromatin results in a compact chromatin structure that prevents an interaction between DNA and regulatory proteins which, in turn, blocks gene expression [76]. Tsankova et al. reported that chronic imipramine treatment reversed this downregulation and increased histone acetylation at BDNF promoters III and VI in the mouse hippocampus [56]. These authors also showed that the hyperacetylation induced by chronic imipramine treatment was associated with the selective downregulation of HDAC5 mRNA levels. Chronic unpredictable stress (CUS) significantly decreased the acetylation rates of H3 at K9 and H4 at K12 and resulted in obvious increases in HDAC expression in the rat hippocampus [57]. However, the administration of sodium valproate, a HDAC5 inhibitor, clearly blunted these decreases in acetylation and blocked the increase in HDAC5 expression [57]. These findings suggest that HDAC5 expression may be involved in the regulation of stress-induced histone acetylation. In the present study, olanzapine blocked the increase in HDAC5 mRNA expression induced by 21 d restraint stress, which indicates that it may affect the epigenetic regulation of HDAC5.

In this study, olanzapine, but not haloperidol, induced epigenetic modifications. Olanzapine is an antipsychotic drug, and the epigenetic modifications that it induces differ from those that may result from haloperidol treatment. It is important to elucidate the molecular mechanisms underlying the epigenetic effects of olanzapine and haloperidol. Although it remains to be confirmed, we suggest that differences in the degree to which dopamine type 2 and serotonin receptors are blocked by olanzapine and haloperidol (the latter principally blocks dopamine type 2 receptors) underlie the differences in histone modification associated with these two agents. In previous studies, clozapine, olanzapine, and sulpiride, but not haloperidol or risperidone, increased GABAergic promoter demethylation. This suggests that dibenzazepine derivatives (e.g., clozapine and olanzapine) may attenuate the dysregulation of GABAergic and glutamatergic transmission by reducing promoter hypermethylation [71].

Although the present study is the first to investigate the effects of olanzapine on the epigenetic mechanisms involved in BDNF gene transcription in the rat hippocampus following 21 d restraint stress, it is not without limitations. First, the protein levels of BDNF, DNMT1, DNMT3a, and HDAC5 were not directly measured; therefore, further studies measuring these proteins using Western blot analyses are required to strengthen the present findings. Second, the behavioral effects of 21 d restraint stress were not evaluated in the rats. If the epigenetic changes induced by olanzapine can be synchronized with behavioral changes, then the results of the present study may be strengthened. Third, although we examined MeCP2 binding to methylated CpG sites, the levels of DNA methylation in BDNF promoter IV were not measured. Increased MeCP2 occupancy reduces BDNF transcription [54], but it is not known if chronic restraint stress-associated increases in MeCP2 occupancy are associated with the hypomethylation of BDNF promoter IV. We also observed an increase in DNMT1 and DNMT3a expression levels following chronic restraint stress. Additional studies on DNA methylation are needed to determine whether there is a causal relationship between DNA methylation and DNMT expression. Fourth, the dosages of olanzapine and haloperidol used in the present study are not applicable to human subjects. Therefore, future studies with clinical doses of antipsychotics are necessary to determine if they will produce the same beneficial effects on epigenetic regulation of the BDNF gene.

In summary, the present study found that 21 d restraint stress and olanzapine treatment both altered the epigenetic regulation of the BDNF gene in the rat hippocampus. More specifically, 21 d restraint stress affected BDNF mRNA expression levels and the epigenetic regulations of BDNF promoter exon IV, HDAC5, DNMT1, and DNMT3a in the rat hippocampus. However, these changes were reversed following administration of the antipsychotic drug olanzapine. Thus, the present findings suggest that antipsychotic drugs can alter epigenetic mechanisms and that epigenetic regulation may represent an additional mechanism underlying the effects of antipsychotic drugs.

Disclosure

Some of the results of this study were presented as poster at the 2017 European Congress of Neuropsychopharmacology (ECNP) in Paris.

Acknowledgments

This research was supported by the Basic Science Research Program through the National Research Foundation of Korea (NRF) grant funded by the Ministry of Education, Science and Technology (NRF-2015R1A6A3A01018922 to Mi Kyoung Seo and NRF-2015R1D1A3A01016360 to Jung Goo Lee) and the Ministry of Science, ICT and Future Planning (NRF-2016R1A2B4010157 to Sung Woo Park).

Supplementary Materials

Figure S1: BDNF expression patterns according to time (2 and 6 h) and duration (1, 7, and 21 d) of restraint stress. Rats ($n = 6$ animals/group) were immobilized for 2 (RS 2 h) or 6 h (RS 6 h) per day over the course of 1, 7, or 21 d. BDNF expression levels in brain homogenates from the hippocampus were detected by SDS-PAGE and Western blot analyses using anti-BDNF antibodies. A representative image and quantitative analysis normalized to the levels of α-tubulin are shown. Results are expressed as a percentage of the corresponding data for the control group (CON; no restraint stress) and represent the mean ± standard error of the mean (SEM) of six animals per group. $^*p < 0.05$ versus control; $^{**}p < 0.01$ versus control. (Supplementary Materials)

References

[1] R. Freedman, "Schizophrenia," *New England Journal of Medicine*, vol. 349, no. 18, pp. 1738–1749, 2003.

[2] D. A. Lewis and J. A. Lieberman, "Catching up on schizophrenia: natural history and neurobiology," *Neuron*, vol. 28, no. 2, pp. 325–334, 2000.

[3] P. V. Gejman, A. R. Sanders, and J. Duan, "The role of genetics in the etiology of schizophrenia," *Psychiatric Clinics of North America*, vol. 33, no. 1, pp. 35–66, 2010.

[4] S. Burton, "Symptom domains of schizophrenia: the role of atypical antipsychotic agents," *Journal of Psychopharmacology*, vol. 20, 6_Supplement, pp. 6–19, 2006.

[5] G. Foussias and G. Remington, "Negative symptoms in schizophrenia: avolition and Occam's razor," *Schizophrenia Bulletin*, vol. 36, no. 2, pp. 359–369, 2010.

[6] R. TANDON, M. KESHAVAN, and H. NASRALLAH, "Schizophrenia, "just the facts" what we know in 2008. 2. Epidemiology and etiology," *Schizophrenia Research*, vol. 102, no. 1-3, pp. 1–18, 2008.

[7] K. R. Shorter and B. H. Miller, "Epigenetic mechanisms in schizophrenia," *Progress in Biophysics and Molecular Biology*, vol. 118, no. 1-2, pp. 1–7, 2015.

[8] T. Archer, "Neurodegeneration in schizophrenia," *Expert Review of Neurotherapeutics*, vol. 10, no. 7, pp. 1131–1141, 2010.

[9] P. Kochunov and L. E. Hong, "Neurodevelopmental and neurodegenerative models of schizophrenia: white matter at the center stage," *Schizophrenia Bulletin*, vol. 40, no. 4, pp. 721–728, 2014.

[10] H. Malkki, "Neurodevelopmental disorders: altered epigenetic regulation in early development associated with schizophrenia," *Nature Reviews Neurology*, vol. 12, no. 1, p. 1, 2016.

[11] A. Cariaga-Martinez, J. Saiz-Ruiz, and R. Alelú-Paz, "From linkage studies to epigenetics: what we know and what we need to know in the neurobiology of schizophrenia," *Frontiers in Neuroscience*, vol. 10, p. 202, 2016.

[12] F. Antequera, "Structure, function and evolution of CpG island promoters," *Cellular and Molecular Life Sciences (CMLS)*, vol. 60, no. 8, pp. 1647–1658, 2003.

[13] P. Zhou, E. Wu, H. B. Alam, and Y. Li, "Histone cleavage as a mechanism for epigenetic regulation: current insights and perspectives," *Current Molecular Medicine*, vol. 14, no. 9, pp. 1164–1172, 2014.

[14] H. Tao, J. J. Yang, and K. H. Shi, "Non-coding RNAs as direct and indirect modulators of epigenetic mechanism regulation of cardiac fibrosis," *Expert Opinion on Therapeutic Targets*, vol. 19, no. 5, pp. 707–716, 2015.

[15] S. Akbarian and H. S. Huang, "Epigenetic regulation in human brain—focus on histone lysine methylation," *Biological Psychiatry*, vol. 65, no. 3, pp. 198–203, 2009.

[16] S. L. Berger, "The complex language of chromatin regulation during transcription," *Nature*, vol. 447, no. 7143, pp. 407–412, 2007.

[17] E. Borrelli, E. J. Nestler, C. D. Allis, and P. Sassone-Corsi, "Decoding the epigenetic language of neuronal plasticity," *Neuron*, vol. 60, no. 6, pp. 961–974, 2008.

[18] C. Dulac, "Brain function and chromatin plasticity," *Nature*, vol. 465, no. 7299, pp. 728–735, 2010.

[19] L. D. Moore, T. Le, and G. Fan, "DNA methylation and its basic function," *Neuropsychopharmacology*, vol. 38, no. 1, pp. 23–38, 2013.

[20] P. L. Jones, G. C. Jan Veenstra, P. A. Wade et al., "Methylated DNA and MeCP2 recruit histone deacetylase to repress transcription," *Nature Genetics*, vol. 19, no. 2, pp. 187–191, 1998.

[21] X. Nan, H. H. Ng, C. A. Johnson et al., "Transcriptional repression by the methyl-CpG-binding protein MeCP2 involves a histone deacetylase complex," *Nature*, vol. 393, no. 6683, pp. 386–389, 1998.

[22] F. Fuks, P. J. Hurd, R. Deplus, and T. Kouzarides, "The DNA methyltransferases associate with HP1 and the SUV39H1 histone methyltransferase," *Nucleic Acids Research*, vol. 31, no. 9, pp. 2305–2312, 2003.

[23] D. A. Collier, B. J. Eastwood, K. Malki, and Y. Mokrab, "Advances in the genetics of schizophrenia: toward a network and pathway view for drug discovery," *Annals of the New York Academy of Sciences*, vol. 1366, no. 1, pp. 61–75, 2016.

[24] A. Guidotti, D. R. Grayson, and H. J. Caruncho, "Epigenetic RELN dysfunction in schizophrenia and related neuropsychiatric disorders," *Frontiers in Cellular Neuroscience*, vol. 10, p. 89, 2016.

[25] I. Negron-Oyarzo, A. Lara-Vasquez, I. Palacios-Garcia, P. Fuentealba, and F. Aboitiz, "Schizophrenia and reelin: a model based on prenatal stress to study epigenetics, brain development and behavior," *Biological Research*, vol. 49, no. 1, p. 16, 2016.

[26] F. Matrisciano, P. Tueting, I. Dalal et al., "Epigenetic modifications of GABAergic interneurons are associated with the schizophrenia-like phenotype induced by prenatal stress in mice," *Neuropharmacology*, vol. 68, pp. 184–194, 2013.

[27] D. A. Lewis, L. A. Glantz, J. N. Pierri, and R. A. Sweet, "Altered cortical glutamate neurotransmission in schizophrenia: evidence from morphological studies of pyramidal neurons," *Annals of the New York Academy of Sciences*, vol. 1003, no. 1, pp. 102–112, 2003.

[28] L. A. Glantz and D. A. Lewis, "Decreased dendritic spine density on prefrontal cortical pyramidal neurons in schizophrenia," *Archives of General Psychiatry*, vol. 57, no. 1, pp. 65–73, 2000.

[29] D. A. Lewis, A. A. Curley, J. R. Glausier, and D. W. Volk, "Cortical parvalbumin interneurons and cognitive dysfunction in schizophrenia," *Trends in Neurosciences*, vol. 35, no. 1, pp. 57–67, 2012.

[30] H. S. Huang and S. Akbarian, "GAD1 mRNA expression and DNA methylation in prefrontal cortex of subjects with schizophrenia," *PLoS One*, vol. 2, no. 8, article e809, 2007.

[31] S. Akbarian, "The molecular pathology of schizophrenia—focus on histone and DNA modifications," *Brain Research Bulletin*, vol. 83, no. 3-4, pp. 103–107, 2010.

[32] M. R. Bennett, "Monoaminergic synapses and schizophrenia: 45 years of neuroleptics," *Journal of Psychopharmacology*, vol. 12, no. 3, pp. 289–304, 1998.

[33] E. Dong, M. Nelson, D. R. Grayson, E. Costa, and A. Guidotti, "Clozapine and sulpiride but not haloperidol or olanzapine activate brain DNA demethylation," *Proceedings of the National Academy of Sciences of the United States of America*, vol. 105, no. 36, pp. 13614–13619, 2008.

[34] Y. Aoyama, A. Mouri, K. Toriumi et al., "Clozapine ameliorates epigenetic and behavioral abnormalities induced by phencyclidine through activation of dopamine D1 receptor," *The International Journal of Neuropsychopharmacology*, vol. 17, no. 5, pp. 723–737, 2014.

[35] M. G. Melka, B. I. Laufer, P. McDonald et al., "The effects of olanzapine on genome-wide DNA methylation in the hippocampus and cerebellum," *Clinical Epigenetics*, vol. 6, no. 1, p. 1, 2014.

[36] J. Mill, T. Tang, Z. Kaminsky et al., "Epigenomic profiling reveals DNA-methylation changes associated with major psychosis," *The American Journal of Human Genetics*, vol. 82, no. 3, pp. 696–711, 2008.

[37] H. M. Abdolmaleky, S. Pajouhanfar, M. Faghankhani, M. T. Joghataei, A. Mostafavi, and S. Thiagalingam, "Antipsychotic

drugs attenuate aberrant DNA methylation of *DTNBP1* (dysbindin) promoter in saliva and post-mortem brain of patients with schizophrenia and Psychotic bipolar disorder," *American Journal of Medical Genetics. Part B: Neuropsychiatric Genetics*, vol. 168, no. 8, pp. 687–696, 2015.

[38] O. Guillin, C. Demily, and F. Thibaut, "Brain-derived neurotrophic factor in schizophrenia and its relation with dopamine," *International Review of Neurobiology*, vol. 78, pp. 377–395, 2007.

[39] G. Favalli, J. Li, P. Belmonte-de-Abreu, A. H. C. Wong, and Z. J. Daskalakis, "The role of BDNF in the pathophysiology and treatment of schizophrenia," *Journal of Psychiatric Research*, vol. 46, no. 1, pp. 1–11, 2012.

[40] T. Ikegame, M. Bundo, Y. Murata, K. Kasai, T. Kato, and K. Iwamoto, "DNA methylation of the *BDNF* gene and its relevance to psychiatric disorders," *Journal of Human Genetics*, vol. 58, no. 7, pp. 434–438, 2013.

[41] D. P. Gavin and S. Akbarian, "Epigenetic and posttranscriptional dysregulation of gene expression in schizophrenia and related disease," *Neurobiology of Disease*, vol. 46, no. 2, pp. 255–262, 2012.

[42] B. S. McEwen, "Stress and hippocampal plasticity," *Annual Review of Neuroscience*, vol. 22, no. 1, pp. 105–122, 1999.

[43] J. Yun, H. Koike, D. Ibi et al., "Chronic restraint stress impairs neurogenesis and hippocampus-dependent fear memory in mice: possible involvement of a brain-specific transcription factor Npas4," *Journal of Neurochemistry*, vol. 114, no. 6, pp. 1840–1851, 2010.

[44] P. Vestergaard-Poulsen, G. Wegener, B. Hansen et al., "Diffusion-weighted MRI and quantitative biophysical modeling of hippocampal neurite loss in chronic stress," *PLoS One*, vol. 6, no. 7, article e20653, 2011.

[45] M. K. Seo, N. N. Ly, C. H. Lee et al., "Early life stress increases stress vulnerability through BDNF gene epigenetic changes in the rat hippocampus," *Neuropharmacology*, vol. 105, pp. 388–397, 2016.

[46] H. Xu, H. Qing, W. Lu et al., "Quetiapine attenuates the immobilization stress-induced decrease of brain-derived neurotrophic factor expression in rat hippocampus," *Neuroscience Letters*, vol. 321, no. 1-2, pp. 65–68, 2002.

[47] S. W. Park, C. H. Lee, J. G. Lee et al., "Differential effects of ziprasidone and haloperidol on immobilization stress-induced mRNA BDNF expression in the hippocampus and neocortex of rats," *Journal of Psychiatric Research*, vol. 43, no. 3, pp. 274–281, 2009.

[48] S. W. Park, V. T. Phuong, C. H. Lee et al., "Effects of antipsychotic drugs on BDNF, GSK-3β, and β-catenin expression in rats subjected to immobilization stress," *Neuroscience Research*, vol. 71, no. 4, pp. 335–340, 2011.

[49] S. Kapur, R. Zipursky, C. Jones, G. Remington, and S. Houle, "Relationship between dopamine D(2) occupancy, clinical response, and side effects: a double-blind PET study of first-episode schizophrenia," *American Journal of Psychiatry*, vol. 157, no. 4, pp. 514–520, 2000.

[50] L. Farde, F. A. Wiesel, C. Halldin, and G. Sedvall, "Central D2-dopamine receptor occupancy in schizophrenic patients treated with antipsychotic drugs," *Archives of General Psychiatry*, vol. 45, no. 1, pp. 71–76, 1988.

[51] V. N. Barth, E. Chernet, L. J. Martin et al., "Comparison of rat dopamine D2 receptor occupancy for a series of antipsychotic drugs measured using radiolabeled or nonlabeled raclopride tracer," *Life Sciences*, vol. 78, no. 26, pp. 3007–3012, 2006.

[52] S. Natesan, G. E. Reckless, J. N. Nobrega, P. J. Fletcher, and S. Kapur, "Dissociation between in vivo occupancy and functional antagonism of dopamine D$_2$ receptors: comparing aripiprazole to other antipsychotics in animal models," *Neuropsychopharmacology*, vol. 31, no. 9, pp. 1854–1863, 2006.

[53] C. Andersson, R. M. Hamer, C. P. Lawler, R. B. Mailman, and J. A. Lieberman, "Striatal volume changes in the rat following long-term administration of typical and atypical antipsychotic drugs," *Neuropsychopharmacology*, vol. 27, no. 2, pp. 143–151, 2002.

[54] W. G. Chen, Q. Chang, Y. Lin et al., "Derepression of BDNF transcription involves calcium-dependent phosphorylation of MeCP2," *Science*, vol. 302, no. 5646, pp. 885–889, 2003.

[55] K. Martinowich, D. Hattori, H. Wu et al., "DNA methylation-related chromatin remodeling in activity-dependent BDNF gene regulation," *Science*, vol. 302, no. 5646, pp. 890–893, 2003.

[56] N. M. Tsankova, O. Berton, W. Renthal, A. Kumar, R. L. Neve, and E. J. Nestler, "Sustained hippocampal chromatin regulation in a mouse model of depression and antidepressant action," *Nature Neuroscience*, vol. 9, no. 4, pp. 519–525, 2006.

[57] D. Liu, H. M. Qiu, H. Z. Fei et al., "Histone acetylation and expression of mono-aminergic transmitters synthetases involved in CUS-induced depressive rats," *Experimental Biology and Medicine*, vol. 239, no. 3, pp. 330–336, 2014.

[58] M. Erburu, I. Muñoz-Cobo, J. Domínguez-Andrés et al., "Chronic stress and antidepressant induced changes in Hdac5 and Sirt2 affect synaptic plasticity," *European Neuropsychopharmacology*, vol. 25, no. 11, pp. 2036–2048, 2015.

[59] J. Turek-Plewa and P. P. Jagodzinski, "The role of mammalian DNA methyltransferases in the regulation of gene expression," *Cellular and Molecular Biology Letters*, vol. 10, no. 4, pp. 631–647, 2005.

[60] J. Feng, Y. Zhou, S. L. Campbell et al., "Dnmt1 and Dnmt3a maintain DNA methylation and regulate synaptic function in adult forebrain neurons," *Nature Neuroscience*, vol. 13, no. 4, pp. 423–430, 2010.

[61] J. B. Ortiz, C. M. Mathewson, A. N. Hoffman, P. D. Hanavan, E. F. Terwilliger, and C. D. Conrad, "Hippocampal brain-derived neurotrophic factor mediates recovery from chronic stress-induced spatial reference memory deficits," *European Journal of Neuroscience*, vol. 40, no. 9, pp. 3351–3362, 2014.

[62] M. Fuchikami, S. Morinobu, A. Kurata, S. Yamamoto, and S. Yamawaki, "Single immobilization stress differentially alters the expression profile of transcripts of the brain-derived neurotrophic factor (*BDNF*) gene and histone acetylation at its promoters in the rat hippocampus," *The International Journal of Neuropsychopharmacology*, vol. 12, no. 1, pp. 73–82, 2009.

[63] K. Yamaura, Y. Bi, M. Ishiwatari, N. Oishi, H. Fukata, and K. Ueno, "Sex differences in stress reactivity of hippocampal BDNF in mice are associated with the female preponderance of decreased locomotor activity in response to restraint stress," *Zoological Science*, vol. 30, no. 12, pp. 1019–1024, 2013.

[64] O. Bai, J. Chlan-Fourney, R. Bowen, D. Keegan, and X. M. Li, "Expression of brain-derived neurotrophic factor mRNA in rat hippocampus after treatment with antipsychotic drugs," *Journal of Neuroscience Research*, vol. 71, no. 1, pp. 127–131, 2003.

[65] F. Fumagalli, R. Molteni, M. Roceri et al., "Effect of antipsychotic drugs on brain-derived neurotrophic factor expression under reduced N-methyl-D-aspartate receptor activity," *Journal of Neuroscience Research*, vol. 72, no. 5, pp. 622–628, 2003.

[66] R. G. Hunter, K. J. McCarthy, T. A. Milne, D. W. Pfaff, and B. S. McEwen, "Regulation of hippocampal H3 histone methylation by acute and chronic stress," *Proceedings of the National Academy of Sciences of the United States of America*, vol. 106, no. 49, pp. 20912–20917, 2009.

[67] H. He and N. Lehming, "Global effects of histone modifications," *Briefings in Functional Genomics and Proteomics*, vol. 2, no. 3, pp. 234–243, 2003.

[68] K. J. McManus and M. J. Hendzel, "The relationship between histone H3 phosphorylation and acetylation throughout the mammalian cell cycle," *Biochemistry and Cell Biology*, vol. 84, no. 4, pp. 640–657, 2006.

[69] S. Cohen and M. E. Greenberg, "Communication between the synapse and the nucleus in neuronal development, plasticity, and disease," *Annual Review of Cell and Developmental Biology*, vol. 24, no. 1, pp. 183–209, 2008.

[70] S. Cohen, Z. Zhou, and M. E. Greenberg, "Medicine. Activating a repressor," *Science*, vol. 320, no. 5880, pp. 1172-1173, 2008.

[71] E. Dong, P. Tueting, F. Matrisciano, D. R. Grayson, and A. Guidotti, "Behavioral and molecular neuroepigenetic alterations in prenatally stressed mice: relevance for the study of chromatin remodeling properties of antipsychotic drugs," *Translational Psychiatry*, vol. 6, no. 1, article e711, 2016.

[72] M. Gehring, W. Reik, and S. Henikoff, "DNA demethylation by DNA repair," *Trends in Genetics*, vol. 25, no. 2, pp. 82–90, 2009.

[73] F. Chédin, "The DNMT3 family of mammalian de novo DNA methyltransferases," *Progress in Molecular Biology and Translational Science*, vol. 101, pp. 255–285, 2011.

[74] G. J. Boersma, R. S. Lee, Z. A. Cordner et al., "Prenatal stress decreases Bdnf expression and increases methylation of Bdnf exon IV in rats," *Epigenetics*, vol. 9, no. 3, pp. 437–447, 2014.

[75] R. Machado-Vieira, L. Ibrahim, and C. A. Zarate Jr., "Histone deacetylases and mood disorders: epigenetic programming in gene-environment interactions," *CNS Neuroscience & Therapeutics*, vol. 17, no. 6, pp. 699–704, 2011.

[76] J. S. Guan, S. J. Haggarty, E. Giacometti et al., "HDAC2 negatively regulates memory formation and synaptic plasticity," *Nature*, vol. 459, no. 7243, pp. 55–60, 2009.

16

Activation of Phosphotyrosine-Mediated Signaling Pathways in the Cortex and Spinal Cord of SOD1^{G93A}, a Mouse Model of Familial Amyotrophic Lateral Sclerosis

Cinzia Mallozzi (ID),[1] Alida Spalloni (ID),[2] Patrizia Longone (ID),[2] and Maria Rosaria Domenici (ID)[3]

[1]*Department of Neuroscience, Istituto Superiore di Sanità, Viale Regina Elena 299, 00161 Rome, Italy*
[2]*Molecular Neurobiology Unit, Experimental Neurology, Santa Lucia Foundation, Via Ardeatina 306/354, 00142 Rome, Italy*
[3]*National Center for Drug Research and Evaluation, Istituto Superiore di Sanità, Viale Regina Elena 299, 00161 Rome, Italy*

Correspondence should be addressed to Cinzia Mallozzi; cinzia.mallozzi@iss.it

Academic Editor: Preston E. Garraghty

Degeneration of cortical and spinal motor neurons is the typical feature of amyotrophic lateral sclerosis (ALS), a progressive neurodegenerative disease for which a pathogenetic role for the Cu/Zn superoxide dismutase (SOD1) has been demonstrated. Mice overexpressing a mutated form of the SOD1 gene (SOD1^{G93A}) develop a syndrome that closely resembles the human disease. The SOD1 mutations confer to this enzyme a "gain-of-function," leading to increased production of reactive oxygen species. Several oxidants induce tyrosine phosphorylation through direct stimulation of kinases and/or phosphatases. In this study, we analyzed the activities of src and fyn tyrosine kinases and of protein tyrosine phosphatases in synaptosomal fractions prepared from the motor cortex and spinal cord of transgenic mice expressing SOD1^{G93A}. We found that (i) protein phosphotyrosine level is increased, (ii) src and fyn activities are upregulated, and (iii) the activity of tyrosine phosphatases, including the striatal-enriched tyrosine phosphatase (STEP), is significantly decreased. Moreover, the NMDA receptor (NMDAR) subunit GluN2B tyrosine phosphorylation was upregulated in SOD1^{G93A}. Tyrosine phosphorylation of GluN2B subunits regulates the NMDAR function and the recruitment of downstream signaling molecules. Indeed, we found that proline-rich tyrosine kinase 2 (Pyk2) and ERK1/2 kinase are upregulated in SOD1^{G93A} mice. These results point out an involvement of tyrosine kinases and phosphatases in the pathogenesis of ALS.

1. Introduction

Amyotrophic lateral sclerosis (ALS) is a fatal neurodegenerative disease characterized by a progressive loss of motor neurons in the cortex, brain stem, and spinal cord [1]. The degeneration of motor neurons leads to skeletal muscle weakness, paralysis, and eventually death, with a mean survival between three and five years after disease onset [2–5]. Despite that the disease has been described since more than a century ago, the exact aetiology is still unknown. About 5–10% of ALS cases are inherited and among those about 20% are associated with missense mutations in the ALS1 locus on chromosome 21, which codes for Cu/Zn superoxide dismutase (SOD1) [6]. As familial and sporadic ALS (fALS and sALS, resp.) are symptomatically indistinguishable, it is likely that they share common pathogenetic mechanisms. Such mechanisms include protein misfolding, inflammation, oxidative stress, and mitochondrial dysfunction (reviewed in [7, 8]). Additionally, there is evidence for the involvement of excitotoxicity, as illustrated by the therapeutic effect of riluzole, a drug that blocks glutamatergic neurotransmission, which is currently the only disease-modifying drug available [9, 10]. Excitotoxicity is defined as an excessive activation of glutamate receptors by excitatory amino acids, such as glutamate, that initiates a series of cytoplasmic and nuclear processes promoting neuronal cell death [11, 12]. Overstimulation of the ionotropic glutamate receptors in neurons causes massive influx of calcium into the cytosol, and numerous enzymes are activated in response to the increase in intracellular calcium [13–15].

Several lines of evidence reported that src family protein tyrosine kinases are involved in excitotoxicity [16–19], pointing to their possible role in the pathogenesis of ALS.

In the present study, we analyzed the activities of src and fyn tyrosine kinases and of protein tyrosine phosphatases (PTP), with particular interest to the striatal-enriched protein tyrosine phosphatase (STEP), in synaptosomal fractions prepared from the motor cortex and spinal cord of a transgenic mouse model of ALS (G93A mice), expressing wild-type human SOD1 (SOD1^{WT}) or overexpressing human mutant SOD1 (SOD1^{G93A}). We found that mutation in SOD1 deeply modulates the activity of tyrosine kinases and phosphatases, influencing the phosphorylation state of several substrates, including NMDA receptor (NMDAR) subunit GluN2B, proline-rich tyrosine kinase 2 (Pyk2), and ERK1/2 kinase.

2. Materials and Methods

2.1. Mice. Adult B6.Cg-Tg(SOD1-G93A)1Gur/J mice expressing high copy number of mutant human SOD1 with a Gly93Ala substitution (SOD1^{G93A}) and adult B6SJL-TgN(SOD1)2Gur mice expressing wild-type human SOD1 were originally obtained from Jackson Laboratories (Bar Harbor, ME, USA). For the mSOD1^{G93A} transgene, the G1 line was used, while for the SOD1^{WT}, the N1029 line was used [20]. The two lines express a different number of copies, with the G1 having more than double the number of gene copies and the N1029 line expressing a comparable number of human SOD1 copies or even greater in the brain [20, 21]. Both lines are maintained and selectively bred in the hemizygous state on an F1 hybrid C57BL6 × SJL genetic background in the animal facility of the Fondazione Santa Lucia (Rome, Italy) by crossbreeding transgenic hemizygous males with C57BL/6 females. The transgenic progeny was genotyped by analyzing tissue extracts from tail tips as previously described [22]. The animals were kept under standardized temperature, humidity, and lighting conditions, with free access to water and food (standard pellets). Animal care and use followed the European Directive 2010/63/EU adopted by the Council of the European Union for animal experiments, and adequate measures were taken to minimize pain or discomfort. The experimental protocol was approved by the Italian Ministry of Health. The mice used in the present study develop degeneration in lower motor neurons and paralysis at about 120 days. The groups were transgenic human wild-type SOD1 mice (SOD1^{WT}), transgenic G93A mice (SOD1^{G93A}), and the age-matched nontransgenic controls. The mice used in the study were all male and all at 120 days of age. Before proceeding to the dissection of tissues for biochemical analyses, mice were deeply anesthetized and then sacrificed by decapitation. The brain, carefully removed, was washed in ice-cold phosphate-buffered saline, and a 1 mm coronal slice containing the motor cortex was dissected using a 1 mm coronal mouse Jacobowitz brain slicer (Zivic Miller). The slice was then carefully laid down on a glass slide under a dissection microscope, and the motor cortex M1 region was dissected as previously described [14]. Whole spinal cords were ejected from the vertebral column by means of

sterile 0.1 M phosphate-buffered saline injection in the vertebral column. Tissues were immediately frozen on dry ice and stored at −80°C until use.

2.2. Materials. We used the following antibodies: polyclonal anti-STEP, anti-Pyk2 (pY402), anti-ERK1/2 (pT202/pY204), and anti-ERK1/2 from Cell Signaling Technology (Danvers, MA, USA); polyclonal anti-Pyk2, monoclonal anti-β-actin, and polyclonal anti-fyn from Santa Cruz Biotechnology (Santa Cruz, CA, USA); monoclonal anti-v-src (Ab1, clone 327) from Calbiochem (EMD Chemical, Merck, Darmstadt, Germany); polyclonal anti-GluN2B (pY1472), anti-GluN2B, and monoclonal anti-phosphotyrosine (pY, clone 4G10) from Millipore Bioscience Research Reagent (Billerica, MA, USA); and peroxidase-conjugated goat anti-mouse and goat anti-rabbit from Bio-Rad (Hercules, CA, USA). Protein A/G PLUS agarose was from Santa Cruz Biotechnology and Trysacryl-immobilized protein A from Thermo Scientific (Waltham, MA, USA). Nitrocellulose was from Schleicher and Schuell Bioscience Inc. (Dassel, Germany); *p*-nitrophenyl phosphate (*p*-NPP) and enolase were from Sigma Chemical (St. Louis, MO, USA). Complete protease inhibitor cocktail was from Roche Diagnostics (Basel, Switzerland). [γ^{32}P] ATP (>3000 Ci/mmol) was obtained from DuPont NEN (Boston, MA, USA).

2.3. Synaptosome Preparation. Crude synaptosomal fraction was prepared from the motor cortex and spinal cord according to a previous report [23]. Briefly, brain tissues were homogenized in 10 vol (*w/v*) of ice-cold buffer A (0.32 M sucrose, 5 mM Hepes-NaOH (pH 7.4), 0.5 mM EGTA, 5 mM NaF, and 1 mM Na$_3$VO$_4$) in the presence of protease inhibitor mixture (Complete; Roche Molecular Biochemicals, Indianapolis, IN, USA) using a Teflon-glass grinder. The homogenate was centrifuged at 1000 ×g for 5 min at 4°C; the resulting pellet (P1), containing nuclei and debris, was discarded whereas the supernatant (S1) was collected and centrifuged at 9200 ×g for 15 min. The supernatant (S2) was removed, and the pellet was washed in homogenization buffer and centrifuged at 10200 ×g for 15 min at 4°C to obtain a crude synaptosomal fraction (P2). The purity of synaptosome was previously evaluated by Western blotting using the markers specific to synaptosome [14]. The samples prepared for determination of PTP and STEP activity were solubilized in buffer A without phosphatase inhibitors. Protein content was determined by bicinchoninic acid assay (BCA kit, Thermo Scientific, Waltham, MA, USA), and synaptosomes were diluted to a concentration of 1 mg/ml.

2.4. Immunoprecipitation and In Vitro Kinase Assay. Immunoprecipitation of src and fyn kinases and *in vitro* kinase assay were performed as previously described [24]. Synaptosomes were solubilized by incubation for 1 hour at 0°C with an equal volume of 4X RIPA buffer (100 mM Tris–HCl (pH 7.5), 0.6 M NaCl, 4% (*w/v*) Triton X-100, 4% (*v/v*) Na-deoxycholate, 0.4% (*v/v*) SDS, 0.4 mM Na$_3$VO$_4$, 20 µg/ml leupeptin, 20 µg/ml aprotinin, and 4 mM PMSF), diluted twice with TBS (50 mM Tris–HCl (pH 7.4) and 150 mM NaCl), and then centrifuged at 12000 ×g for 15 min at 4°C.

After centrifugation, the supernatant was incubated with 25 μl of 50% (wt/vol) protein A/G PLUS agarose beads (Santa Cruz) for 1 hour at 4°C, clarified by centrifugation, and incubated overnight at 4°C in a rotating wheel with the different antibodies (2 μg/ml monoclonal anti-v-src and 2 μg/ml polyclonal anti-fyn). Src and fyn immunocomplexes were precipitated by the addition of 50% (wt/vol) protein G or protein A beads, respectively, and incubated at room temperature for 1 hour under gentle rotation. The beads were collected by centrifugation and washed twice with 1X RIPA buffer, twice with TBS, and once with kinase buffer (25 mM Tris–HCl (pH 7.5), 10 mM $MnCl_2$, and 0.1 mM Na_3VO_4). The kinase reaction was carried out in 20 μl of kinase buffer containing 1 μg of enolase and 1 μCi of $[\gamma^{32}P]$ ATP (>3000 Ci/mmol) at room temperature for 10 min. The reaction was stopped by adding 10 μl of 4X loading buffer, and the samples were subjected to Western blot. The gels were dried and exposed to X-ray film for autoradiography. Dried gels were used for direct determination of radioactivity using a phosphor imager instrument (Packard, Canberra, CO).

2.5. Western Blot Analysis. Samples prepared for Western blot analysis were solubilized in 4X loading buffer, boiled for 5 min, and proteins were resolved on 10% SDS-PAGE. Proteins were transferred to nitrocellulose paper at 35 V overnight. Blots were washed with TBS-0.05% Tween 20 (TTBS) and blocked with 3% BSA in TTBS for 2 hours. Washed nitrocellulose filters were incubated overnight at 4°C with the appropriate antibody. After extensive washes in TTBS, the immunoreactive bands were detected by chemiluminescence coupled to peroxidase activity (ECL), according to the manufacturer's specifications (ECL Kit, Thermo Scientific, Waltham, MA, USA), and quantified using a Bio-Rad ChemiDoc XRS system.

2.6. PTP and STEP Activity. Total PTP activity was detected in synaptosomes using *para*-nitrophenyl phosphate (*p*-NPP) as substrate, according to the procedure previously described [25]. Briefly, synaptosomes were suspended in assay buffer (25 mM Hepes (pH 7.4), 20 mM $MgCl_2$, and 0.1 mM PMSF) containing 15 mM *p*-NPP and incubated at 37°C for 30 min. The reaction was stopped by the addition of 0.1 mM NaOH. Samples were centrifuged, and the release of *p*-nitrophenol from *p*-NPP was measured in the supernatant at 405 nm.

The activity of STEP was measured in the immunocomplexes obtained from synaptosomes as described above using a polyclonal anti-STEP antibody. STEP immunocomplexes were precipitated by the addition of 50% (*w/v*) Trysacryl-immobilized protein A beads. To measure the activity of STEP, the immunoprecipitates were suspended in 200 μl of assay buffer containing 15 mM *p*-NPP and incubated for 60 min at 30°C under gentle stir. The activity was determined in the clarified supernatants by measuring the absorbance at 405 nm of *p*-nitrophenol.

2.7. Statistical Analysis. All data are presented as mean ± SEM. The Mann–Whitney *U* test or Student's *t*-test was used for single comparisons. Differences among multiple groups were analyzed by the Kruskal-Wallis nonparametric analysis of variance (followed by Dunn's test for multiple comparisons). A *p* value ≤ 0.05 indicated statistically significant differences.

3. Results

3.1. Tyrosine Phosphorylation Signal Is Enhanced in the Motor Cortex and Spinal Cord of $SOD1^{G93A}$ Mice. The pattern of phosphotyrosine distribution was assayed by Western blot analysis using an anti-phosphotyrosine (pY) antibody in synaptosomes prepared from the motor cortex and spinal cord of control, $SOD1^{WT}$, and $SOD1^{G93A}$ mice. Synaptosomes retain the elaborated structural specialization of isolated nerve terminals [26] and are a particularly useful model to explore specific proteins modified by physiological oxidants. As shown in Figure 1, tyrosine-phosphorylated proteins increased in $SOD1^{G93A}$ mice, both in the cortex and spinal cord (a and b, resp.). A slight increase was also observed in the $SOD1^{WT}$ cortex when compared to control mice (Figure 1(a)).

3.2. Activation of Src and Fyn Tyrosine Kinases in the Cortex and Spinal Cord of $SOD1^{G93A}$ Mice. The results described above prompted us to investigate the contribution of specific tyrosine kinases and PTP to the modulation of the phosphotyrosine signal. To this end, we performed *in vitro* kinase assays on src family tyrosine kinases src and fyn, immunoprecipitated from synaptosomes of the cortex and spinal cord. We measured the kinase activity as autophosphorylation and phosphorylation of the exogenous substrate enolase. As shown in Figure 2, src and fyn activities were upregulated in $SOD1^{G93A}$ compared with control and $SOD1^{WT}$ mice, both in the motor cortex (Figure 2(a)) and in the spinal cord (Figure 2(b)). When the kinase activities were expressed as percentage variation of the respective controls, a statistically significant increase in the activity of both kinases was evident in the motor cortex and spinal cord of $SOD1^{G93A}$ with respect to control and $SOD1^{WT}$ mice (Figure 2).

3.3. Downregulation of Tyrosine Phosphatase Activity in the Cortex and Spinal Cord of $SOD1^{G93A}$ Mice. We next evaluated the contribution of PTPs. The phosphatase assay revealed a decrease in enzymatic activity of total PTP in $SOD1^{G93A}$ synaptosomes, both in the cortex and spinal cord. When PTP activity was expressed as percentage variation of controls, a statistically significant reduction was observed in the cortex and spinal cord of $SOD1^{G93A}$ with respect to controls and $SOD1^{WT}$ (Figure 3(a)).

Among the brain-specific tyrosine phosphatases that could be modulated by the mutation of SOD1, we focused on STEP. To measure the activity of STEP, we immunoprecipitated the protein by a specific antibody and evaluated the phosphatase activity associated with the immunocomplex. As shown in Figure 3(b), STEP activity was downregulated in $SOD1^{G93A}$, both in the cortex and in the spinal cord (58.7 ± 5.9% and 63.7 ± 7.4% of reduction, resp., $p < 0.05$ with respect to controls, Mann–Whitney *U* test). Western blot analysis revealed that the two major isoforms, STEP61 and STEP46, although differently expressed in the cortex and

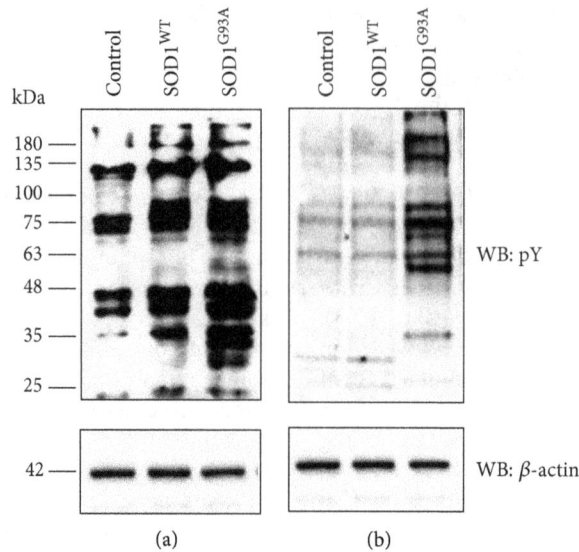

FIGURE 1: Activation of phosphotyrosine signal in the cortex and spinal cord of SOD1^{G93A} mice. Synaptosomes (1 mg/ml) were prepared from the motor cortex (a) and spinal cord (b) of control, SOD1^{WT}, and SOD1^{G93A} animals, and phosphotyrosine content was evaluated in solubilized synaptosomes by Western blot (WB) analysis using an anti-pY antibody. The nitrocellulose was also probed with an anti-β-actin antibody to evaluate the amount of loaded proteins (lower panels). Immunoreactive bands were detected by ECL. Data are representative of four separate experiments.

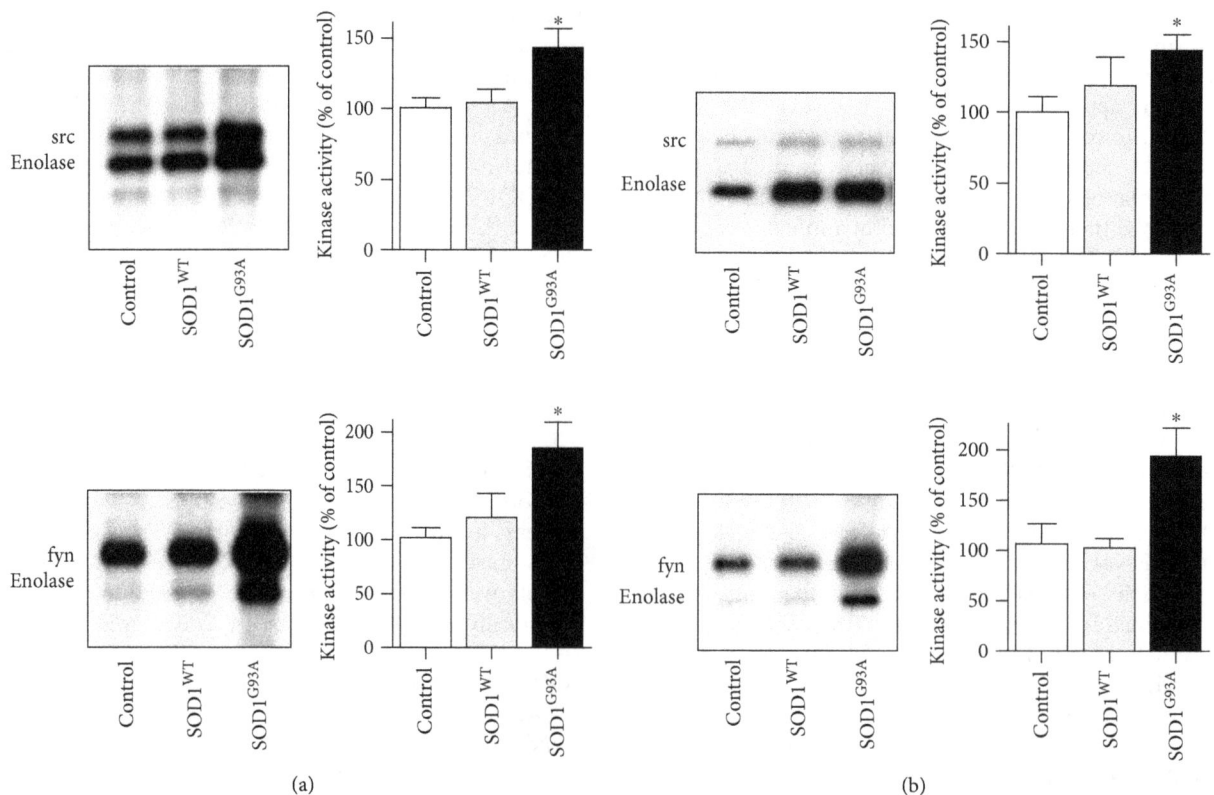

FIGURE 2: The activity of src and fyn kinases is upregulated in the cortex and spinal cord of SOD1^{G93A} mice. *In vitro* kinase activity of src (upper panels) and fyn (lower panels) isolated from the cortex (a) and spinal cord (b) obtained from control, SOD1^{WT}, and SOD1^{G93A} mice. Enolase was used as an exogenous substrate. The [^{32}P]-labelled proteins were revealed on dried gel by exposure to X-ray film, and the extent of [^{32}P] incorporation in the substrate enolase was quantified using phosphor imager instrument and expressed as percentage of the value of the control samples (100%). The bar graphs represent the means ± SEM of four independent experiments. *Significantly different from SOD1^{WT} and control ($p \leq 0.05$, Kruskal-Wallis followed by Dunn's test).

(a)

(b)

(c)

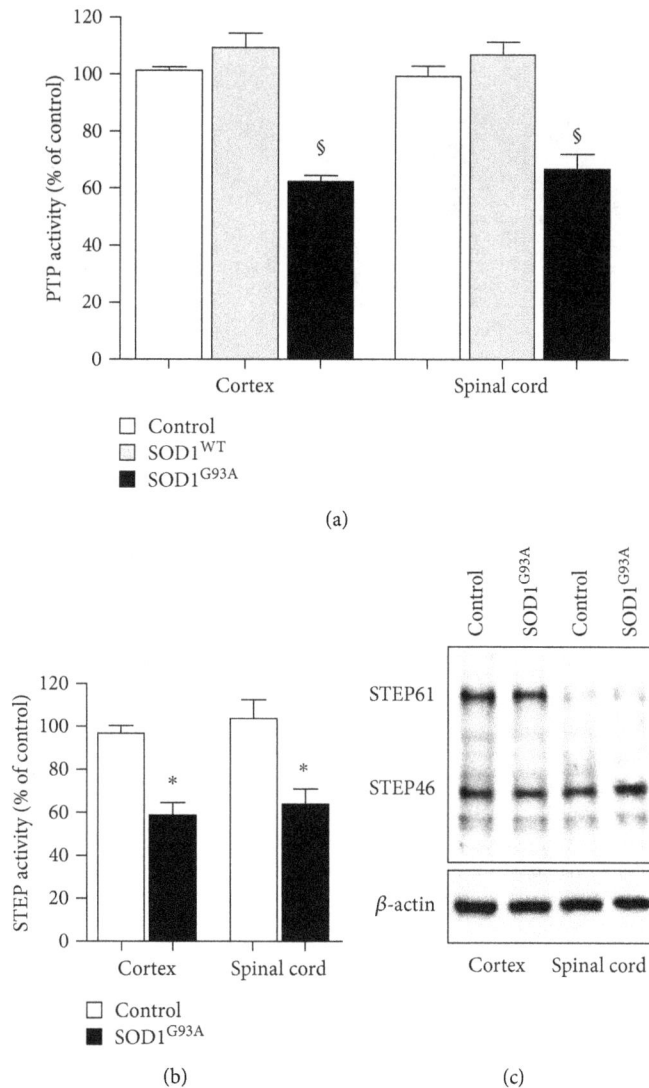

FIGURE 3: Effects of G93A mutation in SOD1 mice on PTP and STEP activities. (a) PTP activity was measured in synaptosomes obtained from the cortex and spinal cord of control, SOD1^{WT}, and SOD1^{G93A} animals. The activity is expressed as percentage variation of control values. The bar graphs represent the means $\pm$ SEM of five independent experiments for each group. §Significantly different from SOD1^{WT} and control ($p < 0.05$, Kruskal-Wallis followed by Dunn's test). (b) STEP protein was immunoprecipitated by a specific polyclonal antibody from solubilized synaptosomes prepared from the cortex and spinal cord of SOD1^{G93A} and control mice. The phosphatase activity of the STEP-immunocomplex is expressed as percentage variation of control values (100%). The bar graphs represent the means $\pm$ SEM of four independent preparations. *Significantly different from control ($p < 0.05$, Mann–Whitney U test). (c) Western blot analysis with an anti-STEP polyclonal antibody of solubilized synaptosomes prepared from the cortex and spinal cord of control and SOD1^{G93A} mice. The nitrocellulose was also probed with an anti-β-actin antibody to evaluate the amount of loaded proteins (lower panel). The immunoreactive bands were detected by ECL. The results shown are representative of four independent experiments.

spinal cord (STEP61 is less expressed in the spinal cord than in the cortex), did not differ between control and SOD1^{G93A} mice (Figure 3(c)).

3.4. Tyrosine Phosphorylation of GluN2B, ERK1/2, and Pyk2.
In order to verify whether the inhibition of STEP activity observed in SOD1^{G93A} mice resulted in the hyperphosphorylation of tyrosine residues of its substrates, we evaluated the phosphorylation status of the GluN2B subunit of the NMDAR, Pyk2, and ERK1/2, three known STEP substrates [27–29]. We found by Western blot analysis that in the presence of a decreased activity of STEP, as in SOD1^{G93A} mice,

GluN2B tyrosine phosphorylation level was significantly upregulated (Figure 4(a)) as well as the phosphorylation level of ERK1/2 and Pyk2 (Figures 4(b) and 4(c), resp.), both in the cortex and in the spinal cord of SOD1^{G93A} mice.

4. Discussion

In the present study, we highlight the impact of phosphotyrosine-mediated signaling in the pathogenesis of ALS. In mice overexpressing the mutant human SOD1 (SOD1^{G93A}), we demonstrate, both in the motor cortex and spinal cord, that (i) the protein-associated tyrosine

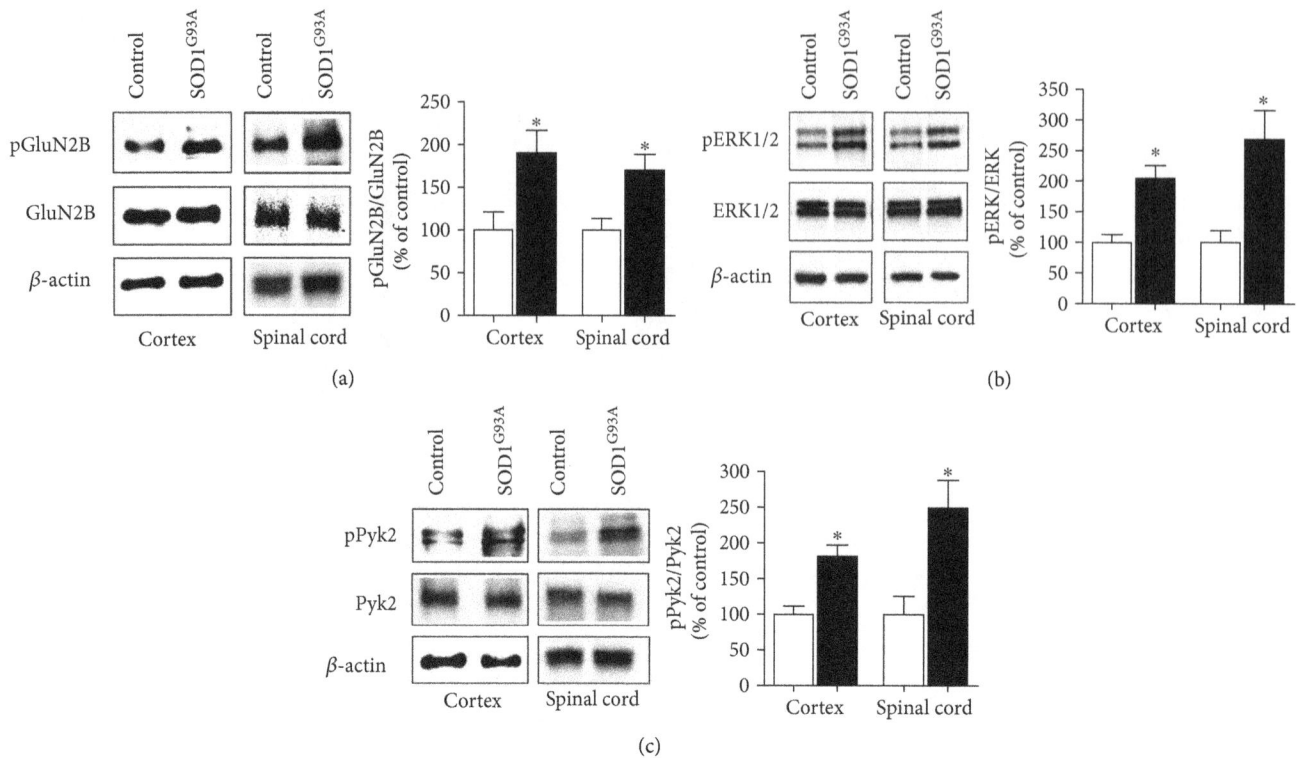

FIGURE 4: Tyrosine phosphorylation of STEP substrates. The tyrosine phosphorylation levels of GluN2B (a), ERK1/2 (b), and Pyk2 (c) were evaluated by Western blot analysis using specific antibodies that recognized the phosphorylated and nonphosphorylated forms of each enzyme in the cortex and spinal cord of control and SOD1^{G93A} animals. Anti-β-actin antibody was used to evaluate the amount of loaded proteins. The immunoreactive bands were detected by ECL. The immunoblots are representative of three independent experiments. The bar graphs represent quantification by densitometric analysis of band intensity relative to the appropriate nonphosphorylated proteins, expressed as percentage of the relative controls. White and black columns: control and SOD1^{G93A} mice. The bar graph represents the means ± SEM of 3 independent experiments. *Significantly different from control ($p \leq 0.05$, Student's t-test).

phosphorylation signal is increased, (ii) the enzymatic activity of two members of the src kinase family, src and fyn, is upregulated, and (iii) the activity of PTP, in particular of STEP, is inhibited. Moreover, we found that the tyrosine phosphorylation of the NMDAR subunit GluN2B, the major tyrosine phosphorylated substrate in the brain, and that of Pyk2 and ERK1/2 are greatly amplified.

SOD1^{G93A} mice develop a syndrome that closely resembles the human disease, but the molecular pathways that cause motor neurodegeneration are still largely debated. The mutations of SOD1 confer to the enzyme a "gain-of-function," leading to increased hydrogen peroxide levels and reactive oxygen species (ROS) [30]. In ALS, various indices of ROS-induced damage have been reported within the specific brain region that undergoes selective neurodegeneration [31]. In addition, oxidative stress and the formation of oxygen free radicals are key components of the glutamate-induced neurotoxicity, a pathogenetic mechanism that has received much attention as a critical player in ALS development and progression [32]. Several lines of evidence reported that src family protein tyrosine kinases are involved in excitotoxicity [16–19], pointing to a possible role in the pathogenesis of ALS. Accordingly, we report the activation of two members of the src family kinases highly expressed in the central nervous system, src and fyn, both in the cortex and in the spinal cord of SOD1^{G93A} mice. We previously

demonstrated that several oxidants are able to activate the src family tyrosine kinases, which are directly implicated in tyrosine phosphorylation of the NMDAR [33–35]. Indeed, NMDARs are particularly vulnerable to the action of free radicals, such as nitric oxide and superoxide anion, which can modulate the activity of tyrosine kinases and phosphatases and then control the functionality of NMDAR [33–38]. In fact, NMDAR activity is governed by a balance between tyrosine phosphorylation and dephosphorylation: the activation of src kinases and/or inhibition of phosphatase activity results in the enhancement of NMDAR function [39, 40]. The NMDAR subunits GluN2A and GluN2B are tyrosine phosphorylated and, in particular, the GluN2B subunit is the main tyrosine-phosphorylated protein in the postsynaptic density, with Tyr1472 as probably the most phosphorylated site in the brain. Thus, the hyperphosphorylation of GluN2B and the consequent increase in NMDAR activity, sustained by ROS-activated src signaling, might represent a causal link between SOD1 mutation and the excitotoxic phenotype characterizing ALS.

STEP is a tyrosine phosphatase highly expressed in the striatum which is also present in several other areas of the central nervous system, including the cerebral cortex and spinal cord [41]. STEP has two major isoforms, the membrane-associated STEP61 and the cytosolic STEP46 [42], differently expressed in the brain regions. STEP has been implicated in

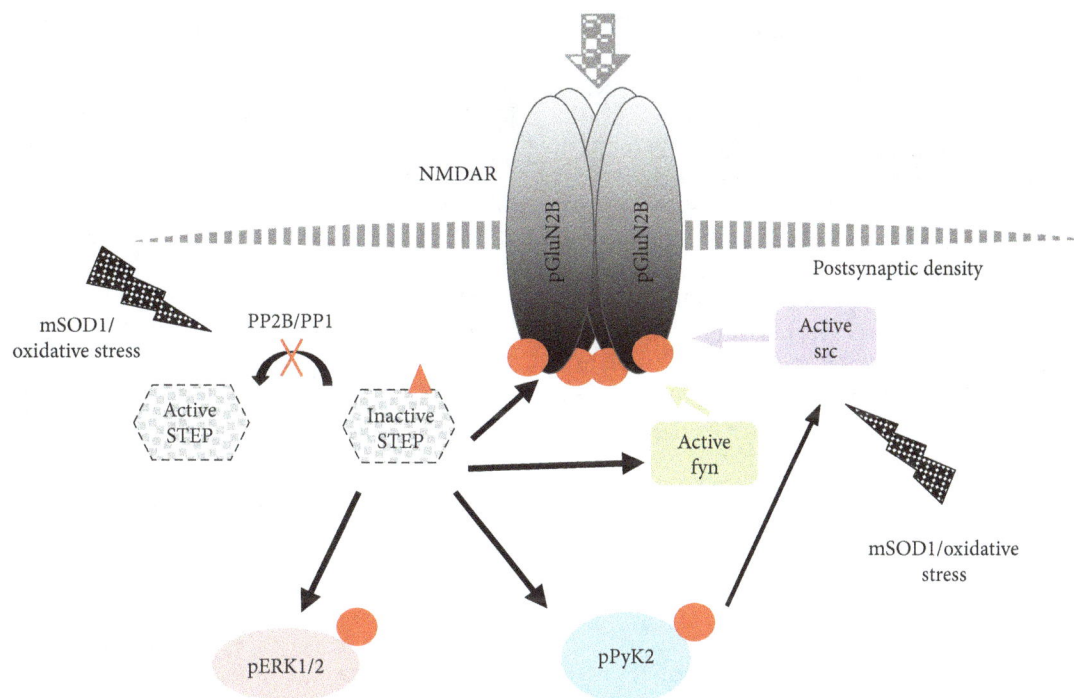

FIGURE 5: Schematic representation of STEP-mediated signaling cascade in ALS. Exposure to mutant SOD1 (mSOD1)/oxidative stress leads to inactivation of STEP, reasonably through inactivation of PP2B (calcineurin)/PP1 pathway, and activation of src kinases, both of which drive the tyrosine phosphorylation of the GluN2B subunit. In addition, as a consequence of STEP downregulation, Pyk2 becomes hyperphosphorylated and activated. Phospho-Pyk2 (pPyk2), in turn, upregulates NMDAR function by further activating src kinase, thus contributing to the potentiation of the activation loop. Red points and triangle represent phosphate groups at tyrosine and serine residues, respectively.

the pathophysiology of several neuropsychiatric diseases, and both high and low levels of STEP disrupt synaptic function and contribute to learning and behavioral deficits [43]. STEP, in its active form, dephosphorylates tyrosine residues on its substrates, causing their inactivation. In the case of glutamate receptor subunits, it dephosphorylates the GluN2B subunit of NMDARs at Tyr1472, counteracting the activity of src kinases, and promotes the internalization from surface membranes of the NMDARs, thus contributing to the homeostatic stabilization of the excitatory synapses [44–46]. In the spinal cord, the role for STEP61 in the modulation of nociception and in the development of inflammatory pain has been demonstrated [47, 48]. Li and collaborators [48] demonstrated that the hyperphosphorylation of GluN2B, fyn, and ERK2, induced by a reduction in the activity of STEP61, was critical to trigger pain hypersensitivity. Our study demonstrates for the first time a dysfunction of STEP activity in a mouse model of ALS and the hyperphosphorylation of its substrates, GluN2B, ERK1/2, and Pyk2. Pyk2 is a member of the focal adhesion kinase family, upstream of src in the signaling cascade through which tyrosine phosphorylation enhances the function of NMDAR [49]. Our results suggest that the reduced STEP activity resulted in the hyperphosphorylation of Pyk2, which may contribute to the potentiation of synaptic activity through activation of src kinase (Figure 5). We speculate that exposure to mSOD1/oxidative stress in SOD1^{G93A} leads to inactivation of STEP. Calcineurin is a phosphatase that regulates the activity of STEP through DARP32/PP1

cascade [41]. It has been recently demonstrated that calcineurin protein level and activity were significantly lower in the SOD1^{G93A} rat spinal cord [50]. In addition, decreased calcineurin enzyme activity in lymphocytes from ALS patients was reported [51]. Even though we did not evaluate calcineurin activity, it is reasonable to think that also in our SOD1^{G93A} mice, a reduced calcineurin activity fails to activate PP1, which in turn contributes to the maintenance of the phosphorylated/inactive status of STEP (Figure 5).

In contrast with previous papers demonstrating that STEP61 was the only isoform expressed in the dorsal spinal cord neurons [48, 52], we found that both isoforms were expressed in the spinal cord, with STEP46 even more expressed than STEP61 (Figure 3(c)). Although methodological differences (fetal versus adult spinal cord, dorsal versus total spinal cord) could be evoked, this discrepancy deserves further investigation.

The hyperphosphorylation of GluN2B at Tyr1472 correlates well with the role played by GluN2B in triggering NMDAR hyperfunctioning during inflammatory pain [53] and could be involved in the mechanisms of neuroinflammation that contributes to motor neuron degeneration in ALS [54, 55]. Interestingly, masitinib, a highly selective tyrosine kinase inhibitor, currently in phase 3 clinical development in ALS patients, modulates the neuroinflammation in the SOD1^{G93A} rat model of ALS and reduces the proliferation, migration, and inflammatory transcriptional profile in microglial cell cultures [56]. The hypothesis that tyrosine kinases could be involved in the pathogenesis of ALS was already suggested by the study of Jiang and collaborators [57] who demonstrated a 4.4-fold increase in the mRNA for c-Abl, a ubiquitous nonreceptor tyrosine kinase, in the motor neurons of sALS patients. Moreover, the c-Abl inhibitor dasatinib demonstrated neuroprotective properties *in vitro* and *in vivo* models of ALS [58]. Our findings are also supported by a recent paper of Imamura et al. [59] that demonstrates a protective role of bosutinib (src/c-Abl inhibitor) in motor neurons derived from iPSC of patients with familial or sporadic ALS. In addition, a tyrosine kinase inhibitor (saracatinib) has been demonstrated to reduce the downstream activation of Pyk2, leading to the restoration of synapse density and a gradual full recovery of behavioral deficits in transgenic mouse models of Alzheimer's disease [60], suggesting a broader exploitation of these drugs in the field of neurodegenerative diseases.

5. Conclusion

Our study demonstrates an increase in the phosphotyrosine-dependent signaling in the SOD1^{G93A} model of ALS and, in particular, identifies STEP as a new actor of the complex pathogenetic mechanisms of the disease. Whether this may help in finding new approaches for the treatment of this disease remains to be examined in depth.

References

[1] D. W. Cleveland and J. D. Rothstein, "From Charcot to Lou Gehrig: deciphering selective motor neuron death in ALS," *Nature Reviews Neuroscience*, vol. 2, no. 11, pp. 806–819, 2001.

[2] J. R.-J. Lee, J. F. Annegers, and S. H. Appel, "Prognosis of amyotrophic lateral sclerosis and the effect of referral selection," *Journal of the Neurological Sciences*, vol. 132, no. 2, pp. 207–215, 1995.

[3] P. M. Preux, P. Couratier, F. Boutros-Toni et al., "Survival prediction in sporadic amyotrophic lateral sclerosis. Age and clinical form at onset are independent risk factors," *Neuroepidemiology*, vol. 15, no. 3, pp. 153–160, 1996.

[4] B. J. Traynor, M. B. Codd, B. Corr, C. Forde, E. Frost, and O. M. Hardiman, "Clinical features of amyotrophic lateral sclerosis according to the El Escorial and Airlie House diagnostic criteria: a population-based study," *Archives of Neurology*, vol. 57, no. 8, pp. 1171–1176, 2000.

[5] O. Hardiman, L. H. van den Berg, and M. C. Kiernan, "Clinical diagnosis and management of amyotrophic lateral sclerosis," *Nature Reviews Neurology*, vol. 7, no. 11, pp. 639–649, 2011.

[6] D. Rosen, "Mutations in Cu/Zn superoxide dismutase gene are associated with familial amyotrophic lateral sclerosis," *Nature*, vol. 364, no. 6435, p. 362, 1993.

[7] L. I. Bruijn, T. M. Miller, and D. W. Cleveland, "Unraveling the mechanisms involved in motor neuron degeneration in ALS," *Annual Review of Neuroscience*, vol. 27, no. 1, pp. 723–749, 2004.

[8] J. P. Taylor, R. H. Brown, and D. W. Cleveland, "Decoding ALS: from genes to mechanism," *Nature*, vol. 539, no. 7628, pp. 197–206, 2016.

[9] A. Doble, "The pharmacology and mechanism of action of riluzole," *Neurology*, vol. 47, Issue 6, Supplement 4, pp. 233S–241S, 1996.

[10] R. G. Miller, J. D. Mitchell, and D. H. Moore, "Riluzole for amyotrophic lateral sclerosis (ALS)/motor neuron disease (MND)," *Cochrane Database of Systematic Reviews*, vol. 3, 2012.

[11] J. Lewerenz and P. Maher, "Chronic glutamate toxicity in neurodegenerative diseases-what is the evidence?," *Frontiers in Neuroscience*, vol. 9, 2015.

[12] A. E. King, A. Woodhouse, M. T. K. Kirkcaldie, and J. C. Vickers, "Excitotoxicity in ALS: overstimulation, or overreaction?," *Experimental Neurology*, vol. 275, pp. 162–171, 2016.

[13] M. Urushitani, N. Tomoki, R. Inoue et al., "N-methyl-D-aspartate receptor-mediated mitochondrial Ca(2+) overload in acute excitotoxic motor neuron death: a mechanism distinct from chronic neurotoxicity after Ca(2+) influx," *Journal of Neuroscience Research*, vol. 63, no. 5, pp. 377–387, 2001.

[14] A. Spalloni, N. Origlia, C. Sgobio et al., "Postsynaptic alteration of NR2A subunit and defective autophosphorylation of alphaCaMKII at threonine-286 contribute to abnormal plasticity and morphology of upper motor neurons in presymptomatic SOD1G93A mice, a murine model for amyotrophic lateral sclerosis," *Cerebral Cortex*, vol. 21, no. 4, pp. 796–805, 2011.

[15] K. A. Staats, L. Van Helleputte, A. R. Jones et al., "Genetic ablation of phospholipase C delta 1 increases survival in SOD1(G93A) mice," *Neurobiology of Disease*, vol. 60, pp. 11–17, 2013.

[16] M. Iqbal Hossain, C. L. Roulston, M. Aizuddin Kamaruddin et al., "A truncated fragment of Src protein kinase generated by calpain-mediated cleavage is a mediator of neuronal death in excitotoxicity," *The Journal of Biological Chemistry*, vol. 288, no. 14, pp. 9696–9709, 2013.

[17] R. Knox, A. M. Brennan-Minnella, F. Lu et al., "NR2B phosphorylation at tyrosine 1472 contributes to brain injury in a rodent model of neonatal hypoxia-ischemia," *Stroke*, vol. 45, no. 10, pp. 3040–3047, 2014.

[18] N. L. Weilinger, A. W. Lohman, B. D. Rakai et al., "Metabotropic NMDA receptor signaling couples Src family kinases to pannexin-1 during excitotoxicity," *Nature Neuroscience*, vol. 19, no. 3, pp. 432–442, 2016.

[19] Y. Sun, Y. Chen, L. Zhan, L. Zhang, J. Hu, and Z. Gao, "The role of non-receptor protein tyrosine kinases in the excitotoxicity induced by the overactivation of NMDA receptors," *Reviews in the Neurosciences*, vol. 27, no. 3, pp. 283–289, 2016.

[20] M. E. Gurney, H. Pu, A. Y. Chiu et al., "Motor neuron degeneration in mice that express a human Cu,Zn superoxide dismutase mutation," *Science*, vol. 264, no. 5166, pp. 1772–1775, 1994.

[21] M. C. Dal Canto and M. E. Gurney, "Development of central nervous system pathology in a murine transgenic model of human amyotrophic lateral sclerosis," *The American Journal of Pathology*, vol. 145, no. 6, pp. 1271–1279, 1994.

[22] S. Apolloni, S. Amadio, C. Montilli, C. Volonte, and N. D'Ambrosi, "Ablation of P2X7 receptor exacerbates gliosis and motoneuron death in the SOD1-G93A mouse model of

amyotrophic lateral sclerosis," *Human Molecular Genetics*, vol. 22, no. 20, pp. 4102–4116, 2013.

[23] W. B. Huttner, W. Schiebler, P. Greengard, and P. De Camilli, "Synapsin I (protein I), a nerve terminal-specific phosphoprotein. III. Its association with synaptic vesicles studied in a highly purified synaptic vesicle preparation," *The Journal of Cell Biology*, vol. 96, no. 5, pp. 1374–1388, 1983.

[24] C. Mallozzi, C. D'Amore, S. Camerini et al., "Phosphorylation and nitration of tyrosine residues affect functional properties of synaptophysin and dynamin I, two proteins involved in exo-endocytosis of synaptic vesicles," *Biochimica et Biophysica Acta (BBA) - Molecular Cell Research*, vol. 1833, no. 1, pp. 110–121, 2013.

[25] C. Mallozzi, A. M. Di Stasi, and M. Minetti, "Peroxynitrite modulates tyrosine-dependent signal transduction pathway of human erythrocyte band 3," *The FASEB Journal*, vol. 11, no. 14, pp. 1281–1290, 1997.

[26] M. E. Burns and G. J. Augustine, "Synaptic structure and function: dynamic organization yields architectural precision," *Cell*, vol. 83, no. 2, pp. 187–194, 1995.

[27] S. S. Jang, S. E. Royston, J. Xu et al., "Regulation of STEP61 and tyrosine-phosphorylation of NMDA and AMPA receptors during homeostatic synaptic plasticity," *Molecular Brain*, vol. 8, no. 1, p. 55, 2015.

[28] J. Xu, P. Kurup, J. A. Bartos, T. Patriarchi, J. W. Hell, and P. J. Lombroso, "Striatal-enriched protein-tyrosine phosphatase (STEP) regulates Pyk2 kinase activity," *The Journal of Biological Chemistry*, vol. 287, no. 25, pp. 20942–20956, 2012.

[29] R. Li, D. D. Xie, J. H. Dong et al., "Molecular mechanism of ERK dephosphorylation by striatal-enriched protein tyrosine phosphatase," *Journal of Neurochemistry*, vol. 128, no. 2, pp. 315–329, 2014.

[30] M. B. Yim, J. H. Kang, H. S. Yim, H. S. Kwak, P. B. Chock, and E. R. Stadtman, "A gain-of-function of an amyotrophic lateral sclerosis-associated Cu, Zn-superoxide dismutase mutant: an enhancement of free radical formation due to a decrease in Km for hydrogen peroxide," *Proceedings of the National Academy of Sciences of the United States of America*, vol. 93, no. 12, pp. 5709–5714, 1996.

[31] Z. Liu, T. Zhou, A. C. Ziegler, P. Dimitrion, and L. Zuo, "Oxidative stress in neurodegenerative diseases: from molecular mechanisms to clinical applications," *Oxidative Medicine and Cellular Longevity*, vol. 2017, Article ID 2525967, 11 pages, 2017.

[32] A. Spalloni, M. Nutini, and P. Longone, "Role of the N-methyl-d-aspartate receptors complex in amyotrophic lateral sclerosis," *Biochimica et Biophysica Acta*, vol. 1832, no. 2, pp. 312–322, 2013.

[33] A. M. Di Stasi, C. Mallozzi, G. Macchia, T. C. Petrucci, and M. Minetti, "Peroxynitrite induces tryosine nitration and modulates tyrosine phosphorylation of synaptic proteins," *Journal of Neurochemistry*, vol. 73, no. 2, pp. 727–735, 1999.

[34] C. Mallozzi, A. M. M. Di Stasi, and M. Minetti, "Activation of src tyrosine kinases by peroxynitrite," *FEBS Letters*, vol. 456, no. 1, pp. 201–206, 1999.

[35] M. Minetti, C. Mallozzi, and A. M. M. Di Stasi, "Peroxynitrite activates kinases of the src family and upregulates tyrosine phosphorylation signaling," *Free Radical Biology & Medicine*, vol. 33, no. 6, pp. 744–754, 2002.

[36] J. Garthwaite and C. L. Boulton, "Nitric oxide signaling in the central nervous system," *Annual Review of Physiology*, vol. 57, no. 1, pp. 683–706, 1995.

[37] T. Nakamura and S. A. Lipton, "Redox modulation by S-nitrosylation contributes to protein misfolding, mitochondrial dynamics, and neuronal synaptic damage in neurodegenerative diseases," *Cell Death and Differentiation*, vol. 18, no. 9, pp. 1478–1486, 2011.

[38] M. I. Hossain, M. A. Kamaruddin, and H. C. Cheng, "Aberrant regulation and function of Src family tyrosine kinases: their potential contributions to glutamate-induced neurotoxicity," *Clinical and Experimental Pharmacology & Physiology*, vol. 39, no. 8, pp. 684–691, 2012.

[39] G. Kohr and P. H. Seeburg, "Subtype-specific regulation of recombinant NMDA receptor-channels by protein tyrosine kinases of the src family," *The Journal of Physiology*, vol. 492, no. 2, pp. 445–452, 1996.

[40] E. B. Ziff, "Enlightening the postsynaptic density," *Neuron*, vol. 19, no. 6, pp. 1163–1174, 1997.

[41] M. Kamceva, J. Benedict, A. C. Nairn, and P. J. Lombroso, "Role of striatal-enriched tyrosine phosphatase in neuronal function," *Neural Plasticity*, vol. 2016, Article ID 8136925, 9 pages, 2016.

[42] A. Bult, F. Zhao, R. Dirkx Jr, A. Raghunathan, M. Solimena, and P. J. Lombroso, "STEP: a family of brain-enriched PTPs. Alternative splicing produces transmembrane, cytosolic and truncated isoforms," *European Journal of Cell Biology*, vol. 72, no. 4, pp. 337–344, 1997.

[43] S. M. Goebel-Goody, M. Baum, C. D. Paspalas et al., "Therapeutic implications for striatal-enriched protein tyrosine phosphatase (STEP) in neuropsychiatric disorders," *Pharmacological Reviews*, vol. 64, no. 1, pp. 65–87, 2012.

[44] Y. Zhang, D. V. Venkitaramani, C. M. Gladding et al., "The tyrosine phosphatase STEP mediates AMPA receptor endocytosis after metabotropic glutamate receptor stimulation," *The Journal of Neuroscience: The Official Journal of the Society for Neuroscience*, vol. 28, no. 42, pp. 10561–10566, 2008.

[45] Y. Zhang, P. Kurup, J. Xu et al., "Genetic reduction of striatal-enriched tyrosine phosphatase (STEP) reverses cognitive and cellular deficits in an Alzheimer's disease mouse model," *Proceedings of the National Academy of Sciences of the United States of America*, vol. 107, no. 44, pp. 19014–19019, 2010.

[46] Y. Zhang, P. Kurup, J. Xu et al., "Reduced levels of the tyrosine phosphatase STEP block beta amyloid-mediated GluA1/GluA2 receptor internalization," *Journal of Neurochemistry*, vol. 119, no. 3, pp. 664–672, 2011.

[47] G. Azkona, A. Saavedra, Z. Aira et al., "Striatal-enriched protein tyrosine phosphatase modulates nociception: evidence from genetic deletion and pharmacological inhibition," *Pain*, vol. 157, no. 2, pp. 377–386, 2016.

[48] L. Li, L. Shi, Y. M. Xu, X. Yang, Z. W. Suo, and X. D. Hu, "GABAergic inhibition regulated pain sensitization through STEP61 signaling in spinal dorsal horn of mice," *Anesthesiology*, vol. 122, no. 3, pp. 686–697, 2015.

[49] Y.-Q. Huang, W.-Y. Lu, D. W. Ali et al., "CAKβ/Pyk2 kinase is a signaling link for induction of long-term potentiation in CA1 hippocampus," *Neuron*, vol. 29, no. 2, pp. 485–496, 2001.

[50] J. M. Kim, E. Billington, A. Reyes et al., "Impaired Cu–Zn superoxide dismutase (SOD1) and calcineurin (Cn) interaction in ALS: a presumed consequence for TDP-43 and zinc aggregation in Tg SOD1G93A rodent spinal cord tissue," *Neurochemical Research*, 2018.

[51] A. Ferri, M. Nencini, S. Battistini et al., "Activity of protein phosphatase calcineurin is decreased in sporadic and familial amyotrophic lateral sclerosispatients," *Journal of Neurochemistry*, vol. 90, no. 5, pp. 1237–1242, 2004.

[52] K. A. Pelkey, R. Askalan, S. Paul et al., "Tyrosine phosphatase STEP is a tonic brake on induction of long-term potentiation," *Neuron*, vol. 34, no. 1, pp. 127–138, 2002.

[53] H. B. Yang, X. Yang, J. Cao et al., "cAMP-dependent protein kinase activated Fyn in spinal dorsal horn to regulate NMDA receptor function during inflammatory pain," *Journal of Neurochemistry*, vol. 116, no. 1, pp. 93–104, 2011.

[54] S. Apolloni, P. Fabbrizio, S. Amadio et al., "Histamine regulates the inflammatory profile of SOD1-G93A microglia and the histaminergic system is dysregulated in amyotrophic lateral sclerosis," *Frontiers in Immunology*, vol. 8, p. 1689, 2017.

[55] G. Morello, A. G. Spampinato, and S. Cavallaro, "Neuroinflammation and ALS: transcriptomic insights into molecular disease mechanisms and therapeutic targets," *Mediators of Inflammation*, vol. 2017, Article ID 7070469, 9 pages, 2017.

[56] E. Trias, S. Ibarburu, R. Barreto-Nunez et al., "Evidence for mast cells contributing to neuromuscular pathology in an inherited model of ALS," *JCI Insight*, vol. 2, no. 20, 2017.

[57] Y.-M. Jiang, M. Yamamoto, Y. Kobayashi et al., "Gene expression profile of spinal motor neurons in sporadic amyotrophic lateral sclerosis," *Annals of Neurology*, vol. 57, no. 2, pp. 236–251, 2005.

[58] R. Katsumata, S. Ishigaki, M. Katsuno et al., "c-Abl inhibition delays motor neuron degeneration in the G93A mouse, an animal model of amyotrophic lateral sclerosis," *PLoS One*, vol. 7, no. 9, article e46185, 2012.

[59] K. Imamura, Y. Izumi, A. Watanabe et al., "The Src/c-Abl pathway is a potential therapeutic target in amyotrophic lateral sclerosis," *Science Translational Medicine*, vol. 9, no. 391, article eaaf3962, 2017.

[60] A. C. Kaufman, S. V. Salazar, L. T. Haas et al., "Fyn inhibition rescues established memory and synapse loss in Alzheimer mice," *Annals of Neurology*, vol. 77, no. 6, pp. 953–971, 2015.

17

Corticospinal Tract Wiring and Brain Lesion Characteristics in Unilateral Cerebral Palsy: Determinants of Upper Limb Motor and Sensory Function

Cristina Simon-Martinez ⓘ,[1] Ellen Jaspers,[1,2] Lisa Mailleux,[1] Els Ortibus,[3] Katrijn Klingels ⓘ,[1,4] Nicole Wenderoth,[2] and Hilde Feys[1]

[1]*Department of Rehabilitation Sciences, KU Leuven-University of Leuven, Leuven, Belgium*
[2]*Neural Control of Movement Lab, Department of Health Sciences and Technology, ETH Zurich, Zurich, Switzerland*
[3]*Department of Development and Regeneration, KU Leuven-University of Leuven, Leuven, Belgium*
[4]*Rehabilitation Research Centre, BIOMED, Hasselt University, Diepenbeek, Belgium*

Correspondence should be addressed to Cristina Simon-Martinez; cristina.simon.martinez@gmail.com

Academic Editor: Michael Borich

Brain lesion characteristics (timing, location, and extent) and the type of corticospinal tract (CST) wiring have been proposed as determinants of upper limb (UL) motor function in unilateral cerebral palsy (uCP), yet an investigation of the relative combined impact of these factors on both motor and sensory functions is still lacking. Here, we first investigated whether structural brain lesion characteristics could predict the underlying CST wiring and we explored the role of CST wiring and brain lesion characteristics to predict UL motor and sensory functions in uCP. Fifty-two participants with uCP (mean age (SD): 11 y and 3 m (3 y and 10 m)) underwent a single-pulse Transcranial Magnetic Stimulation session to determine CST wiring between the motor cortex and the more affected hand ($n = 17$ contralateral, $n = 19$ ipsilateral, and $n = 16$ bilateral) and an MRI to determine lesion timing ($n = 34$ periventricular (PV) lesion, $n = 18$ corticosubcortical (CSC) lesion), location, and extent. Lesion location and extent were evaluated with a semiquantitative scale. A standardized protocol included UL motor (grip strength, unimanual capacity, and bimanual performance) and sensory measures. A combination of lesion locations (damage to the PLIC and frontal lobe) significantly contributed to differentiate between the CST wiring groups, reclassifying the participants in their original group with 57% of accuracy. Motor and sensory functions were influenced by each of the investigated neurological factors. However, multiple regression analyses showed that motor function was predicted by the CST wiring (more preserved in individuals with contralateral CST ($p < 0.01$)), lesion extent, and damage to the basal ganglia and thalamus. Sensory function was predicted by the combination of a large and later lesion and an ipsilateral or bilateral CST wiring, which led to increased sensory deficits ($p < 0.05$). These novel insights contribute to a better understanding of the underlying pathophysiology of UL function and may be useful to delineate individualized treatment strategies.

1. Introduction

Upper limb (UL) function is commonly impaired in individuals with unilateral cerebral palsy (uCP), negatively impacting on daily life activities [1]. The large variability in the clinical presentation of UL function, but also in treatment response, has resulted in increasing interest in understanding the underlying neural mechanisms that determine UL

function and its contribution to further optimize therapy planning for the individual with uCP. A number of neurological factors have been put forward as potential predictors of UL function, i.e., the structural brain lesion characteristics (i.e., lesion timing, location, and extent), and the type of corticospinal tract (CST) wiring [2–6].

The timing of the lesion during gestation is closely related to the type of the damaged tissue and can be classified into three categories: malformations (1st and 2nd trimesters of pregnancy), periventricular lesion (PV, early 3rd trimester), and corticosubcortical lesions (CSC, late 3rd trimester and around birth) [7]. Previous studies investigating the impact of lesion timing on UL function have shown that individuals with a later lesion (i.e., CSC lesions) present with poorer UL motor and sensory functions [2, 3, 5]. Besides lesion timing, lesion location and extent have shown to play an important role in determining UL function, whereby damage to the posterior limb of the internal capsule (PLIC) and the basal ganglia, and a larger lesion extent is related to worse UL motor and sensory functions [2, 3]. However, there is still large variability in UL function that remains unexplained based on these factors.

The unilateral brain damage in individuals with uCP can also result in a partial or complete reorganization of the CST toward the nonlesioned hemisphere [8]. This reorganization of the CST wiring is unique in uCP and refers to the efferent motor input to the affected hand. Researchers have identified three types of CST wiring, i.e., contralateral (CST_{contra}, the affected hand receives input from the crossed CST, originating in the lesioned hemisphere), ipsilateral (CST_{ipsi}, the affected hand receives input from the uncrossed CST, originating in the nonlesioned hemisphere), and bilateral (CST_{bilat}, the affected hand receives input from both the crossed and uncrossed CSTs, originating in the lesioned and nonlesioned hemispheres, respectively) [8, 9]. It has been suggested that the type of CST wiring is the main factor influencing UL function, whereby individuals with CST_{contra} present with more preserved UL function compared to the other groups [6, 10–13]. Nevertheless, assessing the underlying CST wiring with Transcranial Magnetic Stimulation (TMS) in young children might become challenging. Therefore, the identification of either behavioural or brain lesion features that relate to the underlying CST wiring could be useful to define tailor-made interventions in a clinical setting.

Whilst the role of lesion timing, location, and extent has been well investigated [2, 3, 14], only a few studies examined the impact of the CST wiring on UL function and they often have several limitations (i.e., small sample sizes, ordinal scoring of impairments, and limited to motor deficits) [5, 10, 15]. Moreover, studies thus far focused on each factor independently, whereas only one study described the impact of the CST wiring and lesion timing on UL function in uCP [10], and only one study reports the impact of CST wiring and lesion extent in children with PV lesions [4]. Although the authors suggested the relevance of both lesion timing and type of CST wiring in predicting UL function, the small sample size, the lack of a standardized evaluation of motor function, and the merely descriptive nature of the study hampered the possibility of drawing strong conclusions.Furthermore, it has been shown that an intact sensory function is essential to develop an adequate motor function in other neurological disorders (such as adult stroke) [16, 17]. Also in individuals with uCP, sensory and motor functions are highly related [1], although the impact of the CST wiring on this relationship remains unknown.

In this study, we investigated the impact of CST wiring and structural brain lesion characteristics on UL motor and sensory functions in a large group of individuals with uCP, using a systematic and comprehensive evaluation. Our first hypothesis is that the type of the CST wiring pattern in unilateral CP can be predicted based on a linear combination of measures of lesion timing, location, and extent. Second, we hypothesize that the combination of these predictors together with the CST wiring has a stronger predicting value for UL motor and sensory functions than any of these factors alone. Last, we speculate that the relation between motor and sensory functions is disrupted by the type of CST wiring.

2. Materials and Methods

2.1. Participants. Children and adolescents with uCP aged between 5 and 21 years old were recruited via the CP reference center of the University Hospitals Leuven between 2014 and 2017. They were excluded if they (1) received UL botulinum toxin injections six months prior to the assessment, (2) had UL surgery two years prior to the assessment, and/or (3) had other neurological or genetic disorders. All individuals assented to participate; all parents signed the informed consent (participants younger than 18 years old), and participants older than 12 years also signed the informed consent, in accordance with the Declaration of Helsinki. This study was approved by the Medical Ethical Committee of the University Hospital Leuven (S55555 and S56513).

Participants with contraindications for the MRI (e.g., metal implants) or the Transcranial Magnetic Stimulation (TMS; ventricular-peritoneal (VP) shunt, seizure two years prior to the study) did not undergo the respective assessment. All TMS measurements were conducted by two experienced physiotherapists (CSM and EJ), and UL function was evaluated by four experienced physiotherapists (LM, CSM, JH, and EJ) at the Clinical Motion Analysis Laboratory of the University Hospitals Leuven (campus Pellenberg, Belgium).

2.2. Upper Limb Evaluation

2.2.1. Motor Function. Grip strength, unimanual capacity, and bimanual performance composed the motor evaluation. Maximum *grip strength* was assessed using the Jamar® hydraulic hand dynamometer (Sammons Preston, Rolyan, Bolingbrook, IL, USA). The less-affected hand was measured first, and the mean of three maximum contractions was calculated per hand. The ratio between hands was used for further analyses to cancel out the effect of age (grip strength ratio = grip strength less – affected hand/grip strength affected hand, whereby a lower score (closer to 1) indicates a grip strength in the affected hand similar to that of the less-affected hand). *Unimanual capacity* was assessed with the Jebsen-Taylor hand function test (JTHFT). The JTHFT reliably measures movement speed during six unimanual tasks [18, 19]. Similar to other studies, we used a modified version for children and adolescents with uCP in which the writing task was removed and the time to carry out each task was reduced from 3 to 2 minutes to avoid frustration [19, 20]. The time to perform every task was summed up, and the ratio between hands was used for further analyses to cancel out the effect of age (JTHFT ratio = JTHFT affected hand/JTHFT less-affected hand, whereby a lower score (closer to 1) indicates movement speed in the affected hand similar to that of the less-affected hand). *Bimanual performance* was evaluated with the Assisting Hand Assessment (AHA), which assesses how effectively the affected hand is used in bimanual activities [21–23]. The spontaneous use is evaluated during a semistructured play session with standardized toys requiring bimanual handling. Given the age range of the participants of this study, the School Kids AHA and the Ad-AHA were administered [22, 24]. The AHA was scored by certified raters (LM and CSM), using the 5.0 version which includes 20 items that are scored from 0 ("does not do") to 4 ("effective use"), resulting in a final score between 0 and 100 AHA units.

2.2.2. Sensory Function.

Sensory assessments comprised measures of exteroception (tactile sense), proprioception (movement sense), two-point discrimination (2PD, Aesthesiometer®), and stereognosis (tactile object identification), which have been shown to be reliable in this population [25]. Tactile and movement senses were classified as normal (score 2), impaired (score 1), or absent (score 0). 2PD was classified according to the width between the two points that the participants could discriminate: normal (0–4 mm, score 2) or impaired (>4 mm, score 1) [26]. Tactile object identification was used as the number of objects that the children could recognize (0–6). In addition, a kit of 20 nylon monofilaments (0.04 g–300 g) (Jamar Monofilaments, Sammons Preston, Rolyan, Bolingbrook, IL, USA) was used to reliably determine threshold values for touch sensation [27, 28]. Touch sensation was categorized as normal (0.008–0.07 g), diminished light touch (0.16–0.4 g), diminished protective sensation (0.6–2 g), loss of protective sensation (4.19–180 g), and untestable (300 g), according to the manual (Jamar Monofilaments, Sammons Preston, Rolyan, Bolingbrook, IL, USA).

2.3. Structural MRI.

Structural images were acquired using three-dimensional fluid-attenuated inversion recovery (3D FLAIR) (321 slices, slice thickness = 1.2 mm, slice gap = 0.6 mm, repetition time = 4800 ms, echo time = 353 ms, field of view (FOV) = 250×250 mm^2, $1.1 \times 1.1 \times 0.56$ mm^3 voxel size, acquisition time = 5 minutes). In addition, magnetization prepared rapid gradient echo (MPRAGE) was acquired (182 slices, slice thickness = 1.2 mm, slice gap = 0 mm, TR = 9.7 ms, TE = 4.6 ms, FOV = 250×250 mm^2, voxel size = $0.98 \times 0.98 \times 1.2$, acquisition time = 6 minutes). The structural MRI was used to provide a detailed description of the lesion location and extent and to classify the timing of the lesion, which was conducted by a paediatric neurologist (EO).

Timing of the brain lesion was classified according to the predominant pattern of damage as described by Krägeloh-Mann and Horber [7]: malformations (1st and 2nd trimesters of pregnancy), periventricular lesion (PV, early 3rd trimester), corticosubcortical lesions (CSC, late 3rd trimester and term), or acquired brain lesions (between 28 days and two years postnatally).

Lesion location and extent were determined using a semiquantitative scale recently developed by Fiori et al. [29]. The scale consists of a graphical template with six axial slices of the brain and an extra template for the basal ganglia (lenticular and caudate), thalamus, posterior limb of the internal capsule (PLIC), brainstem, corpus callosum, and cerebellum. Firstly, the slices corresponding to the template slices are to be found and the lesion is drawn onto the template. Next, the damage to the periventricular, middle, and corticosubcortical layers of each lobe is scored for both hemispheres separately. The sum of the damage to each lobe results in the lobar score, ranging from 0 to 3 for each lobe. Damage to the basal ganglia (lenticular and caudate), thalamus, PLIC, and brainstem directly is binarily scored from the MRI (affected or nonaffected). Damage to the corpus callosum is scored from 0 to 3, based on the involvement of the anterior, middle, and posterior thirds of the corpus callosum on a sagittal view. Last, the involvement of the cerebellum is based on damage to the vermis (0–1) and each of the hemispheres (0–2), resulting in a total score ranging from 0 to 3. A total ipsilesional score is calculated based on the damage to the lobes (0–3 for each lobe, i.e., total of 0–12) and damage to the subcortical structures (0–5; ranging from 0 to 17). More detailed information about the scale and its scoring procedure can be found in the respective study [29]. This semiquantitative scale has been shown valid and reliable in children with uCP [29, 30].

In the present study, lesion location was indicated by the damage to the frontal and parietal lobes (0–4), damage to the basal ganglia and thalamus (0–3), and damage to the PLIC (0–1). These locations were chosen based on their relation to the sensorimotor system [31]. Lesion extent was indicated by the total ipsilesional score (0–17).

2.4. Transcranial Magnetic Stimulation.

Single-pulse TMS was conducted to assess CST wiring. TMS was applied using a Magstim 200 stimulator (Magstim Ltd., Whitland, Wales, UK) equipped with a focal 70 mm figure-eight coil and a Bagnoli electromyography (EMG) system with two single differential surface electrodes (Delsys Inc., Natick, MA, USA). A Micro1401-3 acquisition unit and Spike software version 4.11 (Cambridge Electronic Design Limited, Cambridge, UK) were used to synchronize the TMS stimuli and the EMG data acquisition. Motor evoked potentials (MEPs) were bilaterally recorded from the muscles opponens pollicis brevis. During the TMS assessment, participants wore a cap that allows creating a grip with a coordinate system to identify the optimal point to stimulate (hotspot) in a standardized and systematic way. The hotspot and the resting motor threshold (RMT, defined as the minimum intensity required to obtain 5/10 MEP of at least 50 μV in the corresponding muscle) were identified by starting the stimulation intensity at 30% with an incremental increase of 5% [4]. For each hemisphere, stimulation started from the assumed "motor hotspot," which is located 5 cm lateral and 1 cm anterior from the scalp middle point (Cz), at 30%. After approximately 2–3 pulses, the stimulation intensity was increased 5% for another 2–3 pulses, until MEPs were found. If no MEP can be elicited after increasing up to 60 to 80%, the coil would be moved to a different location on the scalp grid and the procedure would be repeated until an MEP was elicited. Stimulation up to 100% of the maximum stimulator output was continued until an MEP was elicited. The nonlesioned hemisphere was always stimulated first and allowed to identify contralateral CST projections to the less-affected hand. Stimulation in the nonlesioned hemisphere was continued up to 100% of the maximum stimulator output to search for possible ipsilateral CST projections to the affected hand. Next, the lesioned hemisphere was stimulated to identify possible contralateral CST projections to the affected hand. If only contralateral MEPs from each hemisphere were found, the child was categorized as having a CST_{contra} wiring. If MEPs in the affected hand were evoked from both hemispheres, the child was categorized as having a CST_{bilat} wiring. Lastly, if MEPs in the impaired hand were only evoked when stimulating the nonaffected hemisphere, the child was categorized as having a CST_{ipsi} wiring. TMS measures have been shown to be reliable in adults [32, 33] and in children [34]. In this study, the TMS assessment was used for diagnostic purposes. In cases when high intensities were not tolerated, the stimulation intensity was increased up to at least 80% of the maximum stimulator output and children were asked to hold a pen to ensure precontraction of the evaluated muscle and thereby facilitate the CST and MEP detection. This allowed us to rule out the possibility of miscategorizing the child regarding their CST wiring pattern.

2.5. Statistical Analyses. First, descriptive statistics were used to document the distribution of brain lesion characteristics according to the CST wiring. Next, we investigated the differences in occurrence of lesion timing, location, and extent between the CST wiring groups by using analysis of contingency tables (chi-square and Fisher's exact tests), Kruskal-Wallis test (ordinal data), and ANOVA (lesion extent). Lastly, we used discriminant analysis to explore whether the type of CST wiring would differ depending on the linear combination of lesion timing, location, and extent, in a multivariate way. Cross-validation procedure was included to investigate the accuracy of the model in reclassifying the participants in the original CST wiring groups. Variables related to lesion timing, lesion location (damage to the frontal lobe, parietal lobe, PLIC, basal ganglia, and thalamus), and extent (ipsilesional extent of the lesion) were included in the model, which was fitted using the stepwise selection method.

To investigate the impact of the type of CST wiring and brain lesion characteristics on UL function, we first used linear simple regression and then multiple regression analysis to investigate the combined impact of these factors on UL motor and sensory functions. For the continuous variables related to motor function, normality was first verified by inspecting the histograms and with the Shapiro-Wilk test, showing a normal distribution only for the AHA. For the JTHFT ratio and the grip strength ratio, a logarithmic transformation was applied ($y' = \log 10 (y)$). To investigate the impact of the type of CST wiring and brain lesion characteristics on UL motor function, we computed a multiple regression analysis. Similarly, for UL sensory function, we conducted a simple ordinal logistic regression for stereognosis

and thresholds for touch sensation and a simple logistic regression for 2PD to investigate the impact of each individual neurological factor on the sensory function. Next, we performed multiple regression analyses (ordinal and logistic) to investigate the combined impact of the neurological predictors on the sensory deficits. The predictors included in the multiple regression model were the type of CST wiring, lesion timing, location (damage to the frontal lobe, parietal lobe, PLIC, basal ganglia, and thalamus), and ipsilesional extent of the lesion. To predict both motor and sensory functions, interaction terms were built between the CST wiring and (i) lesion timing and (ii) lesion extent and included in the model. The multiple regression models were fitted with the backward elimination method until a set of variables significantly contributing to the model was identified.

Lastly, to investigate the relation between sensory and motor functions for the whole group and within CST wiring groups, Spearman rank correlation coefficients were used between each of the motor function variables and deficits in stereognosis. Correlation coefficients were considered as little or no correlation (<0.30), low (0.30–0.50), moderate (0.50–0.70), high (0.70–0.90), and very high correlation (>0.90) [35].

In addition, effects sizes were calculated for the comparisons and interpreted according to Cohen, depending on the computed test: η^2 (partial eta squared) for the prediction models (small 0.01, medium 0.06, and large 0.14) [36, 37]. Statistical significance was set at $\alpha < 0.05$ for main tests with Bonferroni correction for post hoc tests. All statistical analyses were computed with SPSS Statistics for Windows version 24.0 (IBM Corp., Armonk, NY).

3. Results

3.1. Participants. Seventy-five children and adolescents with uCP participated in this study (mean age (SD): 11 y and 1 m (3 y and 6 m); 33 girls; 39 left uCP). According to the Manual Ability Classification System (MACS), 25 individuals were classified as MACS I, 25 as MACS II, and 25 as MACS III. Sixteen participants did not have CST wiring data ($n = 1$ panic attack, $n = 2$ hemispherectomy, $n = 3$ VP shunt, $n = 2$ epilepsy, $n = 1$ tumor, $n = 4$ refusals to participate, and $n = 3$ inconclusive TMS results), resulting in a total of 59 participants. The TMS assessment identified 20 individuals with CST_{contra}, 18 with CST_{bilat}, and 21 with CST_{ipsi}. For the analyses in this study, participants with malformations ($n = 1$), acquired lesions ($n = 4$), or no visible lesions ($n = 2$) were excluded due to the very small sample size of these subgroups, resulting in a total group of 52 participants (mean age (SD): 11 y and 4 m (3 y and 10 m); 22 girls; 28 left uCP) with available CST wiring ($n = 17$ contralateral, $n = 19$ ipsilateral, and $n = 16$ bilateral) and data related to the timing, location, and extent of the lesion. A summary of the lesion locations and extent according to the lesion timing is provided in Supplementary Materials (Table 1). Thirty-four individuals had a PV lesion, and 18 had a CSC lesion. Clinical motor and sensory data was missing in one participant (boy, 19 y and 7 m, PV lesion, and CST_{contra} wiring), and sensory data

TABLE 1: Contingency table (count and percentage, descriptive statistics) of the occurrence of lesion timing, location, and extent according to the CST wiring.

| | | | CST wiring | | | |
			Contralateral	Bilateral	Ipsilateral	p value
Timing						
Lesion timing[¥]	PV	N (%)	15 (88.2%)	8 (50%)	11 (57.9%)	0.04
	CSC		2 (11.8)	8 (50%)	8 (42.1%)	
Location						
PLIC[¥]	Not affected	N (%)	8 (47%)	1 (6%)	0 (0%)	<0.001
	Affected		9 (53%)	15 (94%)	19 (100%)	
Basal ganglia and thalamus[◊]		Me (p25–p75)	0 (0–1)	1.50 (0–2.50)	1 (1–2)	0.006[a,b]
Frontal lobe[◊]		Me (p25–p75)	1 (1–1)	1.50 (1–2.25)	1 (1–1.50)	0.004[a,b]
Parietal lobe[◊]		Me (p25–p75)	2 (1–2)	2 (1.25–3)	2 (2–2.50)	0.09
Extent						
Ipsilesional extent[○]		X (SD)	5.18 (3.07)	8.38 (3.95)	9.05 (3.27)	0.004[a,b]

CST: corticospinal tract; PV: periventricular; CSC: corticosubcortical; PLIC: posterior limb of the internal capsule. [¥]Chi-square statistic. [$]Fisher's exact test. [◊]Kruskal-Wallis test. [○]ANOVA. [a]Contralateral vs. ipsilateral. [b]Contralateral vs. bilateral.

was evaluated in a subsample of participants (see Section 3.3.2 for more details).

3.2. CST Wiring and Brain Lesion Characteristics.

Table 1 displays the distribution of lesion timing, location, and extent variables according to the three CST wiring groups. Except for the damage to the parietal lobe, all variables were significantly different between the CST wiring groups ($p < 0.05$) (Table 1).

In the discriminant analysis, we found that the combined value of the damage to the PLIC and the damage to the frontal lobe could significantly discriminate between the type of CST wiring (Wilks' $\lambda = 0.611$, chi-square test $= 23.88$, df $= 4$, canonical correlation $= 0.602$, $p < 0.001$). The two functions extracted accounted for nearly 57% of the variance in the type of CST wiring. The standardized discriminant function coefficients of the two extracted functions indicated the contribution of each retained independent variable (damage to the PLIC and damage to the frontal lobe) to each function, showing how strongly the discriminant variables affect the score. These coefficients can be then used for the classification of a single individual (function $1 = 0.81 *$ damage to the PLIC $+ 0.50 *$ damage to the frontal lobe; function $2 = -0.60 *$ damage to the PLIC $+ 0.88 *$ damage to the frontal lobe).

Cross-validated reclassification of cases based on the new canonical variables was successful in 57.7% of the cases: 89.5% were correctly classified in the CST_{ipsi} group, 47.1% in the CST_{contra} group, and only 31.3% in the CST_{bilat} group (Figure 1).

3.3. CST Wiring, Brain Lesion Characteristics, and UL Function

3.3.1. Motor Function.

Descriptive statistics of the motor function according to the type of CST wiring, lesion timing, location, and extent are presented in Supplementary Materials (Table 2). The simple linear regression analyses to predict motor function based on a single neurological factor showed

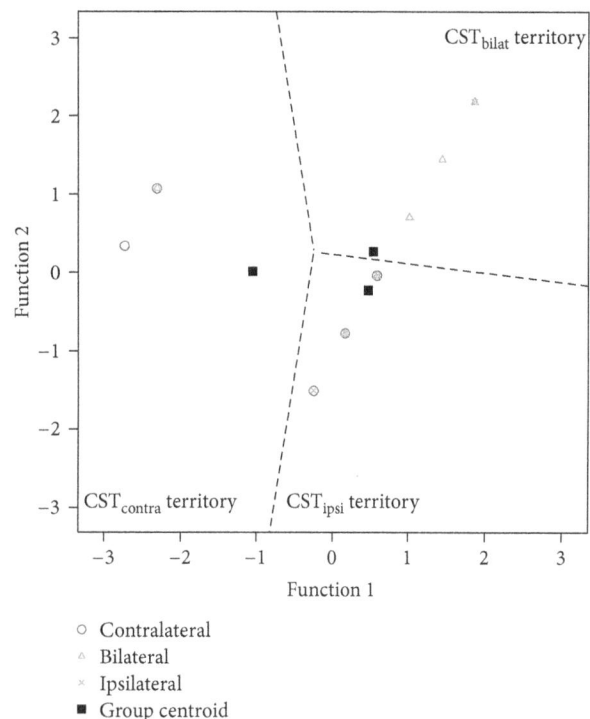

FIGURE 1: Territorial map showing the relative location of the boundaries of each CST wiring category and the location of each of the participants. The group centroids are indicated with a black-filled square (CST_{contra} (−1.05, 0.01), CST_{ipsi} (0.48, −0.23), and CST_{bilat} (0.54, 0.26)).

that every factor had an influence on motor function (grip strength, $p < 0.04$; JTHFT, $p < 0.004$; AHA, $p < 0.01$; see Supplementary Materials Table 2 for detailed information).

When all the neurological factors were included in the same model in a multiple regression analysis, the backward elimination method identified the variables that were significantly contributing to the model. Table 2 documents the estimated marginal means, which represent the mean response

TABLE 2: Descriptive statistics of the observed and estimated marginal means of upper limb motor function according to the CST wiring groups.

	Estimated marginal means and SD		
	CST_{contra} ($n = 16$)	CST_{ipsi} ($n = 19$)	CST_{bilat} ($n = 16$)
Grip strength ratio (log)[a]	0.14 (0.13)	0.55 (0.20)	0.46 (0.24)
JTHFT ratio (log)[b]	0.30 (0.24)	0.67 (0.23)	0.64 (0.22)
AHA (0–100)[c]	79.66 (10.28)	58.70 (9.81)	61.58 (9.67)

CST: corticospinal tract; JTHFT: Jebsen-Taylor hand function test; AHA: Assisting Hand Assessment; SD: standard deviation. [a]The values coincide with the observed values, as there is no significant covariate in the model. [b]Adjustments based on ipsilesional lesion extent mean = 7.67. [c]Adjustments based on ipsilesional lesion extent mean = 7.67 and damage to the basal ganglia and thalamus mean = 1.12.

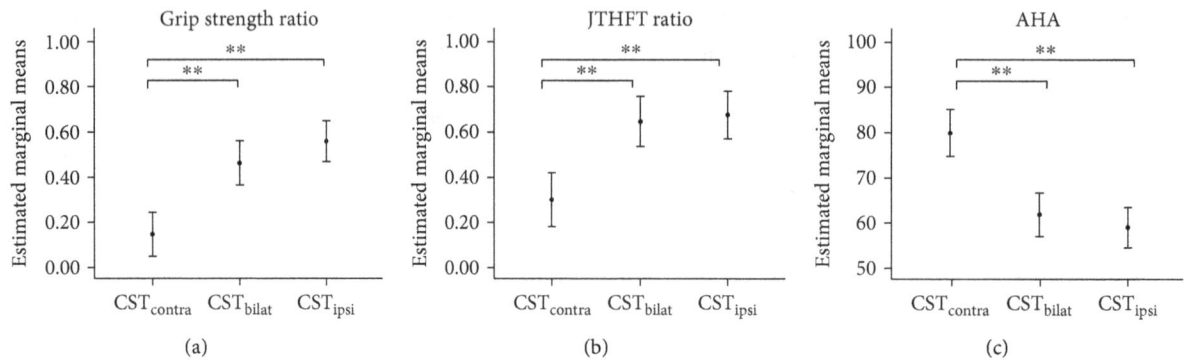

FIGURE 2: Upper limb motor function differs in individuals with CST_{contra} wiring compared to those with CST_{bilat} or CST_{ipsi} wiring. Estimated marginal means and 95% CI per CST wiring type and lesion timing group for (a) grip strength (log ratio, i.e., closer to zero indicates preserved grip strength), (b) JTHFT (log ratio, i.e., closer to zero indicates preserved manual dexterity, measured by speed), and (c) AHA. AHA: Assisting Hand Assessment; JTHFT: Jebsen-Taylor hand function test; CST: corticospinal tract. $*p < 0.01$; $**p < 0.001$. Estimated marginal means are adjusted according to the significant covariates (see Table 2 for details).

in each CST wiring group adjusted by the covariates that significantly contribute to the model. The multiple regression model to predict grip strength deficits only retained the type of CST wiring, explaining 46% of the variance ($F(2, 51) = 20.90$; $p < 0.001$; $\eta^2 = 0.47$). For the JTHFT, 54% of the variance was explained by the type of CST wiring ($F(2, 51) = 12.20$; $p < 0.0001$; $\eta^2 = 0.34$, $R^2 = 46\%$) and the total extent of the lesion ($F(1, 51) = 8.05$; $p = 0.007$; $\eta^2 = 0.15$, $\Delta R^2 = 8\%$). For bimanual performance (AHA), the regression model explained 61% of the variance, with the type of CST wiring ($F(2, 51) = 19.03$; $p < 0.0001$; $\eta^2 = 0.45$, $\Delta R^2 = 52\%$), the total extent of the lesion ($F(1, 51) = 10.65$; $p < 0.001$; $\eta^2 = 0.19$, $\Delta R^2 = 5\%$), and the damage to the basal ganglia and thalamus ($F(1, 51) = 4.90$; $p = 0.03$; $\eta^2 = 0.10$, $\Delta R^2 = 4\%$) significantly contributing to the model (Figure 2). No interaction effects were identified for any of the motor outcome variables.

3.3.2. Sensory Function. Descriptive information of sensory function according to each neurological factor is summarized in Table 3 of Supplementary Materials. Sensory function data (tactile sense, movement sense, stereognosis, and 2PD) and thresholds for touch sensation, as assessed with the monofilaments, were available in 46 and 35 individuals, respectively. Due to the lack of variation in the tactile sense and movement sense modalities, the predictive model was only applied to the stereognosis, 2PD, and the thresholds for touch sensation.

The simple linear analyses to predict sensory function based on a single neurological predictor indicated that every predictor impacted on stereognosis ($p < 0.032$). In contrast, 2PD was influenced by all neurological predictors ($p < 0.04$) except the damage to the PLIC ($p < 0.17$) and touch sensation could be significantly predicted by all factors ($p < 0.01$) except damage to the PLIC ($p = 0.99$) and type of CST wiring ($p = 0.42$).

When all the neurological factors were included in the same model in a multiple regression analysis, the backward elimination method identified predictors that were significantly contributing to the model. For stereognosis, the retained main effects were the CST wiring (Wald chi-square test (2) = 9.09, $p = 0.011$), lesion timing (Wald chi-square test (1) = 4.34, $p = 0.04$), and ipsilesional extent of the lesion (Wald chi-square test (1) = 7.15, $p = 0.008$) (Table 3(a)). These results show that the odds of having better stereognosis function were 5.56 times higher in the group with PV lesions than in the CSC group ($p = 0.04$). Similarly, individuals with a CST_{contra} wiring show 10.23 and 9.7 times higher probability of having better scores in the stereognosis test compared to those with a CST_{ipsi} or CST_{bilat} wiring, respectively ($p = 0.02$), whilst there was no difference between the last two ($p = 0.34$). Lastly, the odds of having higher stereognosis scores decrease by 0.74 for every unit change in the ipsilesional extent of the lesion ($p = 0.01$). No interactions were found between the CST wiring and the brain lesion characteristics to predict deficits in stereognosis ($p > 0.05$).

TABLE 3: Descriptive statistics of the sensory function ((a) stereognosis (number of correctly recognized objects), (b) two-point discrimination, and (c) touch sensation) according to each of the variables significantly contributing to each prediction model.

(a)

		Stereognosis (number of correctly guessed objects)						
		0	1	2	3	4	5	6
Lesion timing								
PV	N (%)	0 (0%)	0 (0%)	1 (25%)	0 (0%)	5 (71%)	6 (67%)	17 (44%)
CSC	N (%)	5 (100%)	2 (100%)	3 (75%)	1 (100%)	2 (29%)	3 (33%)	1 (6%)
CST wiring								
Contralateral	N (%)	0 (0%)	0 (0%)	1 (25%)	0 (0%)	0 (0%)	1 (11%)	13 (72%)
Bilateral	N (%)	4 (80%)	0 (0%)	2 (50%)	0 (0%)	3 (43%)	3 (33%)	3 (17%)
Ipsilateral	N (%)	1 (20%)	2 (100%)	1 (25%)	1 (100%)	4 (57%)	5 (56%)	2 (11%)
Lesion extent								
Ipsilesional	Me (IQR)	13 (2.07)	13 (—)	10 (3.88)	—	6 (3.50)	6 (5.25)	5.25 (3.75)

(b)

		Two-point discrimination	
		Normal (≤4 mm)	Impaired (>5 mm)
Lesion timing			
PV	N (%)	26 (93%)	3 (17%)
CSC	N (%)	2 (7%)	15 (83%)
Lesion extent			
Ipsilesional	Me (IQR)	5.25 (3.88)	12 (5.25)

(c)

		Threshold of touch sensation			
	Normal	Diminished light touch	Diminished protective sensation	Loss of protective sensation	Untestable
Lesion extent					
Ipsilesional Me (IQR)	6 (4.50)	—	10.50 (11.25)	13 (2.41)	12.50 (—)

PV: periventricular lesion; CSC: corticosubcortical lesion; CST: corticospinal tract; N: number of cases; Me: median; IQR: interquartile range.

The logistic multiple regression to predict 2PD showed lesion timing (Wald chi-square test $(1) = 10.62$, $p = 0.001$) and ipsilesional extent of the lesion (Wald chi-square test $(1) = 3.75$, $p = 0.05$) to be significant contributors ($p > 0.05$) (Table 3(b)). The odds of having an impaired 2PD are 31 times higher in the group with CSC lesions than in the PVL group ($p = 0.001$). Secondly, the odds of having impaired 2PD increase by 1.34 for every unit change in the ipsilesional extent of the lesion ($p = 0.05$). No interactions were found between the CST wiring and the brain lesion characteristics to predict deficits in 2PD ($p > 0.05$).

The ordinal logistic multiple regression for touch sensation, as measured by the monofilaments, indicated that only the lesion extent significantly contributed to the deficits in touch sensation (Wald chi-square test $(1) = 10.75$, $p = 0.001$) (Table 3(c)). The odds of having better touch sensation decrease by 0.66 for every unit change in the ipsilesional extent of the lesion. No interactions were found between the CST wiring and the brain lesion characteristics to predict deficits in touch sensation ($p > 0.05$).

3.3.3. Impact of CST Wiring on the Relation between Motor and Sensory Functions. The correlation analyses between the motor and sensory functions for the whole group indicated a moderate association between the stereognosis score and grip strength ratio ($r_s = -0.60$, $p < 0.001$), JTHFT ratio ($r_s = -0.60$, $p < 0.001$), and AHA ($r_s = 0.61$, $p < 0.001$).

After group division according to CST wiring, there was no low correlation between motor function and stereognosis in the CST_{contra} and CST_{ipsi} groups (r_s (range) $= -0.31$–0.36, $p > 0.05$). Interestingly, in the CST_{bilat} group, moderate correlations were found with the JTHFT ratio ($r_s = -0.48$, $p = 0.07$) and the AHA ($r_s = 0.65$, $p < 0.01$), despite a low correlation with grip strength ratio ($r_s = -0.31$, $p = 0.2$). An illustration of the individual data points regarding these results can be found in Figure 3.

4. Discussion

In this study, we explored the predictive value of brain lesion characteristics on the type of CST wiring as well as the impact of these factors on UL motor and sensory functions. A comprehensive and standardized evaluation of both motor (grip strength, unimanual capacity, and bimanual performance) and sensory functions was used to predict UL function in a large cohort of individuals with uCP.

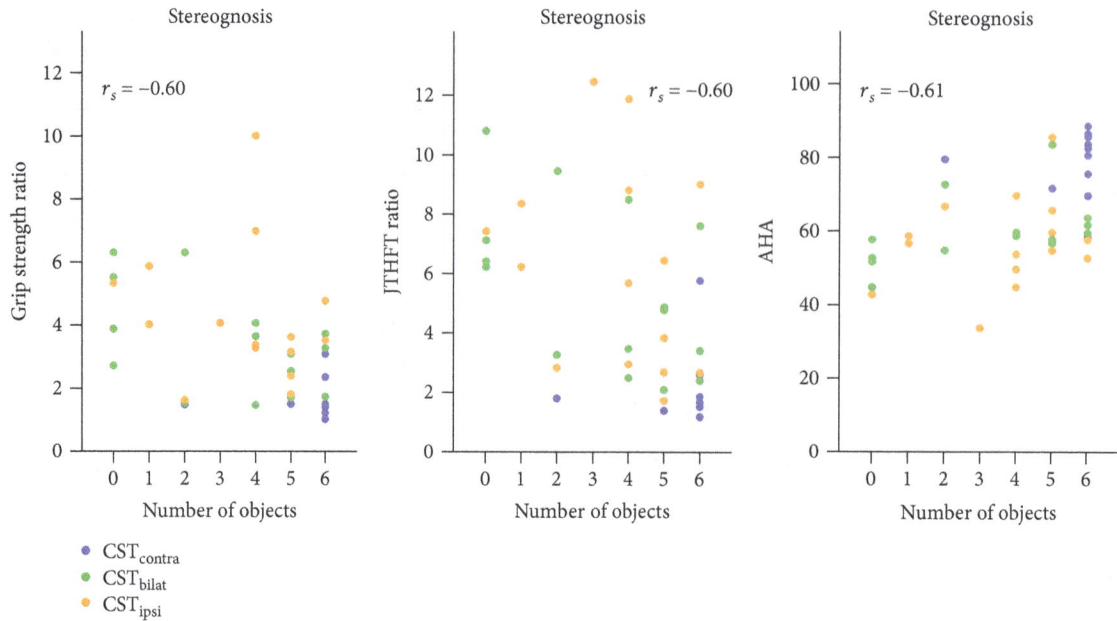

FIGURE 3: The relation between motor and sensory functions seems to vary depending on the CST wiring. Individuals with a CST_{contra} and CST_{ipsi} wiring showed no low correlations, whereas those with CST_{bilat} showed moderate correlations. Each dot represents an individual child, with CST_{contra} (blue), CST_{bilat} (green), and CST_{ipsi} (orange). Correlations between stereognosis with grip strength ratio (ratio, i.e., closer to one indicates preserved grip strength), JTHFT ratio (ratio, i.e., closer to one indicates preserved grip strength), and AHA. Correlation coefficients correspond to the analysis for the whole group.

Our first research question examined the discriminant ability of lesion timing, location, and extent to predict the type of CST wiring. A simple linear analysis demonstrated that lesion timing, location, and extent were significantly different between the CST wiring groups. Our results showed that a CST_{contra} was only seen in 2 out of 18 children with a CSC lesion, compared to 15 out of 34 children with a PV lesion. Current results suggest that damage to cortical and/or subcortical structures (i.e., CSC lesion) reduces the potential of the CST to develop according to its typical contralateral trajectory. We hypothesize that this is likely driven by the reduced neural activity in the motor cortical areas after a CSC lesion, which are crucial for the development of the CST during the postnatal period [38]. However, a contralateral development of the CST is still possible in CSC lesions, and it may occur differently depending on lesion location and extent.

Once all predictors were simultaneously entered in a multiple linear analysis, we found that the combination of the damage to the PLIC and the frontal lobe significantly discriminated between the CST wiring groups. Half of the children in the CST_{contra} group showed damage to the PLIC, in contrast to the 94% and 100% in the CST_{bilat} and CST_{ipsi} groups who showed damage to this white matter bundle. Furthermore, the frontal lobe was also more damaged in the CST_{bilat} and CST_{ipsi} groups, compared to the CST_{contra} group. Although it is not unexpected that the PLIC and the frontal lobe are the two significant predictors in the model, due to their undoubtable relation with the motor cortex and the performance of actions, this is the first time that this interaction with the type of CST wiring is shown. Contrary to the importance of the location, Staudt et al. [4] postulated

that the type of CST wiring depended on the lesion extent. However, as they only included children with a PV lesion, their results cannot be extended to all the uCP populations. Further efforts should be made to underpin whether structural damage of the brain lesion may serve as a biomarker of the underlying CST wiring.

Next to the predictive model, we also investigated how accurate the two functions derived from the discriminant analysis would be to reclassify the individuals in their original categories. Despite the significant contribution of the PLIC and the frontal lobe to the discriminant model, the classification accuracy only reached 57%, suggesting that timing, location, and extent of the lesion (as included in the model) do not provide sufficient accurate information to predict the underlying type of CST wiring. Notwithstanding the validity and reliability of the semiquantitative scale that was used to investigate lesion location and extent, we acknowledge that the semiquantitative character of the scale may have underestimated the predictive value of the structural brain damage. Therefore, these results should be replicated in the future with volumetric measures of the different brain structures. For example, the projections to the PLIC have been shown to be topographically organized with reduced microstructural integrity in children with uCP [39] by using diffusion measures. Investigating the volumetric damage to the frontal lobe and the microstructural integrity of the PLIC may provide with further insights in determining the type of CST wiring in uCP.

For our second research question, we investigated the impact of CST wiring and brain lesion characteristics (timing, location, and extent) on motor and sensory functions. Regarding *motor outcome*, simple linear regression analyses indicated that the CST wiring and all brain lesion characteristics had an influence on the grip strength, manual dexterity, and bimanual performance, which confirmed what previous studies have shown [5, 6, 10]. However, in the multiple linear regression analysis, we found that the underlying CST wiring plays a major, but not unique, role in determining UL motor function, as lesion location and extent also significantly contributed to increasing the explained variance for the JTHFT and AHA. Specifically, the type of CST wiring explained 46% and 52% of the JTHFT and AHA variances, respectively, which was increased up to 54% and 61% by including lesion extent and damage to the basal ganglia and thalamus into the model. In general, our results show that a CST_{ipsi} or CST_{bilat} leads to poorer UL motor function compared to CST_{contra} for all motor outcomes, even when controlling for the significant contribution of lesion extent and location. The importance of the underlying CST wiring is an expected result, as the CST is the main motor drive and its damage causes vast disturbances on voluntary motor control, drastically reducing motor capabilities [38]. Whilst lesion timing, location, and extent have been put forward as a predictor of UL function [2, 3] and were also confirmed in our linear regression analysis, the huge variability in motor function reported by previous studies seems to be mainly explained by the underlying CST wiring. Staudt et al. [10] were the first to report on the relation between CST reorganization potential at different gestational ages and UL motor function. These authors also found that, along with the CST wiring, UL motor function further worsened in later lesions (CSC lesions) [10]. Linear regression analysis also showed that later lesions led to poor motor outcome, but multiple regression analysis revealed that lesion location and extent were key factors, next to the type of CST wiring. Although later lesions seem to be associated to a larger extent [3], it seems that the lesion extent itself plays a more important role in motor outcome, i.e., children with a PV lesion with large extent will also present with poorer hand function. Interestingly, the damage to the basal ganglia and thalamus explained an extra 4% of the variability in the AHA. In accordance with our results, previous studies have reported the negative impact of these subcortical structures on UL motor outcome [2, 5].

It is important to note that we still found large variability in the three motor outcome measures within both the CST_{ipsi} and CST_{bilat} groups, whereas the variability in the CST_{contra} group was rather small (Figure 2, see also Table 2 Supplementary Materials for observed means). In other words, some individuals with a CST_{ipsi} and CST_{bilat} wiring had good motor function, similar to those with a CST_{contra} wiring. This variability could not be completely explained by the location and extent of the lesion, and other factors may play a role. In the CST_{ipsi} group, this large variability may be explained by the amount of overlap of the hotspot within the nonlesioned hemisphere to evoke MEPs in the affected and less-affected hands. Vandermeeren et al. [40] showed that dexterity indeed varies in individuals with ipsilateral wiring depending on the location of the hotspot of the CST innervating the affected hand and less-affected hand; overlapping hotspots resulted in poorer dexterity, whereas distinct nonoverlapping hotspots resulted in a preserved dexterity. Conversely, in the CST_{bilat} group, the large variability may be explained by a predominant contralateral or ipsilateral projection that controls the affected hand, as Jaspers et al. [9] proposed in their theoretical framework. Altogether, this seems to point toward a distinct underlying pathophysiology of the UL motor impairments in these two CST groups (CST_{ipsi} or CST_{bilat}), suggesting that individuals with either a CST_{bilat} or CST_{ipsi} pattern should be treated as two separate groups for future research. To further unravel the underlying mechanisms of the pathophysiology of motor control and motor capabilities in uCP, additional functional measures should be included such as excitatory and inhibitory intracortical circuits based on TMS (e.g., cortical silent period or paired-pulse paradigms) [15, 41] or functional connectivity of the sensorimotor network based on resting-state functional MRI [42, 43].

We also investigated the impact of the CST wiring and brain lesion characteristics on *sensory function*, based on the fact that CST projections also extend from the primary sensory cortex and mediate several sensory functions at the level of the spinal cord (control of nociceptive, somatosensory, and somatic motor functions) [44, 45]. Although our simple linear regression analyses suggested that all neurological factors individually played a role in determining sensory function, the multiple prediction model showed that a larger lesion extent, a later lesion (i.e., CSC lesion), and a CST_{ipsi} or CST_{bilat} led to higher chances of developing sensory deficits. Our results are in agreement with a recent study by Gupta et al. [6], who showed that more than 80% of the children with larger extent and later lesions (CSC) had disrupted somatosensory anatomy and physiology (lack of ascending sensory tracts and lack of somatosensory evoked potentials), consequently leading to a loss of sensory function [6]. If the sensory tracts are present, there is evidence suggesting that their main compensatory mechanism is an intrahemispheric reorganization, i.e., the sensory system reaches the original cortical destination on the postcentral gyrus, regardless of lesion timing (PV or CSC lesion) or CST wiring [11, 46, 47]. Current study results suggest that lesion extent best predicts the sensory deficits in individuals with uCP, although lesion timing and CST wiring also play an important role. Future research focusing on the pathophysiology of the sensory system based on noninvasive neurophysiological techniques (e.g., short-latency afferent inhibition [48] or sensory evoked potentials [11]), as well as functional connectivity measures, may contribute to increase our understanding of the underlying sensory pathways in uCP.

Lastly, we investigated whether the relationship between motor and sensory functions was disrupted by the type of CST wiring. We first confirmed previous study results indicating a significant relation between the motor and sensory outcomes in the total group [1, 25]. However, this association was disrupted by the type of CST wiring, whereby no little association was shown in the CST_{ipsi} and CST_{contra} groups, but a moderate association was found for the CST_{bilat} group. In the CST_{contra} group, the lack of a significant (or high) correlation seems to be due to the fact that these participants show both adequate motor and sensory functions, with little variation in the sensory scale, due to its ordinal nature. This scale used to evaluate sensory function may not be sensitive enough to detect subtle sensory deficits, leading to a possible ceiling effect in the CST_{contra} group. By measuring with more quantitative techniques and devices, e.g., KINARM End-Point Lab (BKIN Technologies) [49], we may be able to discern the potential sensory problems that these individuals may present with. Secondly, the sensorimotor dissociation found in the CST_{ipsi} group may be explained at two different levels of the central nervous system. At the level of the spinal cord, the descending CST fibres entering the dorsal horn play an important role in presynaptic inhibition of primary sensory afferent fibres [45, 50], ensuring smooth execution of a movement. A CST_{ipsi} wiring may have consequences in the presynaptic inhibition at the level of the spinal cord and could, consequently, affect the relation between motor and sensory functions. On the other hand, at the level of the brain, the intrahemispheric communication between M1 and S1 has been shown to be very relevant for adequate processing of sensorimotor information [51–53]. As such, the lack of intrahemispheric corticocortical connections may affect the processing of sensory information, having a negative impact on the motor command. On the contrary, the CST_{bilat} group seems to preserve the relation between motor and sensory functions, as shown by the stereognosis modality. This may be potentially explained by the predominant behaviour that those with a CST_{bilat} wiring hypothetically show [9]. A relation between adequate sensory and adequate motor functions, as seen in the CST_{contra} group, may indicate a more "contralateral" behaviour, whilst a disparate relation may be indicative of rather an "ipsilateral" behaviour. However, this needs further confirmation with neurophysiological tools. Although current data do not allow drawing strong conclusions regarding sensorimotor integration, our results highlight the importance of investigating these aspects in the future to better understand the mechanisms of sensorimotor information processing in uCP. By using more advanced techniques to unravel the coupling between the sensory and motor systems, we will be able to determine the impact of such dissociation on motor control and motor performance. For instance, short-latency afferent inhibition has been put forward as a valuable indicator of the process of bilateral sensorimotor integration [48] and may potentially aid in measuring the reorganization of sensorimotor pathways in uCP.

There might be some important clinical implications based on the results of this study. A better understanding of the underlying mechanisms of motor and sensory impairments will surely contribute to developing new treatment approaches, specifically targeting the individual pathophysiological deficits. First, the type of CST wiring has been investigated as a potential biomarker of treatment response. Although motor improvement does not seem to be CST-type dependent after bimanual training [12, 54], there are conflicting results regarding unimanual training [55–57]. Furthermore, our results highlight the importance of considering the sensory system together with the available motor execution paradigms during UL training. Preliminary results of recent studies have shown the effectiveness of bimanual and sensory training on both motor and sensory functions

in uCP [58, 59]. To further support interventions targeting sensory deficits, there is evidence in healthy adults suggesting that sensory input can modulate the excitability in both motor cortices simultaneously, as well as the communication between hemispheres [60]. In this line, it seems relevant to combine bimanual and sensory training to enhance the excitability of both motor cortices, which may increase intra- and interhemispheric connections between the sensory and motor systems, potentially resulting in long-lasting neuroplastic changes.

Next to the training approaches, it is also important to identify clinically feasible measures to infer the CST wiring and the sensory system. As these assessments are not always pleasant in young children nor practical in a clinical setting, there is a necessity to find tools that are more applicable to daily practice than neurophysiological techniques. To probe the motor system, mirror movements have been put forward as a valid clinical assessment tool that may reflect the underlying individual CST wiring [9, 61]. On the other hand, it seems very challenging to develop an accessible and simple tool to clinically probe the sensory system in uCP. Further research in this field is required to develop quantitative and valid measures of sensory function (e.g., perceptual threshold of touch with electrical stimulation [62] or robotic measures of proprioception [49, 63]) and to link these measures to the underlying mechanisms of the sensory system in uCP.

There are some limitations to be considered for the current study. First, we used scales for the evaluation of lesion location and extent, as well as for assessing sensory function that was based on an ordinal scoring. Although they have been shown to be reliable in uCP [25, 29], such scales may lack sensitivity. Second, our study lacked a neurophysiological technique to probe the sensory system (i.e., sensory evoked potentials) that may contribute to better understand the underlying mechanisms of sensory function in individuals with uCP. Third, the main limitation of the TMS assessment itself lays in the maximum stimulator output intensity that can be reached. This intensity may not have been sufficient to elicit a MEP from either the lesioned or the nonlesioned hemisphere, as the resting motor thresholds are normally higher in children and may be even higher in individuals with uCP. This limitation might have prevented us from finding a CST projection to eventually diagnose the individual as CST_{bilat} or CST_{ipsi} wiring. Furthermore, the MEP data were not analysed, which may provide with useful insights in future studies. Lastly, although our sample size was large and covers the most common lesion timing groups, our results cannot be completely extended to those children with malformations or postnatally acquired brain injuries, as these were not included in the analyses.

5. Conclusions

CST wiring mainly determines UL motor function, although also lesion extent and damage to the basal ganglia and thalamus significantly contributed to the prediction of UL motor deficits. For sensory function, lesion extent, timing, and the type of CST wiring pattern seem to be important to develop adequate sensory function. The underlying CST wiring seems to disrupt the association between sensory and motor functions, pointing toward different mechanisms of sensorimotor integration in uCP. The results of our study contribute to a better understanding of the underlying pathophysiology of motor and sensory functions and highlight the importance of investigating sensorimotor integration in future studies. Subsequently, these insights will aid in developing new intervention strategies tailored to the specific deficits of the motor and sensory systems of the individual child with uCP.

Acknowledgments

We would like to express our deepest gratitude to the children and families who participated in this study. We also specially thank Jasmine Hoskens for her assistance during the clinical assessments. Lastly, we would like to acknowledge the biostatisticians from the Leuven Biostatistics and Statistical Bioinformatics Centre (L-BioStat) of the KU Leuven (Prof. Geert Molenberghs and Dr. Annouschka Laenen) for their advice regarding the statistical analysis. This work is funded by the Fund Scientific Research Flanders (FWO project, grant G087213N) and by the Special Research Fund, KU Leuven (OT/14/127, project grant 3M140230).

Supplementary Materials

Table 1: descriptive information of the distribution of the lesion location and extent according to the lesion timing groups. Table 2: descriptive statistics (X (SD)) and univariate analysis of upper limb motor function according to the CST wiring and the brain lesion characteristics. Table 3: descriptive statistics (Me (IQR)) and univariate analysis of upper limb sensory function (3A, stereognosis and 3B, two-point discrimination and thresholds of touch sensation) according to the CST wiring and the brain lesion characteristics. (Supplementary Materials)

References

[1] K. Klingels, I. Demeyere, E. Jaspers et al., "Upper limb impairments and their impact on activity measures in children with unilateral cerebral palsy," *European Journal of Paediatric Neurology*, vol. 16, no. 5, pp. 475–484, 2012.

[2] H. Feys, M. Eyssen, E. Jaspers et al., "Relation between neuroradiological findings and upper limb function in hemiplegic cerebral palsy," *European Journal of Paediatric Neurology*, vol. 14, no. 2, pp. 169–177, 2010.

[3] L. Mailleux, K. Klingels, S. Fiori et al., "How does the interaction of presumed timing, location and extent of the underlying brain lesion relate to upper limb function in children with unilateral cerebral palsy?," *European Journal of Paediatric Neurology*, vol. 21, no. 5, pp. 763–772, 2017.

[4] M. Staudt, W. Grodd, C. Gerloff, M. Erb, J. Stitz, and I. Krägeloh-Mann, "Two types of ipsilateral reorganization in congenital hemiparesis: a TMS and fMRI study," *Brain*, vol. 125, no. 10, pp. 2222–2237, 2002.

[5] L. Holmström, B. Vollmer, K. Tedroff et al., "Hand function in relation to brain lesions and corticomotor-projection pattern in children with unilateral cerebral palsy," *Developmental Medicine & Child Neurology*, vol. 52, no. 2, pp. 145–152, 2010.

[6] D. Gupta, A. Barachant, A. M. Gordon et al., "Effect of sensory and motor connectivity on hand function in pediatric hemiplegia," *Annals of Neurology*, vol. 82, no. 5, pp. 766–780, 2017.

[7] I. Krägeloh-Mann and V. Horber, "The role of magnetic resonance imaging in elucidating the pathogenesis of cerebral palsy: a systematic review," *Developmental Medicine & Child Neurology*, vol. 49, no. 2, pp. 144–151, 2007.

[8] L. J. Carr, "Development and reorganization of descending motor pathways in children with hemiplegic cerebral palsy," *Acta Paediatrica*, vol. 85, no. s416, pp. 53–57, 1996.

[9] E. Jaspers, W. D. Byblow, H. Feys, and N. Wenderoth, "The corticospinal tract: a biomarker to categorize upper limb functional potential in unilateral cerebral palsy," *Frontiers in Pediatrics*, vol. 3, p. 112, 2016.

[10] M. Staudt, C. Gerloff, W. Grodd, H. Holthausen, G. Niemann, and I. Krägeloh-Mann, "Reorganization in congenital hemiparesis acquired at different gestational ages," *Annals of Neurology*, vol. 56, no. 6, pp. 854–863, 2004.

[11] A. Guzzetta, P. Bonanni, L. Biagi et al., "Reorganisation of the somatosensory system after early brain damage," *Clinical Neurophysiology*, vol. 118, no. 5, pp. 1110–1121, 2007.

[12] A. R. P. Smorenburg, A. M. Gordon, H. C. Kuo et al., "Does corticospinal tract connectivity influence the response to intensive bimanual therapy in children with unilateral cerebral palsy?," *Neurorehabilitation and Neural Repair*, vol. 31, no. 3, pp. 250–260, 2017.

[13] E. Zewdie, O. Damji, P. Ciechanski, T. Seeger, and A. Kirton, "Contralesional corticomotor neurophysiology in hemiparetic children with perinatal stroke: developmental plasticity and clinical function," *Neurorehabilitation and Neural Repair*, vol. 31, no. 3, pp. 261–271, 2017.

[14] E. Arnfield, A. Guzzetta, and R. Boyd, "Relationship between brain structure on magnetic resonance imaging and motor outcomes in children with cerebral palsy: a systematic review," *Research in Developmental Disabilities*, vol. 34, no. 7, pp. 2234–2250, 2013.

[15] A. Mackey, C. Stinear, S. Stott, and W. D. Byblow, "Upper limb function and cortical organization in youth with unilateral cerebral palsy," *Frontiers in Neurology*, vol. 5, p. 117, 2014.

[16] L. Han, D. Law-Gibson, and M. Reding, "Key neurological impairments influence function-related group outcomes after stroke," *Stroke*, vol. 33, no. 7, pp. 1920–1924, 2002.

[17] A. T. Patel, P. W. Duncan, S.-M. Lai, and S. Studenski, "The relation between impairments and functional outcomes poststroke," *Archives of Physical Medicine and Rehabilitation*, vol. 81, no. 10, pp. 1357–1363, 2000.

[18] N. Taylor, P. L. Sand, and R. H. Jebsen, "Evaluation of hand function in children," *Archives of Physical Medicine and Rehabilitation*, vol. 54, no. 3, pp. 129–135, 1973.

[19] A. M. Gordon, J. Charles, and S. L. Wolf, "Efficacy of constraint-induced movement therapy on involved upper-extremity use in children with hemiplegic cerebral palsy is not age-dependent," *Pediatrics*, vol. 117, no. 3, pp. e363–e373, 2006.

[20] J. R. Charles, S. L. Wolf, J. A. Schneider, and A. M. Gordon, "Efficacy of a child-friendly form of constraint-induced movement therapy in hemiplegic cerebral palsy: a randomized control trial," *Developmental Medicine & Child Neurology*, vol. 48, no. 08, p. 635, 2006.

[21] M. Holmefur, P. Aarts, B. Hoare, and L. Krumlinde-Sundholm, "Test-retest and alternate forms reliability of the assisting hand assessment," *Journal of Rehabilitation Medicine*, vol. 41, no. 11, pp. 886–891, 2009.

[22] L. Krumlinde-sundholm and A.-c. Eliasson, "Development of the assisting hand assessment: a Rasch-built measure intended for children with unilateral upper limb impairments," *Scandinavian Journal of Occupational Therapy*, vol. 10, no. 1, pp. 16–26, 2003.

[23] L. Krumlinde-Sundholm, M. Holmefur, A. Kottorp, and A. C. Eliasson, "The Assisting Hand Assessment: current evidence of validity, reliability, and responsiveness to change," *Developmental Medicine & Child Neurology*, vol. 49, no. 4, pp. 259–264, 2007.

[24] A. Louwers, A. Beelen, M. Holmefur, and L. Krumlinde-Sundholm, "Development of the Assisting Hand Assessment for adolescents (Ad-AHA) and validation of the AHA from 18 months to 18 years," *Developmental Medicine & Child Neurology*, vol. 58, no. 12, pp. 1303–1309, 2016.

[25] K. Klingels, P. de Cock, G. Molenaers et al., "Upper limb motor and sensory impairments in children with hemiplegic cerebral palsy. Can they be measured reliably?," *Disability and Rehabilitation*, vol. 32, no. 5, pp. 409–416, 2010.

[26] E. B. Cope and J. H. Antony, "Normal values for the two-point discrimination test," *Pediatric Neurology*, vol. 8, no. 4, pp. 251–254, 1992.

[27] J. Bell-Krotoski and E. Tomancik, "The repeatability of testing with Semmes-Weinstein monofilaments," *The Journal of Hand Surgery*, vol. 12, no. 1, pp. 155–161, 1987.

[28] M. L. Auld, R. S. Ware, R. N. Boyd, G. L. Moseley, and L. M. Johnston, "Reproducibility of tactile assessments for children with unilateral cerebral palsy," *Physical & Occupational Therapy In Pediatrics*, vol. 32, no. 2, pp. 151–166, 2012.

[29] S. Fiori, G. Cioni, K. Klingels et al., "Reliability of a novel, semi-quantitative scale for classification of structural brain magnetic resonance imaging in children with cerebral palsy," *Developmental Medicine & Child Neurology*, vol. 56, no. 9, pp. 839–845, 2014.

[30] S. Fiori, A. Guzzetta, K. Pannek et al., "Validity of semi-quantitative scale for brain MRI in unilateral cerebral palsy due to periventricular white matter lesions: relationship with hand sensorimotor function and structural connectivity," *NeuroImage: Clinical*, vol. 8, pp. 104–109, 2015.

[31] J. Culham, "Cortical areas engaged in movement: neuroimaging methods," in *International Encyclopedia of the Social & Behavioral Sciences (Second Edition)*, Elsevier, 2015.

[32] H. M. Schambra, R. T. Ogden, I. E. Martínez-Hernández et al., "The reliability of repeated TMS measures in older adults and in patients with subacute and chronic stroke," *Frontiers in Cellular Neuroscience*, vol. 9, p. 335, 2015.

[33] M. R. Goldsworthy, B. Hordacre, and M. C. Ridding, "Minimum number of trials required for within- and between-session reliability of TMS measures of corticospinal excitability," *Neuroscience*, vol. 320, pp. 205–209, 2016.

[34] O. Damji, J. Keess, and A. Kirton, "Evaluating developmental motor plasticity with paired afferent stimulation," *Developmental Medicine & Child Neurology*, vol. 57, no. 6, pp. 548–555, 2015.

[35] D. E. Hinkle, W. Wiersma, and S. G. Jurs, *Applied Statistics for the Behavioral Sciences*, Houghton Mifflin, 2003.

[36] F. Gravetter and L. Wallnau, *Statistics for the Behavioral Sciences*, Wadsworth, Belmont, CA, 2004.

[37] J. Cohen, *Statistical Power Analysis for the Behavioral Sciences*, Elsevier Science, 1988.

[38] J. H. Martin, "The corticospinal system: from development to motor control," *The Neuroscientist*, vol. 11, no. 2, pp. 161–173, 2005.

[39] H. Tsao, K. Pannek, S. Fiori, R. N. Boyd, and S. Rose, "Reduced integrity of sensorimotor projections traversing the posterior limb of the internal capsule in children with congenital hemiparesis," *Research in Developmental Disabilities*, vol. 35, no. 2, pp. 250–260, 2014.

[40] Y. Vandermeeren, M. Davare, J. Duque, and E. Olivier, "Reorganization of cortical hand representation in congenital hemiplegia," *European Journal of Neuroscience*, vol. 29, no. 4, pp. 845–854, 2009.

[41] R. A. B. Badawy, T. Loetscher, R. A. L. Macdonell, and A. Brodtmann, "Cortical excitability and neurology: insights into the pathophysiology," *Functional Neurology*, vol. 27, no. 3, pp. 131–145, 2012.

[42] M. Dinomais, S. Groeschel, M. Staudt, I. Krägeloh-Mann, and M. Wilke, "Relationship between functional connectivity and sensory impairment: red flag or red herring?," *Human Brain Mapping*, vol. 33, no. 3, pp. 628–638, 2012.

[43] K. Y. Manning, R. S. Menon, J. W. Gorter et al., "Neuroplastic sensorimotor resting state network reorganization in children with hemiplegic cerebral palsy treated with constraint-induced movement therapy," *Journal of Child Neurology*, vol. 31, no. 2, pp. 220–226, 2016.

[44] Y. Moreno-López, R. Olivares-Moreno, M. Cordero-Erausquin, and G. Rojas-Piloni, "Sensorimotor integration by corticospinal system," *Frontiers in neuroanatomy*, vol. 10, p. 24, 2016.

[45] R. N. Lemon, "Descending pathways in motor control," *Annual Review of Neuroscience*, vol. 31, no. 1, pp. 195–218, 2008.

[46] M. Staudt, C. Braun, C. Gerloff, M. Erb, W. Grodd, and I. Krägeloh-Mann, "Developing somatosensory projections bypass periventricular brain lesions," *Neurology*, vol. 67, no. 3, pp. 522–525, 2006.

[47] G. W. Thickbroom, M. L. Byrnes, S. A. Archer, L. Nagarajan, and F. L. Mastaglia, "Differences in sensory and motor cortical organization following brain injury early in life," *Annals of Neurology*, vol. 49, no. 3, pp. 320–327, 2001.

[48] K. L. Ruddy, E. Jaspers, M. Keller, and N. Wenderoth, "Interhemispheric sensorimotor integration; an upper limb phenomenon?," *Neuroscience*, vol. 333, pp. 104–113, 2016.

[49] A. M. Kuczynski, J. A. Semrau, A. Kirton, and S. P. Dukelow, "Kinesthetic deficits after perinatal stroke: robotic

measurement in hemiparetic children," *Journal of NeuroEngineering and Rehabilitation*, vol. 14, no. 1, p. 13, 2017.

[50] A. J. P. Fink, K. R. Croce, Z. J. Huang, L. F. Abbott, T. M. Jessell, and E. Azim, "Presynaptic inhibition of spinal sensory feedback ensures smooth movement," *Nature*, vol. 509, no. 7498, pp. 43–48, 2014.

[51] B. M. Hooks, "Sensorimotor convergence in circuitry of the motor cortex," *The Neuroscientist*, vol. 23, no. 3, pp. 251–263, 2017.

[52] M. Bornschlegl and H. Asanuma, "Importance of the projection from the sensory to the motor cortex for recovery of motor function following partial thalamic lesion in the monkey," *Brain Research*, vol. 437, no. 1, pp. 121–130, 1987.

[53] H. Asanuma and K. Arissian, "Experiments on functional role of peripheral input to motor cortex during voluntary movements in the monkey," *Journal of Neurophysiology*, vol. 52, no. 2, pp. 212–227, 1984.

[54] K. M. Friel, H.-C. Kuo, J. B. Carmel, S. B. Rowny, and A. M. Gordon, "Improvements in hand function after intensive bimanual training are not associated with corticospinal tract dysgenesis in children with unilateral cerebral palsy," *Experimental Brain Research*, vol. 232, no. 6, pp. 2001–2009, 2014.

[55] N. Kuhnke, H. Juenger, M. Walther, S. Berweck, V. Mall, and M. Staudt, "Do patients with congenital hemiparesis and ipsilateral corticospinal projections respond differently to constraint-induced movement therapy?," *Developmental Medicine & Child Neurology*, vol. 50, no. 12, pp. 898–903, 2008.

[56] M. Islam, L. Nordstrand, L. Holmström, A. Kits, H. Forssberg, and A. C. Eliasson, "Is outcome of constraint-induced movement therapy in unilateral cerebral palsy dependent on corticomotor projection pattern and brain lesion characteristics?," *Developmental Medicine & Child Neurology*, vol. 56, no. 3, pp. 252–258, 2014.

[57] B. Gillick, T. Rich, S. Nemanich et al., "Transcranial direct current stimulation and constraint-induced therapy in cerebral palsy: a randomized, blinded, sham-controlled clinical trial," *European Journal of Paediatric Neurology*, vol. 22, no. 3, pp. 358–368, 2018.

[58] G. Saussez, M. Van Laethem, and Y. Bleyenheuft, "Changes in tactile function during intensive bimanual training in children with unilateral spastic cerebral palsy," *Journal of Child Neurology*, vol. 33, no. 4, pp. 260–268, 2018.

[59] H.-C. Kuo, A. M. Gordon, A. Henrionnet, S. Hautfenne, K. M. Friel, and Y. Bleyenheuft, "The effects of intensive bimanual training with and without tactile training on tactile function in children with unilateral spastic cerebral palsy: a pilot study," *Research in Developmental Disabilities*, vol. 49–50, pp. 129–139, 2016.

[60] O. Swayne, J. Rothwell, and K. Rosenkranz, "Transcallosal sensorimotor integration: effects of sensory input on cortical projections to the contralateral hand," *Clinical Neurophysiology*, vol. 117, no. 4, pp. 855–863, 2006.

[61] E. Jaspers, K. Klingels, C. Simon-Martinez, H. Feys, D. G. Woolley, and N. Wenderoth, "GriFT: a device for quantifying physiological and pathological mirror movements in children," *IEEE Transactions on Biomedical Engineering*, vol. 65, no. 4, pp. 857–865, 2018.

[62] E. Eek and M. Engardt, "Assessment of the perceptual threshold of touch (PTT) with high-frequency transcutaneous electric nerve stimulation (Hf/TENS) in elderly patients with stroke: a reliability study," *Clinical Rehabilitation*, vol. 17, no. 8, pp. 825–834, 2003.

[63] A. M. Kuczynski, S. P. Dukelow, J. A. Semrau, and A. Kirton, "Robotic quantification of position sense in children with perinatal stroke," *Neurorehabilitation and Neural Repair*, vol. 30, no. 8, pp. 762–772, 2016.

18

Impaired Ability to Suppress Excitability of Antagonist Motoneurons at Onset of Dorsiflexion in Adults with Cerebral Palsy

Svend Sparre Geertsen [iD],[1,2] Henrik Kirk,[1,3] and Jens Bo Nielsen[2,3]

[1]*Department of Nutrition, Exercise and Sports, University of Copenhagen, Copenhagen, Denmark*
[2]*Department of Neuroscience, University of Copenhagen, Copenhagen, Denmark*
[3]*Helene Elsass Center, Charlottenlund, Denmark*

Correspondence should be addressed to Svend Sparre Geertsen; ssgeertsen@nexs.ku.dk

Guest Editor: Simona Fiori

We recently showed that impaired gait function in adults with cerebral palsy (CP) is associated with reduced rate of force development in ankle dorsiflexors. Here, we explore potential mechanisms. We investigated the suppression of antagonist excitability, calculated as the amount of soleus H-reflex depression at the onset of ankle dorsiflexion compared to rest, in 24 adults with CP (34.3 years, range 18–57; GMFCS 1.95, range 1–3) and 15 healthy, age-matched controls. Furthermore, the central common drive to dorsiflexor motoneurons during a static contraction in the two groups was examined by coherence analyses. The H-reflex was significantly reduced by 37% at the onset of dorsiflexion compared to rest in healthy adults ($P < 0.001$) but unchanged in adults with CP ($P = 0.91$). Also, the adults with CP had significantly less coherence. These findings suggest that the ability to suppress antagonist motoneuronal excitability at movement onset is impaired and that the central common drive during static contractions is reduced in adults with CP.

1. Introduction

When we move, our nervous system ensures that our muscles are activated to the appropriate extent and at the right time in relation to each other so that the movement may progress according to our intentions and with little or no conscious attention required. This is not something that comes easily and quickly. It takes children 10–12 years to attain the mature characteristics of bipedal gait seen in adults [1–4]. Step-to-step variability of gait is significantly larger than in adults and involves significantly more coactivation of antagonistic muscles [1, 3, 4]. Reaching and grasping follow a similar developmental trajectory, and an adult-like movement pattern is not achieved until around 12–14 years of age [5].

People with early brain lesion (cerebral palsy (CP)) in contrast continue to show very significant coactivation of muscles and high step-to-step variability of gait into adulthood [6–8]. They also lack the normal maturation of gating of sensory feedback at rest [9] and during gait [10, 11]. This may possibly be linked to an impaired development of the ability to predict and therefore suppress sensory feedback, which is linked to adequate prediction of the sensory consequences of the movement [12]. However, little is known about the underlying neural mechanisms that are responsible for the maintained coactivation pattern in adults with CP.

One of the mechanisms known to be important for the coordination of antagonist muscles is Ia reciprocal inhibition. Ia reciprocal inhibition involves a group of interneurons, which are activated through collaterals from descending pathways in parallel with agonist motoneurons and project to antagonist motoneurons [13]. In contrast to what is usually observed in other people with lesion of descending motor pathways, such as stroke and multiple sclerosis [14, 15], Ia reciprocal inhibition appears to be similar at rest in adults with CP as in healthy, age-matched controls [9]. However, pathophysiological changes in transmission in spinal motor circuitries observed at rest may have little relevance for how those circuitries are controlled and modulated during motor activities [16–18]. Indeed, Leonard et al. [19] found that Ia reciprocal inhibition was similar in adults with CP and in healthy adults when measured at rest, but during static agonist contraction, the inhibition was increased in healthy subjects and reduced in adults with CP [19]. Morita et al. have also shown impaired regulation of Ia inhibition at the onset of agonist contraction in adults with multiple sclerosis and suggested that this could explain increased coactivation of antagonists in these subjects [20]. We recently showed that impaired gait function in adults with CP is associated with the ability to perform fast ankle movements [21], but it is not known how reciprocal inhibition is modulated at the onset of contraction in adults with CP.

Here, we consequently hypothesized that impaired descending control of spinal inhibitory circuits is responsible for the inability of adults with CP to adequately suppress antagonist muscle activity in relation to voluntary movement and that this may explain their continued coactivation during functional motor tasks. To assess modulation of spinal reciprocal inhibition, we measured the suppression of the soleus H-reflex at the onset of dorsiflexion, and to assess the central drive to the agonist motor pool (dorsiflexors), we measured the size of coupled oscillations in tibialis anterior motor units.

2. Material and Methods

2.1. Participants. Twenty-four adults diagnosed with CP (age 34.3 years, range 18–57; 15 men, 9 women; GMFCS 1.95, range 1–3) were recruited through the Danish Cerebral Palsy Organization. Fifteen subjects were diplegic, eight hemiplegic, and one quadriplegic. All subjects were described as spastic, and most of the subjects had received antispastic medication for shorter or longer periods. Many subjects had a history of multiple surgeries. See [21] for a detailed description of the participants. Furthermore, 15 age-matched (age 32.9 years, range 23–47; 9 men, 6 women) neurologically healthy adults were recruited to serve as a healthy control group.

The study was approved by the local ethics committee (H-4-2012-107), and all procedures were conducted within the standards of the Helsinki declaration. Prior to the experiments, all the participants received written and verbal information, and a consent form for participation was obtained.

2.2. Testing Procedures. Functional reciprocal inhibition (experiment 1) and central common drive (experiment 2) were assessed on the same day following the application of electromyography (EMG) electrodes and tests of the maximal voluntary contraction strength (MVC) and the rate of force development (RFD).

2.2.1. EMG Recordings. EMG activity was recorded using bipolar electrodes (Ambu Blue sensor N-10-A/25, Ambu A/S Ballerup; recording area 0.5 cm², interelectrode distance 2 cm) placed over the soleus muscle and the proximal and distal parts of the tibialis anterior muscle (TA$_{prox}$ and

TA$_{dist}$, respectively). The skin was gently abraded with sandpaper (3M red dot; 3M, Glostrup, Denmark). A ground electrode was placed on the distal part of the tibia. EMG signals were filtered (band-pass, 5 Hz–1 kHz), amplified (500-2000x), sampled at 2 kHz, and stored on a PC for offline analysis.

All EMG and H-reflex measurements (see below) were normalized to the maximal M-response (M_{max}) evoked in either the TA or soleus muscle by supramaximal stimulation (1 ms rectangular pulses; model DS7A, Digitimer, Hertfordshire, UK) of the common peroneal nerve or the tibial nerve, respectively. In these measurements, the intensity of stimulation of the respective nerves was increased from a subliminal level until there was no further increase in the peak-to-peak amplitude of the M-response with increasing stimulation intensity [22].

2.2.2. Measurement of MVC, RFD, and Cocontraction. The MVC and RFD procedures have been comprehensively described by Geertsen et al. [21]. Briefly, subjects were seated in a chair with their leg fastened to a stationary dynamometer and were carefully instructed to contract "as fast and forcefully as possible" and to hold the contraction for about 3 seconds. During each trial, the subject was verbally encouraged by the experimenter to produce maximal torque. Each subject performed 3 dorsiflexions with maximal effort. If an initial countermovement (identified by a visible drop in the torque trace) was observed, a new trial was performed. Data was recorded with Spike 2.611 software (CED 1401+; Cambridge Electronics Design, Cambridge, UK). Offline, the trial that produced the highest dorsiflexion peak torque (MVC_{DF}) was determined. The MVC_{DF} trial was then used to calculate the RFD at 200 ms following the onset of contraction (RFD_{200}) as a measure of explosive muscle force. The level of cocontraction in the MVC_{DF} trial was calculated as the area of rectified, smoothed soleus EMG (in percent of soleus M_{max}) divided by the area of rectified, smoothed TA$_{dist}$ EMG (in percent of M_{max} in TA$_{dist}$) for the first 1000 ms following the onset of TA$_{dist}$ EMG.

2.2.3. Experiment 1: Functional Reciprocal Inhibition. Functional reciprocal inhibition was evaluated by comparing the size of soleus H-reflexes at rest with H-reflexes elicited at the onset of explosive dorsiflexion contractions. H-reflexes were elicited by stimulation (1 ms rectangular pulses; model DS7A, Digitimer, Hertfordshire, UK) of the tibial nerve using a ball-shaped monopolar electrode (Simon electrode) placed in the popliteal fossa and the anode placed proximal to the patella. All H-reflex measurements were normalized to M_{max}.

To produce comparable afferent input to the soleus motoneuron pool at rest and at the onset of dorsiflexion contraction, the tibial nerve stimulation intensity was adjusted, if necessary, to elicit an M-response of approximately 10% of M_{max} in all trials. However, the actual intensities used were similar at rest (15.78 ± 4.86 mA) and at the onset of dorsiflexion (15.64 ± 4.83 mA). At rest, 15 H-reflexes were elicited with an interstimulus interval of 10 s. The subject was then asked to dorsiflex the ankle as fast as possible every 10 s

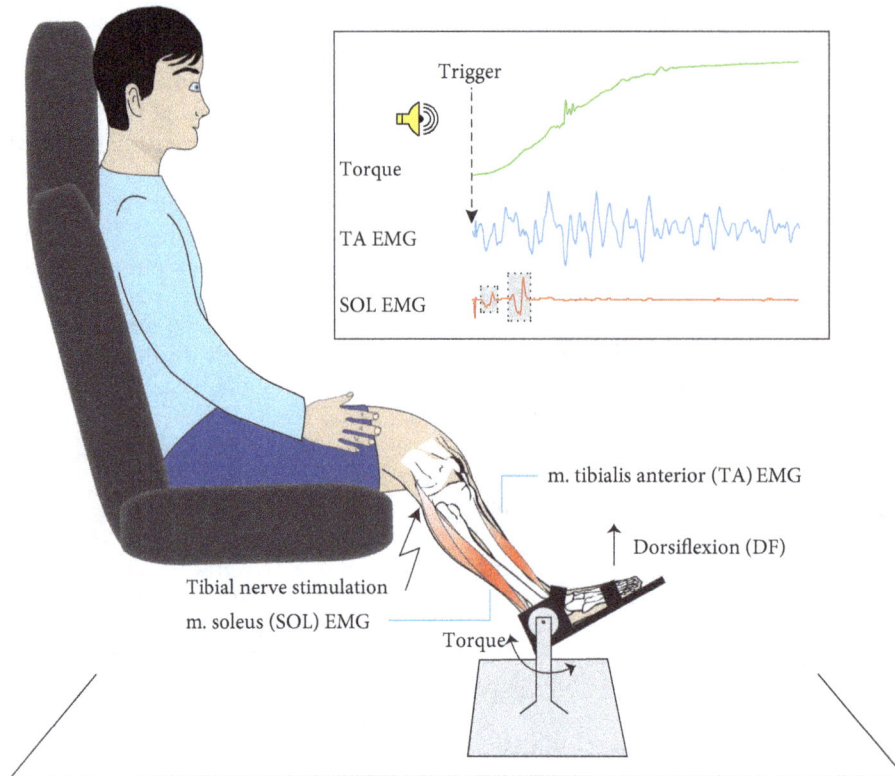

FIGURE 1: Experimental setup. Subjects were seated with their examined leg fastened to a stationary dynamometer. For experiment 1, subjects were instructed to dorsiflex their foot as fast as possible to 50% of MVC in response to an auditory cue. A window discriminator made it possible to time the tibial nerve stimulation to the onset of tibialis anterior (TA) EMG activity. This elicited an M-response (first grey shaded box) and an H-reflex (second grey shaded box) in the soleus (SOL) EMG. At least 45 trials, 15 tibial nerve stimulation and 30 no stimulation trials randomly interspersed, were obtained during dorsiflexion contraction. In experiment 2, subjects were asked to keep a steady dorsiflexion contraction at 10% of MVC for 2 min while given visual feedback of the target torque.

(to 50% of MVC_{DF} to avoid fatigue) following an auditory cue (see Figure 1). A window discriminator made it possible to time the tibial nerve stimulation to the onset of TA EMG activity.

At least 45 trials, 15 tibial nerve stimulation and 30 no stimulation trials randomly interspersed, were obtained during dorsiflexion contraction. Offline, the peak-to-peak amplitude of the H-reflex at the onset of dorsiflexion was then compared to rest (see Figure 2).

In six participants with CP and one participant from the healthy control group, it was not possible to obtain an H-reflex at rest while keeping the M-response at 10% of M_{max}. Also, two participants with CP could not produce a voluntary dorsiflexion contraction. These subjects were therefore excluded from this part of the analyses.

2.2.4. Experiment 2: Central Common Drive. The common drive to the dorsiflexor motoneuron pool was evaluated by coherence analysis of the surface EMG activity from TA_{prox} and TA_{dist} obtained while subjects performed a static dorsiflexion contraction to a torque level of 10% MVC_{DF} for two minutes while given visual feedback. Coherence in the beta band (15–35 Hz) has been shown to be dependent on intact corticospinal activity [23–25] and is therefore thought to reflect central common drive.

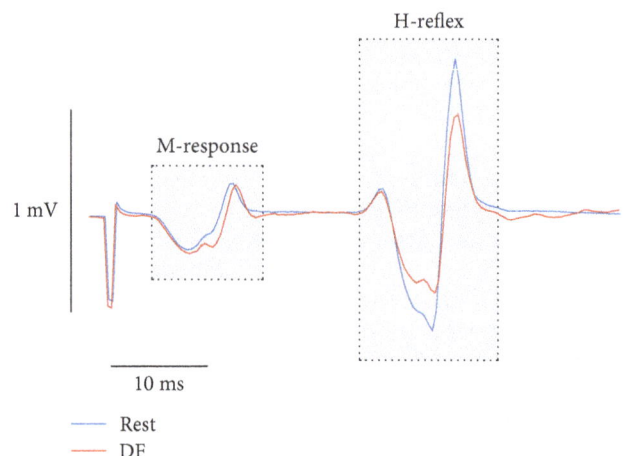

FIGURE 2: Evaluation of functional reciprocal inhibition in a healthy control. To produce a comparable afferent input to the soleus motoneuron pool at rest and during contraction, the tibial nerve stimulation intensity was adjusted to keep the M-response (first shaded box) at approximately 10% of M_{max} both at rest and at the onset of dorsiflexion (DF). The peak-to-peak amplitude of the H-reflex (second shaded box) could then be compared in the two situations, as a measure of the ability to suppress excitability of antagonist motoneurons at the onset of dorsiflexion (i.e., functional reciprocal inhibition).

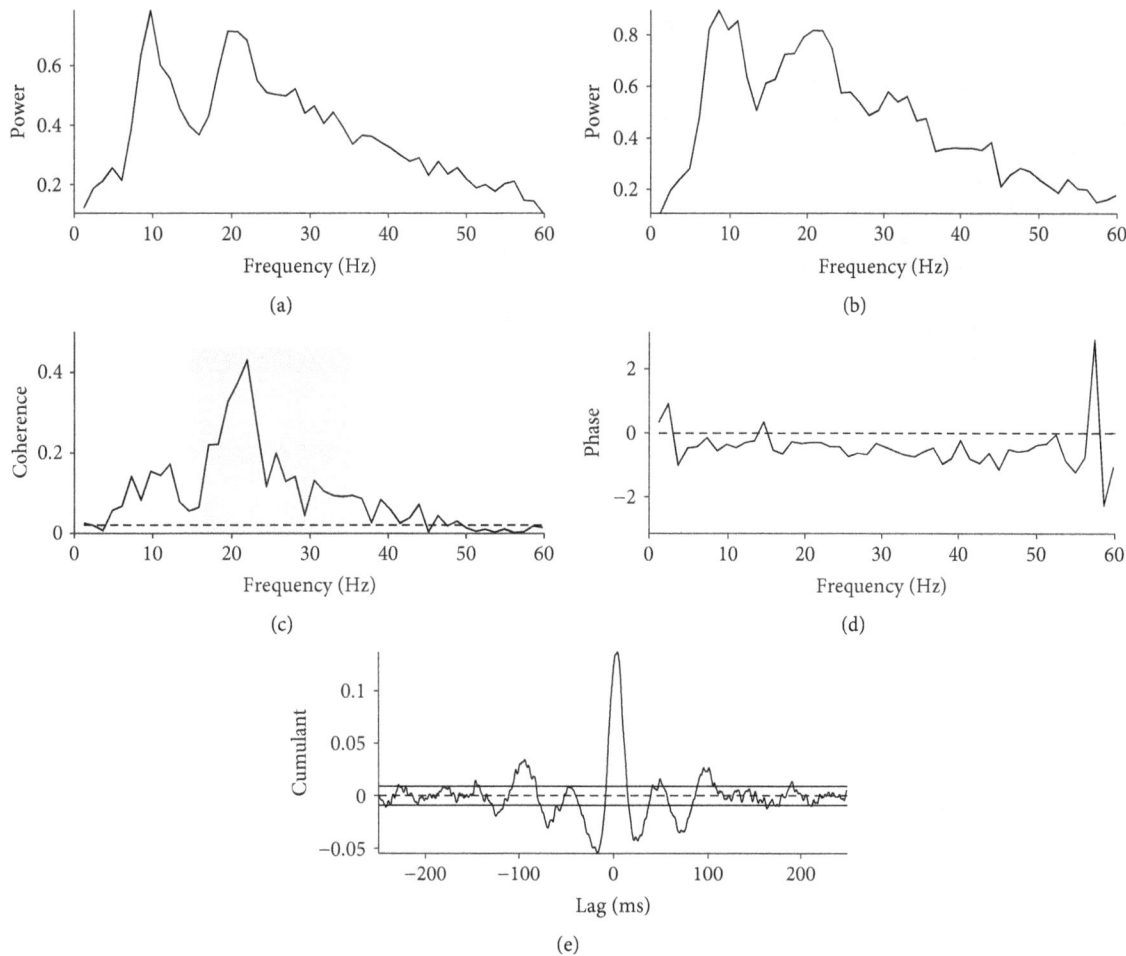

FIGURE 3: Example of intramuscular coherence analyses from a healthy control. (a, b) Autospectra from the proximal (TA$_{prox}$) and the distal (TA$_{dist}$) parts of the tibialis anterior during static dorsiflexion. (c) Coherence at frequencies from 1 to 60 Hz between TA$_{prox}$ and TA$_{dist}$ rectified EMG signals. The dashed horizontal line denotes the upper 95% confidence level, and the grey shaded area highlights the 15–35 Hz frequency band referred to as beta coherence. (d) The phase between the TA$_{prox}$ and TA$_{dist}$ rectified EMG signals indicating the synchronization between coherent EMG frequencies. (e) Cumulant density (range ± 250 ms) associated with the coherence.

Time and frequency domain analysis of the data was performed in MATLAB (version R2016b, MathWorks, MA, USA) using the methods described by Halliday et al. [26] and Farmer et al. [27]. Full-wave rectification of surface EMG signals was performed in order to maximize the information regarding timing of motor unit action potentials while suppressing information regarding waveform shape [28, 29]. The two rectified TA EMG signals were then normalized to have unit variance [30]. Rectified and normalized EMG signals are assumed to be realizations of stationary zero mean time series, denoted by x and y. The analysis of individual records generated estimates of the autospectra of the two EMGs [$f_{xx}(\lambda)$, $f_{yy}(\lambda)$], and their cross-spectra [$f_{xy}(\lambda)$]. Frequency domain analyses were performed with a frequency resolution of 1 Hz. We estimated three functions that characterize the signals' correlation structure: coherence, $R_{xy}(\lambda)^2$; phase, $\Phi_{xy}(\lambda)$; and cumulant density, $q_{xy}(u)$. Coherence describes the linear association between two signals at each frequency of interest and reflects the consistency of phase differences and amplitude ratios between signals across trials.

Coherence estimates are bounded measures of association defined over the range of [0, 1] where 0 indicates no association between signals, and 1 indicates a strong association; cumulant density estimates are not bounded, and phase is defined over the range [$-\pi, +\pi$]. For the present data, coherence estimates provide a measure of the fraction of the activity in one surface EMG signal (TA$_{prox}$) that is correlated with the activity in the second surface EMG signal (TA$_{dist}$). In this way, coherence estimates quantify the strength and range of frequencies of common rhythmic synaptic inputs distributed across the motoneuron pool [27, 31–33]. The timing relations between the EMG signals are estimated from the phase. The cumulant density provides a time-domain representation of the correlation structure analogous to the cross-correlogram. The significance of the individual coherence and cumulant density estimates are assessed by inclusion of an upper 95% confidence limit in coherence plots and upper and lower 95% confidence limits in cumulant density plots (see example in Figure 3), based on the assumption of statistical independence. For details, see [26].

All individual coherence plots were visually inspected for signs of cross-talk, i.e., high coherence across a wide range of frequencies and close to zero lag synchronization in the time domain as evidenced in cumulant density plots [27]. None of the coherence plots displayed these characteristics, so all data from each group were pooled resulting in single group estimates at each frequency of interest for the adults with CP and the healthy controls, respectively. Pooled coherence estimates, like individual coherence estimates, provide a normative measure of linear association on a scale from 0 to 1 [30]. The interpretation of pooled estimates is similar to those for individual records, except that any interference relates to the population as a whole [27]. Group differences were investigated using the χ^2 extended difference of coherence test [34], a nonparametric test that provides the amount of pooled coherence differences between groups at each frequency in relation to an upper 95% confidence interval limit.

As described previously, two participants with CP could not produce a voluntary dorsiflexion contraction. These subjects were therefore excluded from this part of the analyses.

2.2.5. Statistics. Sigma Plot statistical software version 12.5 was used for statistical analysis. A one-way ANOVA was used to investigate differences in the amount of cocontraction between adults with CP and healthy controls. A two-way repeated measure ANOVA with group (CP or CON) and state (rest or onset of dorsiflexion) was applied for H-reflex and M-response analyses. To investigate possible associations between H-reflex modulation and muscle strength in the adults with CP, we used the Pearson product-moment correlations. For experiment 2, the extended χ^2 test was used to calculate the difference of coherence between adults with CP and healthy controls. Coherence was also quantified as the sum (i.e., area) of alpha (5–15 Hz) and beta (15–35 Hz) coherence. These values were transformed logarithmically to symmetrize distributions for statistical analyses [35] and compared using Student's t-test. Associations between H-reflex modulation and coherence area within and across groups were assessed by means of the Pearson product-moment correlations. Statistical significance was given for P values smaller than 0.05. Data are presented as the means ± standard error unless reported otherwise.

3. Results

Data from the test of the dorsiflexion strength has already been reported by Geertsen et al., where we showed that for adults with CP, MVC_{DF} was 42% of healthy controls ($P < 0.001$) and RFD_{200} only 21% healthy controls ($P < 0.001$) [21]. Further analyses performed here showed that during MVC_{DF}, adults with CP exhibited significantly more cocontraction ($10.6 \pm 1.5\%$) than healthy controls ($5.9 \pm 1.2\%$; $P = 0.003$).

3.1. Functional Reciprocal Inhibition. We found a significant group-state interaction when comparing the H-reflex amplitude at rest with the amplitude at the onset of

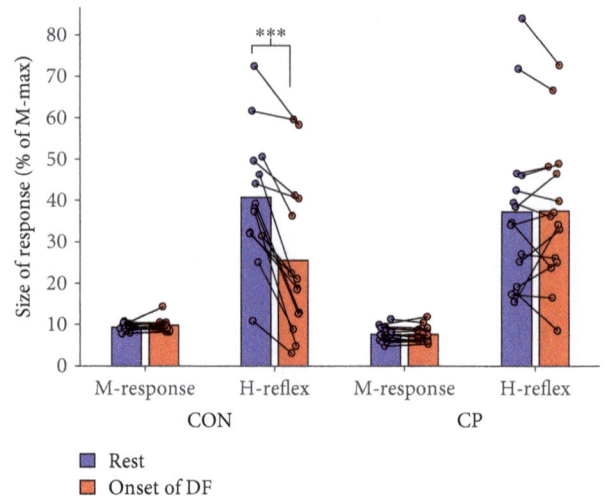

FIGURE 4: Functional reciprocal inhibition in healthy controls and adults with CP. Mean and individual M-response and H-reflex amplitudes in % of the maximal M-responses (M-max) at rest and at the onset of dorsiflexion (DF). The M-response was comparable at rest and at the onset of DF for both healthy controls (CON) and adults with CP. At the onset of DF, the H-reflex was significantly reduced in the healthy controls, whereas it was unchanged in adults with CP. Significant differences between rest and onset of DF are indicated by ***$P < 0.001$.

dorsiflexion for the adults with CP and healthy controls ($F_{1,27} = 22.35$, $P < 0.001$). Post hoc analysis revealed that the healthy control group significantly reduced the H-reflex amplitude by 37% from $40.7 \pm 4.1\%$ of M_{max} at rest to $25.6 \pm 5.0\%$ at the onset of contraction ($P < 0.001$). This functional reciprocal inhibition was not evident in the participants with CP (rest: $37.3 \pm 5.1\%$, dorsiflexion: $37.5 \pm 4.5\%$, $P = 0.91$; Figure 4). There was no significant group-state interaction when comparing the amplitude of the M-response at rest with the amplitude at the onset of dorsiflexion for the adults with CP and healthy controls ($F_{1,27} = 1.32$, $P = 0.26$), indicating a comparable afferent input to the soleus motoneuron pool in the two states for both groups (Figure 4).

In adults with CP, the amount of H-reflex suppression was significantly correlated with both MVC_{DF} ($r = 0.58$, $P = 0.02$) and RFD_{200} ($r = 0.56$, $P = 0.03$).

3.2. Central Common Drive. Figure 3 shows individual coherence data from a healthy control during static dorsiflexion. The autospectra for TA_{prox} and TA_{dist} (Figures 3(a) and 3(b)) illustrate the origin of the elements used for time and frequency domain analysis. Coherence estimates calculated from the autospectra and cross-spectra are shown in Figure 3(c). Here, a clear peak can be seen in the beta (15–35 Hz) frequency band, as well as a small peak in the alpha (5–15 Hz) frequency band. Figure 3(d) shows the phase difference between the two rectified EMGs. The cumulant density constructed from the rectified EMG data is shown in Figure 3(e). Note the clear central peak around 0 ms indicating synchronization between the rectified EMG data from TA_{prox} and TA_{dist}.

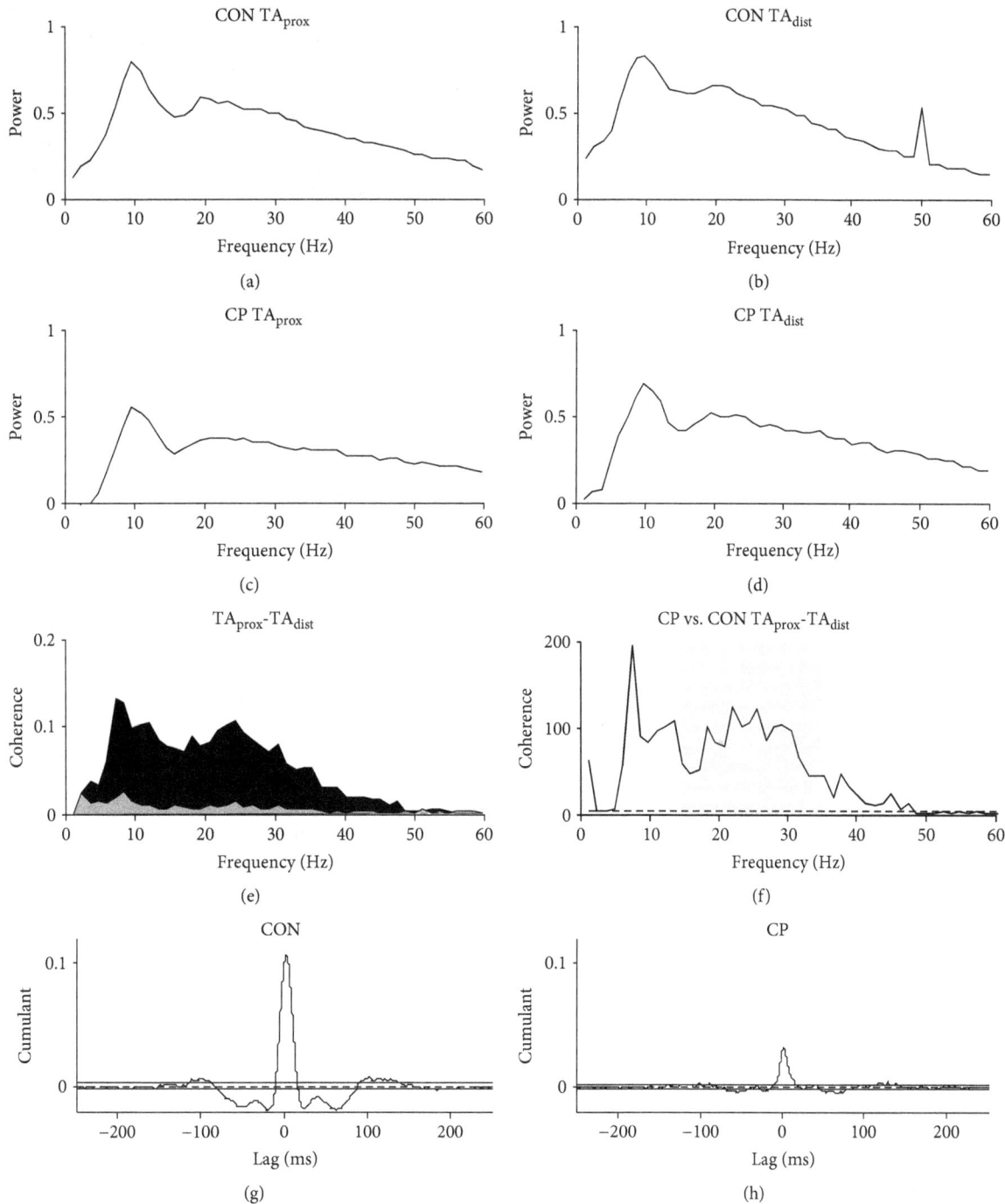

FIGURE 5: Pooled coherence plots and χ^2 analyses. (a–d) Pooled power in the proximal (TA_{prox}) and distal (TA_{dist}) parts of the tibialis anterior during static dorsiflexion for the healthy control group (CON) and adults with cerebral palsy (CP). (e) Pooled coherence between TA_{prox} and TA_{dist} for adults with CP (grey) and CON (black). (f) χ^2 analyses of the difference between adults with CP and the CON group. (g-h) Pooled cumulant density associated with the coherence for the CON and the CP groups.

Pooled TA-TA EMG coherence estimates from adults with CP and healthy controls are presented in Figure 5(a). For both groups, pooled alpha and beta coherence estimates exceeded significance levels, but adults with CP displayed considerably less coherence across all frequencies compared with the healthy adults. This observation was confirmed by the results from the extended χ^2 test of the group coherence estimates displayed in Figure 5(b), which showed a statistical difference at both alpha (5–15 Hz) and beta (15–35 Hz) frequencies.

Reduced TA-TA coherence in adults with CP was also confirmed when comparing the coherence areas at alpha and beta frequencies across individuals (Figure 6). Compared to healthy controls, adults with CP had significantly less

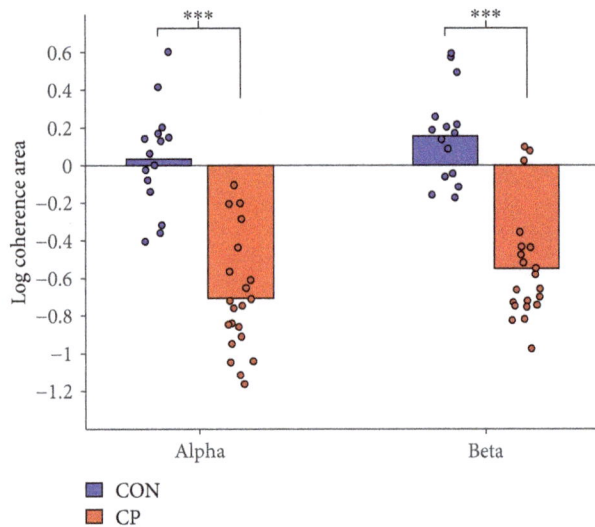

FIGURE 6: Coherence area estimates. Logarithmic coherence area between the proximal (TA_{prox}) and distal (TA_{dist}) part of the tibialis anterior in alpha (5–15 Hz) and beta (15–35 Hz) frequencies during static dorsiflexion for healthy controls (CON; blue) and adults with CP (red). Significant differences between the groups are indicated by $^{***}P < 0.001$.

alpha (-0.705 ± 0.083 vs. 0.034 ± 0.071; $P < 0.001$) and beta (-0.549 ± 0.079 vs. 0.155 ± 0.064; $P < 0.001$) coherence.

We also investigated possible associations between the central common drive to the TA motoneuron pool (log TA-TA coherence area) and the ability to suppress the antagonist motoneuron pool (reduction in soleus H-reflex amplitude at the onset of DF compared to rest). We observed a negative correlation (i.e., more coherence and larger H-reflex reduction) that approached significance in both healthy controls ($r = -0.53$, $P = 0.05$) and adults with CP ($r = -0.43$, $P = 0.13$), and the correlation was significant across groups ($r = -0.74$, $P < 0.001$).

4. Discussion

The main findings of this study are that the central common drive to ankle dorsiflexors and functional reciprocal inhibition of ankle plantar flexors are impaired in adults with CP. This may contribute to the reduced coordination of antagonistic muscles and impaired gait function observed in adults with CP.

4.1. Impaired Functional Reciprocal Inhibition in Adults with CP. The inability of adults with CP to suppress the soleus H-reflex to the same extent as healthy adults at the onset of dorsiflexion is similar to what has been observed in adults who have acquired lesion of descending motor pathways as adults because of multiple sclerosis [20], stroke [36], or spinal cord injury [37, 38]. Our findings indicate that a similar impaired control in adults may also be seen as the result of a lesion early in life and that the intervening years of motor practice and experience apparently do little to change this. We were not able to address the mechanisms responsible for the reduced suppression of the H-reflex further, but based

on previous experiments in healthy subjects [13] and adults with lesion of central motor pathways [20, 39], it appears likely that impaired regulation of spinal interneurons responsible for conveying reciprocal Ia inhibition and/or presynaptic inhibition of Ia afferents is involved. These two spinal interneuronal populations have been shown to be responsible for suppressing stretch reflex activity in antagonist muscles by reducing antagonist motoneuronal excitability and limiting the input from antagonist stretch-sensitive receptors to the motoneurons at the onset of movement [39, 40]. Suppressing transmission in the stretch reflex circuitry through two different populations of interneurons and at two different points may be an efficient safeguard to ensure that stretch of the antagonists does not elicit unwanted stretch reflex activity.

It follows from this that the impaired functional reciprocal inhibition that we have found in adults with CP here could provide an explanation of the inability of the subjects to generate force quickly and efficiently [21]. Previous studies have indicated that people with central motor lesions may move slowly in order to avoid eliciting stretch reflex activity in antagonists when they are stretched at the onset of (fast) movements [15, 16, 41, 42]. However, some caution is required. The adults with CP in our study did not as a group have larger stretch reflexes than healthy subjects at rest (see Figure 4) and the subjects who were the least able to suppress the H-reflex were not those who had the largest stretch reflexes. It should also be kept in mind that the opposite causal relationship is equally likely and that H-reflexes were only slightly suppressed in the adults with CP because they were unable to generate an efficient descending drive to the agonist motoneurons and thereby activate reciprocal inhibitory mechanism efficiently. Our observations of strongly reduced common synaptic drive to ankle dorsiflexors support this interpretation.

4.2. Reduced Central Common Drive in Adults with CP. We used coherence between surface EMG recordings obtained from two different sites over the tibialis anterior muscle as a measure of the central common drive to populations of motoneurons within the same motor pool. This approach requires that the EMG recordings reflected the activity of different populations of motoneurons and that the recordings were not contaminated by cross-talk. Although cross-talk is difficult to rule out definitively, we are confident that we were able to minimize cross-talk to the extent that it cannot explain the findings in the present study: First, we made sure always to position electrodes at least 10 cm apart since muscle fibers in the tibialis anterior muscle have been shown not to exceed 6 cm [43, 44]. Second, cross-talk is easily identified from coherence between the recordings at all frequencies and a large, narrow peak at zero time lag in the cumulant density function [45, 46]. The recordings in the present study only showed coherence within restricted frequency bands (Figures 3 and 5) and peaks of synchronization in the cumulant density function were always found to have a distinct lag with respect to zero. We may therefore safely conclude that the observed coherence and synchronization peaks in the cumulant density function reflect a common central drive to the tibialis anterior motoneurons in the spinal cord [47–49]. The narrow central peak in the cumulant density function and the coherence dominantly in the alpha and beta bands are similar to what has been observed in numerous studies during static contraction in healthy adults previously [31, 47, 49]. There are strong arguments supporting the notion that the narrow central synchronization reflects input to the motoneurons from collaterals of common last order neurons [31, 47, 49], and there is also strong evidence to suggest that the coherence in the beta band reflects activity in corticospinal neurons and that the central drive responsible for these two phenomena therefore originates in the motor cortex and may possibly be explained by activity in the direct monosynaptic corticospinal pathway to the spinal motoneurons [31, 47, 49]. If so, our findings would be consistent with impaired transmission in the corticomotoneuronal pathway in adults with CP, since both coherence and the central short-term synchronization peak in the cumulant density function were reduced in this group. Similar findings with similar interpretation have been reported previously for children with CP [3, 7] and for adults with spinal cord injury [45], stroke [23, 25], and multiple sclerosis [50], but we believe that our findings are the first to demonstrate this for adults with CP. Although the coherence measurements were performed during static contraction rather at the onset of dorsiflexion where reciprocal inhibition was evaluated, the two measures were correlated, and it makes sense from a physiological perspective that the reduced common drive to the dorsiflexors and the impaired reciprocal inhibition at the onset of dorsiflexion are related. The corticomotoneuronal pathway has been shown to be important for the initiation of fast, ballistic movements such as the dorsiflexion we used when testing reciprocal inhibition [51–53]. Corticomotoneuronal cells have also been shown to have collaterals to the Ia inhibitory interneurons responsible for reciprocal inhibition [54–56]. It is therefore, in our opinion, very likely that the reduced coherence between tibialis anterior motor units during static dorsiflexion and the reduced reciprocal inhibition at the onset of dorsiflexion are both linked to impaired transmission in the corticomotoneuronal pathway in the adults with CP.

Petersen et al. [3] found that coherence between tibialis anterior motor units during both static dorsiflexion and gait reached adult levels when children are 10–12 years old in parallel with reduced step-to-step variability of gait and suggested that this was related to the development of the corticospinal tract. In children with CP, this development of coherence was not observed and Petersen et al. [7] therefore suggested that the development of corticospinal drive was impaired. We may now extend these findings to conclude that adults with CP continue to show impaired corticospinal drive to the dorsiflexors and that this also impacts the coordination of antagonistic muscles. It follows that the intervening years of motor practice have not been sufficient to change this.

In children younger than 10 years, 4 weeks of daily treadmill training may increase coherence between tibialis anterior motor units in parallel with improved ability to lift the toes and make ground contact with the heel during gait [57]. This suggests that transmission in the corticospinal pathway is sufficiently plastic in this age group to induce important functional improvements through relatively short-lasting training. However, Willerslev-Olsen et al. [57] also found that such improvements were not found in children older than 10 years and it may therefore be anticipated that this is also the case in adults, although we have at present no knowledge about this. This may be put into the context of current ideas in computational neuroscience, which suggests that motor abilities are the result of a continuous updating of a predictive model that monitors the discrepancy between predicted and actual sensory consequences of movement [58–60]. With 10–12 years of gait experience, a relatively precise predictive model is likely to have been developed and it may therefore be more difficult to alter and require more training than earlier in life. This is consistent with the findings showing that an adult-like gait pattern with little variability (and little cocontraction) is attained around 10–12 years of age [1–4]. It is of interest in this relation that impedance control (i.e., cocontraction of antagonists) and slow movements (i.e., low RFD) have been found to be an optimal control strategy under dynamic conditions that are difficult to predict [61–63]. The characteristics of gait and other movements in adults with CP thus may reflect the most optimal strategy that their nervous system could find under the restrictions imposed by weak muscles and noisy and relatively unpredictable sensory feedback signals. It follows from this that efficient interventions in this group will have to involve "de-learning" of the unwanted movement pattern (cocontraction). This may be followed by learning of a more adequate movement pattern once the prerequisites for this have been established by strengthening muscles, reducing noise in the motor and sensory systems and facilitating relevant sensory signals.

5. Conclusion

We have shown in this study that the central common drive to ankle dorsiflexors and functional reciprocal inhibition of ankle plantar flexors are impaired in adults with CP. This likely reflects the most optimal control strategy under the constraints imposed by an early brain lesion. We suggest that the development of efficient functional interventions in adults with CP will have to take into account that all movements—including "abnormal" movements—may have to be seen as the result of a long learning process involving predictive coding of the sensory consequences of movement.

Disclosure

A preliminary account of these results has been presented as a poster at the 10th FENS Forum of Neuroscience in Copenhagen, Denmark, 2016.

Acknowledgments

The study was supported by a grant from the Elsass Fonden.

References

[1] H. Forssberg, "Ontogeny of human locomotor control I. Infant stepping, supported locomotion and transition to independent locomotion," *Experimental Brain Research*, vol. 57, no. 3, pp. 480–493, 1985.

[2] R. Norlin, P. Odenrick, and B. Sandlund, "Development of gait in the normal child," *Journal of Pediatric Orthopedics*, vol. 1, no. 3, pp. 261–266, 1981.

[3] T. H. Petersen, M. Kliim-Due, S. F. Farmer, and J. B. Nielsen, "Childhood development of common drive to a human leg muscle during ankle dorsiflexion and gait," *The Journal of Physiology*, vol. 588, no. 22, pp. 4387–4400, 2010.

[4] D. H. Sutherland, R. Olshen, L. Cooper, and S. L. Woo, "The development of mature gait," *The Journal of Bone & Joint Surgery*, vol. 62, no. 3, pp. 336–353, 1980.

[5] A. C. Eliasson, H. Forssberg, Y. C. Hung, and A. M. Gordon, "Development of hand function and precision grip control in individuals with cerebral palsy: a 13-year follow-up study," *Pediatrics*, vol. 118, no. 4, pp. e1226–e1236, 2006.

[6] C. T. Leonard, H. Hirschfeld, and H. Forssberg, "The development of independent walking in children with cerebral palsy," *Developmental Medicine & Child Neurology*, vol. 33, no. 7, pp. 567–577, 1991.

[7] T. H. Petersen, S. F. Farmer, M. Kliim-Due, and J. B. Nielsen, "Failure of normal development of central drive to ankle dorsiflexors relates to gait deficits in children with cerebral palsy," *Journal of Neurophysiology*, vol. 109, no. 3, pp. 625–639, 2013.

[8] D. H. Sutherland, "Gait analysis in cerebral palsy," *Developmental Medicine & Child Neurology*, vol. 20, no. 6, pp. 807–813, 1978.

[9] V. Achache, N. Roche, J. C. Lamy et al., "Transmission within several spinal pathways in adults with cerebral palsy," *Brain*, vol. 133, no. 5, pp. 1470–1483, 2010.

[10] M. Hodapp, C. Klisch, V. Mall, J. Vry, W. Berger, and M. Faist, "Modulation of soleus H-reflexes during gait in children with cerebral palsy," *Journal of Neurophysiology*, vol. 98, no. 6, pp. 3263–3268, 2007.

[11] M. Willerslev-Olsen, J. B. Andersen, T. Sinkjaer, and J. B. Nielsen, "Sensory feedback to ankle plantar flexors is not exaggerated during gait in spastic hemiplegic children with cerebral palsy," *Journal of Neurophysiology*, vol. 111, no. 4, pp. 746–754, 2014.

[12] S. J. Blakemore, D. M. Wolpert, and C. D. Frith, "Central cancellation of self-produced tickle sensation," *Nature Neuroscience*, vol. 1, no. 7, pp. 635–640, 1998.

[13] C. Crone and J. Nielsen, "Central control of disynaptic reciprocal inhibition in humans," *Acta Physiologica Scandinavica*, vol. 152, no. 4, pp. 351–363, 1994.

[14] C. Crone, L. L. Johnsen, F. Biering-Sorensen, and J. B. Nielsen, "Appearance of reciprocal facilitation of ankle extensors from ankle flexors in patients with stroke or spinal cord injury," *Brain*, vol. 126, no. 2, pp. 495–507, 2003.

[15] C. Crone, J. Nielsen, N. Petersen, M. Ballegaard, and H. Hultborn, "Disynaptic reciprocal inhibition of ankle extensors in spastic patients," *Brain*, vol. 117, no. 5, pp. 1161–1168, 1994.

[16] V. Dietz and T. Sinkjaer, "Spastic movement disorder: impaired reflex function and altered muscle mechanics," *The Lancet Neurology*, vol. 6, no. 8, pp. 725–733, 2007.

[17] I. K. Ibrahim, W. Berger, M. Trippel, and V. Dietz, "Stretch-induced electromyographic activity and torque in spastic elbow muscles: differential modulation of reflex activity in passive and active motor tasks," *Brain*, vol. 116, no. 4, pp. 971–989, 1993.

[18] T. Sinkjaer and I. Magnussen, "Passive, intrinsic and reflex-mediated stiffness in the ankle extensors of hemiparetic patients," *Brain*, vol. 117, no. 2, pp. 355–363, 1994.

[19] C. T. Leonard, D. Y. Sandholdt, J. McMillan, and S. Queen, "Short- and long-latency contributions to reciprocal inhibition during various levels of muscle contraction of individuals with cerebral palsy," *Journal of Child Neurology*, vol. 21, no. 3, pp. 240–246, 2006.

[20] H. Morita, C. Crone, D. Christenhuis, N. T. Petersen, and J. B. Nielsen, "Modulation of presynaptic inhibition and disynaptic reciprocal Ia inhibition during voluntary movement in spasticity," *Brain*, vol. 124, no. 4, pp. 826–837, 2001.

[21] S. S. Geertsen, H. Kirk, J. Lorentzen, M. Jorsal, C. B. Johansson, and J. B. Nielsen, "Impaired gait function in adults with cerebral palsy is associated with reduced rapid force generation and increased passive stiffness," *Clinical Neurophysiology*, vol. 126, no. 12, pp. 2320–2329, 2015.

[22] S. S. Geertsen, J. Lundbye-Jensen, and J. B. Nielsen, "Increased central facilitation of antagonist reciprocal inhibition at the onset of dorsiflexion following explosive strength training," *Journal of Applied Physiology*, vol. 105, no. 3, pp. 915–922, 2008.

[23] S. F. Farmer, M. Swash, D. A. Ingram, and J. A. Stephens, "Changes in motor unit synchronization following central nervous lesions in man," *The Journal of Physiology*, vol. 463, no. 1, pp. 83–105, 1993.

[24] N. L. Hansen, B. A. Conway, D. M. Halliday et al., "Reduction of common synaptic drive to ankle dorsiflexor motoneurons during walking in patients with spinal cord lesion," *Journal of Neurophysiology*, vol. 94, no. 2, pp. 934–942, 2005.

[25] J. B. Nielsen, J. S. Brittain, D. M. Halliday, V. Marchand-Pauvert, D. Mazevet, and B. A. Conway, "Reduction of common motoneuronal drive on the affected side during walking in hemiplegic stroke patients," *Clinical Neurophysiology*, vol. 119, no. 12, pp. 2813–2818, 2008.

[26] D. M. Halliday, J. R. Rosenberg, A. M. Amjad, P. Breeze, B. A. Conway, and S. F. Farmer, "A framework for the analysis of mixed time series/point process data—theory and application to the study of physiological tremor, single motor unit discharges and electromyograms," *Progress in Biophysics and Molecular Biology*, vol. 64, no. 2-3, pp. 237–278, 1995.

[27] S. F. Farmer, J. Gibbs, D. M. Halliday et al., "Changes in EMG coherence between long and short thumb abductor muscles during human development," *The Journal of Physiology*, vol. 579, no. 2, pp. 389–402, 2007.

[28] D. M. Halliday and S. F. Farmer, "On the need for rectification of surface EMG," *Journal of Neurophysiology*, vol. 103, no. 6, p. 3547, 2010.

[29] L. J. Myers, M. Lowery, M. O'Malley et al., "Rectification and non-linear pre-processing of EMG signals for cortico-muscular analysis," *Journal of Neuroscience Methods*, vol. 124, no. 2, pp. 157–165, 2003.

[30] D. M. Halliday and J. R. Rosenberg, "On the application, estimation and interpretation of coherence and pooled coherence," *Journal of Neuroscience Methods*, vol. 100, no. 1-2, pp. 173-174, 2000.

[31] S. F. Farmer, F. D. Bremner, D. M. Halliday, J. R. Rosenberg, and J. A. Stephens, "The frequency content of common synaptic inputs to motoneurones studied during voluntary isometric contraction in man," *The Journal of Physiology*, vol. 470, no. 1, pp. 127–155, 1993.

[32] D. M. Halliday, B. A. Conway, S. F. Farmer, and J. R. Rosenberg, "Load-independent contributions from motor-unit synchronization to human physiological tremor," *Journal of Neurophysiology*, vol. 82, no. 2, pp. 664–675, 1999.

[33] J. R. Rosenberg, D. M. Halliday, P. Breeze, and B. A. Conway, "Identification of patterns of neuronal connectivity—partial spectra, partial coherence, and neuronal interactions," *Journal of Neuroscience Methods*, vol. 83, no. 1, pp. 57–72, 1998.

[34] A. M. Amjad, D. M. Halliday, J. R. Rosenberg, and B. A. Conway, "An extended difference of coherence test for comparing and combining several independent coherence estimates: theory and application to the study of motor units and physiological tremor," *Journal of Neuroscience Methods*, vol. 73, no. 1, pp. 69–79, 1997.

[35] M. E. Spedden, J. B. Nielsen, and S. S. Geertsen, "Oscillatory corticospinal activity during static contraction of ankle muscles is reduced in healthy old versus young adults," *Neural Plasticity*, vol. 2018, Article ID 3432649, 13 pages, 2018.

[36] Y. Takahashi, T. Fujiwara, T. Yamaguchi et al., "Voluntary contraction enhances spinal reciprocal inhibition induced by patterned electrical stimulation in patients with stroke," *Restorative Neurology and Neuroscience*, vol. 36, no. 1, pp. 99–105, 2018.

[37] G. I. Boorman, R. G. Lee, W. J. Becker, and U. R. Windhorst, "Impaired 'natural reciprocal inhibition' in patients with spasticity due to incomplete spinal cord injury," *Electroencephalography and Clinical Neurophysiology/Electromyography and Motor Control*, vol. 101, no. 2, pp. 84–92, 1996.

[38] S. Cremoux, D. Amarantini, J. Tallet, F. Dal Maso, and E. Berton, "Increased antagonist muscle activity in cervical SCI patients suggests altered reciprocal inhibition during elbow contractions," *Clinical Neurophysiology*, vol. 127, no. 1, pp. 629–634, 2016.

[39] J. B. Nielsen, "Human spinal motor control," *Annual Review of Neuroscience*, vol. 39, no. 1, pp. 81–101, 2016.

[40] C. Crone and J. Nielsen, "Spinal mechanisms in man contributing to reciprocal inhibition during voluntary dorsiflexion of the foot," *The Journal of Physiology*, vol. 416, no. 1, pp. 255–272, 1989.

[41] Y. Okuma and R. G. Lee, "Reciprocal inhibition in hemiplegia: correlation with clinical features and recovery," *Canadian Journal of Neurological Sciences*, vol. 23, no. 01, pp. 15–23, 1996.

[42] Y. Okuma, Y. Mizuno, and R. G. Lee, "Reciprocal Ia inhibition in patients with asymmetric spinal spasticity," *Clinical Neurophysiology*, vol. 113, no. 2, pp. 292–297, 2002.

[43] K. Roeleveld, D. F. Stegeman, H. M. Vingerhoets, and A. Van Oosterom, "The motor unit potential distribution over the skin surface and its use in estimating the motor unit location," *Acta Physiologica Scandinavica*, vol. 161, no. 4, pp. 465–472, 1997.

[44] R. R. Roy, A. Garfinkel, M. Ounjian et al., "Three-dimensional structure of cat tibialis anterior motor units," *Muscle & Nerve*, vol. 18, no. 10, pp. 1187–1195, 1995.

[45] D. Barthélemy, M. Willerslev-Olsen, H. Lundell et al., "Impaired transmission in the corticospinal tract and gait disability in spinal cord injured persons," *Journal of Neurophysiology*, vol. 104, no. 2, pp. 1167–1176, 2010.

[46] A. Ritterband-Rosenbaum, A. Herskind, X. Li et al., "A critical period of corticomuscular and EMG-EMG coherence detection in healthy infants aged 9-25 weeks," *The Journal of Physiology*, vol. 595, no. 8, pp. 2699–2713, 2017.

[47] A. K. Datta and J. A. Stephens, "Synchronization of motor unit activity during voluntary contraction in man," *The Journal of Physiology*, vol. 422, no. 1, pp. 397–419, 1990.

[48] P. A. Kirkwood and T. A. Sears, "The synaptic connexions to intercostal motoneurones as revealed by the average common excitation potential," *The Journal of Physiology*, vol. 275, no. 1, pp. 103–134, 1978.

[49] S. F. Farmer, "Rhythmicity, synchronization and binding in human and primate motor systems," *The Journal of Physiology*, vol. 509, no. 1, pp. 3–14, 1998.

[50] N. L. Hansen, S. Hansen, C. Crone et al., "Chapter 23 Synchronization of lower limb motor units in spastic patients," *Supplements to Clinical Neurophysiology*, vol. 53, pp. 178–186, 2000.

[51] P. D. Cheney and E. E. Fetz, "Functional classes of primate corticomotoneuronal cells and their relation to active force," *Journal of Neurophysiology*, vol. 44, no. 4, pp. 773–791, 1980.

[52] E. E. Fetz and P. D. Cheney, "Functional relations between primate motor cortex cells and muscles: fixed and flexible," *Ciba Foundation Symposia*, vol. 132, pp. 98–117, 1987.

[53] J. Nielsen and N. Petersen, "Changes in the effect of magnetic brain stimulation accompanying voluntary dynamic contraction in man," *The Journal of Physiology*, vol. 484, no. 3, pp. 777–789, 1995.

[54] P. D. Cheney, E. E. Fetz, and S. S. Palmer, "Patterns of facilitation and suppression of antagonist forelimb muscles from motor cortex sites in the awake monkey," *Journal of Neurophysiology*, vol. 53, no. 3, pp. 805–820, 1985.

[55] E. Jankowska, Y. Padel, and R. Tanaka, "Disynaptic inhibition of spinal motoneurones from the motor cortex in the monkey," *The Journal of Physiology*, vol. 258, no. 2, pp. 467–487, 1976.

[56] J. Nielsen, N. Petersen, G. Deuschl, and M. Ballegaard, "Task-related changes in the effect of magnetic brain stimulation on spinal neurones in man," *The Journal of Physiology*, vol. 471, no. 1, pp. 223–243, 1993.

[57] M. Willerslev-Olsen, T. H. Petersen, S. F. Farmer, and J. B. Nielsen, "Gait training facilitates central drive to ankle dorsiflexors in children with cerebral palsy," *Brain*, vol. 138, no. 3, pp. 589–603, 2015.

[58] R. A. Adams, S. Shipp, and K. J. Friston, "Predictions not commands: active inference in the motor system," *Brain Structure and Function*, vol. 218, no. 3, pp. 611–643, 2013.

[59] D. W. Franklin and D. M. Wolpert, "Computational mechanisms of sensorimotor control," *Neuron*, vol. 72, no. 3, pp. 425–442, 2011.

[60] R. Shadmehr, M. A. Smith, and J. W. Krakauer, "Error correction, sensory prediction, and adaptation in motor control," *Annual Review of Neuroscience*, vol. 33, no. 1, pp. 89–108, 2010.

[61] E. Burdet, R. Osu, D. W. Franklin, T. E. Milner, and M. Kawato, "The central nervous system stabilizes unstable dynamics by learning optimal impedance," *Nature*, vol. 414, no. 6862, pp. 446–449, 2001.

[62] D. W. Franklin, E. Burdet, R. Osu, M. Kawato, and T. E. Milner, "Functional significance of stiffness in adaptation of multijoint arm movements to stable and unstable dynamics," *Experimental Brain Research*, vol. 151, no. 2, pp. 145–157, 2003.

[63] D. W. Franklin, U. So, M. Kawato, and T. E. Milner, "Impedance control balances stability with metabolically costly muscle activation," *Journal of Neurophysiology*, vol. 92, no. 5, pp. 3097–3105, 2004.

Permissions

All chapters in this book were first published in NP, by Hindawi Publishing Corporation; hereby published with permission under the Creative Commons Attribution License or equivalent. Every chapter published in this book has been scrutinized by our experts. Their significance has been extensively debated. The topics covered herein carry significant findings which will fuel the growth of the discipline. They may even be implemented as practical applications or may be referred to as a beginning point for another development.

The contributors of this book come from diverse backgrounds, making this book a truly international effort. This book will bring forth new frontiers with its revolutionizing research information and detailed analysis of the nascent developments around the world.

We would like to thank all the contributing authors for lending their expertise to make the book truly unique. They have played a crucial role in the development of this book. Without their invaluable contributions this book wouldn't have been possible. They have made vital efforts to compile up to date information on the varied aspects of this subject to make this book a valuable addition to the collection of many professionals and students.

This book was conceptualized with the vision of imparting up-to-date information and advanced data in this field. To ensure the same, a matchless editorial board was set up. Every individual on the board went through rigorous rounds of assessment to prove their worth. After which they invested a large part of their time researching and compiling the most relevant data for our readers.

The editorial board has been involved in producing this book since its inception. They have spent rigorous hours researching and exploring the diverse topics which have resulted in the successful publishing of this book. They have passed on their knowledge of decades through this book. To expedite this challenging task, the publisher supported the team at every step. A small team of assistant editors was also appointed to further simplify the editing procedure and attain best results for the readers.

Apart from the editorial board, the designing team has also invested a significant amount of their time in understanding the subject and creating the most relevant covers. They scrutinized every image to scout for the most suitable representation of the subject and create an appropriate cover for the book.

The publishing team has been an ardent support to the editorial, designing and production team. Their endless efforts to recruit the best for this project, has resulted in the accomplishment of this book. They are a veteran in the field of academics and their pool of knowledge is as vast as their experience in printing. Their expertise and guidance has proved useful at every step. Their uncompromising quality standards have made this book an exceptional effort. Their encouragement from time to time has been an inspiration for everyone.

The publisher and the editorial board hope that this book will prove to be a valuable piece of knowledge for researchers, students, practitioners and scholars across the globe.

List of Contributors

Aliza K. De Nobrega and Lisa C. Lyons
Department of Biological Science, Program in Neuroscience, Florida State University, Tallahassee, FL 32306, USA

Zhi-Zhi Liu, Jian Zhu, Chang-Ling Wang, Xin Wang, Ying-Ying Han, Ling-Yan Liu and Hong A. Xu
Institute of Life Science, Nanchang University, Nanchang, China
School of Life Sciences, Nanchang University, Nanchang, China
Jiangxi Provincial Collaborative Innovation Center for Cardiovascular, Digestive, and Neuropsychiatric Diseases, Nanchang, China

Jun Han Yoon, Alysia Fogliani, Emmanuel A. Akinpelu, Danii Baron-Heeris, Imke G. J. Houwers, Lachlan P. G. Wheeler, Sarah J. Lovett, Emma Duce, Margaret A. Pollett, Tylie M. Wiseman and Brooke Fehily
School of Human Sciences, The University of Western Australia (UWA), Perth, WA 6009, Australia

Stuart I. Hodgetts, Sreya Santhakumar and Alan R. Harvey
Perron Institute for Neurological and Translational Science, Nedlands, WA 6009, Australia

Bernadette T. Majda
University of Notre Dame Australia, Fremantle, WA 6959, Australia

Arturo Ortega
Laboratorio de Neurotoxicología, Departamento de Toxicología, Centro de Investigación y de Estudios Avanzados del Instituto Politécnico Nacional, Apartado Postal 14-740, 07000 Ciudad de México, Mexico

Donají Chi-Castañeda
Laboratorio de Neurotoxicología, Departamento de Toxicología, Centro de Investigación y de Estudios Avanzados del Instituto Politécnico Nacional, Apartado Postal 14-740, 07000 Ciudad de México, Mexico
Soluciones para un México Verde S.A. de C.V., 01210 Ciudad de México, Mexico

James E. Orfila, Myriam Moreno, Nicholas Chalmers and Nidia Quillinan
Neuronal Injury Program, Department of Anesthesiology, University of Colorado, Anschutz Medical Campus, Aurora, CO 80045, USA

Paco S. Herson
Neuronal Injury Program, Department of Anesthesiology, University of Colorado, Anschutz Medical Campus, Aurora, CO 80045, USA
Department of Pharmacology, University of Colorado, Anschutz Medical Campus, Aurora, CO 80045, USA

Nicole McKinnon and Robert M. Dietz
Department of Pediatrics, University of Colorado, Anschutz Medical Campus, Aurora, CO 80045, USA

Guiying Deng
Department of Pharmacology, University of Colorado, Anschutz Medical Campus, Aurora, CO 80045, USA

Garth J. Thompson, Peter Herman and Maxime J. Parent
Department of Radiology and Biomedical Imaging and Magnetic Resonance Research Center, Yale University, New Haven, CT, USA

Kristian N. Mortensen
Department of Radiology and Biomedical Imaging and Magnetic Resonance Research Center, Yale University, New Haven, CT, USA
Department of Neuroscience, University of Copenhagen, Copenhagen, Denmark

Douglas L. Rothman and Fahmeed Hyder
Department of Radiology and Biomedical Imaging and Magnetic Resonance Research Center, Yale University, New Haven, CT, USA
Department of Biomedical Engineering, Yale University, New Haven, CT, USA

Ron Kupers
Department of Neuroscience, University of Copenhagen, Copenhagen, Denmark

Albert Gjedde
Department of Neuroscience, University of Copenhagen, Copenhagen, Denmark
Departments of Nuclear Medicine and Clinical Research, Odense University Hospital, University of Southern Denmark, Odense, Denmark

Maurice Ptito
Department of Neuroscience, University of Copenhagen, Copenhagen, Denmark
Departments of Nuclear Medicine and Clinical Research, Odense University Hospital, University of Southern Denmark, Odense, Denmark

Chaire de Recherche Harland Sanders, School of Optometry, University of Montreal, Montreal, Canada
Neuropsychiatry Laboratory, Psychiatric Centre, Rigshospitalet, Copenhagen, Denmark

Johan Stender
Department of Neuroscience, University of Copenhagen, Copenhagen, Denmark
GIGA-Consciousness, Coma Science Group, Université de Liège, Liège, Belgium

Steven Laureys
GIGA-Consciousness, Coma Science Group, Université de Liège, Liège, Belgium

Valentin Riedl
Departments of Neuroradiology, Nuclear Medicine and Neuroimaging Center, Technische Universität München, München, Germany

Michael T. Alkire
Department of Anesthesiology, University of California, Irvine, CA, USA

Marcel Irintchev, Orlando Guntinas-Lichius and Andrey Irintchev
Department of Otorhinolaryngology, Jena University Hospital, Am Klinikum 1, 07747 Jena, Germany

Edith Durand, Pierre Berroir and Ana Inés Ansaldo
Centre de Recherche de l'Institut Universitaire de Gériatrie de Montréal (CRIUGM), École d'Orthophonie, Faculté de Médecine, Université de Montréal, Montreal, QC, Canada

Qi Zhang, Ying-Ying Tan and Xiao-hua Liu
Shaanxi Key Laboratory of Chinese Medicine Encephalopathy, Shaanxi University of Chinese Medicine, Xianyang, Shaanxi 712046, China

Fan-Rong Yao
Department of Pharmacology and Toxicology, Brody School of Medicine, East Carolina University, Greenville, NC 27834, USA

Dong-Yuan Cao
Key Laboratory of Shaanxi Province for Craniofacial Precision Medicine Research, Research Center of Stomatology, Xi'an Jiaotong University College of Stomatology, Xi'an, Shaanxi 710004, China

Juan Hong
ENT Institute and Otorhinolaryngology Department of Affiliated Eye and ENT Hospital, State Key Laboratory of Medical Neurobiology, Fudan University, Shanghai 200031, China

Department of Otorhinolaryngology-Head and Neck Surgery, Huashan Hospital, Fudan University, Shanghai 200040, China

Yan Chen, Yanping Zhang, Jieying Li, Liujie Ren, Lin Yang, Tianyu Zhang and Peidong Dai
ENT Institute and Otorhinolaryngology Department of Affiliated Eye and ENT Hospital, State Key Laboratory of Medical Neurobiology, Fudan University, Shanghai 200031, China
NHC Key Laboratory of Hearing Medicine, Fudan University, Shanghai 200031, China

Huawei Li
ENT Institute and Otorhinolaryngology Department of Affiliated Eye and ENT Hospital, State Key Laboratory of Medical Neurobiology, Fudan University, Shanghai 200031, China
NHC Key Laboratory of Hearing Medicine, Fudan University, Shanghai 200031, China
Institutes of Biomedical Sciences, The Institutes of Brain Science and the Collaborative Innovation Center for Brain Science, Fudan University, Shanghai 200032, China
Shanghai Engineering Research Centre of Cochlear Implant, Shanghai 200031, China

Lusen Shi and Ao Li
Department of Otolaryngology Head and Neck Surgery, Affiliated Drum Tower Hospital of Nanjing University Medical School, Jiangsu Provincial Key Medical Discipline (Laboratory), Nanjing 210008, China

Cristine de Paula Nascimento-Castro, Ana Claudia Wink, Victor Silva da Fônseca, Claudia Daniele Bianco, Elisa C. Winkelmann-Duarte and Patricia S. Brocardo
Department of Morphological Sciences, Center of Biological Sciences, Universidade Federal de Santa Catarina, 88040- 900 Florianópolis, SC, Brazil

Marcelo Farina and Ana Lúcia S. Rodrigues
Department of Biochemistry, Center of Biological Sciences, Universidade Federal de Santa Catarina, 88040-900 Florianópolis, SC, Brazil

Andreza Fabro de Bem
Department of Biochemistry, Center of Biological Sciences, Universidade Federal de Santa Catarina, 88040-900 Florianópolis, SC, Brazil
Department of Physiological Science, Institute of Biological Science, University of Brasilia, Brasília, DF, Brazil

Joana Gil-Mohapel
Division of Medical Sciences, UBC Island Medical Program, University of Victoria, Victoria, BC, Canada V8W 2Y2

Navah Ester Kadish, Michael Siniatchkin and Vera Moliadze
Institute of Medical Psychology and Medical Sociology, University Hospital of Schleswig-Holstein (UKSH), Campus Kiel, Christian Albrechts University, Kiel, Germany

Hannah Brauer
Institute of Medical Psychology and Medical Sociology, University Hospital of Schleswig-Holstein (UKSH), Campus Kiel, Christian Albrechts University, Kiel, Germany
Department of Child and Adolescent Psychiatry and Psychotherapy, School of Medicine, Christian Albrechts University, Kiel, Germany

Anya Pedersen
Clinical Psychology and Psychotherapy, Christian Albrechts University, Kiel, Germany

Shiquan Shuai, Zhiwei Guo, Huaping Chen and Morgan A. McClure
Department of Imaging and Imaging Institute of Rehabilitation and Development of Brain Function, The Second Clinical Medical College of North Sichuan Medical College, Nanchong Central Hospital, Nanchong 637000, China

Lan Zhang
Department of Imaging and Imaging Institute of Rehabilitation and Development of Brain Function, The Second Clinical Medical College of North Sichuan Medical College, Nanchong Central Hospital, Nanchong 637000, China
Department of Radiology, Langzhong People's Hospital, Nanchong 637000, China

Guoqiang Xing
Department of Imaging and Imaging Institute of Rehabilitation and Development of Brain Function, The Second Clinical Medical College of North Sichuan Medical College, Nanchong Central Hospital, Nanchong 637000, China
Lotus Biotech.com LLC., John Hopkins University-MCC, Rockville, MD 20850, USA

Qiwen Mu
Department of Imaging and Imaging Institute of Rehabilitation and Development of Brain Function, The Second Clinical Medical College of North Sichuan Medical College, Nanchong Central Hospital, Nanchong 637000, China

Peking University Third Hospital, Beijing 100080, China

Xiaojuan Chen
North Sichuan Medical College, Nanchong 637000, China

Hannes Aftenberger
Institute of Physiotherapy, University of Applied Sciences FH-Joanneum, Graz, Austria

Monica Christova
Institute of Physiotherapy, University of Applied Sciences FH-Joanneum, Graz, Austria
Otto Loewi Research Center, Physiology Section, Medical University of Graz, Graz, Austria

Eugen Gallasch
Otto Loewi Research Center, Physiology Section, Medical University of Graz, Graz, Austria

Raffaele Nardone
Department of Neurology, Franz Tappeiner Hospital, Merano, Italy
Department of Neurology, Christian Doppler Clinic, Paracelsus Medical University, Salzburg, Austria

Mi Kyoung Seo and Ah Jeong Choi
Paik Institute for Clinical Research, Inje University, Busan, Republic of Korea

Jung Goo Lee
Paik Institute for Clinical Research, Inje University, Busan, Republic of Korea
Department of Psychiatry, College of Medicine, Haeundae Paik Hospital, Inje University, Busan, Republic of Korea
Department of Health Science and Technology, Graduate School, Inje University, Busan, Republic of Korea

Sung Woo Park
Paik Institute for Clinical Research, Inje University, Busan, Republic of Korea
Department of Health Science and Technology, Graduate School, Inje University, Busan, Republic of Korea
Department of Convergence Biomedical Science, College of Medicine, Inje University, Busan, Republic of Korea

Young Hoon Kim
Department of Psychiatry, Gongju National Hospital, Gongju, Republic of Korea

Yena Lee and Nicole E. Carmona
Mood Disorders Psychopharmacology Unit, University Health Network, University of Toronto, Toronto, ON, Canada

Roger S. McIntyre and Rodrigo B. Mansur
Mood Disorders Psychopharmacology Unit, University Health Network, University of Toronto, Toronto, ON, Canada
Department of Psychiatry, University of Toronto, Toronto, ON, Canada

Gyung-Mee Kim
Department of Psychiatry, College of Medicine, Haeundae Paik Hospital, Inje University, Busan, Republic of Korea

Cinzia Mallozzi
Department of Neuroscience, Istituto Superiore di Sanità, Viale Regina Elena 299, 00161 Rome, Italy

Alida Spalloni and Patrizia Longone
Molecular Neurobiology Unit, Experimental Neurology, Santa Lucia Foundation, Via Ardeatina 306/354, 00142 Rome, Italy

Maria Rosaria Domenici
National Center for Drug Research and Evaluation, Istituto Superiore di Sanità, Viale Regina Elena 299, 00161 Rome, Italy

Cristina Simon-Martinez, Lisa Mailleux and Hilde Feys
Department of Rehabilitation Sciences, KU Leuven-University of Leuven, Leuven, Belgium

Ellen Jaspers
Department of Rehabilitation Sciences, KU Leuven-University of Leuven, Leuven, Belgium

Neural Control of Movement Lab, Department of Health Sciences and Technology, ETH Zurich, Zurich, Switzerland

Katrijn Klingels
Department of Rehabilitation Sciences, KU Leuven-University of Leuven, Leuven, Belgium
Rehabilitation Research Centre, BIOMED, Hasselt University, Diepenbeek, Belgium

Nicole Wenderoth
Neural Control of Movement Lab, Department of Health Sciences and Technology, ETH Zurich, Zurich, Switzerland

Els Ortibus
Department of Development and Regeneration, KU Leuven-University of Leuven, Leuven, Belgium

Svend Sparre Geertsen
Department of Nutrition, Exercise and Sports, University of Copenhagen, Copenhagen, Denmark
Department of Neuroscience, University of Copenhagen, Copenhagen, Denmark

Henrik Kirk
Department of Nutrition, Exercise and Sports, University of Copenhagen, Copenhagen, Denmark
Helene Elsass Center, Charlottenlund, Denmark

Jens Bo Nielsen
Department of Neuroscience, University of Copenhagen, Copenhagen, Denmark
Helene Elsass Center, Charlottenlund, Denmark

Index

www.ingramcontent.com/pod-product-compliance
Lightning Source LLC
Chambersburg PA
CBHW080515200326
41458CB00012B/4213